The Story of Orthopaedics

The Story of Orthopaedics

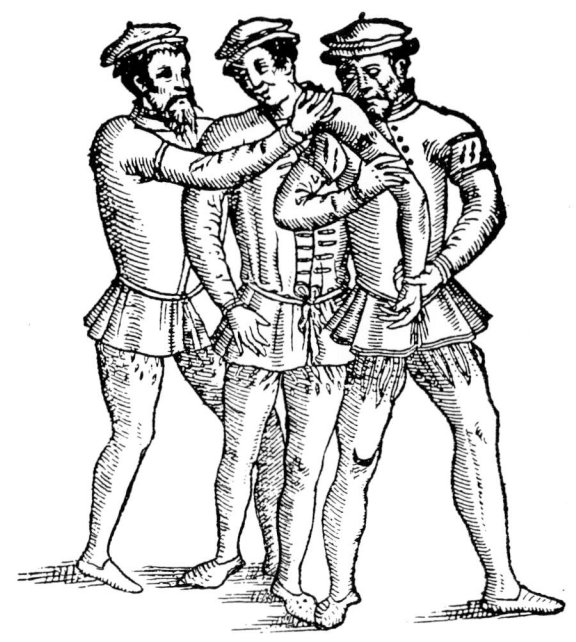

Mercer Rang

MB BS, FRCS (Eng), FRCSC
Professor of Surgery, University of Toronto
Pediatric Orthopaedic Surgeon,
The Hospital for Sick Children and
The Bloorview MacMillan Centre
Toronto, Canada

W.B. SAUNDERS COMPANY
A Harcourt Health Sciences Company
Philadelphia   London   Sydney   Toronto

W.B. SAUNDERS COMPANY
A Harcourt Health Sciences Company

The Curtis Center
Independence Square West
Philadelphia, Pennsylvania 19106

Library of Congress Cataloging-in-Publication Data

The story of orthopaedics/Mercer Rang.

p.   cm.

Includes bibliographical references.

ISBN 0-7216-7141-1

1. Orthopedics.   2. Fractures.   3. Musculoskeletal system—Diseases.
   4. Sports medicine.   I. Title.   [DNLM: 1. Orthopedics.
   2. Fractures.   3. Musculoskeletal Diseases.   WE 168 R196s 2000]

RD705.R36 2000   616.7—dc21

DNLM/DLC   99-088684

Editor: Richard H. Lampert
Editorial Assistant: Beth LoGiudice
Book Designer: Jonel Sofian
Production Manager: Natalie Ware
Project Manager: Edna Dick
Illustration Coordinator: Peg Shaw

THE STORY OF ORTHOPAEDICS   ISBN 0-7216-7141-1

Copyright © 2000, 1977, 1966 by W.B. Saunders Company

All rights reserved. No part of this publication may be reproduced or transmitted in any form or by any means, electronic or mechanical, including photocopy, recording, or any information storage and retrieval system, without permission in writing from the publisher.

Printed in the United States of America.

Last digit is the print number: 9   8   7   6   5   4   3   2   1

To Helen and all the family in appreciation

◆ PREFACE

GALAPAGOS—that's where Darwin learned about the origin of species. Where do you go to learn about the origin of Orthopaedics? Here. Read about the survival of the fittest, good and bad mutations, and even a few big bangs. This book had its origin thirty years ago when I was a Registrar to Lipmann Kessel. He ran a Fellowship course and enlivened it with historical questions: such as "Who was Colles?" or "What did Trendelenburg really describe?" Curiosity drove me to dig out the original information. I wrote *The Anthology of Orthopaedics,* a collection of classic papers and short biographies. For many years nothing seemed to change and there was no point in updating it. Since then, fringe subjects have become mainstream and a lot of the orthopaedic canon has become archaic. The focus of history has changed. Hence a new book.

The interest of history is not just *who* and *when*. History is human behavior in action—it tells us about ourselves. We all find ourselves in situations today that seem new and without precedent: for example, day surgery and outcome studies. Yet these two ideas were vigorously debated at the beginning of the century, but neither caught on. The leader of outcome studies lost his job because his colleagues didn't want their failures revealed. How are we going to deal with this possibility today?

History is the evidence for evidence-based behavior.

Past experience often goes unknown, unstudied, ignored, or discarded as the reminiscences of the elderly, who cannot keep up with new wonders, but the stories of the past have parallels in the present and the future.

History gives us the opportunity to see the natural evolution of disease. Today, we are treating disease early and have lost the day-to-day familiarity with its untreated course that physicians formerly required. Are we treating paper tigers? History shows us the reality of untreated club feet and osteomyelitis.

When a condition has a favorable outcome without treatment, we see that all kinds of prescriptions are credited with cure. Examples are acute back pain and flat feet in children. Once a non–evidence-based prescription has been taught to a generation of doctors, it is almost impossible to eradicate.

The transformation of orthopaedics to its current form has been achieved by prevention more than by treatment. We are no longer a specialty based on TB/osteomyelitis/polio/rickets. This is a pointer to the continuing importance of prevention in the future for trauma, arthritis, and genetic problems. There is room for research on the pathology of prevention as well as the pathology of disease and trauma—why does prevention go wrong? Prevention of polio is giving shots, but prevention of trauma is more complicated. It means changing attitudes to risk taking and lifestyle changes.

Preventive orthopaedics is better than reactive orthopaedics!

Prevention is wholesale and treatment is retail!

Many major advances that have shaped orthopaedics were made by nonorthopaedists—for example, X-rays, sterile surgery, antibiotics, and biomaterials. We have to be ready to research in fields far from what seems relevant to patients. These advances have produced paradigm shifts; nothing is the same after them. They completely change the way we see the world. Paradigm shifts are more and more common, making it difficult to keep up. Examples are CT and MRI. Paradigm shifts produced by orthopaedic surgeons include arthroscopy and joint replacement.

Necessity is sometimes the mother of invention. For example, the modern treatment of wounds began when Paré ran out of boiling oil 400 years ago. History provides all kinds of clues to creative strategies in your thinking.

Many advances are produced outside the university setting. The arrival of science, of questioning, of research funding, and of academic organizations transformed orthopaedics, yet many advances have been produced without grants by doctors in practice, working outside universities—like John Charnley. The productive time a university position is supposed to provide may be used by committees on downsizing.

Nontechnical advances have been as important as technical advances. History taking, physical examination, classification of disease, registries, organizations, and outcome studies have evolved over centuries. There is a lot of room for making advances through nontechnical work.

Many advances were initiated by people who are not credited with them. If you read enough old journals you will always find someone who invented or described it first. The moral is that writing is not enough. You have to run a coast-to-coast promotion.

There is a time when progress can be made and a time when it cannot. For example, the chemical dysplasias of bone took great leaps forward when chemical analysis of tissues started but then came to a standstill until the search for the gene and bone marrow transplantation. These are the waves of discovery.

We have something to offer that is not provided by our medical colleagues/rivals. The first orthopaedists took deformed patients from the bracemakers, infections from the general surgeons, and fractures from bone setters. Today our case mix is different, but we have to be empire builders rather than empire losers.

One famous patient can do a lot for a disease. Roosevelt promoted the March of Dimes for polio. Terry Fox started the Marathon of Hope for cancer—he started unknown and his campaign made him famous. Perhaps we should be encouraging our patients to start campaigns.

History turns up a lot of eccentric, persistent, nonconformist characters. This may be a quality to foster rather than squelch. Today it is said that research requires team work, but somewhere there has to be someone who does not listen to conventional wisdom.

Orthopaedic history may change the way you think and it goes some way to explaining the present.

Orthopaedics is a large part of the history of medicine because musculoskeletal disease is so prevalent in the population.

As you read about some of the human misery of the past, you may think, "If I had been there I could have made such a difference. I wish I could step back in time with the tools of today." You can. See living history—visit the Third World with your doctor's bag.

Good Reading!

MERCER RANG

◆ ACKNOWLEDGMENTS

With grateful thanks to my teachers and colleagues in London, Jamaica, and Toronto who have been so full of ideas and support over the years: Lipmann Kessel, John Golding, Robert Salter, John Hall, Donald Gibson, Walter Bobechko, Norris Carroll, Robert Gillespie, Colin Moseley, Ivan Krajbich, Deborah Stanitski, Peter Armstrong, John Wedge, Douglas Hedden, William Cole, James Wright, Benjamin Alman, Andrew Howard. And to Mihran Tachdjian, Eugene Bleck, Dennis Wenger, Edward Blair, Gordon Hunter, Lew Reines, and a generation of Residents and Fellows.

◆ CONTENTS

- 1 Chapter 1 Introduction

33 Part One—Orthopaedics
- 35 Chapter 2 Adult Hip
- 65 Chapter 3 Child's Hip
- 93 Chapter 4 The Foot
- 115 Chapter 5 Hand and Forearm
- 143 Chapter 6 Deformity of the Spine
- 173 Chapter 7 Spinal Pain
- 195 Chapter 8 Cervical Spine and Whiplash
- 203 Chapter 9 Infection
- 221 Chapter 10 Neuromuscular Disease
- 241 Chapter 11 Arthritis
- 261 Chapter 12 Tumors
- 277 Chapter 13 General Bone Diseases
- 293 Chapter 14 Amputations and Prostheses
- 307 Chapter 15 Orthopaedic Treatment

345 Part Two—The Story of Fractures
- 347 Chapter 16 Injury
- 373 Chapter 17 Lower Limb Fractures
- 395 Chapter 18 Upper Limb Fractures
- 411 Chapter 19 Spine Fractures and Traumatic Paraplegia
- 423 Chapter 20 Fracture Treatment

473 Part Three—The Story of Sports Medicine
- 475 Chapter 21 Sports and Medicine
- 487 Chapter 22 Knee
- 511 Chapter 23 The Shoulder

519 Part Four—Finale
- 521 Chapter 24 Hospitals and the Organization of Care
- 537 Chapter 25 Conclusions
- 543 Chapter 26 References
- 573 Credits
- 579 Index

◆ Chapter One

Introduction

Go into Orthopaedics? "Don't. You will be wasting your surgical talent. Flat feet, crooked backs, and a few cases of joint tuberculosis."
Advice given in 1910.

More orthopaedic surgeons are alive today than in all recorded history. More papers and books are published in a single day than were produced during the thousand-year-long Dark Ages. More operations are done in a day now than were done in these thousand years.

Infection killed children, war maimed the young men, and arthritis made previous generations miserable during their last 20 years of life—but not today. Now, every citizen can be treated—not just the rich and important.

There is more and more effective treatment. These are wonderful times. Never has there been progress at such a rate. There is an orthopaedic culture that separates us from other specialties. We encompass screening newborn hips, going to the games of our team, the excitement of all-night trauma surgery, and the leisurely pace of rehabilitation.

How has this come about? Will it continue? What are our roots? Where did we come from?

History tells us why the specialty of orthopaedics exists and how knowledge about bones and joints was won—sometimes by great leaps forward, but mostly at glacial speed. It explains the

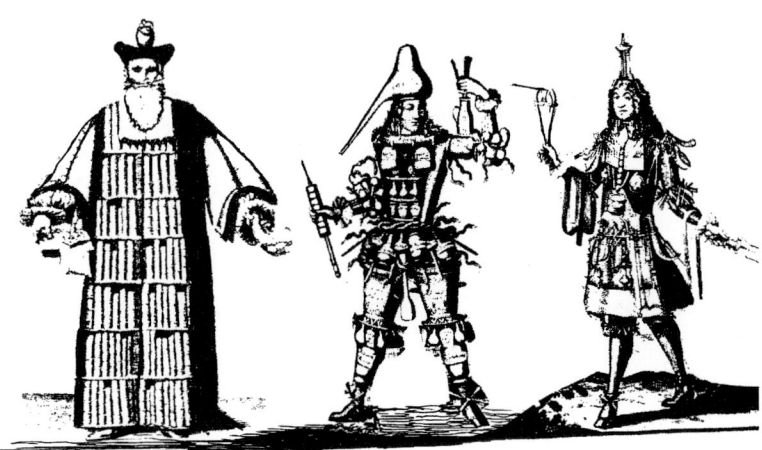

An 18th century cartoon of the doctor as a man of books, as a man of science, and as a surgeon festooned with instruments.

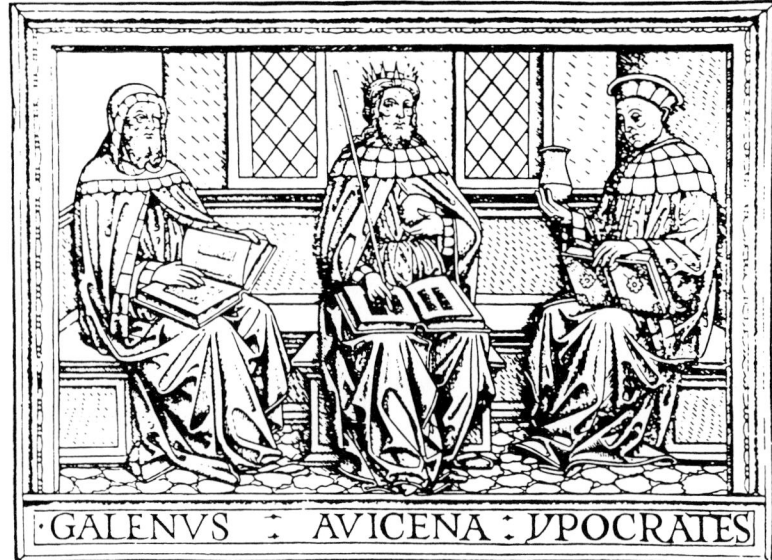

Galen, Avicenna, Hippocrates. You could say these three men wrote everything that a doctor needed to know for more than a thousand years. Or that the unquestioning respect shown by their readers held back progress for a thousand years.

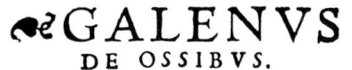

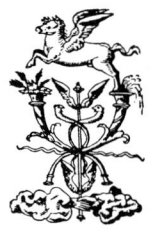

Galen's title page.

development of ideas and technology. It explains why orthopaedics, which was founded on rickets and tuberculosis, had a predilection for immobilization and alignment. Only now, with joint replacement, do we take movement seriously.

Orthopaedics is a success story.

But there is a dark side to history too.

Progress was stagnant for a thousand years during the Dark Ages because doctors looked backward at historical precedents. Faced with a problem, they said, "What did Galen write?" Now, we know they should have been looking forward and using experiments to seek new information. They could have been using outcome studies and clinical trials to guide their practice. There is nothing high tech about this. Instead, "Galen worship" prevailed. Things only looked up when we stopped reading dead languages and started to look at dead bodies.

"We have not taken the quickest and most direct route to our present position. One of the main values of a historical story is that one sees how the growth of knowledge is hampered by prejudice and the failure to recognize one's own ignorance, as well as the misuse of words and the mixing up of facts and theories. Having seen that, one resolves to do better in the future." Macfarlane.

History of Orthopaedics

History Is Not Just Dates

The purpose of history is not to provide a lot of useless facts to be remembered—a game of Trivial Pursuit. History can easily become an addiction to "quaintness." It is fun to hold a famous surgeon's notebook in an old library and see the brown ink and the italic writing done with a quill pen. Pictures of comical splints and old operating scenes bring a chuckle. New technology likes to gloat over old ways. Then, when we see that these pioneers got something right, we say "Wow! Fancy them knowing that so long ago."

We have some pretty strange ancestors who did some strange things in the past. But in the future, after the scalpel is abandoned for something better, we too will be seen as quaint and slightly stupid.

Handwritten Letter in the Royal College of Surgeons Library

Correspondence to Sir Astley Cooper:

"Sir, I have been informed you are in the habit of purchasing bodies and allowing the person a sum weekly, knowing a poor woman that is desirous of doing so I have taken the liberty of calling to know the truth. I remain your humble servant."

Cooper answered:

"The truth is that you deserve to be hanged for such an unfeeling offer. AC"

History Tells Us About Our Rich Heritage

Orthopaedics did not start with AO and hip replacements. We started about 250 years ago in name. But we really only got going at the turn of the century when surgery became safe and X-rays made diagnosis possible. At this time there were very few full-time orthopaedic surgeons; most work on the musculoskeletal system was done by general surgeons. These early part-time orthopaedists were a keen bunch and had amassed about 15,000 papers by 1905, when the first index of the orthopaedic literature was published. By 1935 there were about 84,000 articles. Now there must be several thousand more each year.

If you think you have invented something new, there is more than a slight chance it has been tried before.

History Tells Us About Opportunities Missed

If a simple idea like the randomized control trial had been part of Hippocrates' thinking, I believe progress would have been much faster. He could have done it. He did not need unavailable technology—like electricity—to put medicine on the right track. But why didn't he? Could it be that he had no effective treatment—so that the results for controls would have been no different from those for the treated group?

Another surprise is that physical examination took a back seat to considerations of the weather in making a diagnosis. When people believed that disease was due to sin or an excess of black bile, examination was irrelevant.

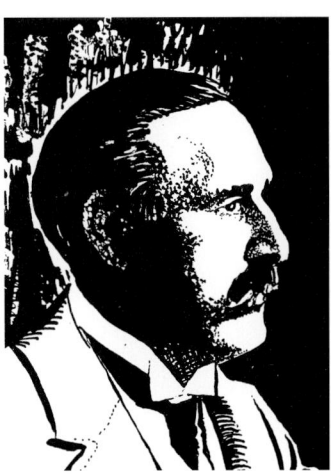

◆ **Albert Hoffa (1859–1908)**
Born in South Africa, the son of a German physician, he started a clinic in Wurzburg and became Professor in Berlin. He is known for his writings, Hoffa's disease, and an early bibliography of 1905.

Medical treatment was quickly trapped by prevailing ideas—particularly medieval morality. The view was that good intentions are enough. For example, the good intention of bloodletting was to remove bad humors. This practice lasted 2000 years. The best of intentions killed George Washington because he was bled by his doctors.

The idea that the end justifies the means was religious heresy, yet this notion is the basis of outcome studies today. Does the treatment work? Only a good outcome justifies a method of treatment.

We tend to think that orthopaedics took a long time to get started because we had to wait for magnetic resonance imaging and computed tomography scans and arthroscopes and hip replacements. But progress was slow because of shoddy thinking. Diagnosis was often uncertain. Imagine a time when the cause of pain in the hip could not be sorted out, when the doctor had no idea whether a patient's pain arose from the spine, from infection, from osteoarthritis, or from a metastasis. For centuries hip disease meant only one thing—tuberculosis of the hip joint. How could progress be made? How could any conclusions be reached about the efficacy of treatment?

The flowery language of case reports, lack of precision, and inclusion of gossipy details used in 18th century descriptions of disease make it difficult for me to read them and make a diagnosis today given a knowledge of bacteria, pathology, and differential diagnosis. But these poor, ignorant 18th century doctors knew only about white swelling (TB), and pus, and they thought they knew about gout, scurvy, and rickets—and that was about it. They stood no chance of diagnosing a torn meniscus or osteoarthritis because they had never heard of either.

Even when a patient came in with complaints about a torn meniscus—as they must have—our forebears did not recognize it as something different. Perhaps this is because the patients were poor historians. We have all had the experience of trying to take a history from an unsophisticated patient—they don't know when it started, they don't know where it hurts, and cannot give much information at all. "It just isn't right, Doc." Is this what our forebears had to live with? At least we know what questions to ask to draw out these patients: Does your knee lock? Did you twist it? And we know a few physical signs. But our forebears asked only whether anyone had cast a spell on them or whether they had forgotten their devotions.

Reading ancient Asian and Oriental descriptions reveals the same problem—inclusion of extraneous information and lack of relevant information. Diagnosis was different then, and so there is little here from those sources.

Looking at Orthopaedic History

History is a bowl of spaghetti, with all the strands being all tangled together. Writing about history is like lifting up one strand

and trying to find the end without having it break. Just as pasta aficionados go for the sauce, so readers of history want a few juicy bits.

We can focus on the people. There are stories of unusual people and wonderful people who would make role models. Many innovators succeed because they persist and persist and disregard the conventional image of a doctor.

We can try to make sense of the past—like Karl Marx. He went further than anyone else in looking at historical events as illustrating laws of human behavior. Like Karl Marx, we can make generalizations based on orthopaedic history, such as "War has led to many of the innovations in trauma care" and "Back ache was ignored until Pott's disease was controlled," and so on.

We can trace the strands of discovery from past to present. For example, surgical sterile technique starts with Pasteur and Lister and goes on to steam sterilization, gloves, masks and gowns, and then to Charnley's operating room greenhouse* and gamma sterilization.

We can try to find parallels in the past to events occuring today. The monks of the 12th century had a monopoly on medicine, just as some governments have today. The monks had to give it up because it was too expensive and because they became so busy with private practice that they neglected their religious duties. This is the stuff of old men's reminiscences.

We can try to provide a schoolboy history, obsessed with dates and names. There are lots of facts arranged as timelines. Some expect a history book to answer arguments posed over a drink. This is why the *Guinness Book of Records* was written. Who was first to describe an operation? A disease? Was neurofibromatosis first described in 1882 by von Recklinghausen—after whom it is often known—or by R. W. Smith in 1849? Or was it someone else? Early descriptions are often vague and poorly organized. There is much irrelevant information but little about systematic examination. The first doctor is usually forgotten, with good reason.

We can try to name the eras of the past just as the layers of the earth's rock are given names. Some people see history as layered and give each layer a name, such as the Renaissance, the Age of Enlightenment, and the Dark Ages. Orthopaedics can be divided into different ages, such as the Age of Nonoperative Orthopaedics, the Age of Implants, and Molecular Orthopaedics.

History is a great field for speculation and the writing of fiction. Why did Fleming take so long to follow up on his observation that bacteria were inhibited around the growth of penicillin? What if Hippocrates had taken a bit more interest in drugs and discovered anesthesia?

If you look at portraits of our eminent forebears, you may think that the greatest innovation was the marketing of the safety razor in 1903. Facial hair was the rule until then.

---

*A glass enclosure inside an operating room used to lessen the chance of infection.

History Is Natural History

Why do you wash out an open fracture? To prevent gas gangrene and tetanus. Have you ever seen these conditions? Probably not. You really have to take it on faith that the washout is necessary—the only evidence is history, working in the Third World, or malpractice by a colleague.

History Is the Story of Stupid Mistakes

For centuries it was thought that air was the cause of inflammation after operation and not dirt, so it was a long time before cleanliness became a part of practice. Suppuration was thought to be beneficial, and so applications that would guarantee infection were favored over those that did not. Wounds were burned and tissue was killed to make a culture medium.

Bleeding was the treatment for shock and many life-threatening conditions—conditions now treated with transfusion.

History Is the Story of Creativity

Why think? Why not try the experiment? John Hunter

Why are we not more creative? It is easy to regard Charnley or Lister or Fleming as a genius as if that explained everything—but why doesn't everyone come up with a good idea? Why did it take so long?

I think the reason is that we are sheep much of the time. No one wants to be first. We all attend seminars so that we fill our heads with the ideas of other people and leave no space for uncertainty and admissions of ignorance—the springboard of innovation.

Many creative people reject conventional answers and may spend their lives on the edge of being fired because they are not team players. History explodes the idea that progress is neat and orderly—eccentrics and antiauthoritarians have made the changes. Perhaps this is changing as massive projects such as the human genome become more important than the work of small laboratories.

Many inventions that have changed the face of orthopaedics are not due to the work of orthopaedists—Pasteur, Fleming, Salk, and Roentgen were not orthopaedists. So much of what passes for research by orthopaedic surgeons today is no more than auditing results and making modifications. The chance of a new concept being uncovered by an orthopaedist is less than the chance of an outsider doing it. We should always be looking at other fields to see whether there is anything that we could incorporate into our practice. The best chance of making a big contribution comes from looking at any field—so long as it is not orthopaedics!

History shows us why we should be creative and independent when we are young. Most original work is done by people under the age of 30 years.

Many Breakthroughs Result from Using New Tools, such as MRI, arthroscopy, and chemotherapy. A researcher is more likely to make an advance from playing with a new tool than from looking more deeply at something we have been doing for years—for example, reviewing the results of an operation.

Many new ideas have taken long to be accepted. They are often laughed at. We must be tolerant. We must not be the last to accept new ideas nor try to stamp them out.

The road of an innovator is not easy. If you, the reader, hope to be an innovator, this book will prepare you for the problems you must face. Innovators are tenacious; they are strong advocates for their ideas; they are not content to commit an idea to paper and then sit back. If they do, the idea will die.

Are Wrong Ideas a Bigger Block to Progress Than Ignorance? There are plenty of examples of principles promoted by vocal authorities that time has proved wrong. One can cite the policy that acute nerve injuries should never be sutured primarily, that joint injuries should be immobilized, and that blood letting was good for many severe problems. Ignorance is more easily dealt with than a strongly held erroneous belief.

The Work of an Orthopaedist Has Changed and Will Continue to Change. The diseases that dominated orthopaedics in the past are not the problems we see today. Yesterday's orthopaedist knew about rickets, chronic osteomyelitis, tuberculosis, polio, and malunited fractures. Today's orthopaedist knows about osteoarthritis, back ache, and knee injuries. Natural history is a thing of the past.

When orthopaedics was starting around 1850, the life expectancy for a blue collar worker was 23 years (hardly long enough to be affected by the diseases that fill our time today).

The repertoire of treatment has changed as much as the repertoire of disease.

As diseases that we treat change, so we develop new concepts that we use in everyday speech, which carry a wealth of meaning to us. Stem loosening, creeping substitution, iatrogenic disease—each of these ideas had to make a start and then be updated as we learned more about each. Some concepts, such as range of movement, muscle strength, reflexes, ligamentous instability, were not there from the beginning, and early accounts of disease suffer from lack of these basics. It is as if they had lousy residents then. The sense of time, in the days before watches and calendars, is vague. However, even today in the Third World, many people don't know their age because birthdays are not celebrated.

Just to list all that we take for granted would be a big task. The longer this history book becomes, the more incomplete it seems.

What Was Orthopaedics Like in Victorian London?

In 1855, Edward Lonsdale reported on the diagnosis of 3000 patients that he and Dr. Adams treated during 3 years at the Royal Orthopaedic Hospital in London.

Bowlegs and knockknees   1663 (dietary rickets was common)
Clubfeet   495
Deformities of the spine   465
Contraction of joints, etc   243
Paralysis   45
Fractures, dislocations, and diseased joints   65
Congenital malformations   24

What Was American Orthopaedics Like 100 Years Ago?

The major interest of orthopaedics at the turn of the 20th century can be gauged from the papers presented during the first 10 years of the American Orthopaedic Association—40% were on tuberculosis, 15% on clubfeet, and another 15% on developmental dysplasia of the hip, rickets, and polio combined.

Knight's book *Orthopaedia* was one of the first published in the United States in 1884. The chapter titles are interesting. He includes hernia, procidentia, varicose veins, and ectopia of the bladder. The musculoskeletal topics are clubfoot, scoliosis, polio, tuberculosis, and rickets. There is nothing about back ache, osteoarthritis, or the knee. There is nothing about operating!

Lovett and Bradford's textbook, published in 1915, has 406 pages: 113 are on tuberculosis, 34 on polio, 24 on rickets. Only two pages each are devoted to meniscal tears, back pain, osteoarthritic hip, and osteoarthritic knee, and there is one page on tumors—such are the changes in practice.

What Is Third World Orthopaedics Like Now?

I collected some figures in a poor part of Africa recently. I was looking after about 100 beds because there were big delays in treatment and inpatient care was cheap. The inpatients were not impatient. Most were there with injuries—mostly from the road, but some were due to war and animal bites. Osteomyelitis, tuberculosis, and joint infections arrived late and stayed long. If you want to see history today, go to the Third World.

This is very different from First World orthopaedics—joint replacement, polytrauma, fractures in elderly people, and arthroscopic surgery—conditions hardly considered part of orthopaedics in the past.

When Did Orthopaedics Really Begin?

You need the word before you can think the thought.   George Orwell in *New Speak*

Was it in 1741, when the first book with the word "Orthopaedia" was published?

Orthopaedics was little more than a word invented by an 83-year-old grumpy Parisian pediatrican, Nicholas Andry (Nicolas André). *Orthopaedia* was the title of a self-help book written for

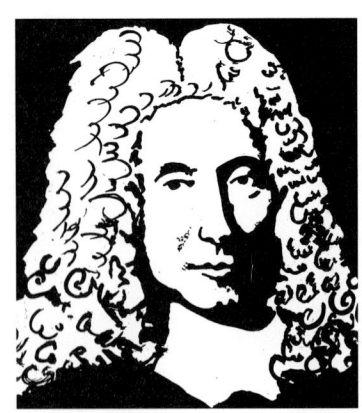

◆ Nicholas Andry

Orthopaedia title page.

Orthopaedia preface.

parents. Today every bookstore has a self-help section, and at the end of the 18th century they would have had medical books. Self-help was popular because doctors were costly and had little effective treatment, transportation was rudimentary, and communication was difficult—there were no Yellow Pages. Doctors were university-trained internists; they were few and too expensive for ordinary folks. They did no surgery. They moved into the home for the duration of an illness and then moved to the next patient's home. Herbalists or apothecaries knew a little medicine and sold drugs. A surgeon who had apprenticed with a master surgeon would treat wounds and infections. A bonesetter looked after fractures. A bracemaker took care of deformities. A lot of medical care was provided by wise women without any training, because they were near at hand and cheap.

Was it in 1780, when the first orthopaedic hospital was founded? Was it at the beginning of the 19th century, when intellectual curiosity was expanding horizons or was it at the end of the century when anesthesia, asepsis, and X-rays made it possible to change the subject from orthopaedics to orthopaedic surgery?

Was it at the beginning of the 19th century, when we began the correction of soft tissue deformities by tenotomy and splinting and exercises? Or was it at the end of the last century, when we began the correction of bony deformities by osteotomy? Or was it because outbreaks of cholera and other infectious diseases stopped being the main preoccupation of doctors and patients?

Or was it joint replacement in the middle of the 20th century that defines us?

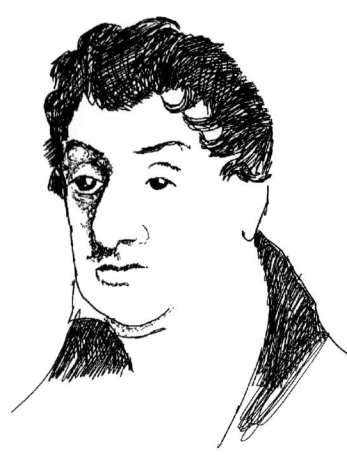

◆ Robert Chessher

Where Was the First Orthopaedic Hospital?

There is no easy answer, and I am expecting lots of readers to write in with suggestions.

Was it an inpatient scoliosis institute in Holland in the 1660s, run by the Schott brothers?

Was it the Royal Mineral Water Hospital at Bath, founded in 1740, which treated arthritis?

Was it an institute opened by Jean-André Venel in 1780 in his home in Orbe, Switzerland? (He used splints and braces for clubfeet and scoliosis. Soon after he died the institution closed).

In the United Kingdom there is a shadowy Robert Chessher who ran a hospital at Hinckley, in the Midlands, for similar problems from 1778. This died with Dr. Chessher.

Was it the Royal Sea Bathing Hospital at Margate, England, founded in 1791 and still in operation? This was a publicly funded hospital dedicated to the healing qualities of sea bathing for many diseases. Gradually the focus came to be bone and joint tuberculosis.

On the continent of Europe, orthopaedics meant correcting deformities by nonoperative means, and many institutes rose to the challenge. They were separate from the general hospitals where fracture repair, treatment of osteomyelitis, and amputation surgery were carried out.

Many orthopaedic institutes began in the 1820s, with a few before this.

At Morley, Meuse, France, François Humbert founded an Établissement Orthopédique in 1817, mostly for spinal deformity.

Jacques-Mathieu Delpech started a hospital in Montpellier in 1825. The surgical treatment of deformity was ushered in when he did a tenotomy of the tendo Achillis in 1816. His peers thought badly of the plan and persuaded him to give it up.

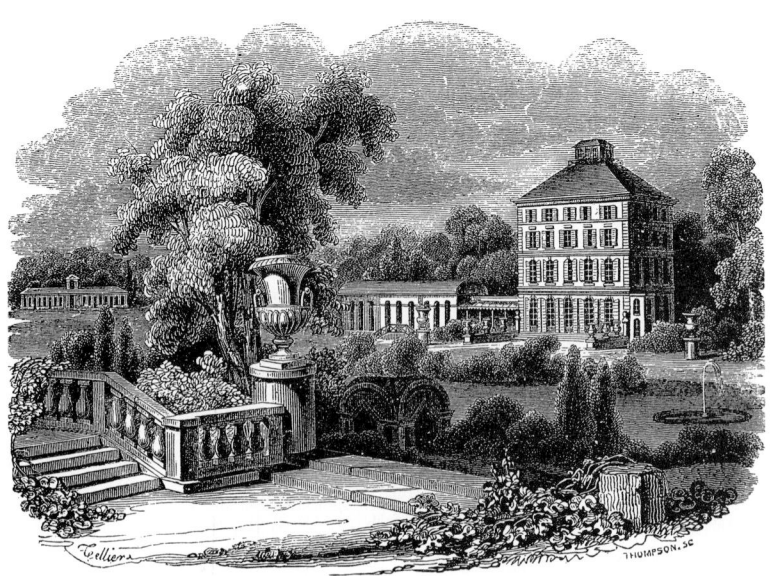

Guerin's Hospital outside Paris in 1837.

Guillaume Jalade-Lafond founded an Institute at Chaillot, outside Paris, in 1823.

Charles-Gabriel Pravaz started an Institute outside Paris at Passy in 1826, and Jules Guérin took it over.

Johann Georg Heine started an Orthopaedic Institute in Wurtzburg, Germany, in 1816. Jacob Heine started the Orthopaedic Institute in Cannstatt, near Stuttgart, in 1829. In Hanover, Germany, Stromeyer opened an Orthopaedic Institute in 1829 and did a tenotomy in 1831.

In Italy, Bartolommeo Borella founded an Institute at San Donato in 1823.

William Little, born with a clubfoot in Britain, went to Germany to be treated by Stromeyer by tenotomy. He went on to found an Orthopaedic Hospital in London in 1837. Stromeyer had another student, Detmold, who emigrated to the States and began orthopaedics in New York City in 1837.

John Ball Brown started an orthopedique infirmary in Boston in 1838.

John Rhea Barton worked at the Pennsylvania Hospital, Philadelphia, when he did the first osteotomies in 1826.

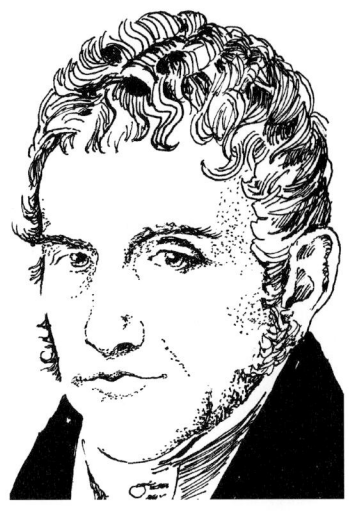

◆ Johann Georg Heine

What Is the Family Tree of an Orthopaedic Surgeon?

Before there were orthopaedists, musculoskeletal disease was looked after by several groups:

- Bracemakers took care of deformities.
- General surgeons drained pus, treated open wounds, and did amputations. They were said by Thomas Fuller to need "an Eagle's eye, a Lady's hand, and a Lion's heart."
- Bonesetters treated fractures. Robert Turner took a book started by a friar in 1539 and published *The Compleat Bone-Setter* in 1654.

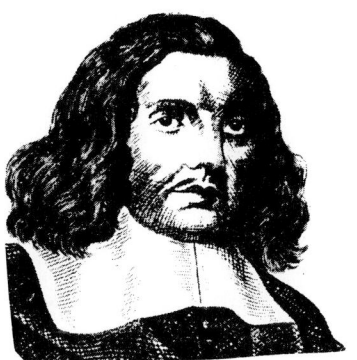

◆ Robert Turner

Where Did Orthopaedics Start?

Orthopaedics started in many countries. In Egypt there were papyri about fractures 5000 years ago. In India, it started with Suśruta in 800 BC, who was a sort of Indian Hippocrates. In Greece there was the original Hippocrates who wrote much about fractures, tuberculosis, and deformities. He broke away from attributing disease to the gods. He pointed out that there were diseases with specific characteristics and names—others had thought that there were no patterns.

The Chinese were held back by Confucius, who held that the body was sacred and should not be mutilated. This sabotaged a scientific approach, and their early books are hard to understand. However, Hua t'o, a surgeon in 190 AD, was worshipped as a god! He emphasized the value of exercise and movement. The Imperial medical college in 1076 published a book on fractures.

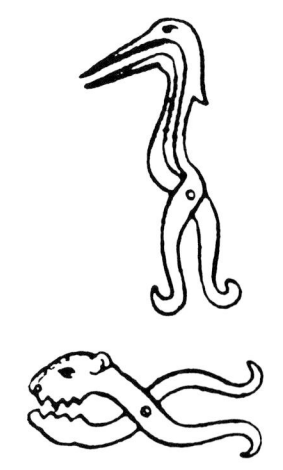

Suśruta's forceps. Heron and lion forceps: 800 BC.

Title page of book, by Bauer and Barthelmess, 1854.

In Japan, the Chi so ki book on wounds and fractures was produced in 834 AD. More recently, in 1808, the Seikotzu han book on manipulation of fractures and dislocations was published.

During the Dark Ages in Europe, knowledge was kept alive in the Arab world. Avicenna (980–1036) wrote a *Canon of Surgery* in Bokhara, and Albucasis in Cordova wrote that "Surgical operations are of two kinds: those that benefit the patient and those that kill him." Also in Cordova, the great Jewish physician Moses Maimonides wrote his aphorisms in 1497.

In Europe in the 18th and 19th centuries, the spirit of the Industrial Revolution fired an explosion of medical progress. People realized that discovery and the application of science to technology were the pathway to continuing progress. Just arguing about what Hippocrates really meant was not going to produce results. This was a revolution of thought.

In the United States in the 19th century, orthopaedics was established when it was still fighting for recognition in Europe.

Though orthopaedics started in many places with different ideas, today the world is a village and ideas flash round.

False Trails and Timing of Discoveries

Positive and negative events have shaped orthopaedics—pushing it forward or holding it back. The discovery of anesthesia, sterilization, X-rays, antibiotics, stainless steel, and polio vaccine are the biggest positive events. But the many wrong ideas could be argued to have had as big an effect as positive influences. They held orthopaedics back as much as the others had pushed it forward. Examples are deliberately infecting wounds, neglecting anatomy, believing long-dead authorities over verifiable fact, and all kinds of useless operations—sacroiliac fusion for back ache, bleeding for shock, colectomy for arthritis. Outcome studies and randomized trials should guard us from these in the future. Elsewhere the question has been asked: Why did these simple low-tech checks take so long to be applied?

The Rise of the Specialties

Surgery has always been separate from medicine—surgery was regarded as a gross occupation, not much different from butchery, whereas medicine was a clean profession, resembling law. About the beginning of the 20th century, both medicine and surgery began to fragment into specialties. Why? Because, for the first time, treatment began to produce a better outcome than natural history alone. Honed skills, an organization, specialist journals, and a library began to pay off. Specialists were no longer regarded as failed generalists. Doctors accepted that they couldn't manage everything and began to refer patients to specialists.

Then, as treatment became more and more effective and mass transportation allowed patients to travel to the best doctor instead of just the closest doctor, specialists became the rule rather than the exception. Fragmentation increased with the growth of technology, which is unfriendly to the casual user.

The idea of being an orthopaedic surgeon did not attract followers quickly—at first there were no more than a handful of people who could say that they earned a living doing orthopaedics full-time. Orthopaedics did not become an operative specialty until after the advent of the Three Amigos: anesthesia in 1846, asepsis in 1867, and X-rays in 1895. Before the Three Amigos, everything that was not fatal was treated nonoperatively.

By the beginning of the 20th century, a lot had been learned about locomotor diseases.

Gradually the organization to care for these conditions came together, but on a small scale. Then the First World War turned the world upside down. Out of the war came many people trained in trauma and with organizational skills. Suddenly it was realized that orthopaedics was not just about crippled children but about real men and women as well. A critical mass of orthopaedists was achieved.

Orthopaedics Nearly Didn't Make It as a Specialty

We had a battle to separate from general surgeons. In the United States there was more freedom and less tradition and orthopaedics took off early. In Britain, there was more difficulty. General surgeons were opposed to fragmentation. The British Orthopaedic Society was founded and started a journal. It floundered—most surgeons said they didn't know what orthopaedic meant and those who did believed it had the German meaning of nonoperative treatment. Different words were tried out—such as orthomorphy—but they worked no better. The journal was failing until it changed its name from *Journal of Orthopaedic Surgery* to *Journal of Bone and Joint Surgery*—a permanent testimony to the importance of plain words.

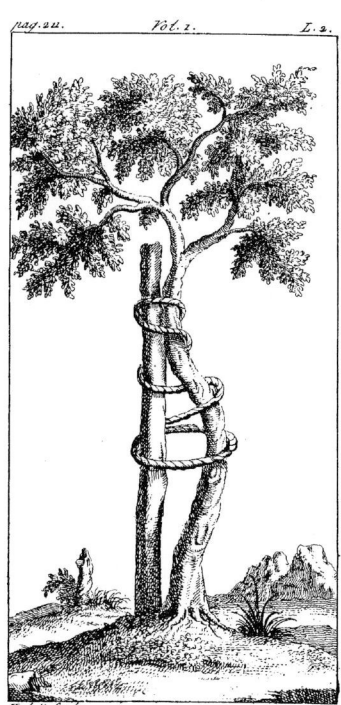

Andry's Tree—the symbol of orthopaedics. He was trying to keep the legs of rickety children straight, hence the analogy to a young tree. Now that our motto is "Movement is life," we need a better symbol.

Today we have community orthopaedists, and in the big city there are subspecialists in sports medicine, spine, hand, pediatrics, joint replacement, and so on.

After 2000 years of being a part of general surgery, the general orthopaedist has had a life of only 50 years before disappearing into subspecialties.

The Growth of Knowledge

Injury and disease were first looked on as the result of divine punishment or an evil spell—this led to prayer and magic and incantation. There was no need to understand anatomy and pathology. In poor countries this is still the case—think of Voodoo in Haiti.

Hippocrates took the first step away from magic/religious tradition by objective descriptions of disorders and their outcome. Galen pushed knowledge forward by dissecting animals but gave up before discovering the circulation of the blood. Today's surgeons find it hard to imagine that this piece of information took so long to be discovered. Galen and Hippocrates might as well have written the Bible because their views were unquestioned for 1500 years—the Dark Ages. This was a time when people believed what they were told over what they saw for themselves.

The written word was respected over personal experience. Today, a paper contains a brief review of the literature and a lot of new experimental data. But during the Dark Ages, a paper had an exhaustive review of the literature and no new data.

Why were ideas static?

Poverty. The world was poor due to strife—much like parts of Africa today. No one expects scientific breakthroughs from Rwanda.

New Ideas Seen as Heresy. The Church and priests controlled the information highway and regarded any new idea as heresy after Constantine made Christianity the official religion of the Roman Empire in 313. The early Church came close to being broken by factions; they clung to old authoritarian ideas and discouraged experiments. Priests had a monopoly on medicine and saw human dissection as desecrating the body. They were concerned with the health of the soul and viewed the body as packaging. Medicine did not have the same prestigious position as it does today. Lack of knowledge made medicine too ineffective to be useful. Uselessness discouraged interest.

The experimental approach was discouraged. Knowledge was based on revealed information and resulted in faith. It was not to be questioned. Only in Victorian times did Galton test the value of religious prayer using the experimental method. He pointed out that in Britain the National Anthem was frequently played, which includes the words "God Save the King/Queen." Large numbers of people sing this. As a result, far more people are praying for the longevity of the King/Queen than for the average person. Galton found that royalty does not live longer than the average person—indeed a little shorter because of assassinations. He argued that prayer did not pass the test of science.

The grip of the Church on medicine softened in the 12th and 13th centuries when it was found that the financial drain was too great and that the staff were neglecting their religious duties in the pursuit of private practice. This is a state of affairs not without parallel today. Lay doctors filled the gap. All kinds of Hospital Societies sprang up.

With the Renaissance, the artists wanted to be able to paint more realistic saints. Artists started dissecting criminals to know what made the skin bulge and crease. They were not concerned with the theory of the four humors; they drew what they saw. Within a few years, anatomic knowledge went from a little to a lot—with Vesalius' *Atlas* of 663 pages in 1543. The paintings that fill the Louvre were the reason for anatomic studies!

Knowledge So Small That It Was Not Useful. A basic infrastructure of knowledge is needed before the scientific approach provides useful technology. For example, it has been known for centuries that hip fractures often fail to unite. But nothing could be done to improve outcome until aseptic surgery, anesthesia, X-rays, and implants were developed.

Then there was a lot of wrong information that was counterproductive.

The real advances came from the invention of new tools—the microscope, arthroscope, gait analysis, and MRI—because they provide so much information that knowledge can progress fast.

Stages of Knowledge. A feature of orthopaedics in the past century has been the rise and fall of many orthopaedic diseases, for example tuberculosis, polio, rickets. It is instructive to look at the evolution of ideas for a disease.

First someone provides an early clinical description, so flawed that the disease in question is confused with other diseases. Interest is created. All kinds of ineffectual treatment are proposed and argument starts. Little progress is made until an advance in another field sheds light—argument lessens. Perhaps special facilities are built, such as the tuberculosis sanataria. The disease becomes treatable. Then methods of prevention become known and the disease fades in importance—special facilities become redundant.

We are now treating diseases that have not gone through this evolutionary process, for example scoliosis, clubfeet, and osteoarthritic hip. We do not understand why they happen. We accept that they cannot be prevented or restored to normal, but we can treat them empirically. We hope that they will disappear the way of the others.

Surgeons knew only a few physical signs in the past to make a diagnosis. There were no investigations. Now we know about 2000 signs. These have been overtaken in the 20th century by investigations, which are used to make or confirm just about every diagnosis. Often the diagnosis is the product of the test, such as dark disc disease seen on MRI.

It is only in the modern era that doctors can do more good than harm. The turning point varies with each disease. For open fractures it was Lister in the 1860s. For carpal tunnel it was in the 1950s. For malignant tumors it was the late 1970s.

We have reached the end of an orthopedic adolescence—we are no longer the poorly paid, little skilled, low status straighteners of crippled children. Now we are members of the techno-industrial complex. Hurrah! Enjoy it before the Health Maintenance Organizations and oversupply spoil everything.

The Scientization of Orthopaedics

There is the perception that the olden day doctors looking after orthopaedic problems just did what the ancients told them. They had neither the means nor the desire to change. Today we disbelieve anything told us by a person aged more than 50 years or written more than 5 years ago. New ideas are the key to promotion—not parroting old ones.

Until the 1850's, healing was held in low esteem. The movers and shakers went into cathedral building and engineering, or exploration, or the Army, where great advances and conquests could be made.

What has changed? Science works. We are organized along scientific lines.

We have research groups. We value objective over subjective data. We believe what we see over what we read.

We look forward for information and not backward. We spend no time trying to interpret some observation in terms of what

Galen or Charnley or anyone else would say. Confronted by a problem, we consult Medlines, and if this does not have the answer we may do some research ourselves. We do not try to find a hidden meaning in Galen's works.

We question rather than accept—Journal clubs look beyond the summary to see whether the data support the conclusion.

We try to see things in mathematical, biomechanical, or biologic terms.

Information is used for a hypothesis that can be tested and put to use. For example, with the hypothesis that chemotherapy prevents most metastases from osteosarcoma, a research question was this: Does limb-sparing surgery give as good a survival rate as amputation? Each new piece of information is the stepping stone to another.

The scientization of orthopaedics begins with the discoveries of anesthesia, asepsis, and X-rays and continues with molecular orthopaedics.

The Three Amigos

Only after anesthesia, aseptic surgery, and X-rays were discovered did we make much progress. Prior to these discoveries, remarkable doctors had done remarkable things, but the patient in the street did not have much chance of diagnosis and successful treatment.

The Invention of Anesthesia

An editorial in the *Lancet* (1836) was written before anesthesia was invented:

Fear During Operations

"Unsteadiness in a patient, during an operation, is one of the many trying things which disturb the tranquility of a surgeon in extensive practice. In an operation vast responsibility rests on the composure of the sufferer. Much also depends on the steadiness, and mild, though confident manner, in which the surgeon himself sets about his painful duty, inspiring his victim with reliance on a certainty of relief at the expense of a temporary amount of suffering."

The novelist Fanny Burney had a mastectomy in 1810 and wrote a chilling account of her experience.

None of us would have been surgeons 150 years ago. It was too unpleasant—operations were like torture. Operating rooms

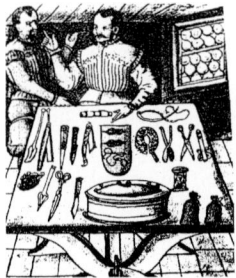
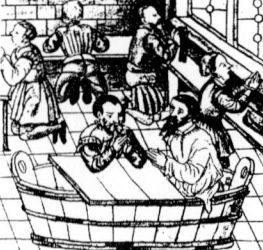
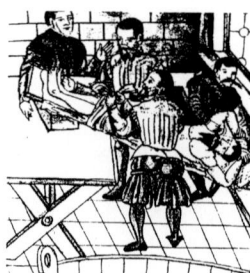

Stages of an operation in 1559. (A) Checking the instruments. (B) Pray with the patient. (C) Tie the patient down. From a book by Caspar Stomayr. Lake Leman.

October 17, 1846. This is the second operation done with ether anesthesia at Massachusetts General Hospital. The photographer was too upset to record the first operation. Drs Morton, Warren, and Bigelow were present.

were invented because patients in one bed could not stand the horror of an operation going on in the next bed.

Hypnotism was tried.

Attempts at narcosis using drugs and alcohol are of great antiquity but were of little use until street drugs were brought into the hospital.

Joseph Priestley lived next to a brewery in England and became interested in smells and gases. Self-taught, he discovered nitrous oxide in 1772 and oxygen in 1774. His political views led to his house being vandalized in 1791, and he left for Pennsylvania. He suggested that oxygen would help people with breathing problems. While testing this, a young chemist, Humphry Davy, discovered the high from breathing nitrous oxide. Soon there were laughing gas orgies. In Georgia a general practitioner, Dr. Crawford Long, was asked in 1841–1842 for nitrous oxide for a party. All he had was ether. Some of the party revelers injured themselves without feeling pain. One of them, who had moles on his neck, returned and asked Dr. Long to remove them while he was breathing ether. Dr. Long did this on March 30, 1842 but did not publicize it.

In Boston, two dentists, Horace Wells and William T. G. Morton, were visiting a fair in Hartford where a showman put on a display of laughing gas in December 1844. Horace had a painful tooth so he bought some of the gas and had his tooth pulled painlessly—"A new era of tooth pulling," he said. They tried a demonstration at Massachusetts General Hospital, but it failed. Wells committed suicide three years later.

Morton experimented with ether and put on a demonstration at Massachusetts General Hospital on October 16, 1846; a neck tumor was removed—a triumph. "Gentlemen, this is no humbug," said the patient. The dark side of Morton appeared—he didn't tell anyone what he had used and wanted to patent it. However, the secret was discovered and Morton died in poverty in 1868. Anesthesia spread to Europe on the first boat. Liston used it first at University College Hospital, London, and said, "Gentlemen, this Yankee dodge beats mesmerism hollow."

A miserable time followed the invention of anesthesia. Anesthesia stimulated the volume of surgery and the invention of operations, but operations became infected and there were many deaths because the idea of sterility was still years away.

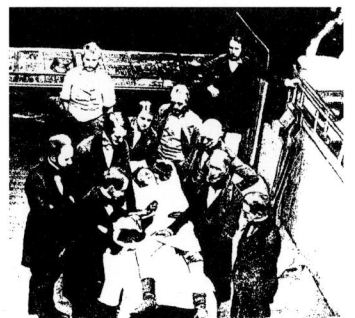

◆ **Henry Jacob Bigelow, 1818–1890.**

He was the son of a Harvard professor and qualified there. Affected with lung disease, he traveled to Cuba and Europe to recuperate. He visited all the leaders of orthopaedics and at age 27 years wrote about what he had learned in a manual of orthopaedic surgery—In What Cases and to What Extent Is the Division of Muscles, Tendons, or Other Parts Proper for the Relief of Deformity or Lameness? This won a prize in 1844 and was one of the first American works on orthopaedics. He heard about TG Morton pulling teeth under ether and persuaded him to come to Massachusetts General Hospital to demonstrate while the chief, Dr JC Warren, operated on Oct 16, 1846. His paper about this operation was published (Boston Med Surg J 1846, 35, 309, 379).

He described the importance of a Y-shaped ligament in the front of the hip in a 1869 book on hip dislocation and was rewarded by having his name attached to it.

TIMELINE

- 1853 Hollow needle. Alexander Wood, Scotland
- 1853 Hypodermic syringe. Charles-Gabriel Pravaz, early French orthopedic surgeon
- 1871 Gas cylinders. Johnstone brothers, USA
- 1874 Intravenous anesthesia: Pirre Ore
- 1878 Endotracheal anesthesia. Macewen, an early Scottish general/orthopedic surgeon
- 1904 Procaine. Alfred Einhorn, Germany
- 1909 Intravenous block. August Bier, Germany

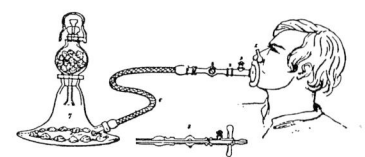

Ether equipment in 1847.

Chlorurets: This was an 1827 attempt to rid hospitals of infection.

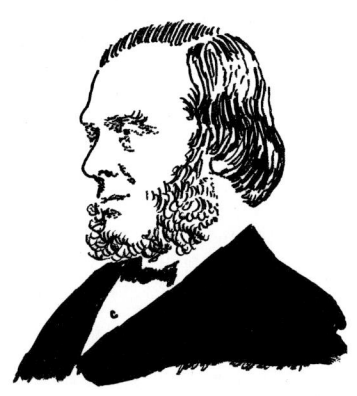

◆ Joseph Lister

The Control of Infection

"The man laid on the operating table in one of our surgical hospitals, is exposed to more chances of death than the English soldier on the field of Waterloo (1815)."—Comment on operating 150 years ago.

Wound infection

Three errors made any kind of operation a death trap.

1. **Pus is good**. Perhaps this idea came from the observation that draining pus is better than undrained pus. But it led to all kinds of things, which promoted the formation of pus, being applied to wounds. Dung brought in organisms and boiling oil cooked the tissues to be feasted on by bacteria.
2. **Air carries in contagion**. The miasma theory. This was correct in the sense that bacteria are in the air, but they are present in much larger numbers on unwashed hands and instruments. This led to subcutaneous tenotomy, an operation that didn't let the air in—the operation which was the jumping-off point for orthopaedics.
3. **Spontaneous generation of contagion**. Prevention was not possible. This idea meant that there was no separation of septic cases and no attempt to clean equipment used on one patient after another.

There had been attempts to prevent infection before Lister. Wards were sprinkled with bleach to destroy "miasmata."

Lister in Glasgow was trying to find an answer to infection. A chemistry professor told him to read a paper by Pasteur that was several years old; Pasteur had found that microorganisms made grapes ferment, and Lister saw a similarity between putrefaction of grapes, food, and flesh. Lister and his wife converted their kitchen into a small laboratory and tested carbolic acid, which was used to stop sewage from smelling. He tried it on wounds and published a paper in 1867 describing success in 9 of 11 patients.

ON THE ANTISEPTIC PRINCIPLE IN THE PRACTICE OF SURGERY

JOSEPH LISTER, FRS, 1867

"I arrived at the conclusion that the essential cause of suppuration in wounds is decomposition. . . . It has been shown by the researches of Pasteur that the septic property of the atmosphere depended on minute organisms suspended in it . . . It occurred to me that decomposition in the injured part might be avoided . . . by applying some material capable of destroying the life of the floating particles.

The material which I have employed is carbolic or phenic acid.

The first class of cases to which I applied it was that of compound fractures. . . . Limbs which would otherwise unhesitatingly be condemned to amputation may be retained with confidence of the best results.

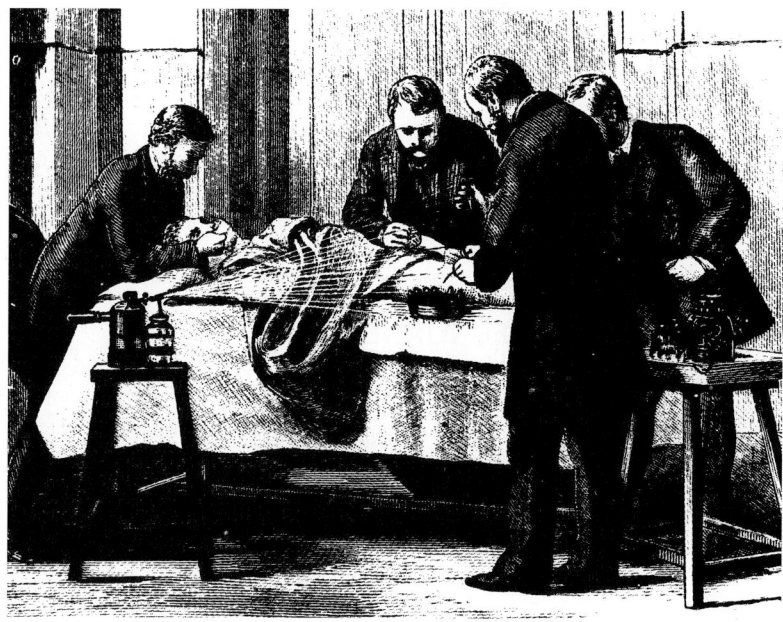

Lister's Spray in action. His students said at the beginning of an operation, "Now let us spray." This looks very different from an operation scene today.

I am prepared to go so far as to say that a solution of carbolic acid in twenty parts of water, may be relied on for destroying any septic germs that may fall upon a wound during the performance of an operation.

Previous to its introduction, the two large wards in which most of my cases of accident and of operation are treated were amongst the unhealthiest in the whole surgical division of the Glasgow Royal Infirmary. I have felt ashamed, when recording the results of my practice, to allude to hospital gangrene or pyaemia. Whenever all, or nearly all, the beds contained cases with open sores, these grievous complications were pretty sure to show themselves: so that I came to welcome simple fractures, though in themselves of little interest either for myself or the students, because their presence diminished the proportion of open sores among the patients. But since the antiseptic treatment has been brought into full operation, and wounds and abscesses no longer poison the atmosphere with putrid exhalations, my wards . . . have completely changed their character; so that during the last nine months not a single instance of pyaemia, hospital gangrene, or erysipelas has occurred in them."

Lister traveled widely, describing antiseptic surgery, and progressive surgeons started spraying carbolic acid. It was a simple system, needing no elaborate equipment. However, it didn't catch on universally. Statisticians have said that this is because he used historical controls, and Lister himself said that 75 patients was not enough to draw a statistical conclusion. However, if he had known about the chi squared test, he would have known that a difference between 43% mortality in the untreated group and 15% in the treated group was highly significant, and his paper might have carried more weight. Many surgeons angrily opposed Lister's ideas. For twenty years battles prevented patients benefiting—until the emphasis changed to aseptic surgery with the invention of boilers by Neuber in Kiel in 1885 and steam sterilizers by Bergmann and Schimmelbusch later.

TIMELINE OF SAFE SURGERY

1775 Claude Pouteau in Lyon emphasized handwashing to prevent the spread of infection. In 1744 he had pricked his finger, and quickly his finger began to resemble the wounds he continued to dress in the hospital.

1795 Epidemic of puerperal fever in Aberdeen reported by Alexander Gordon.

1843 A paper by Oliver Wendell Holmes of Harvard describes how he stopped an epidemic of puerperal fever in 1835 by washing his hands between cases. He provoked more opposition than agreement.

1836-1837 Theodor Schwann (1810-1882, Berlin, Liège, Louvain) beat Pasteur to the theory of infection and its control. He showed that putrefaction was due to living cells that could be killed by heat. Fermentation due to yeasts could be prevented by heat. But for some reason his vision was dwarfed by Pasteur later.

1848 Ignaze Semmelweis introduces handwashing to a delivery ward in Vienna, reducing maternal mortality after childbirth from 18.3% to 1.3%. His idea was the result of doing many autopsies on dead mothers. His pathology teacher died after sustaining a laceration in the autopsy room, which showed the same changes as those of the mothers. Semmelweis concluded that small particles on the hands caused these deaths.

His ideas were not accepted; he became psychotic and died (possibly of a head injury) in an asylum in 1865.

1857-1859 Pasteur publishes the result of fermentation experiments: wine spoiled by particles that are destroyed by heat.

"In the field of observation, chance favours the prepared mind."

1864 T. Spencer Wells: *Some causes of excessive mortality after surgical operations.*

A mortality in the Paris Hospitals from 1836 to 1841 of 39%, including amputations of the fingers and toes (thigh, 62; leg, 55; arm, 45; forearm, 28) was, when announced by M. Malgaigne, regarded as a startling revelation.

He then referred to the work of Pasteur and germs in the air, Davaine's work on "bacteria" in the blood, and Polli's observation in Milan that sulfuric acid had an

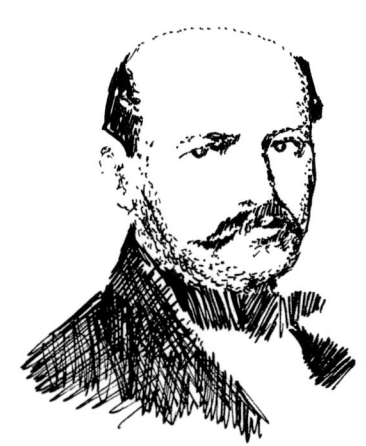

◆ Ignaz Semmelweis

"antiseptic" action. He tried using various sulfites by mouth in cases of septicemia but never had the insight of Lister to sterilize the surgical field.

1865 Glasgow's Professor of Chemistry reads Pasteur's paper and talks to Lister about it. Lister repeats the experiments, aided by his wife in their home laboratory. He decides to use carbolic acid (which is used to prevent sewage from smelling) on an open fracture of the tibia on an 11 year old boy, James Greenlees. The leg healed. He met with success in other open fractures. He started to use handwashing and carbolic dressing and sprays for amputation, and published his results in Lancet, January 8, 1870. Before antisepsis—16 deaths in 35 cases; after asepsis—6 deaths in 40 cases.

1874 Volkmann becomes a convert to asepsis, and the idea catches on quicker in Germany than in Britain.

1876 Robert Koch identifies a specific bacterium as the cause of a specific disease.

1878 Koch: Investigations show that wound infection is produced by bacteria.

1881 Chamberland built an autoclave for Pasteur's laboratory, and in 1886 Redard in Paris introduced it to the operating room.

1883 Lister's ideas begin to catch on—after more than 10 years of controversy.

1883 Gustav Neuber of Kiel: Gown and cap, dust-free ventilation.

1884 Macewen, in Glasgow, had been a medical student when Lister was doing his experiments and became an enthusiast for asepsis. It was the time when industrial smoke made rickets endemic. In this year he reported 1800 osteotomies without major sepsis.

1886 Ernst von Bergmann of Berlin introduced steam sterilization.

1887 Lister stops using the spray.

1889 W. S. Halsted introduces rubber gloves in Baltimore. He invented these for his fiancée in the operating room whose hands were being ruined by carbolic acid.

1890 Until the invention of anesthesia and asepsis, surgeons spent only a few minutes a year actually operating. They took on only cases facing death. Operations lasted only a minute or two—the length of time a person could be held down. Only the simplest kind of operation could be done. The average number of operations done in a year at the Massachusetts General Hospital before ether anesthesia was 38. Shortly after ether was invented the number was 190; before Lister, 770; and shortly after Lister, 1012. In the 1890s, it was 2500.

1892 Neuber builds a closed operating room. Until this time operating theaters were literally theaters, with up to 400 students gathered in tiers around the operating table, coughing and and shaking their street clothes.

1972 John Charnley develops the greenhouse operating room enclosure, exhaust system, impermeable gown fronts and double gloving and reduces infection.

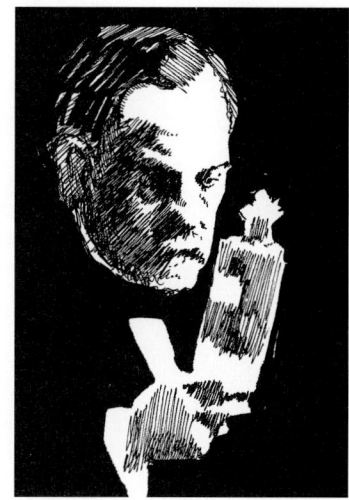

◆ **Louis Pasteur, 1822–1895**

He was born in Dole, France, and graduated in chemistry. Research on crystals in Paris led to sugar crystals and research on fermentation. He found that microorganisms in the air were responsible for fermentation and that they could be killed by heat. Still there were believers in the spontaneous generation of organisms, so Pasteur organized a shoot out experiment in 1864. The vinegar makers of Dijon and later the wine makers were having problems that Pasteur solved by pasteurization. He wrote studies on wine, beer, and diseases of silkworms before inventing vaccines for cholera, anthrax and rabies. He had a left-sided stroke at age 46 but continued to be as productive as ever until his death at the age of 73.

With these two tools—aseptic surgery and anesthesia—the number of conditions amenable to operation increased enormously. Patients began to see surgery as an option compatible with survival. The complexity of operations increased. Surgeons at the end of the 19th century were like little boys given a new toy.

Antibiotics and Immunization

Preventing operative infection made surgery safe, but if infection occurred there was no way to treat it. Penicillin is a mold and various moldy dressings were found to be effective for infected wounds in early times. But the systemic administration of antigerm substance began with quinine for malaria, and then there was salvarsan—the magic bullet— for syphilis in 1907, synthesized by Paul Ehrlich. Gerhard Domagk began with the dye industry, which produced a huge number of organic compounds. He tested many substances for activity against bacteria and came up in 1932 with Prontosil Red, which killed streptococci in mice. This was a sulfonamide first synthesized in 1907. This shows that the things we seek are always around us but only need to be seen in a different light. His daughter, Hildegarde, developed an infection in 1935 and was dying when, as a last-ditch measure, he gave her Prontosil and she came through. He was awarded the Nobel Prize, but Hitler prevented him from accepting it.

In 1938, a British drug company was testing related compounds and found that sulfadiazine had antibacterial properties, and this came to be widely used. It saved Winston Churchill's life when he had pneumonia during World War II.

Alexander Fleming had worked on wounds during World War I and then worked as a bacteriologist at St. Mary's Hospital in London. Returning from a holiday in August 1928, he found that a contaminant on a Petri dish had killed a culture of staphylococci. This turned out to be penicillin. He published this result but did not pursue it.

At Oxford, Harold Florey, a pathologist, and Ernst Chain, a refugee biochemist from the Nazis, came across Fleming's report as they searched for antibacterial substances and found in 1940 that this penicillin worked against streptococci in mice. Drug companies in the United States and later in Britain mass-produced it, and by 1945 they all shared a Nobel Prize.

With the advent of antibiotics, the risks of surgery, an open wound, an open fracture, tuberculosis, and osteomyelitis began to disappear.

Although immunization had begun before penicillin was discovered, it was not until more than ten years later that polio was conquered.

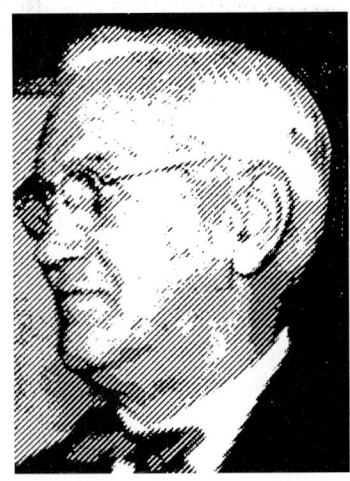

◆ Alexander Fleming

The Invention of X-rays

Everyone knows that Konrad Roentgen discovered X-rays in 1895. What is little known is the reason why they were not found a year or two earlier.

William Crookes used the same rays and found that a piece of film left nearby was fogged. He sent the film back to the manufacturers as defective.

Another researcher, Goodspeed in Philadelphia, had the same experience but thought no more about it. The lesson to be learned is that observing something unusual is not the key to success. The key is to interpret it and find a use for it.

Roentgen had been experimenting with these rays but had to give up research because he was appointed Rector in 1894. Only when this administrative job came to an end could he get back to research—we can only be glad this was not a permanent appointment.

Roentgen was a man who only just made it. When he was 3 years old, his family left Prussia for Holland as political refugees. Expelled from high school because he wouldn't tell who had drawn a caricature of the teacher on a blackboard, he studied at home but failed the University entrance examination. After going to technical school in Zurich, he tried to become a teacher but was turned down. His fortunes improved, and he eventually became Professor of Physics at Würzburg in 1888. In 1895 he had his laboratory in total darkness to see whether a cardboard box was lightproof. He sent a high-tension current through a vacuum tube in the box and noticed that some nearby chemicals glowed. He knew this was something unusual and moved a campbed into the laboratory so that he could work uninterrupted.

Putting his hand between the chemical screen and the tube, he could see the bones of his hand. He substituted a photographic plate for the screen. These were the master strokes that took his discovery from a piece of research that would have been ignored in a journal to something of instant utility. He dashed off a paper to the local scientific community on December 28, 1895. At a dinner with friends a week later, one of his fellow guests was the son of a newspaper editor. The next day the story was in *Die Presse*.

Soon after, he wrote to his friends, *"On the first of January I sent off the photographs I had taken with X-rays and then all hell broke loose. First it was the Vienna newspapers, and then the rest followed suit. After a few days I was sick of the whole affair: I could no longer recognize my work from references in the paper."*

His wife wrote, *"When Willi told me in November that his work was going well, we had no idea of the consequences it would bring. But scarcely had he published the results of his research than our peace of mind was at an end.... It is no small matter to become a great man."*

Roentgen won the Nobel Prize in 1901 and then turned down honors and titles and returned to teaching and research.

X-rays took off fast. Big hospitals obtained a machine within months. Fairgrounds had them. Cartoonists had a field day. Only later were the dangers of radiation appreciated.

Surgical Use of X-rays, March 1896

"The employment of the Roentgen radiations in surgery continues to meet with many applications, but it will be well if surgeons at once

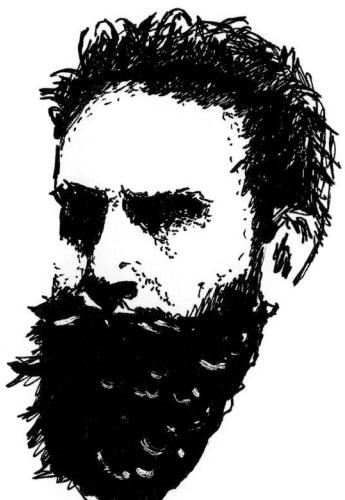

◆ Konrad Roentgen

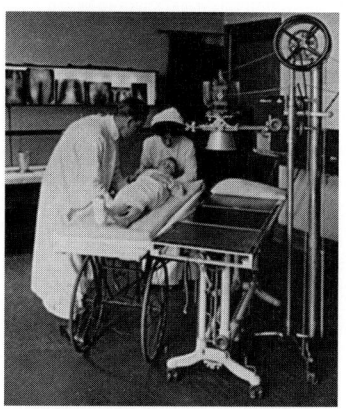

The X-ray department at The Hospital for Sick Children, Toronto, in the 1920s. The equipment was simple.

appreciate the fact that their new ally may possibly become a tacit witness against them. An instance of such an unfortunate contretemps lately came under our notice.

A gentleman had the misfortune, when a youth, to break his forearm, and break it badly too. The limb was duly set; the arm never regained its normal strength, and exhibited a deformed appearance. He had an X-ray done by a friend and the malunion was clear.

"It's a good thing for him," said the victim," that the surgeon who set my arm is dead, otherwise I would certainly take action against him." Let surgeons be careful in recommending to their patients the use of a Crookes tube, in case the revelations it affords should recoil upon their own heads."

This quote from the *British Journal of Photography* appeared within three months of the invention of X-rays. In the same journal is an account of X-rays being produced in court to obtain compensation for a foot injury.

Unlike the practice of internal medicine, orthopaedics is so very dependent on the Three Amigos. One would have thought that internal medicine would have been much farther ahead of surgery in the 19th century because it lacked the brake that surgery suffered until anesthesia and asepsis were discovered. Not so. Pathology, history taking, physical examination, preventive medicine, and real drugs were just as far behind and just as essential. People died of cholera because the mode of spread was unknown and because rehydration had not been invented.

The brakes to progress in surgery are just more obvious than the brakes in medicine. In the 19th century there was a speed of progress on all fronts that had never been seen before. The development of pathology suddenly increased the menu of diseases from which the clinician could choose. Diseases became partitioned off from one another—a swollen knee that discharged tuberculous pus was recognized as different from a swollen knee due to a torn meniscus. At first diseases could be distinguished only by fairly gross physical signs. Now with our sophisticated systems disease can be recognized and distinguished earlier and earlier.

Other imaging technology is of recent origin:

Computed Tomography

The struggle to create three-dimensional images began with stereoscopic pictures and blurring tomography in the 1920s. Many manufacturers produced machines. However, CT originated from people who had nothing to do with any of this.

In 1967, Dr. Godfrey Hounsfield, an engineer, was working in the research laboratories of the EMI Company in Middlesex, England. The company had a great deal of money for research because they recorded the musical group The Beatles.

Godfrey Hounsfield was interested in pattern recognition and had just finished working on face and fingerprint recognition; unfortunately, the police were not interested and the project was a commercial failure. He moved on to consider how to recognize the size, shape, and position of objects in a closed box; he decided to use X-rays aimed from many different directions.

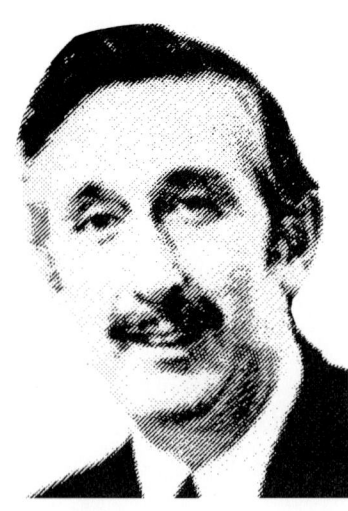

◆ **Godfrey Hounsfield**

One of his great breakthroughs in thinking was to stay away from photographic film for recording. Photographic film had always been so much a part of radiology, but the scale between black and white on film covers only a small range. By using a crystal to record he could extend the scale 100 times. He used a computer to print out the measurements.

His first image took 9 hours to complete, and later he cut it down to minutes. He wondered whether this could be applied to human radiology and was told that only the human brain stayed still for long enough to image at this rate. So a machine was built and used in a neurosurgical hospital in Wimbledon. The first article about it was published in 1973. In 1979, he and Allan M. Cormack shared the Nobel Prize.

Alan Cormack was Lecturer in Physics in Cape Town, South Africa, in 1956 and became interested in radiotherapy planning. This led to working out the mathematics that underlie CT. He published the work in 1963, but the only interest was expressed by the Swiss Avalanche Research Center as a method of measuring the depth of snow. His interest waned until other developments got him going again in the early 1970s.

Magnetic Resonance Imaging

In 1952, Felix Bloch of Stanford and Edward Purcell of Harvard received the Nobel Prize in Physics for their discovery of nuclear magnetic resonance, which was applied to analytic spectroscopy. It became useful for the chemical analysis of biologic tissues. In 1971, Raymond Damadian found he could distinguish a test tube of tumor tissue from a test tube of normal tissue, and with great foresight he filed a patent in 1972 for the medical application of this concept. The first image, of two tubes of water, was produced by P. C. Lauterbur in 1973. An image of a dead mouse was produced the next year. Several centers worked on the idea. In July 1977, Raymond Damadian produced the first primitive live human image of himself in Brooklyn, New York. The word "nuclear" has been dropped from the name because no radiation is involved and the word needlessly scared the public.

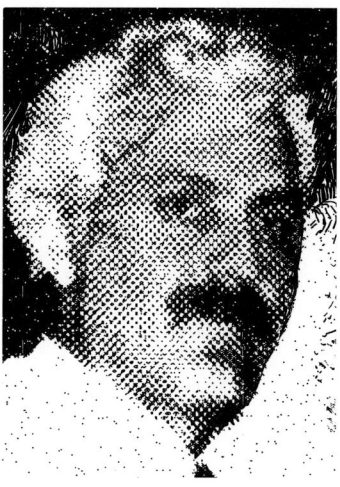

◆ Raymond Damadian

Bone Scans

Today everyone has a digital watch with back lighting. But in days gone by, telling the time at night using a watch with hands was impossible. Then luminous paint was invented. It was radioactive. The dial painters used to point their brushes with their tongue, thereby shortening their lives because the minute amounts of paint they swallowed went to the bones and caused radiation cancer.

Autoradiography was done on their bones in 1924, and the bone itself was found to be radioactive. These were the first scans. In 1961, Fleming introduced strontium-85 to localize areas of osteoblastic activity. But the isotope had a high radiation dose, and its use was largely restricted to patients with malignant disease. Other substances were tried but were difficult to obtain. Attention turned to the polyphosphates, which were known to bind to hydroxyapatite crystals; these were labeled with phosphorus-32, but again, the problem of high radiation dosage came up. Then in 1971 Subramanian and McAfee solved this by using technetium-99m-labeled diphosphonates—a nearly ideal labeling compound. Only then did it become possible to use scanning to study benign bone pathology safely. Since then, bone scanning has taken off.

There are many investigative methods that have not stood the test of time: dunking witches, feeling the pulse, and The Oracle Bones of Shang popular in 1200–1050 BC. This was an ancient Chinese method of deciding on an action. The leaders wrote on bones such words as ATTACK, or DON'T ATTACK and then put the bones in the fire. They looked to see where the bone cracked—if it was through ATTACK they knew what to do. Many of these bones have been preserved.

What Happened to the Patient with—

A Closed Colles' Fracture

Until 150 years ago, distal radial fractures were thought to be a wrist dislocation, and a bonesetter would try to snap it back without an anesthetic. Doctors before this time were more like internists of today and considered fractures beneath them. Probably most patients went untreated. With anesthesia and X-rays came closed reduction.

An Open Tibial Fracture

Most came to amputation without anesthesia. The chance of death from infection was high, particularly under military conditions.

When amputation was done in hospitals with more than 330 beds, the death rate was 41%. In country hospitals, the rate was 11%. In Paris, it was 60%; Zurich, 46%; and Massachusetts General Hospital, Boston, 26% (James Simpson, 1867).

Lister showed that spraying antiseptic everywhere dramatically reduced infection, but it was some time before he was believed.

A Closed Tibial Fracture

This was treated by lying down in bed on a splint until the fracture united. About 1900 came the realization that an ambulant cast was possible. And only in 1950 did a weight-bearing cast come into fashion.

After anesthesia came along, there was no rush to operate so there was no sudden increase in mortality from infection—as happened in osteotomies for deformity. Operative treatment did not begin until after the invention of X-rays and was safe (from the point of view of infection) though the implanted metals used were not very good.

A Closed Ankle Fracture

Before X-rays, the ankle was patted back into shape and the patient was not able to walk again because of malunion. X-rays displayed the injury, and open reduction soon became popular.

Carpal Tunnel Syndrome

This waited until 1944 to be recognized and operated so that the discoveries of the Three Amigos made no difference.

Prolapsed Disc

Nontuberculous back ache and sciatica were hardly worthy of consideration until the 1930s, when the disc was discovered.

Joint Replacement

The first joints to be replaced in the 1880s were damaged by tuberculosis, and infection caused failure. X-rays enabled later doctors to select joints that were free of infection. Success depended more on materials and design than on the Amigos. Painful arthritis of the hip was treated with canes, tablets, and spas. Patients became crippled. They were homebound. In the 1930s, intertrochanteric osteotomies were used to correct deformities and were found by chance to relieve some of the pain. Unilateral arthritis was treated by fusion. Bilateral arthritis was treated by joint excision.

Joint replacement did not become widely available until the 1970s and 1980s.

The Eras of Orthopaedics

1. **The Era of Nonoperative Orthopaedics.** This lasted 2000 years and came to an end with the introduction of anesthesia in 1846.
2. **The Era of High-Risk Operative Orthopaedics.** Anesthesia made elective surgery possible, but the risk of dying from infection was great. This stage lasted about 40 years and should have come to an end with the first paper on aseptic surgery in 1867.
3. **The Era of Operative Orthopaedics.** Sterility took nearly 20 years to be accepted. This era has lasted about 110 years and we are still there. It can be broken up into stages:

    Stage of Uncertain Diagnosis: This ended when X-rays were discovered in 1895, but the films were not very good for at least 10 years.

    Stage of Deformity Correction: About half the early elective operations were done for rachitic deformity. When Vitamin D was discovered in 1922, rickets was eradicated.

    Stage of Implantless Surgery: Implants were not widely used until stainless steel, invented in the 1920s, made them safe.

Stage Without Antibiotics and Vaccines: Infection was a huge problem—staphylococci, tuberculosis, polio—until the 1950s.

Stage of Minimally Invasive Endoscopic Orthopaedics and Joint Replacements: Started in the mid-1960s.

The Success of Orthopaedics

There are few cripples on the streets outside the Third World.

There are no long-stay orthopaedic hospitals.

Orthopaedics has coped with the aging population better than other specialties.

There are more orthopaedists alive now than there have been in the whole of history.

EARLY BOOKS ON ORTHOPAEDICS

300 BC Hippocrates on Fractures

1601 Geronimo Mercuriale: *De artis Gymnastica.* First book on sports medicine. There are extracts in Clinical Orthopaedics, 1985, Volume 198, 21.

1705 Jean-Louis Petit: *The Art of Curing Diseases of Bone.* Paris

> *"In general I will write a book that will be useful both for surgeons and patients. The surgeons will find sure methods to win the confidence of those beginning treatment and patients will find the evidence to distinguish between a methodical surgeon who knows the cause of the disease he is treating from quacks who are all pretence and bluster, pretending that a bruise or twist is a dislocation and then causing grief with unnecessary traction, making the pain worse than before they had put their hand to it."*

1742 Nicholas Andry's book was written for parents and not for doctors.

1810 Johann Christian Gottfried Jorg, a German obstetrician, wrote the first orthopaedic text in 1810: *On the Distortions of the Human Body and a Rational and Certain Method of Curing the Same.*

1828 Delpech: *L'Orthomorphie*

1844 One of the first American books was *A Manual of Orthopedic Surgery,* by Henry J. Bigelow. It was a dissertation that won the Boylston Prize for 1844 on the following question: In what cases and to what extent is the division of muscles, tendons, or other parts proper for the relief of deformity or lameness?

1844 Many short tracts were written by Guérin, Pravaz, St. Hilaire, and Anthony White about this time, and since then the exuberance of orthopaedists has made them leaders in the author stakes.

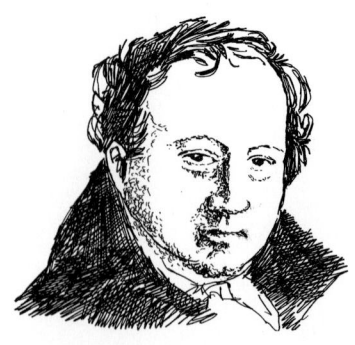

◆ Johann Christian Gottfried Jorg

The American Pioneers

Orthopaedics began in Philadelphia, in New York, and in Boston, where the Medical Schools were founded in 1765, 1767, and 1783, respectively.

In Philadelphia, Dr. Philip Syng Physick was the leader and had studied with John Hunter. An inventive surgeon followed him, John Rhea Barton, 1794-1871, of whom more later.

In contrast, New York was soon taken over by an anti-surgeon—James Knight. The early emphasis was on nonoperative or minimally invasive surgery because the specialty was established before aseptic surgery was accepted. To elect surgery was to tempt death. Failures of interpersonal relations were common but did not stop New York from becoming the starting place of a national organization, the American Orthopaedic Association, in 1887.

In New York were to be found:

Valentine Mott (1785-1865). He studied with Astley Cooper in London and returned a bold surgeon. His health failed and he spent 10 years recuperating in Europe. While there he visited Guérin in Paris and saw his tenotomy practice. He returned to set up an institute on the same lines but was crushed by collegial opposition.

Murray Carnochan (1817-1887), author of an early monograph on congenital dislocation of the hip.

Gurdon Buck (1807-1877) of femoral traction fame.

James Knight (1810-1887). He started the first orthopaedic hospital in his own home—calling it the Hospital for the Ruptured and Crippled. He banned operating, banned plaster, and provided trusses for the ruptured and braces for the crippled. When he died the staff breathed a sigh of relief, for they could now operate, and they later renamed the place The Hospital for Special Surgery. Knight is turning over in his grave. Knight's book, *Orthopaedia*, is an interesting read.

William Ludwig Detmold (1808-1894). He was raised in Germany and studied with Stromeyer in Hanover before emigrating to New York in 1837 as an orthopaedic surgeon. He did many tenotomies and opened the first children's clinic in New York. He became surgeon to the Union Army, and at Bull Run battlefield he did 75 amputations in a morning. Detmold invented a combined knife and fork to assist amputees.

Louis Bauer (1814-1898). Another Stromeyer trainee, he left Germany as a political refugee, came to New York where he wrote an early textbook and founded institutions, before moving on to St. Louis as a medico-political refugee.

Henry Gassett Davis (1806-1896). He worked in Massachusetts and in New York. He used traction for fractures and deformities. He developed an elastic scoliosis brace. Buck improved on his traction for fractures. He drained and used an irrigation system for septic arthritis, writing a paper on 59 years' experience with the method. He wrote a book in 1867 on "Conservative surgery as exhibited in remedying mechanical causes that operate injuriously both in health and disease." A giant, but low key.

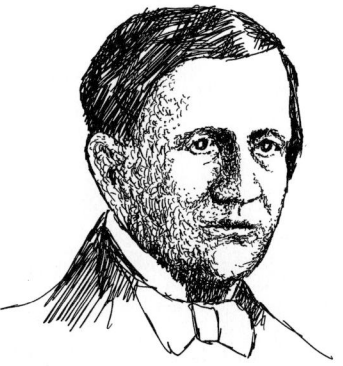
◆ James Knight

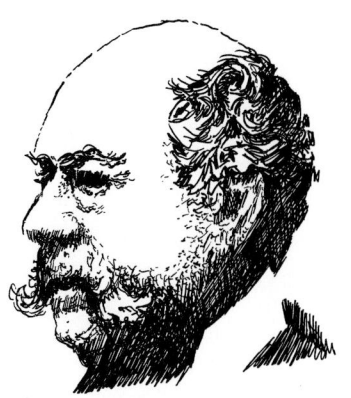
◆ William Ludwig Detmold

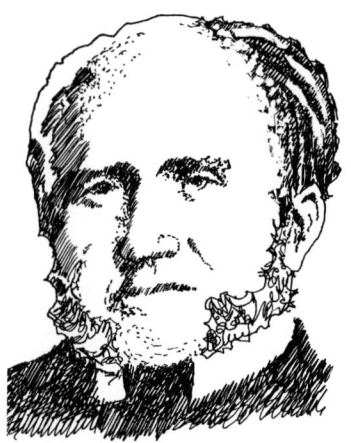

◆ Henry Gasset Davis

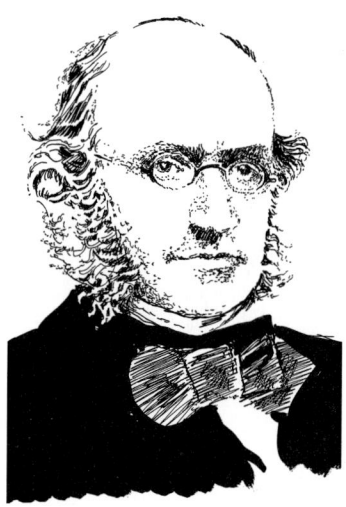

◆ Buckminster Brown

In Boston:

John Ball Brown (1784-1892). He was the son of a Massachusetts physician, became a surgeon at Massachusetts General Hospital, and restricted practice to orthopaedics at the age of 54. He founded the Orthopedique Infirmary in 1838, which became the Boston Orthopaedic Institution. He was an early tenotomist for scoliosis, torticollis, and limb deformities and wrote:

"Having lost my eldest son by inflammation of the great spinal cord, and having my second son confined to his bed by lateral curvature of the spine, my attention has been forcibly drawn to the study and treatment of spinal diseases generally and to the correction of other deformities of the human body." Boston Med Surg J 1838, 18, 139.

His son, Buckminster Brown (1819-1891), had Pott's disease and was bedfast for 8 years. He joined his father in orthopaedic practice after studying in Europe with Guérin, Bouvier, Little, and Stromeyer in 1845-1846. He was the first purely orthopaedic surgeon in the United States. He wrote a textbook and is regarded as the father of children's orthopaedics in the United States.

Early Hospitals

These names show how we have struggled for the right identity:

The General Institution for the Relief of Persons with Bodily Deformities. Birmingham England, 1817.

The Hospital for the Cure of Deformities of the Human Frame, Boston. This was the successor to the Orthopedique Infirmary founded in 1838.

House of the Good Samaritan. Boston, 1861.

The New York Surgeon's Bandage Institute, 1830s.

The Hospital for the Ruptured and Crippled. New York City, 1863.

About References

Very old books are put together with sentences like this: "According to Hippocrates, Galen, and Aristotle, the blood does not circulate." The reason for putting in their names is that these people are AUTHORITIES; you must not question their ideas. They were like laws. Heresy, imprisonment, and burning at the stake were the punishments for suggesting anything else. Servetus, one of the first to suggest the circulation of the blood, was burnt at the stake for his opinions. We have come a long way. Yet in some ways we have not—listen to a detail man exclaiming the virtues of an implant—often it comes down to the fact that a big name is using it; this may count for more than science.

Then references served another purpose—to avoid accusations

of stealing ideas. Academics did not want their ideas plagiarized. Like credits on a movie, their names must be mentioned.

Nowadays references are largely a paper trail for researchers.

The convention for referencing goes back to the days when universities were offshoots of the Church. Doctors writing a paper are at one with a vicar preaching a sermon: "I will take as my text 'Mehitabel smote the Ephesian,' which comes from Leviticus, chapter 3, verse 4."

Keeping track of recent references is just a matter of unloading them from Medlines, and today everyone can appear learned. But older literature is a challenge; it has to be found and photocopied. Often the reference is wrong. Only a few libraries have ancient journals, and often they charge a lot for mail enquiries.

Copies take up space and need time to file. A friend of mine rented an apartment to store his reference collection and employed someone to keep it in order. I store mine in files until I have used them and then toss them into a box for refiling. This is not to be recommended if you have a cleaning lady. Many of the references for this book disappeared into landfill one day, and you will have to put up with some sketchy references until I have time to find them all again. I was not trying, thank goodness, to write a bibliography. I hope you understand. There are a number of chronologies and timeline books on the market that do not reference any of the information, and I took heart from this.

Further Reading

The History of Orthopaedics

There are a number of general books for further reading or for references:

- Bick EM: Source Book of Orthopaedics, 1948
- Bick EM: Classics of Orthopaedics, 1976 (a collection of classics from Clinical Orthopaedics)
- Boyes, Joseph: On the Shoulders of Giants, 1976 (notable names in hand surgery)
- Cooter, Roger: Surgery and Society in Peace and War. Orthopaedics and the Organisation of Modern Medicine 1880-1948. University of Manchester, 1993. (orthopaedics in the context of social change—written by a historian)
- Keith, Arthur: Menders of the Maimed, 1919. The first and in many ways this is still the best, because it tells the story of the evolution of ideas. Robert Salter says everyone should read this—his interest in cartilage and research was fired by reading this when he was a Fellow.
- Le Vay, David: The History of Orthopaedics, 1990. An excellent book that is very complete and has much translated material. It is arranged in large part as national histories.
- Morlacchi, Carlo: Orthopedia e Arte. Rome: Delfino, 1997 (a collection of works of art, which includes orthopaedic patients—good pictures for slides)

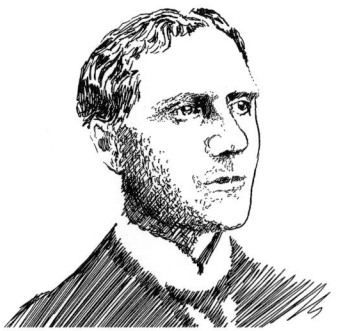

◆ **Arthur Keith**

Peltier, Leonard: Fractures, 1990, and Orthopaedics, 1993, San Francisco: Norman Publishing Company. These are very beautifully produced and well illustrated.

Peltier, Leonard: His "Classics" in the journal Clinical Orthopaedics have included over 300 biographies, portraits, and reprints of papers over recent years, but there is no cumulative index.

Valentin, Bruno: Geschichte der Orthopaedie, 1961 (an excellent book in German)

These books have a focused interest:

Barry H: Orthopaedics in Australia. Sydney: Australian Orthopaedic Association, 1994

Beighton P, Beighton G: The Man Behind the Syndrome. London: Springer-Verlag, 1986

Beighton P, Beighton G: The Person Behind the Syndrome. London: Springer-Verlag, 1997

Cholmeley JA: History of the Royal National Orthopaedic Hospital. London: Chapman and Hall, 1985

McHenry LC: Garrison's History of Neurology, Springfield, Ill: Charles C Thomas, 1969

Strange FG St C: The History of the Royal Seabathing Hospital, Margate 1791-1991. Kent: Meresborough Books, 1991

Waugh W: A History of the British Orthopaedic Association. London: BOA, 1993 (many orthopaedic organizations and hospitals have produced a history)

Most of the literature has been found in the libraries of the Wellcome Foundation in London, The Royal College of Surgeons of England, and the University of Toronto, and I am very grateful for the help their staff have provided.

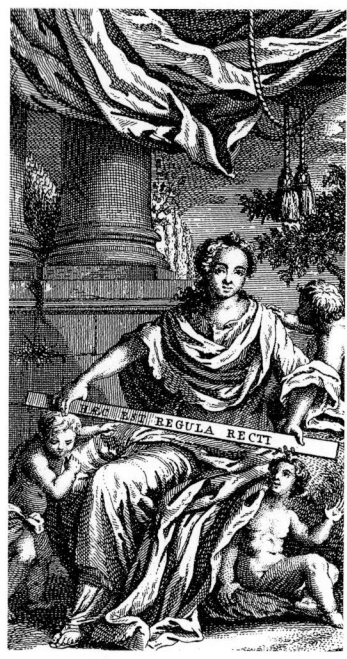

Andry: Haec Est Regula Recti. The latin phrase means "This is the straight rule."

References

Chapter references are located in Chapter 26.

◆
◆
◆ PART ONE

Orthopaedics

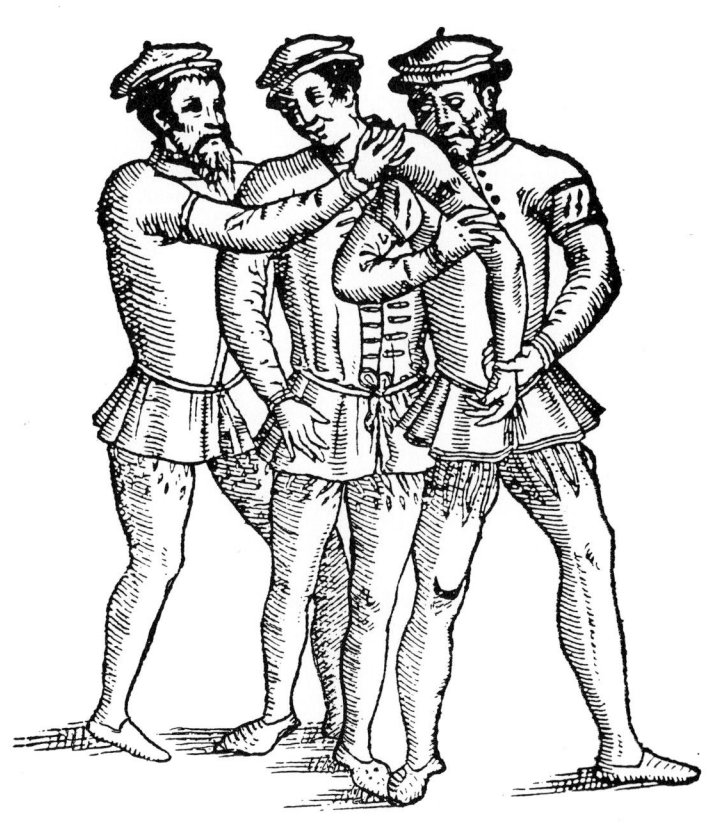

◆ Chapter Two

Adult Hip

"Young medical men find it so much easier to speculate than to observe. Nothing is known to our profession by guess. There is no short road to knowledge. Observations on the diseased living, examinations of the dead, and experiments upon living animals are the only sources of true knowledge." Astley Cooper on Fractures; 1824

The hip is the biggest joint in the body and causes much grief when it malfunctions. In the past, arthritis used to make the last years of life miserable for many citizens, and fracture led many of the rest to their grave. The meaning of old age has been changed by nailing fractures, which began in the 1930s, and by replacing joints since the 1950s. However, in the future, an aging population may need more hip care than the working population can afford.

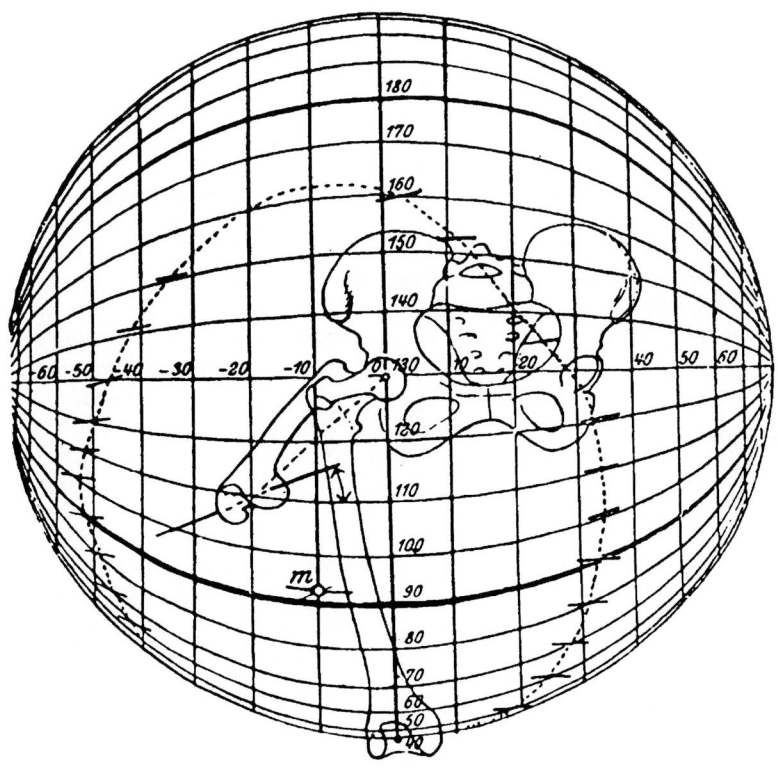

The range of movement of the hip: Strasser, 1893. From Steindler A: Human Locomotion. Springfield, Ill: Charles C Thomas, 1955.

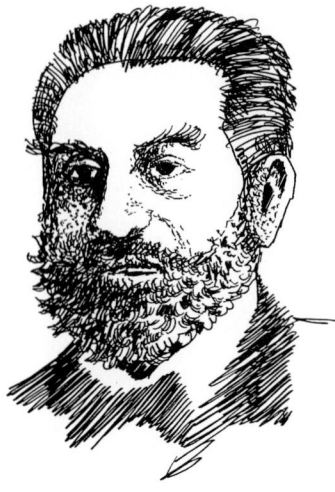

The shape of the proximal femur makes it biomechanically interesting. It cannot be understood quickly. Julius Wolff was one of the first to discover the implications of its shape in health and disease.

Osteoarthritis

TIMELINE:
Pathology of Osteoarthritis

- 400 BC Hippocrates describes arthritis
- 1793 Edward Sandifort provides a nice illustration of the pathology
- 1819 Brodie—book on the diseases of joints
- 1835 R. W. Smith coined the phrase *morbus coxae senilis*
- 1839 Colles describes new bone formation and destruction
- 1857 Adams distinguishes rheumatoid arthritis from osteoarthritis
  John Kent Spender (1829–1916) coined name "osteoarthritis"
- 1910 A. E. Garrod convincingly distinguishes osteoarthritis from rheumatoid arthritis
- 1973 Friedrich Pauwels' concept that a big load over a small area destroys the joint. His book is translated into English, *Biomechanics of the Normal and Diseased Hip*, 1976

◆ **Julius Wolff (1836–1902)**
A native of East Prussia, he studied bone growth at the suggestion of Langenbeck. His scientific career was interrupted by one of the many European wars and by his founding a Hospital. He became a Professor at age 54 years and in 1892 published *The Law of Bone Transformation* prior to the invention of X-rays. He used thin sections of bone to relate form to function according to mathematical laws. "Structure is the physical expression of function." Others had done this before but never with such thoroughness.

Pauwels' Principles

Pauwels taught us to think about load per unit area on the articular cartilage of the hip and on the femoral neck.

"Theoretical reasoning and biomechanical analysis clearly show that three hip diseases, congenital coxa vara, pseudarthrosis of the neck of the femur, and osteoarthritis, are caused and maintained by different types of mechanical stress. Treatment of these three diseases must attack the biomechanical stress. It is astonishing that treatment can be achieved only by an appropriate change of the neck/shaft angle of the femur.

Closing the neck/shaft angle (coxa vara) reduces the load supported by the hip joint and the upper end of the femur but greatly increases the stressing of the femoral neck."

Friedrich Pauwels wrote *Biomechanics of the Normal and Diseased Hip* in 1973, and it was translated and published in English in 1976. Summarizing 40 years' work, this apotheosis of hip osteotomy was published when hip replacement was the main focus of interest. Its value today lies in the wonderful series of radiographs of individual patients taken over many years, showing the response to osteotomy. Pauwels wrote that Wolff's theory—bone reacts to changes in stress—had not been proven until his work.

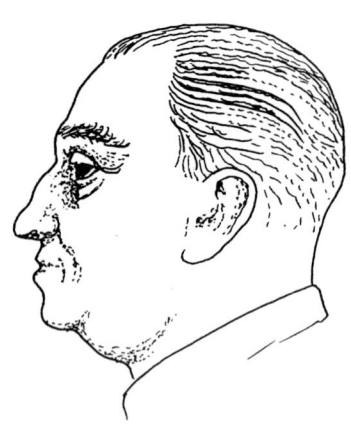

◆ **Friedrich Pauwels (1885–1980)**
He studied with Lorenz and Schanz and founded an Orthopaedic Institute in Aachen in 1913. He focused on biomechanical factors that influenced bone growth and repair. He classified hip fractures and worked until retiring at age 75 years.

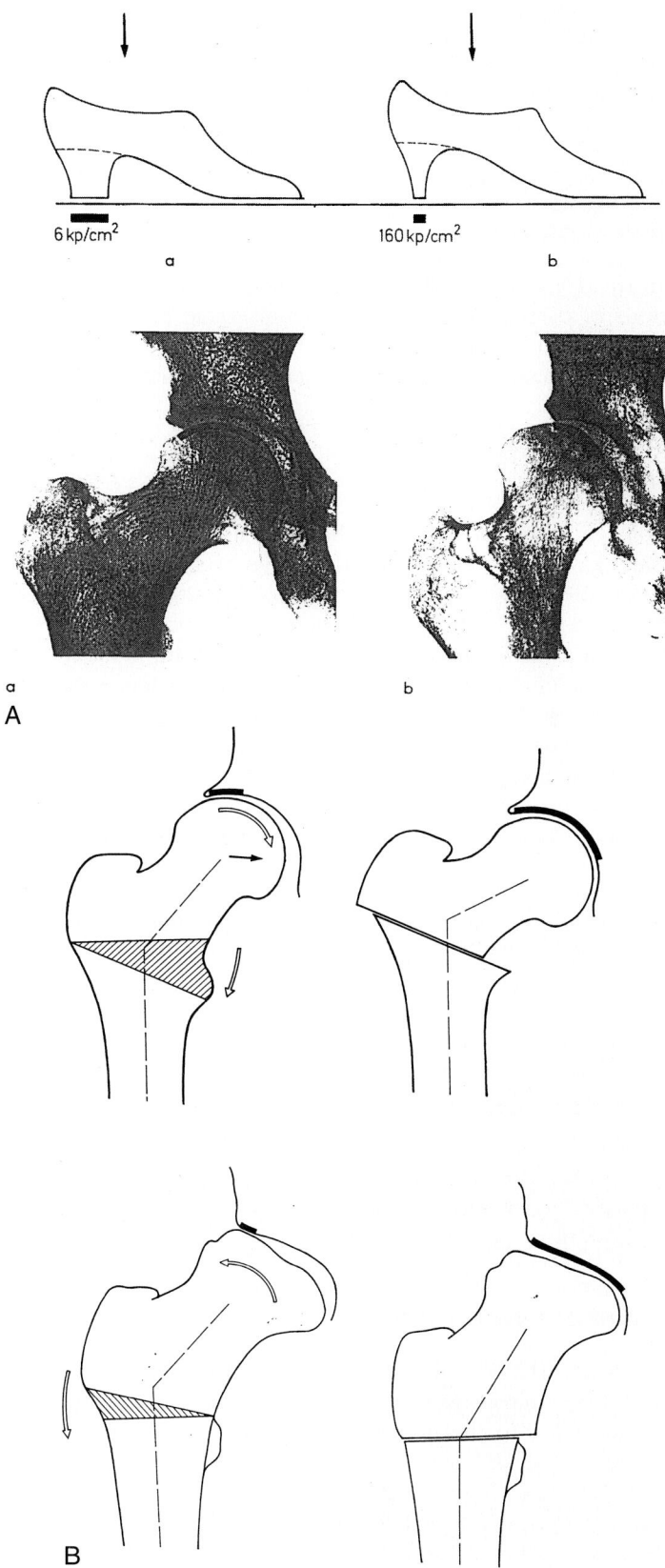

(A) and (B), Pauwels illustrates the effects of pressure. Loading a small area is detrimental to the hip and can be helped by osteotomy. From Pauwels F: Biomechanics of the Normal and Diseased Hip. Berlin: Springer-Verlag, 1976. Reproduced with permission.

He influenced a whole generation of European orthopaedic surgeons, but his book is remarkable for the complete lack of mention of pelvic osteotomies, for the obsession with the anteroposterior appearance of the hip, for lack of interest in clinical results, and for a case-by-case approach without any statistics.

Clinical Features

In the 19th century, hip disease meant tuberculosis. The first mentions of osteoarthritis call it "malum coxae senilis"—hardly a name to appeal to today's seniors. In the first part of the 20th century, orthopaedic textbooks merged osteoarthritis and rheumatoid arthritis.

Treatment

For centuries nothing could be done for the few people who were lucky enough to live beyond the age of 40. They used canes and frequented a spa. In the first half of the 20th century, every family had a lame relative using a cane. Only a few surgeons operated on arthritic hips. If there had been multiple choice questions for residents at this time they would not select "operation" as the right answer for the treatment of osteoarthritis hip. A choice of fusion, osteotomy, joint excision, and various types of primitive arthroplasty—interposition, cup, unipolar—were the unattractive alternatives, and surgeons did not want to take on patients with this problem. Joint replacement has changed everything.

"It is sad and depressing that there are virtually no half measures in treatment. The patient has to grin and bear it, adapting his life as best he can, until such time as symptoms become intolerable."
Philip Wiles, 1957

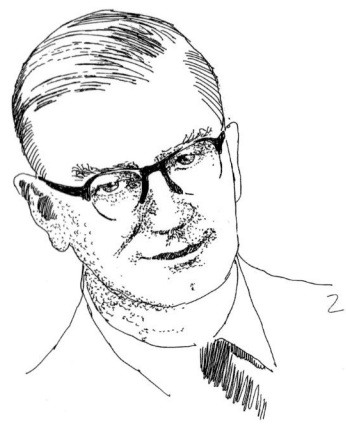

◆ **Philip Wiles (1899–1967)**

Wiles' father was a successful businessman in the city of London and a Member of Parliament. After flying in World War I, Wiles went into the family business but decided at the age of 24 years to study medicine. He went on staff at the Middlesex Hospital in 1935 as a bold surgeon with left wing politics. In 1938 he inserted 3 total hip replacements. He excised a hemivertebra, and he studied the growth of periosteum. By 1940 he was in the Army again. On return to civilian life he wrote two textbooks and underwrote the British volume of the Journal of Bone and Joint Surgery when it started.

He retired early at age 60 and went to live in Jamaica. I knew him there because he used to teach the medical students and was chairman of the Scientific Research Council.

Arthrodesis

Eduard Albert of Vienna is usually credited with inventing arthrodesis in 1881, but all claims to be first are always a challenge to find something earlier still.

Park and Moreau, 1806

H. Park of Liverpool and Moreau in France started to excise joints for tuberculosis. Moreau's son published some cases, and his publication fell into the hands of Park. The result was a 200-page book of the work of both of them, with notes by the professor at Glasgow, Dr. James Jeffray, published in 1806.

The operation included "the entire removal of the extremities of all the bones which form the joint: with the whole, or as much as possible, of the capsular ligament, thereby," says Mr Park, "obtaining a cure by means of callus, or by uniting the femur and tibia, when practiced on the knee: and the humerus, radius, and ulna, when at the elbow, into one bone, without any movable articulation."

Hip arthrodesis was never a common operation because pseudarthrosis was frequent. Brittain, in Norwich, wrote *Architectural Principles in Arthrodesis,* before biomechanics had a name and provided a rational basis for surgical planning.

Charnley developed a compression method. It is hard to think he would do this. In 1946, J Charnley started to do an arthroplasty based on Judet's idea, but the results were so bad he changed direction and devoted his efforts to developing a better arthrodesis. He found that the best results were from a failed central displacement arthrodesis, and this encouraged him to try arthroplasty again.

Arthroplasty

The idea is to restore movement to a painful, stiff joint. This is different from excising a joint in order to get rid of infection.

Several approaches were used:

1. The first idea of Barton was to use an osteotomy to produce a false joint in 1827.
2. Various interposition membranes were used, starting with Verneuil in 1860, to separate the damaged joint surfaces and delay ankylosis. Little bone was removed. Soft tissues, bladder, fascia lata, rubber, metals—almost everything was tried. Then came Smith-Petersen and his great lateral chassé in a counterproductive direction with a rigid mold interposition.
3. Joint replacement started with ivory joints in 1894. At first, just the head was replaced and then the whole joint.
4. Biologic repair—encouraging a new, smooth cartilage surface with allografts.

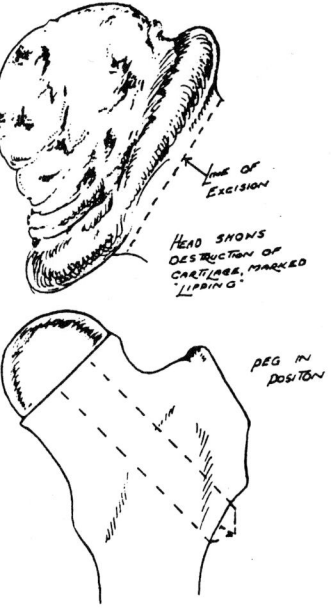

Hey Groves' ivory hip arthroplasty, 1926. From Hey Groves: Brit J Surg 1926, 14, 501.

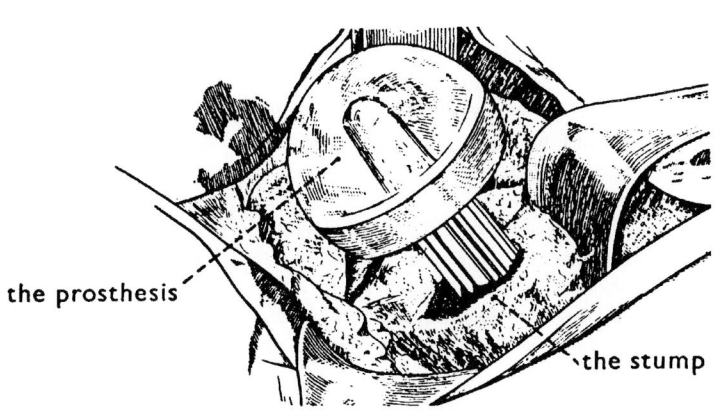

The Judet prosthesis was first implanted in September 1946. Four years later he had done 600—or 3 a week. "The point of view of the surgeon is often very different from the patient. The surgeon is impressed by the range of movement of the new joint, whereas the patient is grateful for the relief of pain and for the improvement of gait. As the years pass, however, the patient is apt to forget his former state and to dwell upon the remaining inconveniences, no matter how slight." From Judet J, Judet R, Lagrange J, Dunoyer J: Resection Reconstruction of the Hip (edited by K Nissen). Edinburgh: Livingstone, 1954. Reproduced with permission.

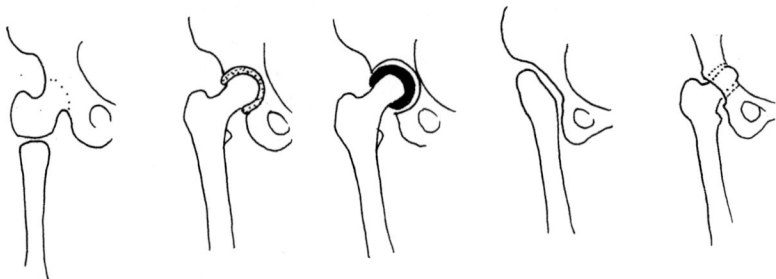

The evolution of hip arthroplasty. Barton 1826, Ollier 1885, Smith-Peterson Cup 1937, Girdlestone 1943, Charnley central-dislocation 1950.

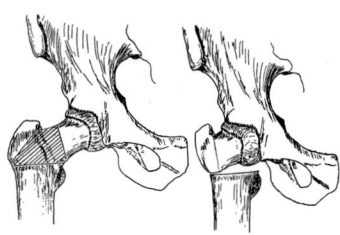

Jones' pseudarthrosis of the hip joint. From McMurray TP: A Practice of Orthopaedic Surgery, 3rd ed. London: E. Arnold, 1949, Figs. 18-71a, b. Reproduced with permission.

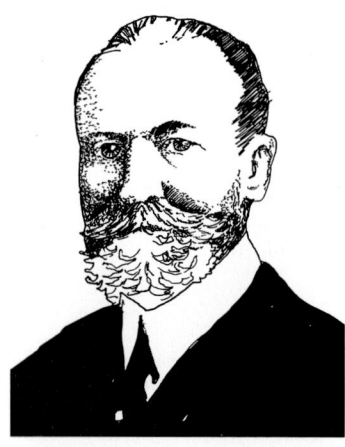

◆ John B. Murphy (1857–1916)

Of Irish parents, he studied at Rush Medical College in Chicago. He was a general surgeon of great energy and innovation. At a time when many orthopaedists were members of the brace and buckle brigade, Murphy was a surgeon. After animal studies, he introduced fascial arthroplasty for joints. He used reamers to shape the head and the acetabulum. He nailed ankle fractures and wired olecranon fractures.

TIMELINE OF HIP ARTHROPLASTY

1827 John Rhea Barton moved a subtrochanteric osteotomy early to create a false joint.

1867 Louis Ollier studied joint repair after damage.

1885 Ollier's book on joint resection raises much interest in interpositional arthroplasty, and many tissues and materials are tried without much success.

1894 Themistocles Gluck: ivory replacement of upper tibia and hip with an ivory ball

1894 Jules Pean: prosthetic replacement of tuberculous shoulder. Toulouse-Lautrec did a drawing of him operating. Pean went on to design hip and knee replacements.

1902 John Murphy uses fat and fascia as an interposition for arthroplasty and goes on to use this for hip, knee, elbow, and jaw.

1903 Delbert: hip replacement

1917 William Baer reports on 100 patients using allograft interposition; in Baltimore.

1921 Putti uses all kinds of interposition in Italy.

1923 Hey Groves replaces hip with ivory ball and stem.

1923 Marius Smith-Petersen starts developing a mold arthroplasty, first using glass and later Vitallium on the advice of his dentist.

1937 Methyl methacrylate marketed as Plexiglass

1938 Philip Wiles replaces both the femoral head and the acetabulum with a metal prosthesis in six patients with juvenile rheumatoid arthritis; 13 years later one patient was walking without pain.

1940 McKee makes models of a hip prosthesis but war stops him from trying it out. In 1951 he reports on three patients. He continues to improve the design of his metal-on-metal prosthesis until he retires and the advantages of metal on plastic become clearer.

1943 Austin Moore and Harold Bohlman: femoral head replacement for tumor. The original design has side plates, but later they introduce the idea of an intramedullary stem.

1946 Robert and Jean Judet develop a mushroom-shaped femoral head prosthesis. The material is acrylic, which breaks, and the stem—following the axis of the neck—is biomechanically unsound.

1950s Charnley starts to develop hip replacement but gives up in favor of arthrodesis. Finds that a failed central dislocation arthrodesis provides painless movement and advocates this for a short time.
1951 McKee and Farrar describe a metal-on-metal replacement in Norwich.
1952 F. R. Thompson: femoral head replacement
1953 Edward Harboush in New York uses dental cement to hold a hip prosthesis and a cup in place.
1954 John Charnley hears a squeaking Judet prosthesis and hits on the idea of low-friction arthroplasty.
1961 Charnley's report in the Lancet
1962 High-density polyethylene
1964 Peter Ring: metal-on-metal cementless replacement with a screw in the acetabulum
1968 The Hip Society established under the leadership of Frank Stinchfield
1970 Ceramic surfaces are introduced by Hulbert.
1973 Porous coating (Cameron, Macnab, and Pilliar, also Tronzo, Lord, and Hahn). Food and Drug Administration approves use of acrylic cement, opening the way for general use of hip replacements.

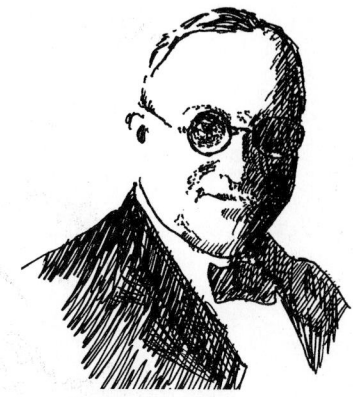

♦ **William Stevenson Baer (1872–1931)**

He graduated from Johns Hopkins and became chief of orthopaedics there. He traveled widely in the pursuit of new ideas. He was known for using membrane from pig bladder for interposition arthroplasty, manipulating the sacroiliac joint, using maggots to clean infected wounds, and using vaccines for arthritis.

Hemiarthroplasty

METAL HIP JOINT

MOORE AND BOHLMAN, 1940

Their obese patient presented with an un-united fracture of the neck of the femur, which was treated with Moore's pins. It united, but 2 years later the patient was back with a previously unrecognized giant cell tumor. It was treated with repeated curettage, grafting, and radiotherapy. He sustained a pathologic fracture and the mass increased in size. The conventional choice lay between doing an amputation or doing nothing.

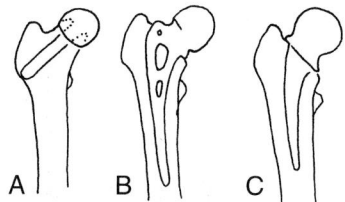

Hemiarthroplasty. (A) Judet, (B) Moore, (C) Thompson.

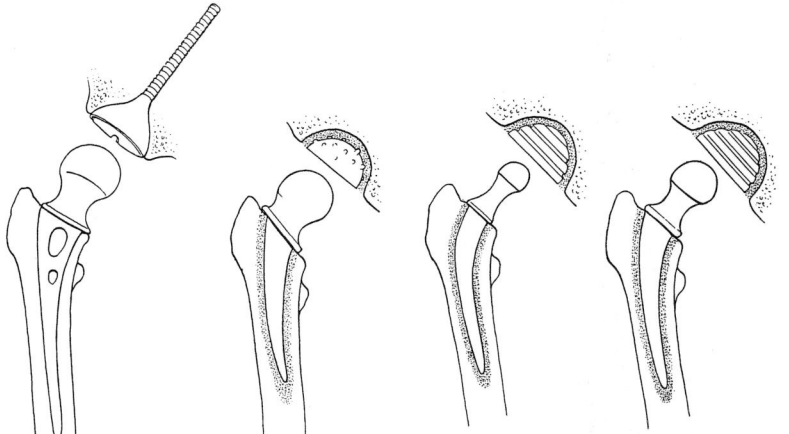

Total hip joint replacement—Ring, McKee-Farrar, Charnley, Müller. From Eftekhar NW: Total Hip Arthroplasty. St. Louis: Mosby, 1963. Reproduced with permission.

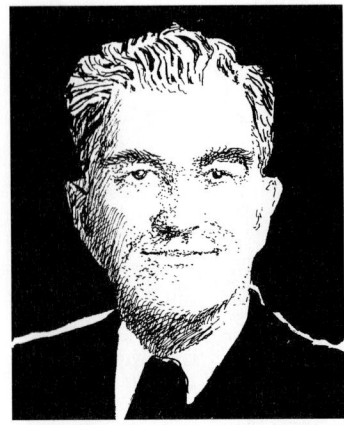

◆ **Austin T. Moore (1899–1963)**
He was born in Ridgeway, South Carolina, and studied in the state. He founded the Moore Clinic in Columbia in 1939 and lived on the international stage after pioneering a successful femoral head prosthesis.

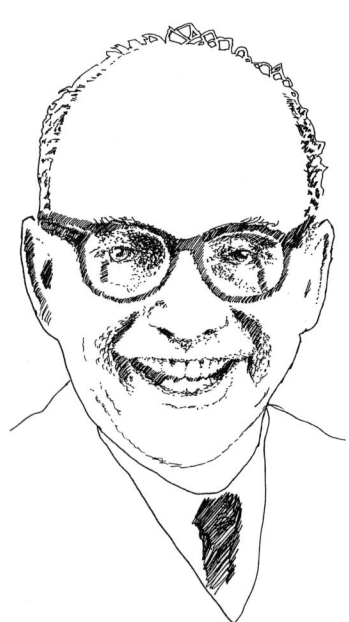

◆ **Frederick R. Thompson (1907–1983)**
Born in Texas, the son of a Professor of Surgery. His three brothers became surgeons and a sister married a surgeon. His orthopaedic life was spent at St Luke's Hospital in New York where he developed his hip prosthesis.

"In an effort to do something for him, it was decided to resect the entire tumor region and to replace this portion of bone with a metal appliance made in the form of the natural bone, and having in it various loops through which the various muscles and tendons could be attached, so that some reasonable postoperative function of the hip might be expected. Apparently no one had ever had the opportunity previously to replace such an extensive amount of bone as this case demanded. Calculations were made from the roentgenograms of the bone, wax models were fashioned and from these models a mold was made, and a Vitallium model of the upper femur was finally produced. The appliance was about twelve inches long. It had a smooth, rounded head to fit in the acetabulum. The lower end was fashioned so that it could be slipped over and be bolted to the lower fragment of the femur."

The patient had a problem with a fracture. But he regained 75% of normal movement and walked without a cane; indeed, he could walk about carrying a 215-pound man. He died of heart failure about 2 years later. The specimen was retrieved. The capsule and synovium were near normal. There was an involucrum around the stem but they do not say if there was loosening.

The self-locking prosthesis was introduced in 1952.

THOMPSON PROSTHESIS, 1950

Thompson reported a 2.5-year follow-up of 35 patients in 1953. The indications were nonunion, avascular necrosis after fracture, and bilateral arthritis.

"The simplicity of the operative procedure and the rapid recovery of function without the necessity of elaborate rehabilitation measures is striking."

This prosthesis offers valuable salvage possibilities. A viable head after a successful nailing, however, is still a more desirable result.

The Cement Story

Methacrylate had been known for 20 years before acrylic cement was used by neurosurgeons for cranial defects and to fill aneurysms in the early 1950s. Kiaer and Jansen reported using it to attach plastic cups to the femoral head in 1951. In 1953, Harboush described using cement to bed a femoral prosthesis in the femur. In the early 1950s Charnley was having trouble with his furnace and went to the laboratory of the dental hospital for advice on measuring the flue temperature. He met D. C. Smith, a chemist writing a Ph.D. thesis on acrylics. This led to the first patient having a stem cemented in for fracture in 1958. Then cement becomes standard for low-friction arthroplasty in Britain after studies showed an excellent bone-cement interface.

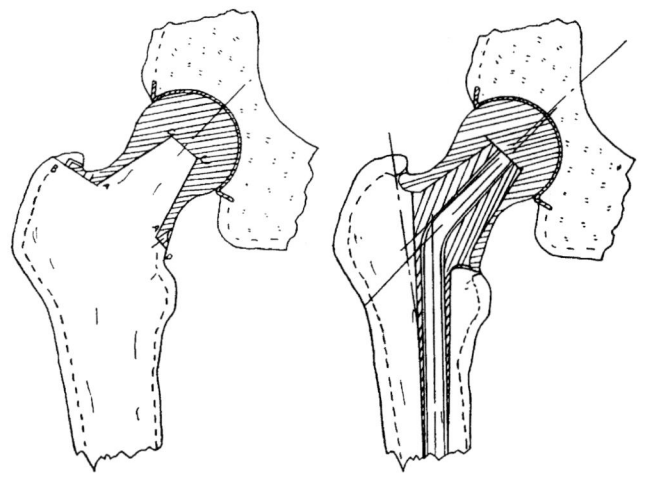

In 1940 Harboush implanted a prosthesis for the femoral head. As time went by it eroded the acetabulum. "There should be, not only a false head and neck, but a false acetabulum as well. Just as an edentulous individual needs a set of both uppers and lowers, so it is with arthroplasty". He made a Vitallium acetabulum and femoral head: both were cemented with acrylic. "The use of fast setting dental acrylic, relatively non-toxic, is introduced in this paper. This may open a new avenue in definitive orthopaedic surgery". From Harboush EJ: Arthroplasty of the hip based on biomechanics, photo-elasticity, fast setting acrylic cement and other considerations. Bull Hosp Joint Dis 1953, 14, 242-77, Figs. 53 and 54. Reproduced with permission.

Cement was licensed for use in the Mayo Clinic in March 1969. Low-viscosity cements were licensed before Charnley's CMW cement was licensed for general use in 1984. In 1970 Charnley published his book on cement. Pressurizing becomes important.

ON PROSTHETIC METHODS INTENDED TO REPAIR BONE FRAGMENTS, 1894

Jules Emile Pean, M.D.

"In recent years, surgeons have endeavored to find prosthetic methods for inducing repair and cicatrization of rigid parts of the organism by unquestionably ingenious methods. It is sufficient to observe with what facility one can maintain resected bones of the extremities or those fractured by accident or surgical intervention, to see all the advantages which one can derive by external means such as aluminum plates and screws applied to each side of the bone, by twisted silver wires passed across their lamina comparta or the diploë. One will find similar examples in our practice reading clinical volumes in which are published the observations of patients which we have treated at the hospital

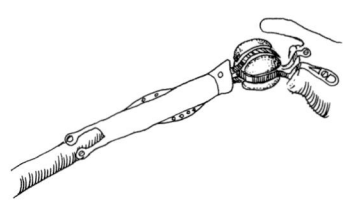

Pean's prosthesis, 1894. The head was made of boiled rubber and shaped to allow movement in two planes. Rotation was through a swivel on the shaft.

◆ **Jules Emile Pean (1830–1898)**
"One of the leading surgeons of Paris during the latter half of the 19th century. Among his credits was the invention of the haemostat, the first gastrectomy for carcinoma, and the introduction of the American ovariectomy into continental Europe. The present paper describes the first attempt at articular prosthesis with metal. Before this, as he notes, Gluck and others had tried ivory and animal bone, all of which were quickly absorbed. Pean not only used metal but, recognizing the corrosive qualities of steel, iron, and other metals, used platinum as least affected by tissue fluids. The concept was good but, of course, not until the classic work of Venable and Struck in 1938 did the non-electrolytic quality of Vitallium and certain steel alloys raise the standard of success for all metal implantations.

"Pean was associated with the Hospital St. Louis for most of his career. Later in life he founded his own hospital, the International. After his death it was renamed the Hospital Pean." E. M. Bick, Clin Orth Rel Res 1973, 94.4. Reproduced with permission.

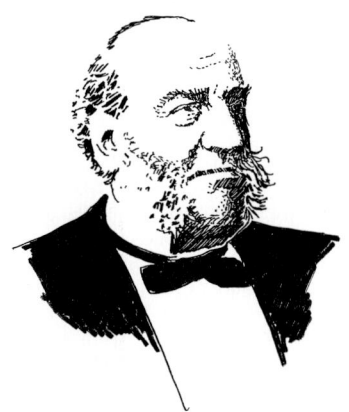

◆ **Jules Emile Pean (1830–1898)**

of St. Louis. Like Ollier and several of his colleagues at Lyon, we have succeeded in replacing the bone structure of the nose by thin and fenestrated plates of platinum, and the results have been satisfactory in several patients in whom the bridge of the nose could not have been otherwise supported.

"A year ago a patient was brought to the International Hospital almost dying with tuberculosis of the humerus involving the shoulder joint. It was complicated by a vast abscess under the muscles and such severe difficulties that we thought there was no alternative to a disarticulation; we found ourselves embarrassed by his firm refusal. The extent of the disease was such that the joint and the humerus seemed as one; an extensive resection would not yield a satisfactory functional result. At this point we thought of a prosthesis. We would be able to remove all the diseased parts and manage all the sound parts.

"We made a vertical incision through the anterior aspect of the arm crossing the acromion and descending vertically to the junction of the middle and lower third of the arm, passing the sinus of a previous incision to incise an abscess. This incision involved the skin, the subcutaneous tissue, and penetrating the intermuscular space which separates the deltoid from the biceps and exposed the anterior face of the bone and the scapulohumeral joint. We released considerable fetid pus and detritus.

"The vessels were clamped and the periosteum was opened with the raspatory for the entire length of the diseased bone from the joint to the mid portion of the bone. Opening the capsule showed the joint filled with pus. The head of the humerus was partly hypertrophied, and partly destroyed. The synovium was lined by thick fungiform tissue which extended to the glenoid cavity. The glenoid cavity was altered but slightly except in a few areas where the cartilage was lightly rarefied. Around the joint and the periosteum of the upper end of the humerus, the many centers of submuscular suppuration were lined similarly by luxuriant fungiform tissue. All of this was removed by scraping with a curette. Then we removed the superior extremity of the humerus with the aid of our forceps and gouges, and seeing that the osseous tissue was infiltrated with yellowish and softened tubercles, we continued to remove the bone from the top to where we met healthy bone. The superior part of the humerus was removed. The synovium was dissected and removed. Nothing remained of the joint structure but the glenoid cavity, the fibrous capsule and the periosteum in the form of a sleeve in all the places where it had not been destroyed.

"Fortunately the loss of substance was big enough for exploration of the infected area. An incision was made through the posterior aspect of the joint to excavate the pus and scrape the lining of an abscess which extended under the deep surface of the deltoid and dorsal musculature toward the spine of the scapula.

"Resection of bone was very important if healing and movement of the limb were not to be compromised. We therefore decided to use a device constructed according to the designs of Gluck: we first consulted M. Mathieu, our skillful mechanic. We

♦ **Themistocles Gluck (1853–1942)**

A Roumanian, he studied in Leipzig and Berlin. He worked in Bucharest and then Berlin. He experimented with nerve suture, synthetic interposition materials to guide nerves to bridge gaps, and synthetic substitutes for tendons and other tissues. He used nickel plated screws and plates for fractures in 1885 and ivory intramedullary pegs in 1890.

He developed ivory joint replacements for the wrist, knee, shoulder, and hip for joints excised because of tuberculosis or tumors. They were secured by intramedullary stems. They failed because of infection.

wanted him to make an interarticular artificial joint at the end of a stem long enough to fill the loss of substance of the humerus. The joint part was able to reach the glenoid cavity with a surface permitting full movement. He was able to give us one of Gluck's pieces. This device was too weak, made of ivory, a substance too easily resorbable, with an articulation too little movable. We then asked Dr. Michaels (who had been clever enough to construct an ingenious apparatus intended to replace the 3 maxillary bones in a patient we presented to the Academy January 14, 1890) whether he would work with us to design a prosthetic device made of an unalterable material and capable of lending itself to an artificial joint with all its motions. This mechanism, a model of which we are presenting today to the Academy, was constructed by him with a speed and facility worthy of commendation. In the construction of this piece, of which the illustration is attached, the hardened rubber and iridescent platinum are the sole materials incorporated. To render the rubber stable in contact with tissue fluids, the pieces of which it was formed were boiled for 24 hours in paraffin. When the prosthesis had been solidly fixed to ensure its stability, the periosteum and articular capsule were attached around it. Catgut sutures closed the shaft within a sort of periosteal case. The wound was then closed with interrupted horsehair sutures. A rubber tube was sutured in place posteriorly to assure drainage of fluids by gravity. A soft iodoform dressing, lightly compressive, kept the arm and shoulder immobilized.

"It was feared that a mechanism so complex would not be tolerated by tissues which had already been the seat of serious disorders, and had not yet recovered from an acute inflammation, aggravating the chronic inflammation which put the days of our patient in danger. Nothing happened. At the end of a few days not only was he relieved, but his fever subsided, his appetite increased with his physical strength, he raised himself and could walk about the ward 12 days after operation, and on the twentieth day, he visited his family for a day on the outskirts of Paris. Finally, since the operation he had gained 35 pounds, and his health would have been excellent had he not been troubled by several recurrences of a small localized abscess which reformed above the epicondyle. We had to open this small abscess on 4 different occasions. It had attacked the lining in several days but in spite of all the care which we gave, and the repeated injections attempted: phenol, chloral, oxygenated water, potassium permanganate, camphorated naphthol, etc., we could not dry the fistula completely. Such is the case history which we submit.

"Is it of a nature to make one believe, as Gluck has said, that foreign bodies as large as those which we have used can definitively replace so considerable loss of skeletal substance? We may respond in the affirmative after seeing the actually surprising result obtained in this patient, if it were not for the occasional recurrence of a small abscess 12 months after the operation. It is true that from this point of view one cannot accuse the prosthesis exclusively, since we daily see small abscesses following simple excision of bone in tuberculosis that fistulae are produced, at-

testing to the fact that the local involvement of the diaphysis was not completely removed. At the least it is remarkable to see that, several weeks after the operation, the patient had regained his health, that the old foci had disappeared, that he had recovered movement in the joint, that he could use the extremity for most of the usual needs of his life. To those who consider that in a similar case, it would have been preferable to immediately disarticulate at the shoulder at the moment the patient presented himself to us, we reply first that it is entirely the opposite; that his state of weakness at that time was such that he would have probably succumbed to so serious an operation as the complete amputation of a limb. Secondly, if the resection as extensive as that which we performed would not have been followed by recovery and would not have allowed the patient to use the extremity, the disarticulation would have become practical and with less danger today.

"*Concluding the preceding observations:*

1. *It is possible to replace an important part of the skeleton and even an enarthrodial joint;*
2. *That this device, to be well tolerated, should be not only aseptic, but made of nonresorbable material;*
3. *That it is tolerated by the organism when one takes the required precautions;*
4. *It permits one to substitute for an immediate disarticulation when the patient refuses such intervention;*
5. *Large resections have the advantage of preventing the destruction of the soft parts;*
6. *Finally that they can be provided with a mechanism permitting the joints to preserve their movement.*"

ARTHROPLASTY OF THE HIP: A NEW OPERATION

JOHN CHARNLEY, 1961

"*In considering how arthroplasty of the hip can be improved, two facts stand out: 1. After replacement of the head of the femur by a spherical surface of inert material, the failures are essentially long-term. At first the patient may notice no difference between the artificial head and the living one which preceded it. Our problem is to make this temporary success permanent. 2. Objectives must be reasonable. Neither surgeons nor engineers will ever make an artificial hip-joint which will last 30 years and at some time in this period enable the patient to play football.*

Deductions from Past Experiences

"*The methods from which we have learned most are those of Smith-Petersen and Judet.*

"*The Smith-Petersen method was a refinement of the oldest of all forms of arthroplasty, in which a membrane, or some kind of tissue, is interposed between the head of the femur and its*

◆ **John Charnley (1911–1982)**

Anyone who thinks that Charnley had a good idea one afternoon and reaped the rewards for the rest of his life should read the excellent biography by William Waugh. Charnley was a man consumed by hip arthroplasty. He wrote in his entry in Who's Who: "Recreation—*Other than surgery, nothing*".

Charnley grew up in the industrial north of England. His father ran a drugstore and his mother was a nurse. He won medals at Manchester Medical School and then trained in General Surgery until the outbreak of World War II. He volunteered and was posted as medical officer to the disastrous evacuation from the beaches of Dunkirk. He later served in Egypt, became an orthopaedic specialist, and was given charge of an orthopaedic workshop, inventing an adjustable fracture brace. He never had any training in engineering but always had a workshop where he created prototypes. In the Army, he gained much experience of trauma. After his demobilization, he went to an Orthopaedic Hospital to learn the rest of orthopaedics in 6 months before he became a staff orthopaedic surgeon. In 1948, he was one of the traveling fellows to North America. At one time he was encouraged to move to the United States, but he did not think that he would be so free to try out new methods of treatment on human beings.

In 1950, *The Closed Treatment of Common Fractures* was published. This is still good reading because it details the principles of reduction—usually left unexplained, to residents. In 1953 came *Compression Arthrodesis*, which described the basic science of bone healing and new operations. In the preface, he wrote "How like the captain of a windjammer is an orthopaedic surgeon: daily he is pestered by his patients to say when they might reasonably expect to arrive at their longed-for destination: how expert he becomes at evading the question". Although considered one of the great books of orthopaedics, the sales in 2 years were only 800 copies. Today no publisher would have taken this on. He wrote a lot of papers, letters to journals, book chapters for medical students, and book reviews. He did general orthopaedics and was trying to focus on the hip.

He probably tried hip arthroplasty in 1946, when Judet's method became known, but gave it up in favor of arthrodesis. He began to think about joint lubrication and friction after a patient reported that his hip squeaked so loudly after a Judet prosthesis had been implanted that his wife had to leave the room. Charnley's experiments showed that cartilage was more slippery than ice, and he looked for a plastic with the same properties. In the mid fifties he started to test Teflon (polytetrafluoroethylene) and implanted some double cups that failed. He went on to cement in a Moore's femoral head prosthesis and press fit a Teflon acetabulum. To decrease friction further, he made the head smaller.

He married at the age of 46 years. A few years afterwards his wife, Jill, had sciatica, and he operated on her disc with complete success.

When he was 49, in 1959, the Centre for Hip Surgery was opened at Wrightington. He studied every step of joint replacement methodically—materials, design, wear, infection, technique—nothing was left unscrutinized. He followed his patients to the grave. In 1960 he reported on 97 low-friction arthroplasties. The results were dramatic. By 1962, 452 hip operations of various kinds were done. Then disaster hit. The Teflon wore badly and produced granulomas. Charnley became profoundly depressed. There was nothing he could offer the patients. At this point a technical representative came in with a sample of high density polyethylene that was used to make gears. Charnley had no time for him and walked out. His workshop manager, Craven, thought he would put the high density polyethylene on the wear testing machine anyway. After 2 days it showed minimal wear. After more tests, Charnley could say "We were on again". The first high molecular weight polyethylene hip went in in November 1962. The operation gradually became routine.

When I visited in 1964, the greenhouse and the multiple trays were already in place. The records were standardized and there were patients everywhere. Charnley retired at the age of 64 and went to work in a private clinic, carried on his research, and wrote his book, *Low Friction Arthroplasty of the Hip,* which was published in 1979. He was knighted. He died of a myocardial infarct—still working—in 1982.

His achievement should be considered in the light of the fact that he did no animal research, he did no randomized controlled trials, and he was not in a University. He should have had a Nobel Prize.

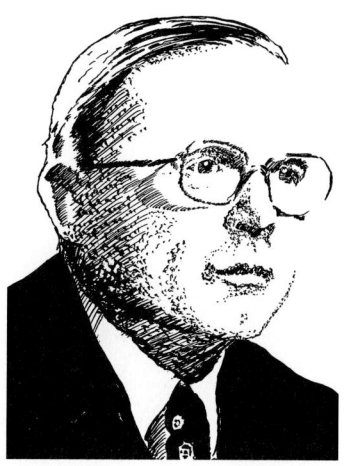

◆ **John Charnley (1911–1982)**

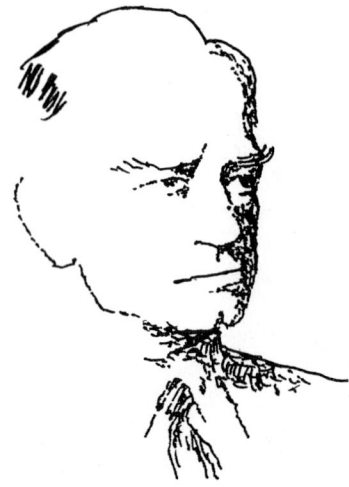

◆ Marius Smith-Petersen
(1886–1953)

◆ Marius Smith-Petersen (1886–1953)

Born in Norway, he was 17 when he arrived in the United States. He graduated in medicine at Harvard and eventually became chief at Massachusetts General Hospital. He was a perfectionist, singleminded, a slow and meticulous surgeon, with a great capacity for friendship.

As a resident he was appalled by the blood loss that occurred during exposure of the hip joint, and this led to the anterior Smith-Petersen approach to the hip in 1917, which is used to this day, and to the triflanged nail in 1925.

Arthroplasty of the hip seemed to yield poor results in his view. He saw that a piece of glass embedded as a foreign body in a child produced a smooth shiny membrane, and this stimulated the cup arthroplasty. Starting with glass, he tried all kinds of materials until he settled on Vitallium. Vitallium arthroplasty had enough drawbacks to prevent it from becoming universally popular, but it had a lifetime of 30 years.

He made a lot of fusions of the sacroiliac joint for back pain. Osteotomy of the spine for flexion deformity due to ankylosing spondylitis was a bold operation he invented. During a sleepless night on a train, traveling back from a clinic filled with failed hip fractures, the idea of a triflanged nail occurred to him. This would fix the fracture and prevent rotation.

He never retired.

◆ Robert Judet

Robert and Jean Judet were brothers, sons of an orthopaedic surgeon, and they dominated French orthopaedics during the postwar period with their strong personalities and interesting ideas.

socket. *A metal cup, loosefitting and polished, was placed between the femoral head and the acetabulum, after the femoral head had been reduced in size and the acetabulum had been enlarged by removal of the eburnated lining. The polished hemispherical surfaces of this metal cup induced changes in the fibrous tissue on the exposed surfaces of cancellous bone, which were transformed into a form of articular cartilage.*

"Smith-Petersen repeatedly emphasized that the moving parts should be made to fit loosely together; in no sense, therefore, could the mechanical arrangement at the finish of this operation be regarded as a mechanically stable ball-and-socket joint. The femoral head inside the cup is capable of slight displacement, and the cup also is capable of displacement inside the socket. In course of time the spaces between the cup and the femoral head and the cup and the acetabulum become filled with fibrocartilaginous material and the hip can thus become stable; but unfortunately the periarticular soft tissues often become thick and stiff, and mobility is lost.

"In the Judet operation the head of the femur is replaced by a prosthesis bearing a polished hemispherical surface. In the original Judet operation the prosthesis was like a gigantic tintack with a hemispherical bead and it was fixed to the femur by driving the spike down the center of the stump of the femoral neck. The joint formed by this procedure was much more stable than that formed by the Smith-Petersen procedure, because a prosthesis was chosen which was a close fit in the acetabulum. Very soon afterwards many patients could perform circumduction of the hip under full muscle control, against the force of gravity and without pain.

"The capacity of the living organism to react favorably to sound mechanical design, and its capacity to reveal incipient mechanical failure by deterioration of function, even before the appearance of frank pain, is a fundamental guide in developing any arthroplasty.

Joint Lubrication

"The starting-point of the present research was the well-known observation that after the Judet operation the hip sometimes squeaks. This does not last more than a few weeks and the final result is neither better nor worse than in cases without a squeak. In our experience the squeaks have occurred in the hips of osteoarthritics, but never when the acetabulum was lined with normal articular cartilage as in the treatment of subcapital fractures of the neck of the femur.

"A squeak indicates that frictional resistance to sliding is so high that the surfaces are seizing together. Hence it seemed likely that the plastic of the original Judet prosthesis had adverse frictional properties when sliding against the bare bone encountered in an osteoarthritic acetabulum. It seemed possible, too, that the cessation of squeaking might be a sign not of improved lubrication but of loosening of the attachment of the prosthesis to the neck of the femur. In these circumstances the head of the prosthesis would be stationary in the acetabulum and all movement would be taking place between the femoral neck and the stem or spike by which it was originally attached to the bone. Clearly, the mechanical bond between the prosthesis and the neck of the femur could be broken by a twisting strain, or torque, resulting from high frictional resistance to the turning of the prosthesis in the acetabulum. If there were no such frictional resistance, the mechanical attachment to the femoral neck would be spared any such strains.

Laboratory Experiments

"I could find only two references to measurements of the coefficient of friction of normal animal joints, and my own experiments closely confirmed the figure of $\mu = 0.02$ reported by Jones, with the possibility that in certain conditions μ might be much less than this. For a skate sliding on ice, μ has been estimated at 0.03, which indicates that an animal joint is rather more slippery than ice. Engineering science knows no way of approaching such low figures for μ in a "plain" bearing when the application concerns reciprocating motion, at slow speeds, and under heavy loads. Nature has solved completely the most difficult set of lubricating conditions which ever face the engineer.

"These investigations on lubrication suggested that synovial fluid is not an essential lubricant but rather a product of the activity of joints—a view taken for granted by Sir Arthur Keith in 1919. Emphasis was transferred from the synovial fluid to the properties of articular cartilage, and attention was drawn to the engineering concept of "boundary lubrication" between dry solid surfaces, or between solid surfaces separated by a film of fluid too thin to behave as a fluid. A boundary lubricant reduces friction by entering into physicochemical combination with the surfaces, and diminishes the free molecular attraction which may seize the surfaces together. Hence there must be a physicochemical affinity between the lubricant and the solid material of the rubbing surfaces; the lubricant is effective only with certain combinations of solids. Even if synovial fluid is a lubricant in an animal joint, it will not necessarily lubricate a prosthesis.

"This was confirmed by experiment on the effect of ox synovial fluid on the frictional resistance between steel and bone and between 'Perspex' and bone. The coefficient of friction for plastic and steel against bone, moistened with ox synovial fluid, was high ($\mu = 0.4$). On the other hand, when the plastic or steel was tested against normal articular cartilage, the frictional resistance was almost as low as in a normal joint ($\mu = 0.02$).

Prosthesis and Socket

"These investigations indicated that to give an artificial hip-joint the same kind of slipperiness as a natural joint, we should need a substance with a low coefficient of friction which at the same time could be tolerated in body tissues. For this purpose I chose polytetrafluoroethylene—a plastic which looks not unlike articular cartilage (being white and semitranslucent, and capable of being cut with a knife) and is chemically the most inert plastic so far discovered.

"The first idea was to use this low-friction material as 'synthetic articular cartilage.' I lined the eburnated acetabulum of the arthritic hip-joint with a thin shell of polytetrafluoroethylene and covered the reshaped head of the femur with a hollow cup of the same material firmly pressed into position. The absolute relief of pain, and the range of active movement under muscular control, were impressive in the first 3 months; but the most conservative feature of this design was its undoing. Adhering to the conservative principle which Smith-Petersen called 'conservation of stock,' I had retained the femoral head and refashioned it as a spigot on which to press the inner plastic sphere; but this resulted in ischemic necrosis of the bone inside the inner sphere. As soon as the early good function started to fail, radiological examination always indicated that the head of the femur was necrotic and was becoming loose inside the inner sphere. The poor results of this kind of prosthesis thus resembled the poor results of the Smith-Petersen cup.

Cementing the Prosthesis to the Femur

"My next step was to replace the head of the femur with a metallic prosthesis in combination with a low-friction plastic socket. I had for some time been interested in improving the mechanical bond between prosthesis and bone, by using a cement to transfer the weight of the body from the metallic stem of the prosthesis uniformly to the cancellous bone of the interior of the neck and upper end of the femur (Charnley, 1960). My object was to get over the defect of the Moore and Thompson types of prosthesis, which is that they have no resistance against stresses tending to twist them in the medullary cavity on its long axis. (Twisting forces of this kind will in particular be experienced when a patient is rising from a sitting position with the femoral shafts horizontal.) In 3 patients in whom the arthroplasty was reexplored, because of mechanical defects in the socket, I found that the cemented prosthesis had remained absolutely rigid in the femur after taking the full weight of the body during 10 or 11 months. Furthermore, experience of over 2 years, with more than 100 patients, led me to believe that, as regards infection, this technic is safer than the original one. Infection of an arthroplasty will probably start with multiplication of bacteria in blood-clot within the cavity of the joint. If the prosthesis is loose in the medulla, the infection will be pumped into the medullary canal at every muscular movement. But where the prosthesis is cemented in position I imagine that the joint might contain pus, and the stump of the femoral neck might be bathed in pus, without any spread of infection to the medullary canal.

Design of the Socket

"Though the results of using the arrangement previously mentioned were gratifying, it was pointed out to me that the best engineering practice would be to use the smallest diameter of ball which would cope with the expected load. Up to then I had used a standard Moore prosthesis with a ball 1 5/8 inches in diameter, believing that polytetrafluoroethylene, being a relatively soft material, would wear longer if the load per unit area of bearing surface were the smallest possible. The recommendation of my engineering colleagues enabled me to make a big improvement in the anchorage of the plastic socket in the bony acetabulum. Resistance to movement of the head in the socket is greatly reduced by reducing the radius of the ball and therefore reducing the 'moment' of the frictional force. If at the same time the radius of the exterior of the polytetrafluoroethylene socket is made as large as possible, the 'moment' of the frictional force between socket and bone will be increased, and this will lessen any tendency for the socket to rotate against the bone. The small remaining shearing force can be resisted easily by the fibrous tissue occupying the deep irregularities on the outer surface of the socket.

Present Operation

"The operation is performed through a lateral exposure by elevating the great trochanter. At the end of the operation the trochanter is reattached to the outer surface of the femur in order to enhance the leverage of the abductor muscles. Though this delays rehabilitation, it is of paramount importance in preventing adduction, external rotation, and dislocation.

"When the head of the femur has been resected, the acetabulum is deepened and then reamed with special tools to an exact diameter for receiving the polytetrafluoroethylene socket. To enhance the precision of the reaming, the sequence of tools all operate on a 1/2- inch pilot hole which is made in the center of the floor of the acetabulum, the exact center being found by a self-centering device. The polytetrafluoroethylene socket carries a spigot 1/2 inch in diameter which engages with the pilot hole and ensures correct orientation. The socket is hammered into the acetabulum with a punch, its external surface being deeply serrated to receive the ingrowth of fibrous tissue or bone.

"The prosthesis carries a head which at present is no more than 7/8 inch in diameter. Several lengths of neck are available, so that during the operation the one which best suits the depth of the socket can be chosen.

"After a trial reduction has shown that everything is satisfactory, the prosthesis is cemented in position and the great trochanter is reattached with wire. The patient is splinted with the leg in abduction for 3 weeks, and is allowed to take full weight on the hip 5 weeks after the operation. Recent experiences suggest that plaster is not essential.

Results So Far

"Though my experience of using polytetrafluoroethylene for arthroplasty of the hip extends over 3 years, the technic in its present form has been in use only since January, 1960. Since then 97 hips have been operated on. There have been no deaths, except a coronary occlusion 6 weeks after operation, and the only serious complication encountered has been deep venous thrombosis.

"While the long-term results are still awaited, the method has been restricted to cases of gross disablement by (1) rheumatoid arthritis, (2) severe osteoarthritis in patients over 65, and occasionally (3) bilateral arthritis in middle age. The only disappointing results have been in very difficult 'salvage' cases where the absence of normal structures made it impossible to carry out a technically sound procedure. With one exception, the only cases of infection have been those in which there have been previous attempts at arthroplasty by other methods.

"On removal of the splints, after 3 weeks, most patients can execute a "straight-leg raise" and have no pain or spasm on passive movement. After a week out of plaster, they have recovered the pre-operative range of movement. If the hip has previously been very stiff the final range may be no greater than 30 degrees, but it will be painless and under muscular control. The average stay in hospital is 8 weeks, and before they go home most patients can walk the length of the ward without sticks and with only a slight limp.

"As regards wear and tear of the socket, working against the metal head of the prosthesis, close scrutiny of the radiographs of patients who have been transmitting the full weight of the body through this implant for 10 months has shown negligible wear. The stresses imposed on the hip-joints of patients disabled by arthritis are only a fraction of those borne by the hip-joints of normal subjects or athletes: but even if the method should prove unsuitable for robust patients in middle life, it may have a permanent place in the treatment of the rheumatoid and elderly, for whom it is particularly suitable because it requires almost no rehabilitation. Even in the early stages there is no pain on movement, and the procedure is therefore appropriate for subjects with the poor muscles and relatively feeble morale which so often accompany long-continued ill-health or old age."

Excision Arthroplasty

Girdlestone's name is given to this salvage operation. He was following a long line of surgeons who excised infected joints in the preantibiotic era, when infection was almost impossible to eradicate.

Excision of the hip for infection could be a lifesaving operation, but operating for deformity, in the days before infection control, was to take a big gamble. Operating for deformity started in 1822 with Anthony White in London. By 1876, the literature contained descriptions of 472 operations, with a mortality of 44%.

Ironically, Girdlestone wrote up the operation in 1943, just as penicillin began to be manufactured, and his operation was later modified for use in osteoarthritis. Girdlestone was dissatisfied with the results of treating chronic hip infections; many were old World War I gunshot wounds. The operation he described was designed to saucerize the acetabulum to permit healing. He made a transverse incision just above the greater trochanter and removed most of the gluteus medius and greater trochanter.

"The whole upper and outer aspect of the capsule of the hip lies exposed. The capsule and synovia are removed and the underlying portions of the neck, head, and acetabular rim are seen. The neck is then divided near its base by a 1 1/2 in. chisel, and the femoral head removed. The removal of the head is greatly facilitated (as it is also in performing pseudarthrosis for osteoarthritis) by the oblique removal of the upper acetabular rim by a 1 1/2 or 2 in. gouge of suitable curvature. All the

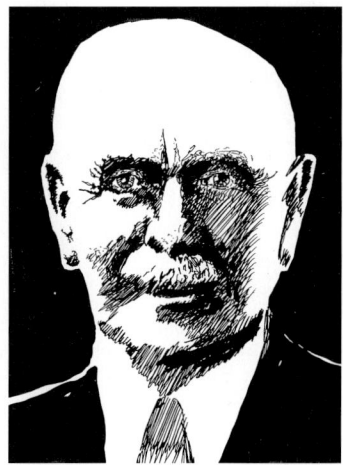

◆ **Gathorne Robert Girdlestone (1881–1950)**

◆ Gathorne Robert Girdlestone (1881–1950)

He went to work as a general practitioner close to the Orthopaedic Hospital at Oswestry. Robert Jones visited the nearby hospital, and Girdlestone quickly came under his spell and became an orthopaedic surgeon. In World War I he was sent to Oxford where the general hospital became more and more of an orthopaedic hospital for the wounded. Following the war, he and Robert Jones proposed a national scheme to care for crippled children based on army organization. Outside Oxford was a large automobile factory run by a man who had started making bicycles, William Morris (Lord Nuffield). One day Nuffield was anesthetized by Dr MacIntosh for dental work, the same anesthetist who worked with Girdlestone. The three men started to play golf together. After one game that Girdlestone won, Nuffield asked "What were we playing for?" Girdlestone named an amount that would pay for his new Hospital. Nuffield wrote out the check.

Girdlestone was a man with strong religious convictions and organizational skills. The Oxford program allowed him to put into operation a plan for the comprehensive care of the crippled child. There were peripheral clinics and outpatient services with a central hospital and research facility. Girdlestone had no children—the Hospital was his family.

He wrote a book on tuberculosis of the bone, and there is a biography of him by Trueta.

The operation of resection of the femoral head and lip of the acetabulum is named after Girdlestone, and it remains the end of the line for hip patients. (In fact, joint resection was one of the first orthopaedic operations to be invented, and if it is known after anyone it should be Charles White of Manchester, who proposed the operation in 1769, or PF Moreau, who reported joint excision in 1782, or Anthony White of London who did it in 1822).

In 1940, Girdlestone resigned but wanted to continue his academic work. Herbert Seddon was appointed, and the two quarrelled until Seddon left for London in 1948. Trueta then took over the Chair.

cartilage is gouged or scraped out of the acetabulum and the rotten bone curetted. It is the rule in this operation to leave no cartilage, no diseased bone, no dead tissue and no dead spaces. The erasion [sic] of the acetabulum should leave raw surfaces of vascular cancellous bone.

"The incisions are analogous to the first cuts in a shoulder or leg of mutton.

"After removal of the head and most of the neck, upward displacement of the femur in relation to the innominate must not be permitted, for such movement would close the opening, spoil the saucerization, and bottle neck the acetabulum. The position is maintained by fixed traction on a frame."

Hip Osteotomy

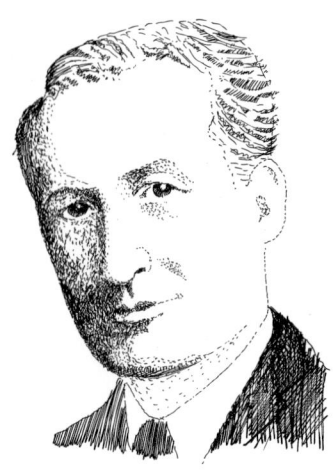

◆ **Sydney Alan Stormer Malkin (1892–1964)**

A pioneer of hip osteotomy for osteoarthritis. Nottingham, in the industrial heartland of England, was known for its slums and poverty at the turn of the century. In 1906, the Duchess of Portland started the Nottingham Cripples Guild, which began with a clinic and her Rolls-Royce as transportation. She found someone who would build an 80-bed hospital for free and soon afterward Malkin, who was a product of the Shepherd's Bush Military Hospital, was appointed as Surgeon. The hospital subsequently became Harlow Wood Orthopaedic Hospital. Here Malkin developed osteotomy for osteoarthritis of the hip and knee.

While President of the British Orthopaedic Association in 1948, he started the ABC traveling fellowships.

Today osteotomy is used for younger patients to improve hip coverage. In the past it was used to relieve improved congruity, decrease loads across the hip, or reduce deformity while preserving the range of motion. There was a certain mystique attached to reasons for the benefits noted—did cartilage heal? Was it a vascular effect?

THE McMURRAY OSTEOTOMY FOR OSTEOARTHRITIC HIP, 1929

"For osteo-arthritis the author has used oblique osteotomy. After division of the shaft of the bone, the upper sharp end of the shaft of the femur is transferred inward until its upper inner border lies directly under the cotyloid ligament of the acetabulum.

"The operation is performed with two objects in view: first, the transference of some of the body weight from the pelvis directly through the shaft of the femur; thus relieving the hip-joint; and, second, the rotation of the head of the femur, so that in weight-bearing a new portion of the articular surface takes the remaining weight."

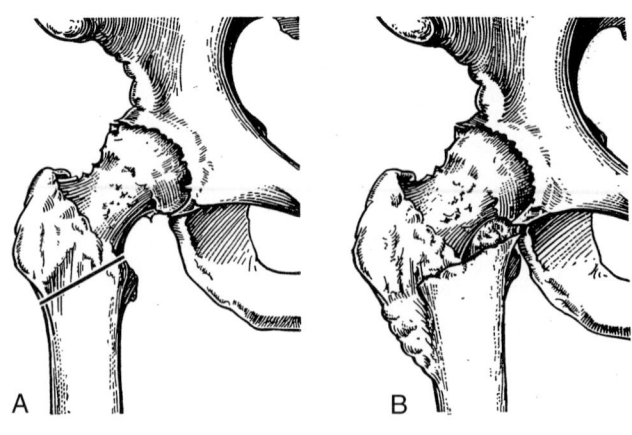

The McMurray osteotomy. An answer to osteoarthritis before joint replacement. The idea was that deformity was corrected, a new part of the head was exposed to wear, the pressure was reduced, and hypervascularity stimulated repair. Fixation was later added. The results were unpredictable and poor. (A) Oblique osteotomy showing site of osteotomy. (B) Showing position of fragments after successful oblique osteotomy. From McMurray TP: A Practice of Orthopaedic Surgery, 3rd ed. London: E. Arnold, 1949, Fig. 18, 72 a, b. Reproduced with permission.

The operation could easily be performed in 10 to 15 minutes, McMurray writes. After the operation the position was held in a cast for 4 months. He expected to retain 50% of hip movement.

Hip Fractures

If he escapes with his life he has to be content with loss of function.   Bissell, 1903

A lot was known about hip fractures because they were so often fatal and could be studied in the autopsy room. They are not hard to diagnose in the absence of radiographs, but separating trochanteric fractures, which would unite, from intracapsular fractures, which would not unite, had to wait not just for the discovery of X-ray in 1897 but for machines good enough to take a lateral radiograph of the hip.

Although today hip fractures are treated by internal fixation, intracapsular fractures used to be treated by rest until the pain decreased enough to permit resumption of activity. Extracapsular fractures were treated with traction and casts.

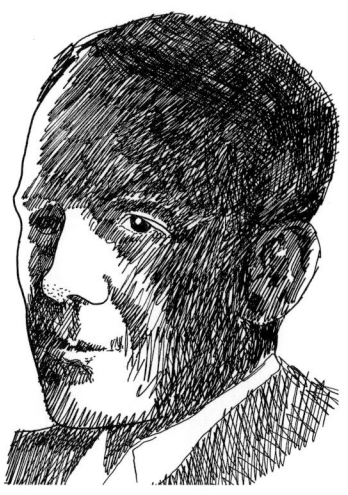

◆ **Thomas Porter McMurray (1887–1949)**
He came from Belfast in Northern Ireland and worked with Robert Jones in Liverpool, where he spent the rest of his life. He was a speedy surgeon and could take out an entire meniscus with the posterior horn in 5 minutes.

He gave his name to a test for a torn meniscus and to femoral osteotomy for osteoarthritis of the hip.

This was a different age—for the last 20 years of his life he did not use a plate or screw or pin.

He was largely responsible for running the Master of Orthopaedic Surgery course from its beginnings in 1921. He was President of the British Orthopaedic Association and would have been President of the British Medical Association if he had not died of a heart attack in Ealing Broadway Station.

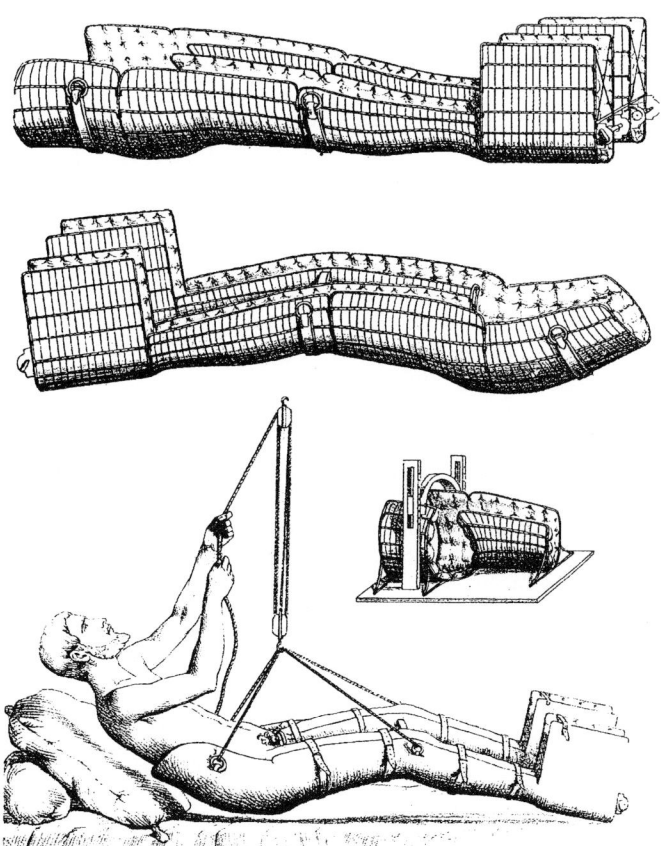

Before the use of internal fixation for hip fractures, they were treated by bed rest, by traction, with huge splints like this, or with plaster casts. This is the Grand Appareil of Bonnet, used for fractures but mostly for tuberculosis of the hip (1845).

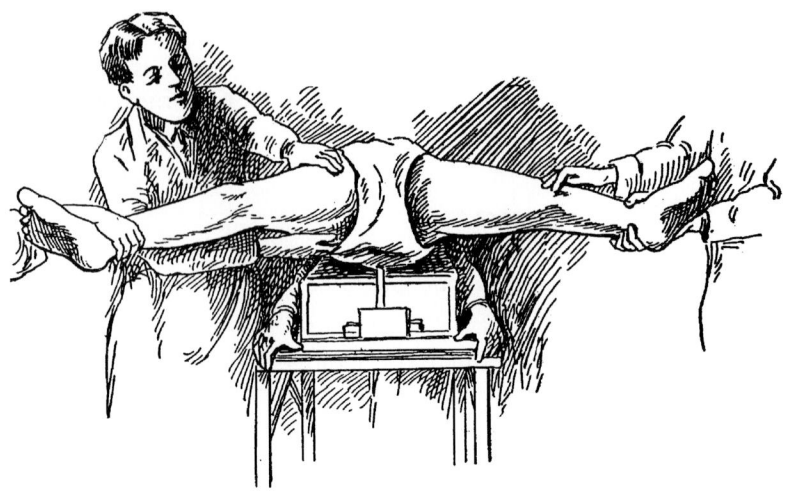

Reduction of a fracture of the femoral neck—the Whitman technique of forced abduction before application of the cast. From Scudder in 1922.

TIMELINE OF HIP FRACTURES

1575 Ambroise Paré describes intracapsular fractures and says that they go on to nonunion because they are bloodless.

1822 Astley Cooper says of intracapsular fractures, "I have never met with one in which bony union had taken place." He did animal experiments—intracapsular fractures went to nonunion while extracapsular fractures united.

1850 B. R. C. Langenbeck, inventor of the retractor, nailed a hip fracture.

1870 Langenbeck's ivory pegs failed.

1878 König: first successful open reduction with internal fixation for hip fracture.

1883 Senn's experiments on animals with hip fractures show that the union rate is better with internal fixation than with cast. However, he meets with such opposition that he continues to treat patients with a cast.

1898 Broeckmann and Gillette use open reduction and bone peg.

1898 Gillette's ivory pegs

1904 Whitman's plaster is the standard.

1907 Delbert begins to use closed reduction and screw fixation using only an anteroposterior radiograph and a jig.

1912 Albee: open reduction and bone peg

1914 Preston adds a side plate to a screw to prevent varus.

1922 Martin and King of New Orleans introduce closed fixation with nail and X-ray.

1930 Hey Groves uses bone pegs.

1930 Commission on hip fractures.

1931 Smith-Petersen uses a triflanged nail combined with open reduction.

1932 Leadbetter devises a method of closed reduction.

1932 Westcott of Virginia performed closed nailing with a solid triflanged nail.

1932 Sven Johansson uses a cannulated nail and closed reduction. Although various kinds of nail had been tried for 30 years,

the results were not good enough to be generally used. The cannulated triflanged nail and closed reduction captured the imagination of most orthopaedic surgeons.
1934 Thornton bolts a plate onto a triflanged nail to prevent varus.
1935 Telson and Ramsohoff: multiple thin pins
1936 Knowles' pins
1937 Moore's pins
1941 Jewett's one-piece nail plate
1955 Pugh's sliding nail plate
1957 Charnley's compression hip screw

A CLINICAL CASE

ASTLEY COOPER, 1822

"The transverse fracture of the cervix femoris within the capsular ligament does not unite by bone. This is a most essential point as the reputation of the surgeon hinges upon it.

"I was called to a case of this fracture in which the medical attendant had been promising, week after week, a union of the fracture, and the restoration to the patient of a sound and useful limb. After many weeks the person became anxious for further advice; I did all in my power to lessen the impression which the mistake of this gentleman had made, by telling the patient she might ultimately walk, although with some lameness; and taking the surgeon into another room, asked him upon what grounds he was led to suppose there would be union; to which he replied he was not aware but that the fracture of the neck of the thighbone would unite like those of other bones of the body; the case, however, proved unfortunate for his character.

"Young medical men find it so much easier a task to speculate than to observe, that they are too apt to be pleased with some sweeping conjecture, which saves them the trouble of observing the processes of nature.

"Nothing is known in our profession by guess. There is no short road to knowledge."

EXPERIMENTAL HIP FRACTURES

NICHOLAS SENN, 1883

Senn noted that for centuries the books had said that unimpacted intracapsular fractures would never unite. But he found that when these fractures were held in accurate contact they healed by callus, providing the scientific basis for current treatment.

"In the animals the fracture was produced by making multiple punctures with a small drill through the neck of the femur entirely within the limits of the capsular ligament and fracturing the balance of the bone by forcibly rotating the femur inwards.

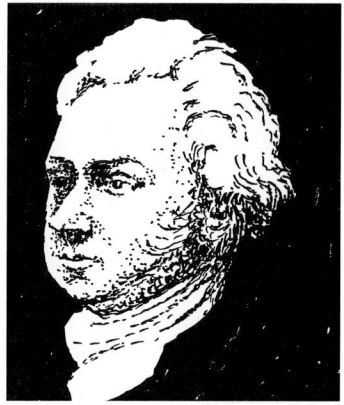

◆ **Sir Astley Cooper (1768–1841)**

He was apprenticed to his uncle and went on staff at Guy's Hospital, where he developed a large practice. Why was he knighted? Because he removed a sebaceous cyst from the king, George IV.

He described disarticulation of the hip (Lancet 16 Jan 1828) and used catgut to tie vessels. He is best known for his *Atlas of Fractures*. He believed that non-union of the femoral neck was due to poor blood supply.

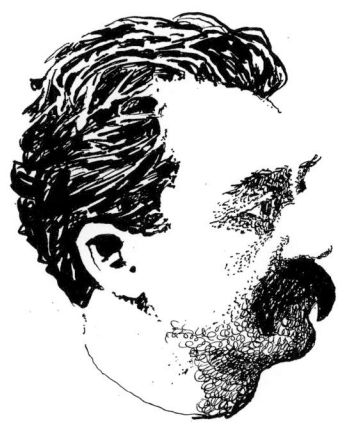

◆ **Nicholas Senn (1844–1908)**

Born of Swiss parents in Wisconsin, he studied in Chicago and became Professor at Rush Medical College. He was energetic. He served in the Spanish American War, became President of the American Medical Association, and was Chairman of the editorial board from the very beginning of the journal *Surgery, Gynecology and Obstetrics,* in addition to writing many books and papers.

He did many animal experiments on fractures of the neck of the femur and proposed nailing intracapsular fractures in 1883, but he received such a hostile reception that he was forced to continue to use casts for treatment.

"Twenty three fractures thus produced were treated on the expectant plan, or by simple fixation with a plaster of Paris dressing. The animals were killed from 4 weeks to 3 months after fracturing the bone. In none of them was I able to find any evidences of bony union. Discouraged by the many failures, I finally resolved to secure accurate coaption of the fragments by drilling a hole from the trochanter major through the entire length of the neck and well into the head and fastening the fragments together with an aseptic iron, bone, or ivory nail. Eight such experiments were made on cats. In two, suppuration followed the operation. In the rest, bony union or union by an exceedingly short ligament without any displacement was obtained."

TREATMENT OF FRACTURES OF THE NECK OF THE FEMUR BY INTERNAL FIXATION
M. N. SMITH-PETERSEN, 1931

"In 1931 a method of internal fixation of fractures of the neck of the femur by means of a flanged nail was published by the author. A series of 24 cases treated over a period of 6 years was reported. This trial period was deemed sufficient to justify publication of experience gained and results obtained. A new method of treatment is never perfect at the time of its inception but it improves as errors are eliminated; at the time of the publication we did not feel that the method of introducing the nail had been perfected since it was an extensive procedure, requiring wide experience with hip joint surgery; this necessarily limited its usefulness. Results obtained, however, were far superior to those obtained by other methods in our clinic.

"After publication we continued the open reduction because the operative findings were such that closed reduction seemed doomed to failure in many cases. Interposition of synovia, capsule or fragments of bone was interpreted as a barrier to bony union. Later developments proved us to be wrong in this conclusion. Apparently the principle of the nail appealed to surgeons in different parts of the world but not the method of insertion. Modifications, simplifying the surgical procedure, soon appeared in the literature and excellent results were reported. Westcott of Roanoke, Virginia, advocated closed reduction, followed by nailing through subtrochanteric incision, using protractors and anteroposterior x-ray films to guide the course of the nail. He reported a very successful series. Johansson of Gothenburg, Sweden, introduced a centrally cannulated nail which was threaded over a Kirschner wire introduced under roentgenographic control by means of a rather complex instrument of precision. Again a series of excellent results was reported. King of Melbourne, Australia, independently of Johansson, proposed the use of a centrally cannulated nail, two wire guides being introduced under the fluoroscope. He also reported a successful series. The interesting point about these three pioneers in the field of closed reduction, followed by nailing through a small lateral incision, is that they all depended upon roentgenographic control.

The Nail

"The nail seemed an ideal means of fixation; it displaced a minimum amount of bone and effectively prevented motion in all planes. However, substitutes for the nail, in the form of wires, pins, screws and bolts soon appeared; their method of introduction was said to be simple, they apparently immobilized the fracture, and good results were reported. No procedure for internal fixation of fractures of the neck of the femur should be termed 'simple'; it may appear so to the originator, but the novice will always find it complex. As to their efficiency: The mechanical principle of the nail is sound, more sound than that of any of the substitutes.

"As to the good results reported: Bony union in fractures of the neck of the femur sometimes does not occur for a year or even more than a year. Roentgenographic evidence in this respect is unreliable. There is little or no external callus, and the amount of internal callus is difficult to estimate; more than once have we interpreted roentgenograms as showing bony union, withdrawn the nail, and obtained nonunion. In 2 cases this occurred over a year following operation.

"The serious objection to the nail has been raised that it slips out or becomes extruded into the soft parts in the subtrochanteric region.

Should the Open Reduction Be Abandoned?

"After publication of the first 24 cases, encouraged by our results, we continued using the open reduction in 26 more cases. The results were not quite so good as in the original series: In only 70 per cent was bony union obtained, although function was most satisfactory. In the total series of 50 cases, 12 were old, ununited fractures at the time of operation; duration of nonunion varied from 6 to 24 months. In 9 or 75 per cent, of these, bony union with excellent function was obtained by open reduction and nailing. The average age was 45 years, considerably younger than in the fresh fracture cases. Just one case is reported to illustrate this series: . . .

"In cases of nonunion, without absorption of the neck, the open reduction is necessary in order to remove scar tissue and to freshen fracture surfaces; the nailing procedure is justified by the results obtained in a relatively high percentage of cases. The operation is extremely difficult and lengthy; it should not be undertaken in the aged.

Present Technique of Inserting Nail

"The procedure used in our clinic at the present time is a combination of the technique as published by Westcott, by Thornton and Sandison, and by White. There is no emergency about the operative procedure; the patient can be made comfortable by suspension of the affected extremity with 5 to 10 pounds of traction. There is very commonly a mild temperature reaction to the injury and resulting hematoma; the temperature runs between 99 and 100 degrees. Thorough physical examination, ac-

companied by the usual clinical laboratory tests, should always precede the operation; on the basis of such an examination the anesthesia is decided—local, spinal, or general.

"The method of reduction is essentially that advocated by Leadbetter.

"A satisfactory reduction does not necessarily mean an anatomical reduction; a slight valgus position of the head is to be desired because it represents a stable relationship for transmission of weight bearing. (It should be remembered, however, that if the head does go into valgus, the nail should be started lower in the subtrochanteric region in order to strike the center of the head.) A varus position of the head is to be avoided; it represents an unstable position which does not stand up under weight bearing. Rotation of the head, either anteriorly or posteriorly, should not be accepted, since they both will result in limitation of hip motion.

"Having obtained a satisfactory reduction, an incision 4 to 6 inches long is made over the trochanter, extending downward parallel with the shaft of the femur. Exposure of the lateral aspect of the trochanter is necessary in order that the superior attachment of the vastus externus to the inferior border of the trochanter may be defined. The vastus externus is reflected subperiosteally, exposing the subtrochanteric region. The central axis of the neck corresponds to a point three-fourths of an inch to one inch below the ridge representing the superior attachment of this muscle. At this point the nail starter is driven in at an angle previously determined by means of a protractor from the roentgenogram taken after reduction. Westcott first described this method of directing the course of the nail from the subtrochanteric region.

"The nail starter is intended for the purpose of going through the cortex without dulling the edges of the nail; it is advisable to direct it in the correct course. As soon as the starter has penetrated the cortex, it is removed and the nail is inserted in its place; again the direction of the nail with the lateral aspect of the femur is usually between 40 and 50 degrees. The nail is now driven in; it is kept in the horizontal plane unless the lateral roentgenogram was made. As the nail enters the medulla, if it is correctly directed, it will enter the central axis of the neck with very little resistance. If it is found that there is resistance to the progress of the nail, roentgenograms should be taken, since resistance usually indicates that the course of the nail is incorrect and that it is striking either the superior or inferior cortex of the neck. Roentgenogram, then, will decide whether the aim is right; if there is any question about its being incorrect, the nail should be withdrawn and started in the corrected direction. It is at this point that White's instrument is particularly valuable; in the past we found it extremely difficult to extract the nail once it was started on its course. With White's instrument it is very easily extracted and started over again. This instrument also serves as an extension to the nail and facilitates aiming it in the right direction.

"With the hip in the abducted position the central axis of the neck of the femur intersects the femoral artery as it passes under Poupart's ligament. A lead marker placed at this point is helpful in directing the nail; I use both the protractor and the lead marker, checking one against the other.

"After the nail has been driven home, anteroposterior and lateral roentgenograms are taken. If these are satisfactory, the fracture is gently impacted. I still feel that impaction is important in apposing and interlocking the fragments, but it should not be overdone.

"Teamwork is essential in any method depending upon radiographic control of the course of the nail. Faulty x-ray technique means loss of time and loss of the surgeon's temper. This is particularly true in the method outlined, which requires the use of one portable x-ray unit only; this means shifting of the x-ray machine for the anteroposterior and lateral films, which increases the chance of error. Relatively few hospitals can boast of two portable units, however; such equipment increases technical accuracy and greatly facilitates the introduction of the nail.

"As already stated, many methods have been developed for closed reduction, followed by lateral nailing; the surgeon must select the one that appeals to him the most and visualize every step before he undertakes it. Our own experience with this method is limited to less than 20 cases, over a period of less than 2 years, so we cannot report end-results. The experience of other surgeons is much more extensive; their results are decidedly favorable.

Postoperative Treatment

"Postoperative treatment remains essentially the same as that described for open reduction. The extremity is suspended with 5 pounds of traction; exercises are started in a few days after operation, for the foot, knee, and hip. At the end of 4 weeks the patient is allowed up; crutches are used for a period of 4 to 6 months, with partial weight bearing at first. A bivalved spica is used for walking for the first 4 to 8 weeks in order to maintain abduction. If the relationship of the fragments remains satisfactory at the end of 6 months, full weight bearing may be allowed. In cases of old nonunion, crutches are used for a longer period, sometimes for as much as a year. The nail is never removed in less time than a year; it may be left in for years without doing harm.

"Five years have elapsed since the first report on internal fixation of fractures of the neck of the femur by means of the flanged nail was published. The principle of the nail has been widely accepted, not so the open reduction. In view of the good results reported from the use of the closed reduction, followed by nailing through a small incision, we have come to the conclusion that the open reduction is unnecessary in fresh fractures; in old ununited fractures open reduction is indicated and good results are obtained in selected cases."

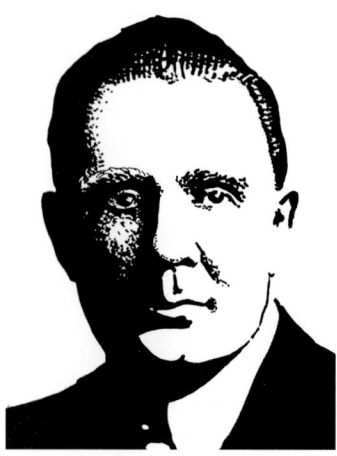

◆ Guy Whitman Leadbetter
(1893–1945)

Leadbetter was born in Bangor, Maine, and studied at Bowdoin College, where he established a record for throwing the hammer, before graduating from Johns Hopkins School of Medicine in 1920. While a student he decided to become an orthopaedic surgeon and after 3 years' training set up in private practice in Washington, D.C. He quickly established his reputation, one of his principal interests being fractures of the neck of the femur. Later he became Professor of Surgery at George Washington Medical School.

He was a man of stern appearance and serious mind, a man with a wide range of interests, efficient and modest. He was a pianist, a linguist, an amateur archaeologist, and he also gave lectures on the background of the Nation's Parks.

REDUCTION OF A FRACTURE OF THE NECK OF THE FEMUR

THE LEADBETTER MANEUVER, 1933

"Anatomical reposition of the fragments is the only position which insures good union and good function.

"The manipulation suggested here is simple, anatomically sound, non-shocking, and offers opportunity for 100% reduction. The patient is first anaesthetised, usually with ethylene gas, on the fracture table. The uninjured leg is harnessed to the foot stirrup. The injured leg is then flexed at the hip at ninety degrees, with the lower leg at ninety degrees to the thigh. Direct manual traction in the axis of the flexed thigh is then made, together with slight adduction of the femoral shaft. In this position the thigh is internally rotated approximately forty-five degrees. The leg is slowly circumducted into abduction, the internally rotated position being maintained. The amount of abduction varies with the individual and can be measured accurately, representing the difference in degrees of the angle made by the fractured neck with the shaft and the angle between the neck and the shaft on the normal side, as evidenced by the roentgenogram.

"The test which in our experience has indicated that the fracture has been completely reduced is as follows. After the leg has been brought down in the measured degree of abduction and internal rotation, the heel of the injured leg is allowed to rest on the outstretched palm. If the reduction, is complete, the leg will not evert itself. Should there be no interlocking of the fragments, however, the leg will slowly rotate externally. This has been found to be an invariable test."

Leadbetter read this paper in 1932 in the days before these fractures were usually nailed. After reduction, patients were encased in plaster from nipple to toe. It is interesting to notice his results. Of 31 intracapsular fractures, 4 patients died (one pulmonary embolus, one diabetic coma, one cellulitis of the neck, and one renal infection), 22 united, 7 went to nonunion, and 2 underwent absorption. Most people today would be pleased if 70% of their intracapsular fractures united.

A METHOD OF INTERNAL FIXATION OF TRANSCERVICAL FRACTURES OF THE FEMUR

H. HEYWOOD WESTCOTT, ROANOKE, VIRGINIA, 1934

Westcott used a protractor as a guide to assist blind percutaneous nailing.

"The internal fixation of transcervical fractures of the femur is possible through a small incision over the lateral aspect of the femur. With the Smith-Petersen nail as the fixing instrument, the total operating time is from 6 to 15 minutes. The operation

produces a minimum amount of shock and allows immediate active use of the joint, preventing the usual complications expected from the prolonged period of fixation and recumbency. After but a few hours the patient is ready for a wheelchair or, if so disposed, may at once enjoy the use of crutches."

CANNULATED NAIL
SVEN JOHANSSON, CHIEF SURGEON, GOTEBORG, SWEDEN, 1932

"The author has now worked out a method intended to make use of the advantages of Smith-Petersen osteosynthesis without exposing the fracture. The principle consists in using a thin metal wire as a guide for the Smith-Petersen nail, which is furnished with a longitudinal canal. Roentgen control in two directions is necessary."

End Results: 1930

In 1928 Fred Albee, incoming president of the American Orthopaedic Association was told to produce figures showing the end results of hip fractures.

In the 1929 report of 201 fractures largely treated with a Whitman cast, the mortality was 28.6%, and only 30.4% of fractures were united at 1 year. In a second report the next year, the combined death/nonunion rate dropped to 14.1% in patients treated by "open surgical attack," but the commission avoided favoring this method because only a small number of cases were treated by a few surgeons. Politics?

"I think that I have never attended a council meeting of the Medical Defence Union without hearing a case of fractured neck of femur discussed, the doctor usually accused of negligence either in diagnosis or treatment." E. W. Hey Groves, 1930

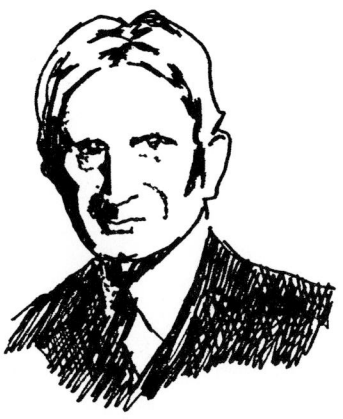

◆ **Royal Whitman (1857–1946)**
Chief at the Hospital for Special Surgery (formerly the Ruptured and Crippled). He was one of the crusaders against flatfeet and invented those abominable Whitman plates. He campaigned against talectomy and then did thousands for neurogenic foot deformities. He did fascial arthroplasty of the hip combined with distal displacement of the greater trochanter. Then he became known for the Whitman cast for hip fracture—a huge hip spica.

References

Chapter references are located in Chapter 26.

◆ Chapter Three

Child's Hip

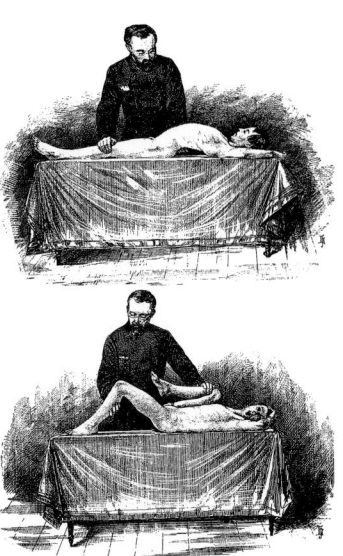

Thomas demonstrating his test for fixed flexion, 1876.

The child's hip has to last through life, and even a slight biomechanical imperfection is likely to cause osteoarthritis. Despite intense study for 150 years, developmental dysplasia of the hip (DDH), Perthes' disease, and slipped epiphysis still present big challenges.

Developmental Dislocation of the Hip

Congenital dislocation of the hip is very commonly overlooked until the child begins to stand and attempts to walk.   Bernard Brodhurst, 1896

The treatment of congenital dislocation of the hip-joint results in a complete cure if reduction is made early enough.   George Perkins, 1928

In the days of Hippocrates, DDH was ignored because the disease produced nothing more than a limp at a time when many people limped because of life-threatening conditions—such as tuberculosis. DDH did not threaten life and seldom caused pain. Until X-rays were discovered, doctors had little idea of what they were treating and little idea of what they achieved.

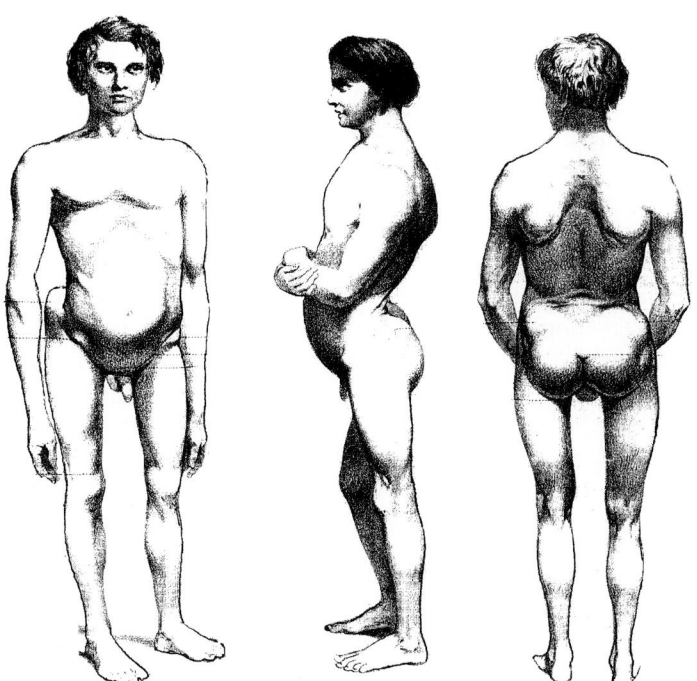

The appearance of bilateral developmental dysplasia of the hip (DDH). From Carnochan JM: A Treatise on the Etiology, Pathology and Treatment of Congenital Dislocation of the Head of the Femur. New York: Wood, 1850.

Ironically, it would have been just as easy for Hippocrates to use the Ortolani sign and apply a Pavlik harness as it is for us today. The modern-day treatment is very low tech and has been reached only by trying to treat DDH the hard way first. Simple treatment without complications has been called the thin chart method of treatment in contrast to elaborate, complication-ridden treatment—the thick chart method.

The first attempts were made on school-aged children. Long periods of traction, special carts, and then all kinds of operations were used. Commissions pontificated on what should be done. Acres of forest have been cut down for articles and books. Miles of cord have been used for traction, and I can remember whole wards full of toddlers strung up in very indecent positions so that the femoral head would dock with the acetabulum. Only later was the simplicity of neonatal treatment allowed to prevail.

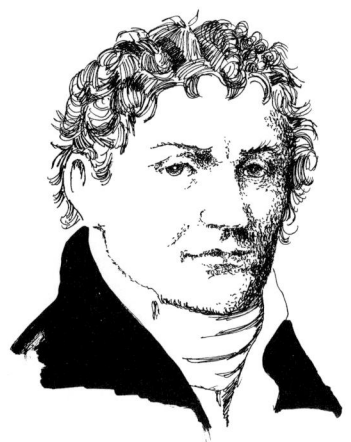

◆ **Giovanni Paletta (1748–1832)**
A surgeon anatomist of Milan who described the autopsy changes of DDH in a 15 day old patient and later advocated subtrochanteric osteotomy for deformity.

TIMELINE FOR DDH

Pathology

- 300 BC Hippocrates—a joint dislocated in utero
- 1564 Paré—"A shallow socket with stretched ligaments"
- 1783 Paletta describes pathology in a 15 day old child
- 1826 Dupuytren writes much about the changes seen
- 1839 Gerard Vrolik—illustration of pathology of DDH in book

Signs

- 1742 Andry describes the waddling gait and uses a girdle to treat
- 1864 Roser described a test for neonatal instability
- 1895 Trendelenburg sign of abductor insufficiency

Screening

Treatment in the newborn period is simpler and better than delayed treatment. This was appreciated and put into action by Roser in 1864 and by Le Damany in Rennes, France, in 1912. The idea did not catch on. In the 1950s, the Ortolani and Barlow tests were applied to all children in some regions. Although many children were found to have dislocatable hips at birth, some skeptics showed that the number of late cases was not greatly changed. Some children thought to be normal initially were later found to have dislocations. Ultrasound examination is an improvement upon clinical examination because ultrasound will pick up hips with shallow sockets that are at risk of late dislocation. These are hips that are passed as normal on clinical examination.

Diagnostic Ultrasound or Sonography

Ultrasound (US) was put to use for submarine detection during wartime, when it was known as sonar, and to detect flaws in industrial materials. Dr. Douglas Howry began to use US in medicine while he was an intern in Denver in 1947. Leftover naval equipment was used for his later experiments, which involved submerging the patient in a cattle trough of water.

At about the same time, Dr. John J. Wild in Minneapolis used US to distinguish benign from malignant breast lesions. Dr. Ian Donald met him in London and began to investigate US when he went to Glasgow as an obstetrician. With an engineer, Donald developed a hand-held contact scanner in the mid-fifties, which has transformed obstetrics.

Ultrasound is better than radiology for the diagnosis of the infant with DDH because it shows the cartilaginous head and acetabulum and because it is free of radiation. R. Graf of Austria has done much in recent years to classify dysplasia. Graf sat on a Swiss mountainside and wondered whether the hip could be viewed like the fetus—vastly improving diagnostic skills.

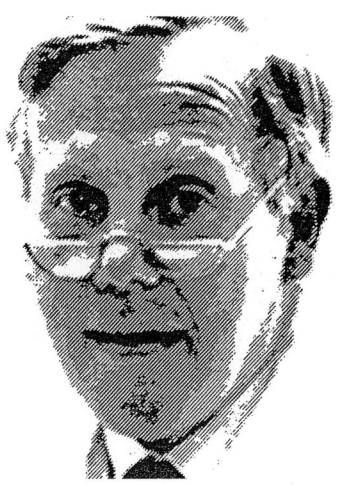

◆ Dr John J. Wild

Diagnosis
1900 Mar Schede of Bonn writes monograph on X-ray appearances
1902 Shenton—a pioneer London radiologist—publishes his line
1923 Le Damany—newborn tests
1925 Heinrich Hilgenreiner, orthopaedist of Prague—describes transverse line on X-ray
1928 George Perkins, orthopaedic surgeon of London—describes vertical line on X-ray
1937 Ortolani's sign of reduction
1962 Barlow's sign of dislocation

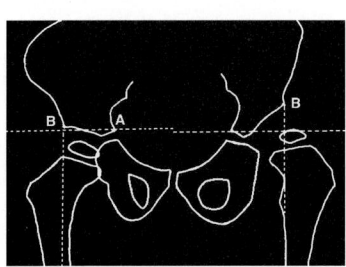

Perkins is remembered for Perkins' X-ray lines to help make the diagnosis of DDH. *"Congenital dislocation of the hip joint is not diagnosed early enough because the general practitioner does not know how to make the diagnosis."* Lancet 1928, 214, 648-50.

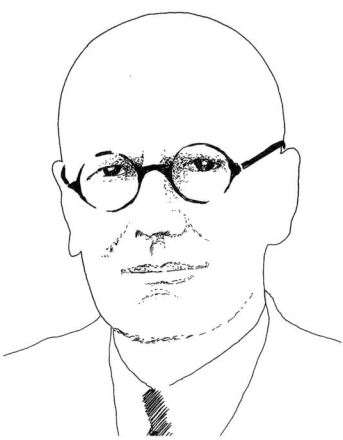

◆ **George Perkins (1892–1979)**
He studied at Oxford and came under the spell of Robert Jones at the Military Orthopaedic Hospital, Shepherd's Bush, where the World War I wounded were treated. He became Chief at St. Thomas' Hospital, London, and President of the British Orthopaedic Association. He wrote a thick textbook and promoted the treatment of fractures by early movement. I once had an anesthetist who, as a medical student, had been taught by Perkins. It was almost impossible to get him to give an anesthetic to reduce a fracture—"splint and move" was his advice to me.

◆ **Edward Warren Hine Shenton (1872–1955)**
He was a pioneer of radiology in Britain—with the title of Surgical Radiographer to Guy's Hospital. Described Shenton's line in *Guy's Hospital Gazette* in 1902 and wrote a book, *Disease in Bone and Its Detection by X-Rays*, in 1911. He was a skilled musician, composer of children's music, and violin maker.

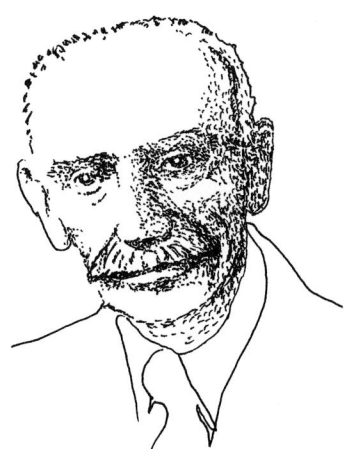

◆ **Heinrich Hilgenreiner (1870–1953)**
Surgeon at Prague, his main interest was in DDH: he described his X-ray lines in 1925 to aid early diagnosis and treatment. He was imprisoned during World War II and suffered from X-ray skin damage like many pioneers. A warning to us all to keep our fingers out of reach of the image intensifier.

SCREENING FOR HIP DISLOCATION

LE DAMANY
1923

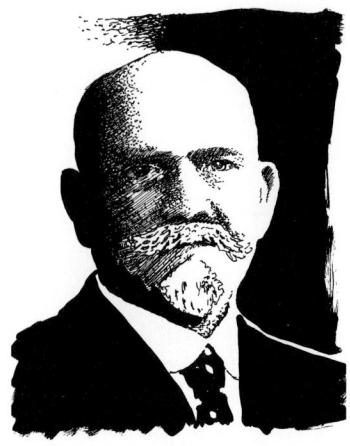

◆ **Pierre Le Damany (1870–1963)**
He screened neonates at the Rennes maternity hospital in 1908, using his thumb and index finger to displace and replace the femoral head—just as Ortolani suggested 20 years later. He distinguished between hips that stabilized quickly and easily and those that were resistant.

"*Any pressure on the knee levers the femur against the edge of the pelvis and tends to distract the femur from the acetabular fossa.*

"*We have observed, by animal experiments, chiefly in dogs and rabbits, that if one diminishes the pressure of the head on the acetabular fossa, one decreases its depth.*

"***Dislocatable Hips of Newborns.*** *How does one prove that congenital dislocation exists or is absent in the newborn? Instead of resuming the fallacious arguments advanced for or against each of these opinions, we have found it far more simple to examine sufficient numbers of live newborns. The results to which we were led were markedly different from those which we hear. We have certainly found complete subluxations of the hips in newborns who have died, and in whom we have observed at autopsy multiple malformations incompatible with life. But in normal, healthy infants we have never encountered this.*

"*Here is how one must proceed. The positioning and maneuvers which we describe are summarized in* [the following illustrations]. *The child is placed on his back, on a table. The examiner positions himself facing the child. Gently, with no force, he grasps each of the legs of the newborn with the opposite hand, in such a way that the cleft of the thumb cradles the child's knee. The pulp of the thumb holds the medial aspect of the thigh, the index*

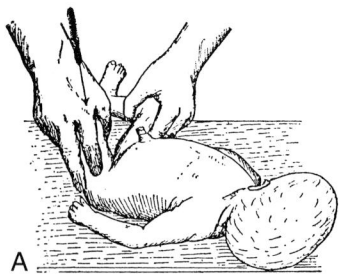

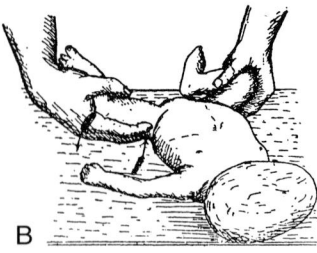

These two diagrams, (A) and (B), were published in a small book in 1923 and illustrate the methods Le Damany used for large-scale screening. They are identical to the Ortolani and Barlow tests described so much later.

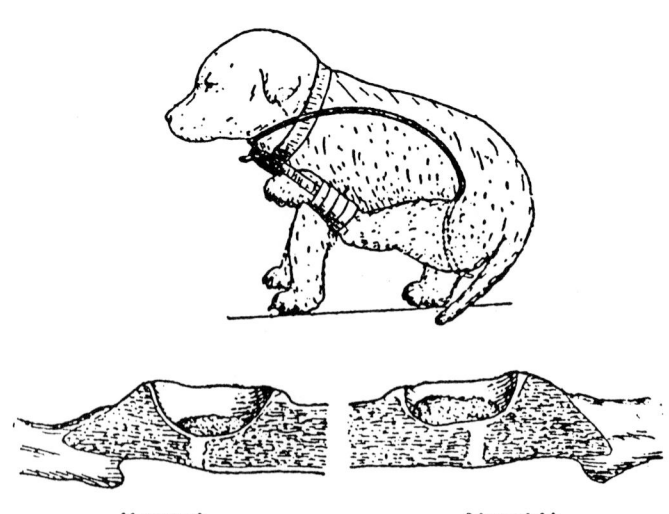

Le Damany found that he could produce acetabular dysplasia by splinting a puppy's knee out straight. This too was rediscovered later.

finger the anterior aspect, and the long finger is extended the length of the lateral aspect with the pulp pressing on the trochanteric region. The ring and small fingers flexed circle the calf. The thigh is held flexed at a right angle to the pelvis, the leg is also flexed to a right angle on the thigh. The examiner uses one lower extremity to stabilize the pelvis while he examines the other.

"***First Time.*** *The thigh, held as described, is moved into adduction while the pulp of the thumb pushes lightly from above to below the end of the thigh, while the cleft of the thumb pushes on the knee. If the hip is dislocatable, sometimes one feels a release caused by the subluxation of the femoral head, sometimes one feels nothing, no more than in normal subjects.*

"***Second Time.*** *The examiner performs on the thigh displacements the inverse of those above. The pulp of the long finger pushes the greater trochanter from behind forward (in relation to the child) and from without to within, while the thigh is taken briskly into abduction. By this maneuver, if it was subluxed, the head returns to the acetabular cavity over the posterior edge, and this return is always accompanied by a bump. Sometimes light, often very distinct, there are times when the bump may be loud enough that one hears it.*

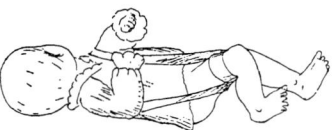

Le Damany's splints in flexion sound a modern note.

"*The double movement of adduction and flexion which subluxes the head, then abduction and flexion which returns it to the articular cavity, can be repeated as many times as one wants. Done gently, as it must be, it is not painful. It is in fact necessary that it must not be painful, because if the infant contracts or moves, the sensations lose their distinctness. The simple preparation of occupying the child by giving him something to drink during these maneuvers suffices to prevent crying and muscle contraction from discomfort.*

"***Future of Subluxable Hips.*** *Spontaneous curability is the most important characteristic of the dislocatable hip. Sometimes it is extremely fleeting and may disappear in a few days. We have encountered cases which have persisted for several weeks and ended by becoming altogether normal. Sometimes one does not find it in the first few days of life, it does not appear until near the end of the first week, becomes very distinct, then diminishes and disappears in one or two months more.*

"*The spontaneous cure of these dislocatable hips is demonstrated by clinical observation. We have followed for a sufficient time eight children who presented with this anomaly. In seven of them, the signs of dislocatability have completely disappeared. Once they lasted more than three months, but resolved nonetheless. Only one of the dislocatable hips we were able to follow ended by becoming a fixed dislocation. Then, instead of the disappearance of the bumps that we have described, we saw appearing little by little the well known signs of congenital dislocation.*

"*This defect was found in one infant in 149 at the Maternity Hospital of Paris, and in one infant in 26 at the same time at Maternity Hospital of Rennes; it is three or four times more common in girls.*" Translation: Dr. Andrew Howard

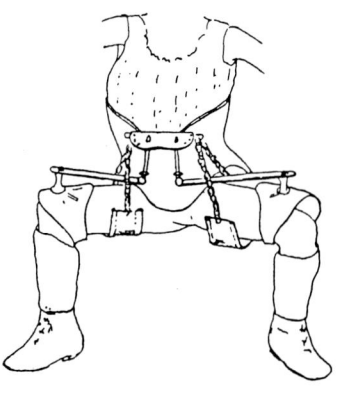

Le Damany's splint.

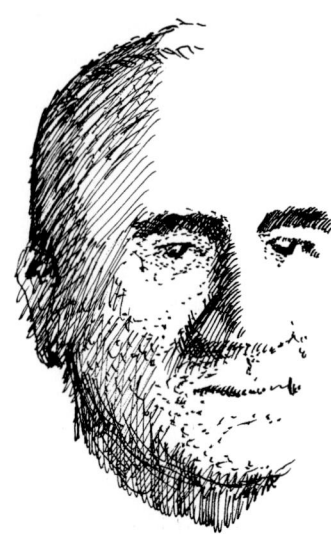

◆ Marino Ortolani

◆ **Marino Ortolani (1904–1987)**

Professor of Paediatrics and Child Health and Director of the Provincial Institute of Infant Welfare at Ferrara. The mother of a 5 month old baby complained to him that the baby's hip clicked when she washed the baby. She showed him how to produce the click. X-ray film showed a dislocated hip. He reported this in a local journal in 1936 and began testing all newborn hips and treating unstable hips with extra diapers. In 1946, the Italian Government made him director of an institute dedicated to DDH.

The same sign had been described years earlier by Le Damany. Why did early diagnosis take so long? Partly because Ortolani was writing in a little-read Italian journal of pediatrics and partly because he presented it as just another sign for examining suspicious hips between the ages of 3 months and 1 year. It was only later that the idea arose that testing hips should be routine in the examination of newborn infants. Then some cynics noticed that despite splinting large numbers of newborns, the same number of late cases was seen. The addition of ultrasound is the latest round in the battle against DDH.

ORTOLANI'S SIGN OF CONGENITAL DISLOCATION OF THE HIP
1937

"The sign of 'scatto,' or snapping, as described by the author, makes the diagnosis a certainty, even in babies. It is probably produced when the head enters or leaves the acetabular cavity, when it jumps over the rim of the acetabulum. This snapping has the same origin as the popping that is usually heard when the hip is reduced during the Paci-Lorenz manoeuvre in the older child under anaesthesia. The 'snapping' sign is much more accurate and early than the X-rays or even the arthrogram.

"This sign is elicited with the patient lying supine; the hips are flexed to a right angle and internally rotated slightly; the knees are flexed. Holding the knees in the palms of the hands, with the thumbs on the inner aspect of the knees, abduction and external rotation of the hips is carried out. At the same time the fingers press the greater trochanters medially. This manoeuvre, which is quite similar to the manoeuvre of reduction, is not painful and is easily performed when the muscles are relaxed.

"Once the 'snapping' has been produced, the head of the femur has returned to the acetabular cavity, and the limitation of abduction of the thigh is released.

"This sign is due to the fact that from the very first there is an anomalous relationship between the head of the femur and the acetabulum when the leg is flexed on the pelvis. When the thighs are abducted the head comes to jump over the labrum and this gives the sensation of snapping.

"The child must be relaxed, otherwise the snapping sign may be missed altogether. This sign may be present even during the child's first month of life."

BARLOW'S TEST
1962

"... The test consists in applying pressure backwards and outwards with the thumb on the inner side of the thigh. If the femoral head slips out over the posterior lip of the acetabulum and back again immediately the pressure is released, the hip is 'unstable'—that is to say the hip is not dislocated but is dislocatable."

◆ **T. G. Barlow**
British orthopaedic surgeon at the Hope Hospital, Salford.

TRENDELENBURG'S TEST
1895

"Both earlier and more recent authors say only that the cause of the swaying gait is caused by the abnormally mobile femoral head sliding up the ilium when the foot is put down—Dupuytren's 'glissement vertical.' A few mention the lordosis of the spine as a contributory cause, and all repeat the old comparison of the swinging gait to the waddle of a duck, which, to some extent, describes this type of gait, but does not explain it.

"This idea that the abnormal mobility of the head of the femur across the ilium is the cause of the waddling gait is so firmly rooted that the first attempts at surgical treatment did not aim at reduction of the dislocation, but only at fixing the head of the femur to the pelvis (König), and operations of this kind are, even now, performed at times.

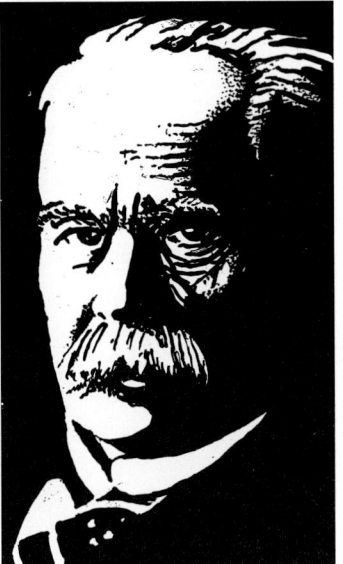

◆ **Friedrich Trendelenburg (1844–1924)**

Born in Berlin, Trendelenburg studied medicine in Glasgow and in Berlin, graduating in 1866. He worked as assistant to Langenbeck, later filling the Chairs of Surgery at Rostock, Berlin, and finally Leipzig.

A prolific writer and leader in practical surgery in many fields, he devised the heroic operation of pulmonary embolectomy, but met with no success. When Trendelenburg was aged 80, Kirschner, one of his pupils, demonstrated a successful case to him.

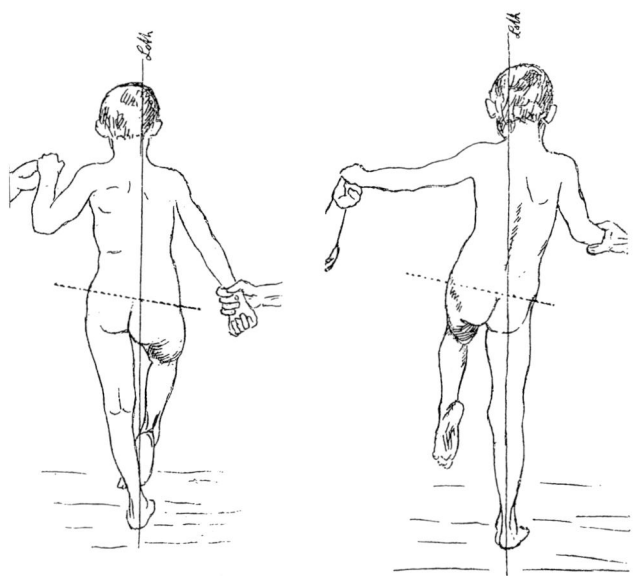

Trendelenburg's drawing—how the test should be done.

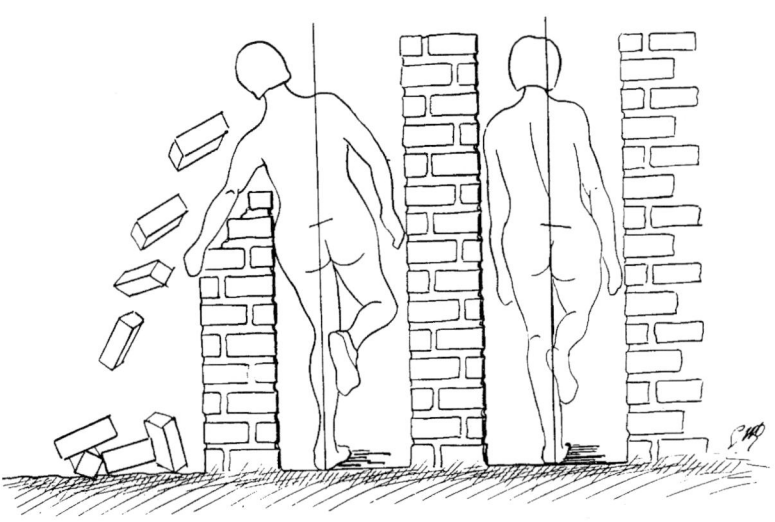

Comparison between the antalgic gait and the pure Trendelenburg gait. The figure on the left has coxalgia and goes beyond the frame and knocks down the wall. The figure on the right with DDH remains well-encased. From Calvé J, Galland M, de Cagny R: Pathogenesis of limp due to coxalgia. J Bone Jt Surg 1939, 21, 12-25. Used with permission.

"If the gait is carefully observed in naked patients it is soon realised that this view is not correct.

"A child or, better, an adolescent or adult girl with bilateral congenital dislocation of the hip is told to walk alternately away and towards us. What do we see? Let us look first at the upper part of the body. At every step it swings to and fro, and it does, in fact, fall at each step to the side on which the weight is carried. If the right foot is put down while the left is raised the upper part of the body leans to the right and vice versa. If we call the side of the body with the foot down the standing side and that with the leg swinging the swinging side, the body thus always swings to the standing side. This fact seems to fit the idea that the head of the femur, sliding up when the foot is put down, is the cause of the swaying.

"But now let us watch the pelvis. This also sways in such a way that the right and left sides alternately fall and rise. The pelvis swings on a horizontal axis running from front to back in the sagittal plane at about the level of the first sacral vertebra. But the swing is not in the same direction as the movements of the upper part of the body, but opposite to them. If the right foot is put down, it is not the right anterior superior spine in front and the right buttock at the back which sink, but the left. In other words the pelvis does not, like the upper part of the body, sink on the standing side, but sinks on the swinging side. Now if the swinging movement of the pelvis were caused by the pelvis sliding down past the insufficiently fixed head of the femur the pelvis would sink, like the upper part of the body, on the standing side, and not on the swinging side.

"It is precisely the opposing swings of the upper part of the body and the pelvis which is characteristic and peculiar in this gait, as the observer will now realise. He may also remember having seen this gait in only one affection other than bilateral dislocation of the hip, that is, progressive muscular atrophy.

"The opposing swings meet between the sacrum and the lumbar spine: this is the pivot of the movements.

"There is another way of demonstrating that the swinging movements are not due to the head of the femur sliding on the ilium. If the patient is told to walk past, or if one walks alongside her and carefully watches the relation of the trochanter to the edge of the pelvis, or feels it with the fingers, it is exceptional to find any distinct rise in the trochanter on putting down the foot.

"Now how are these peculiar swinging movements produced? The answer need only deal with the swinging of the pelvis, since it is obvious that the movements of the spine in the opposite direction are only compensatory, and that they perform the task of bringing the centre of gravity, which shifts sideways, back to a point vertically over the standing foot, or, in short, restoring balance.

"Let us observe first the gait of a normal person and ascertain in detail how it differs from that in dislocation of the hip. If we make a naked person stand with his back to us behind a plumb line, and make him walk a few steps away from us, we see that the whole body leans alternately a little to the right and

left, and always to the side of the foot on the ground. The pelvis does not swing, but moves evenly forward without swaying.

"These to and fro movements of the body can easily be fixed photographically by making the subject examined stand behind a plumb line and raise first one leg and then the other. (I owe Dr. Perthes, Assistant in the Clinic, my special thanks for his help and advice in the sometimes tedious photographic work preliminary to this study.) The first glance shows that the swing of the body occurs in order to bring the centre of gravity vertically above the point of support, i.e., the sole of the standing foot. The fact that the pelvis remains horizontal and does not drop on the side of the swinging leg is due to the action of the abductors of the hip joint, the gluteus medius, the gluteus minimus and partly the gluteus maximus. In the standing leg they are stiffly contracted, in the swinging leg they are relaxed. It is easy to ascertain in oneself that this is true by putting the hands on the region of the gluteus medius while walking. The alternating play of the muscles can then be felt distinctly.

"Let us compare this with a girl with bilateral dislocation; this girl had to support herself slightly with her hands in order to stand quite still. The difference leaps to the eye. The pelvis hangs down on the swinging side, and the upper part of the body leans far over to the standing side to restore balance.

"From what has been said, the cause of the pelvis hanging down can only be that the abductors of the standing leg cannot keep the pelvis horizontal.

"If, therefore, the cause of the swaying gait is the absence of active abduction, it is easy to understand the similarity of this gait with that in progressive muscular atrophy. The pelvis cannot be held up by the abductors of the hip joint on the standing side and falls towards the swinging side, and the upper part of the body swings in compensation to the other side.

"Very defective or entirely absent function of the gluteus medius and gluteus minimus, with the consequent lack of active abduction at the hip, is the cause of the waddling gait in congenital dislocation of the hip.

"After treatment, the two tests described above—standing on the treated leg and raising the buttock of the other side up to or above the horizontal line and raising the treated leg from the bed while lying on the opposite side—are a good measure of what has been gained by the operation, and the result can also be recorded photographically in this way."

CONGENITAL DISLOCATION OF THE HIP

DUPUYTREN
1826

Dupuytren gives an excellent account of congenital dislocation of the hip. He considered its etiology, drawing attention to its familial tendency, described its pathology very accurately, and gave several case histories.

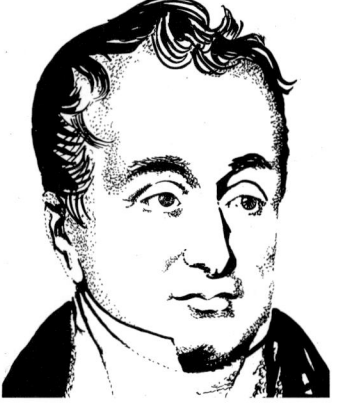

◆ **Baron Guillaume Dupuytren (1777–1835)**
The "Brigande of the Hôtel Dieu" was born in Central France. The son of a poor advocate, he was kidnapped as a boy by a rich lady from Toulouse on account of his good looks, and, after reclamation, was taken to Paris and educated by a rich cavalry officer. As a medical student he endured poverty, allegedly reading books by the light of oil prepared from dissecting cadavers. He became surgeon-in-chief at the Hôtel Dieu at the age of 36, and worked tremendously hard at teaching, operating, and seeing 10,000 private patients a year. He became very rich, and was probably a most unpleasant person to meet, but his writings are delightful to read for their lucid, accurate descriptions and deductive reasoning. Like many of those who are mentioned here, he combined accurate clinical observation with a tremendous interest in pathology. His works are easily readable, and very informative, and he is quoted in this collection more than any other author.

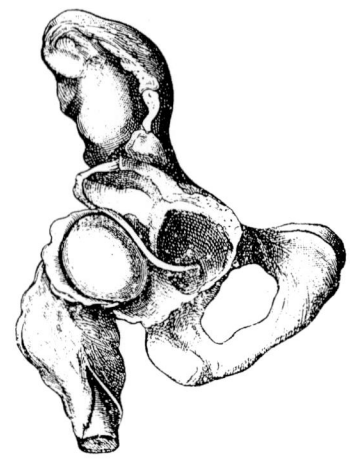

Lorenz dissection of a false acetabulum.

After considering several possible causes, such as violence, intrauterine disease, or faulty development of the ilium, he wrote:

"The position of the lower extremities of the foetus in utero is such, that the thighs are very much bent on the belly, from which it follows that the heads of the thigh-bones are continuously pressing against the lower and back part of the capsular ligament—a circumstance which, though without effect in well-formed individuals, might, I apprehend, have an injurious influence in such as are weak, or of lax, unresisting fibre. If this premise is conceded, there is not much difficulty in imagining that dislocation may result; and the supposition is further strengthened by the fact that the most powerful of the muscles surrounding the articulation have a constant tendency to draw upwards the heads of the thigh-bones, as soon as they escape from the acetabula.

"I must remark that original or congenital dislocation of the thighbones is not so rare as may be supposed. I have met with as many as twenty cases in the course of eighteen years. Almost all the individuals who are affected with this deformity are females: indeed, out of twenty-six cases which I have examined, not more than two or three at most were males.

*"**Original Dislocation of the Ossa Femoris.** Retention of urine, terminating fatally. A man, 74 years of age, suffering from retention of urine, was admitted into the Hôtel-Dieu in February 1828.*

"On the admission of this patient, it was anticipated that he would not long survive, and as there were several features which suggested the probability of there being congenital dislocation of the thigh-bones, I felt considerable interest in the examination of the body, which the patient's death shortly afterwards afforded me an opportunity of prosecuting.

*"**Autopsy.** In the first place it was observed that the thighs could not be separated as in abduction, without making them describe a segment of a large circle: the trochanters were much nearer to the crests of the ilia and higher than natural; the heads of the bones were very much elevated, the knees inverted and the thighs shortened; in fact, there was a total change in the relations, direction and length of the limb. This was the consequence of the cavity destined by nature to receive the head of the bone being almost effaced, and of the latter being deformed. The upper part of each thigh was enlarged, the trunk curved backwards, and the belly protruded; the pelvis had almost lost the oblique bearing which is natural to it; the thighs were shortened, and the buttocks soft and flabby, which was explained by the approximated attachments of the great gluteal muscles, and the consequently relaxed conditions of their intermediate bellies. The gluteus medium was, on the contrary, distended and raised up, the gluteus minimus entirely wasted, and the pyramidalis, instead of being oblique in its direction as is normally the case, was quite horizontal: the gemelli and quadratus were distended, and the adductors were abridged of their natural length.*

"On the left side, the original cavity did not measure more

than an inch at its greatest diameter; it was very shallow, rugged, and filled with a fatty substance of a yellowish colour, and almost of the fluidity of oil; its form was nearly an oval. The external iliac fossa presented, in front of the sciatic notch, a broad, shallow depression, lined by a thick glistening periosteum, which had almost the appearance of articular cartilage; it was on this that the head of the femur rested. The last-mentioned process itself was diminished in volume, a little flattened, irregular, and without any vestige to mark the attachment of the round ligament; it was, nevertheless, invested by articular cartilage which was thinner than natural. The fibrous capsule of the joint, which was in form exactly like a purse, was attached to the upper and lower borders of the original acetabulum, and was in place of an osseous cavity on the side it covered; its length was sufficient to allow the ascent of the head of the femur to the depression I have just described: the space over which it extended amounted to about three inches. This capsule was very thick, and almost as dense as the cartilage.

"On the right side, the original cavity was a little larger, but its interior presented the same appearance as the other. The external iliac fossa, instead of exhibiting, as on the opposite side, a simple depression, presented, in front of the great sciatic notch, and nearly on a level with the space between the two anterior iliac spines, a broad and deep depression, with an osseous margin which was strongly marked, rough, and irregular. The head of the femur, which was larger than that of the other side, had likewise more nearly preserved its natural shape; but it was, as the left, invested by an imperfect articular cartilage, and both surfaces of the articulation were covered by synovial membrane. The orbicular ligament was not so thick as that of the opposite side, although its extent was not strictly limited to that of the circumference of the abnormal cavity. On this (the right) side, the head of the femur was supported by the osseous margin, whereas, on the left, the fibrous capsule was the only structure which, by its great strength and resistance, was effectively opposed to the weight of the body.

"In addition to the above peculiarities there was very unusual mobility at the lumbosacral articulation, so that when the lower extremities and pelvis were fixed, the vertebral column could be moved freely upon the latter. The lax state of the intervertebral fibrocartilage was the only recognisable cause of this singular mobility."

Treatment

Ironically we try to treat DDH nonoperatively by methods that Hippocrates could have safely used. But because of late diagnosis for centuries, our ancestors made an unnecessary detour through traction, forceful manipulation, and all kinds of operations before getting back to safe simplicity.

From the time of Hippocrates until the invention of anesthesia in 1846—2000 years—there was no progress beyond describing the clinical features of DDH. DDH was one of many conditions

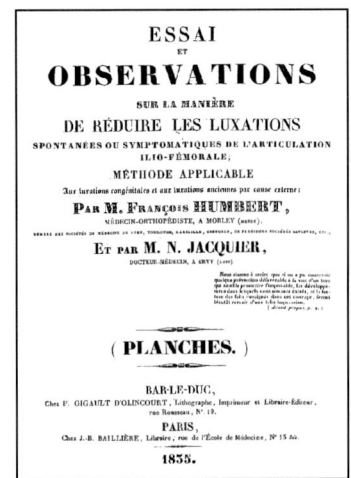

Humbert was one of the first (in 1835) to reduce DDH.

which would cause a limp, but it did not stop a person working and did not shorten life—so there was no drive to treat it—some thought that only a fool would try.

Initially, congenital hip dislocation was not recognized until a child started to limp, and by this time simple methods of treatment were ineffective. Then, as traction methods improved, some success was claimed from prolonged traction treatment. A Commission was struck in Paris in 1840 to look at patients who were said to have been cured. There was not much enthusiasm for the results, and traction was largely given up because the femoral head rarely stayed in the shallow acetabulum.

Brodhurst wrote in 1896, "*It seems to me useless to undertake lengthy treatment—merely to substitute one form of lameness for another.*" With the advent of aseptic surgery all kinds of operations were tried—on the femur and on the pelvis. The age of diagnosis went down. Radiographs contributed to earlier diagnosis and a more critical appraisal of the results. Gradually the interest changed from treating old cases to screening and neonatal splinting.

◆ **Bedrich Frejka (1890–1972)**
He modified Ortolani's splint and became known for a pillow splint, which he reported in 1941.

Splints
1923 Le Damany
1929 Putti abduction pillow
1941 Frejka abduction pillow
1956 Von Rosen aluminum splint
1958 Pavlik harness is successful in 84% of 1912 children treated. It held the hip flexed and allowed movement.

◆ **Sophus Von Rosen (b 1898)**
Swedish—introduced an aluminum splint. He was a strong proponent of screening (1957) and early treatment to rid a country of the need for open reduction of the hip.

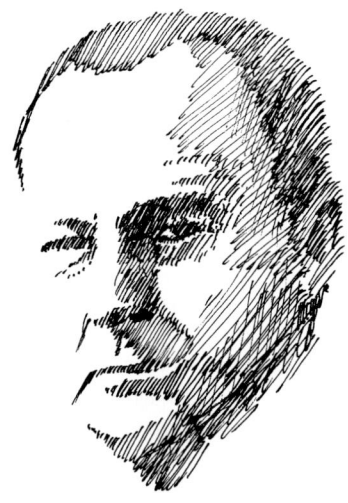

◆ **Arnold Pavlik (1902–1962 or 1965)**
Czechoslovakian orthopedic surgeon, who developed a harness for DDH. The idea was that controlled movement was better than fixed immobilization. He had started as an assistant to Frejka. In 1958 he reported the results of treating 1912 children. Years passed before the harness became standard in the rest of the world.

◆ **Guillaume Jalade-Laford (1805–?)**
He founded an orthopaedic institute in 1823 and used an extension chair and an oscillatory bed to reduce DDH. He developed a garden with equipment for scoliosis exercises in 1827. Jalade-Laford's son-in-law, Vincent Duval, wrote on clubfoot. Flaubert used this book to write about the tragedy of gangrene following a clubfoot operation in the novel *Madame Bovary*.

Reduction by Traction
1710 Verduc: "*Traction applied to a person lame from birth exposes the ignorance of the doctor.*"
1805 Guillaume Jalad-Laford tries to reduce with rocking bed.
1828 Caillard-Biloniere, Amsterdam: treatment of 8 year old by an extension bed in a single case succeeds.
1835 François Humbert (1776–1850) tries to reduce with acute pull.

Chapter 3 ◆ Child's Hip   77

◆ **François Humbert (1776–1850)**
He founded perhaps the first orthopaedic institute in France at Morlaix, Meuse, in 1817. This was mostly concerned with scoliosis, but in 1835 he co-authored a book on manipulative reduction of DDH in an 11 year old girl. There was no way of proving that the hip was reduced before radiography, and his skeptical colleagues damned it with faint praise—"a bold initiative."

The apparatus used by Humbert in 1835 was not simple.

1838 Pravaz reduces with prolonged traction, and reports are presented to Academy of Science in 1838–1839. A Commission of Enquiry is struck which reports success but with persisting problems in 1840. This is really the first time that DDH is reduced. Previous attempts had failed, and doctors knew not to try.
The idea spreads to Heine in Würzburg, to Brodhurst in the United Kingdom, but then traction alone was given up and all kinds of other methods tried because of the introduction of aseptic surgery.

Box continued on following page

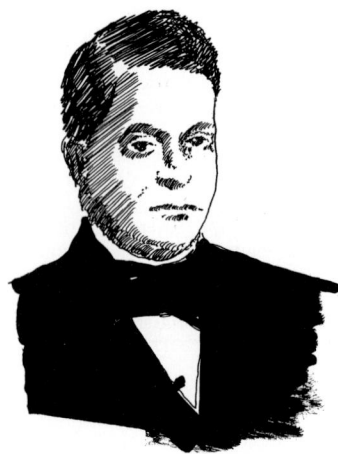

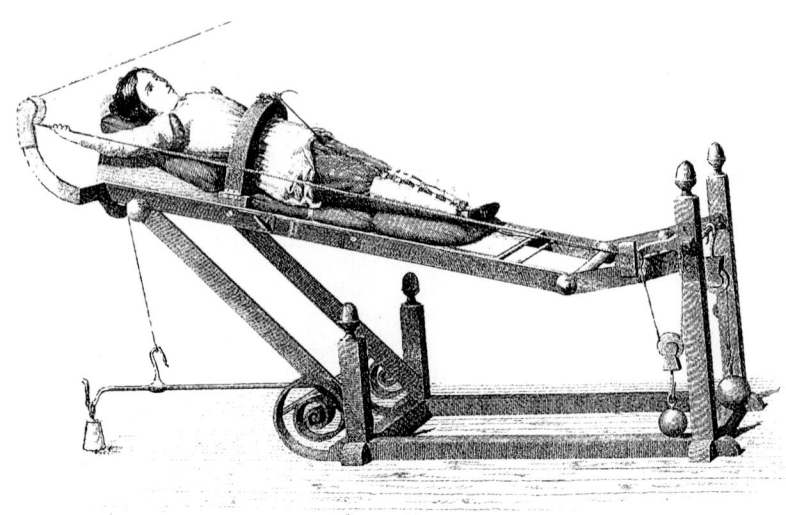

Pravaz used this traction system in 1838 and claimed success. There were skeptics. Today we would not expect a closed reduction to be achieved in an older child.

◆ **Charles Gabriel Pravaz (1791–1853)**
Pravaz is a little-known orthopaedic great. The son of a doctor, he started an orthopaedic institute in 1826 at Passy, just outside Paris. He was joined by Guérin, and they developed many largely useless methods of treating scoliosis that are visually attractive. (The balancing machine is shown on page 158. He left the quarrelsome Guérin to go to Lyons in 1836 and developed traction methods for DDH, which was really the beginning of efforts to reduce the head successfully. He invented the hypodermic syringe and the electrocautery.

1841 Guérin does research on DDH. Book published in Paris. Guérin adds tenotomy and later scarifies the lip of the acetabulum to make the head adhere to the acetabulum. Buckminster Brown studies with him and takes the idea to the United States.

1850 Carnochan's book is published in the United States. It is a review of knowledge but adds nothing new.

1858 Bouvier writes book on disorders of the locomotor system.

1866 Brodhurst in the United Kingdom uses muscle release, and open reduction for older children because traction is ineffective.

1885 W. Adams does it too. Albert Hoffa believed that surgery was best done younger. His operation is described in Bradford and Lovett.

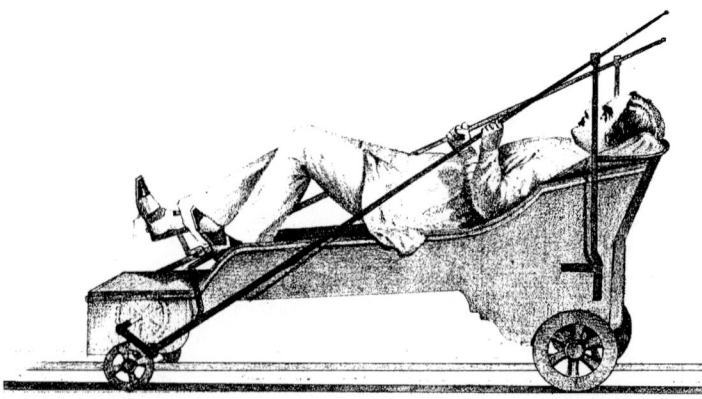

The Pravaz Chariot was used to mobilize the hip after reduction of DDH. Both the arms and feet of the patient crank the wheels. From Carnochan JM: A Treatise on the Etiology, Pathology, and Treatment of Congenital Dislocation of the Head of the Femur. New York: Wood, 1850.

◆ **John Murray Carnochan (1817–1887)**
He was born in Georgia and studied in Edinburgh and Paris. A Professor of Surgery, New York College, he wrote the first American book on DDH in 1850.

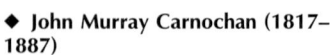

Chapter 3 ◆ Child's Hip

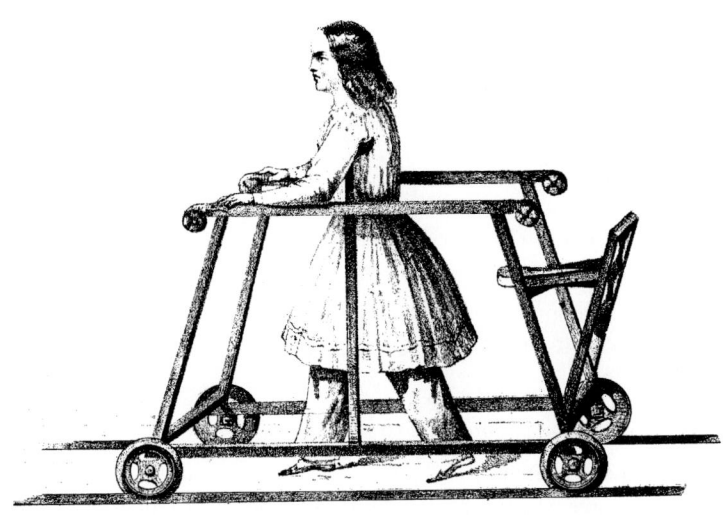

The walking frame of 1850 is little different from that used today. From Carnochan JM: A Treatise on the Etiology, Pathology, and Treatment of Congenital Dislocation of the Head of the Femur. New York: Wood, 1850.

1885 Buckminster Brown visits Guérin and reports a successfully treated case.

Manipulative Reduction

1888 Augustino Paci of Pisa described closed reduction.

1902–1903 Adolf Lorenz does a tour of the United States to demonstrate closed reduction of congenital dysplasia of the hip. He writes an autobiography, displaying a Santa Claus–like countenance.

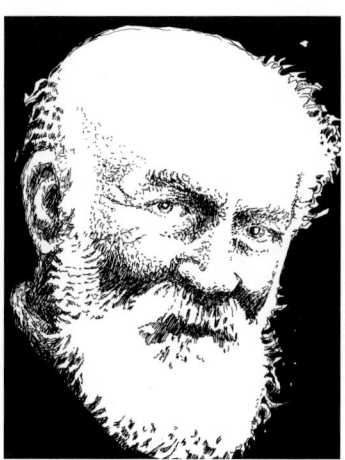

◆ Adolph Lorenz (1854–1946)

He trained as a general surgeon in Austria and then became sensitive to the carbolic acid used as an antiseptic rinse. He could no longer operate and took up nonoperative orthopaedics. He changed from being an advocate of open reduction of DDH to closed, or bloodless, reduction. This name was closer to the truth than he may have intended. The forced abduction caused avascular necrosis. He went on tours around the States, attracting large audiences. He wrote books on DDH in 1895, 1905, and 1920, a book on scoliosis in 1884, and an autobiography. His son, Konrad Lorenz, is best known for his study of animal behavior, "On Aggression."

◆ Bernard Edward Brodhurst (1822–1900)

St. George's Hospital, London. In 1866 he wrote about DDH and loose bodies in the knee.

◆ Albert Hoffa (1859–1907)

He was born in South Africa and worked in Würzburg and Berlin. He popularized surgery for DDH.

◆ Agostino Paci (1845–1902)

Pisa. A leading surgeon of his day. Advocate of closed reduction of DDH. Disputes with Lorenz about who did it first.

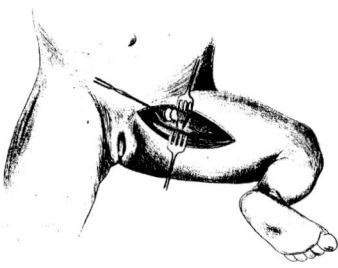

Ludloff's medial approach to the hip. From Am J Orthop Surg 1912, 10, 438.

◆ **K. Ludloff**

Professor at Breslau. He reported the medial approach to the hip in 1908.

◆ **Paul Colonna (1892–1966)**

American orthopaedic surgeon who deepened the acetabulum and carried out a capsular arthroplasty.

TIMING OF TREATMENT

1902 Lorenz—late treatment better than early
1923 Early treatment better than late—Le Damany and followers:
1925 Hilgenreiner
1929 Vittorio Putti
1935 Ortolani
1962 T. G. Barlow

Open Reduction

1890 Poggi reports open reduction and deepening of acetabulum in 12 year old girl.
1896 Hoffa
1908 Ludloff medial approach
1923 Goldthwait Commission to look at results

Acetabular Surgery

The saucer-shaped acetabulum could be made cup-shaped by removing the cartilage. Stiffness was the price paid for stability and length.
1884 Margary in Italy deepens the acetabulum.
1928 Krida
1936 Paul Colonna reamed the acetabulum and sutured the redundant capsule over the head to form a fibrocartilaginous neoacetabulum.

Shelf Operations

Shelf operations are an intuitive approach to the shallow acetabulum. They are easy to do without much risk of making things worse. However, the shelf tends to disappear again. Much ingenuity went into their design in the hope of producing something that would last. Interest died when it was found that acetabular cover is better increased by moving the whole acetabulum than by trying to add to it. Ingenuity then focused on different ways of moving the acetabulum. Here is a list of some surgeons who designed a shelf:

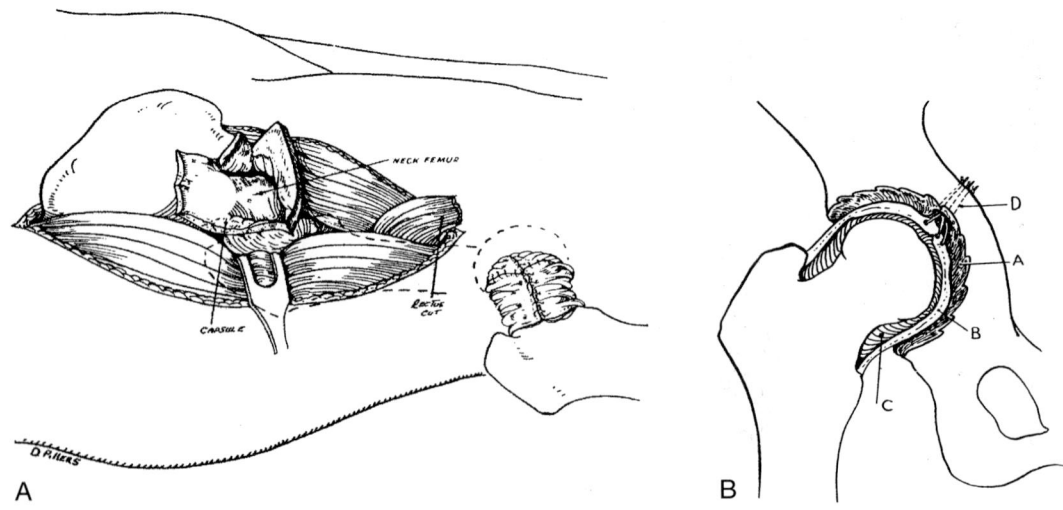

(A) and (B) Capsular arthroplasty of the hip. This was popularized later by Colonna but never worked well. From Hey Groves: Br J Surg 1926, 14, 486.

1871 König
1877 Hueter
1915 Fred Albee
1925 Lance
1927 Hey Groves
1928 Bruce Gill
1930 Soutter
1931 Ghormley
1935 Dickson
1936 Smith-Petersen
1941 Ryerson—acetabulum is redirected.
1955 Karl Chiari—a transiliac osteotomy extends bone above the capsule so that the head is covered by fibrocartilage rather than articular cartilage.

Pelvic Osteotomies

Redirecting the acetabulum has proved to be the safest way of increasing coverage.

1961 Salter—the whole acetabulum is rotated over the femoral head.
1965 Pemberton—the roof of the acetabulum alone is pushed down.

Contemporary names: Steele—triple osteotomy, 1973; Sutherland—double osteotomy, 1977; Eppright—dial osteotomy, 1981; Tonnis, Dega, Wagner, Ganz

Femoral Osteotomy

Osteotomy was originally used to correct deformity and later used to aid reduction

Abduction Osteotomies for Irreducible Hips

1835 Bouvier
1847 Pravaz
1919 Lorenz
1922 Schanz

Femoral Shortening

1926 Hey Groves advocates femoral shortening to assist reduction.
1976 Klisic popularizes the same thing.

◆ **Franz König (1832–1910)**

Surgeon at Göttingen. He described forcible correction of clubfoot, a shelf operation, and hemophilic arthropathy.

◆ **Dietrich Tonnis**

Orthopaedic surgeon at Dortmund, Germany. Organizer of the German multicenter trial and author of a comprehensive book on DDH.

◆ **Alfred Shanz (1870–1932)**

Dresden. Wrote an orthopaedic textbook in 1905. Invented abduction osteotomy for irreducible dislocation of the hip. Pauwels was a student of his.

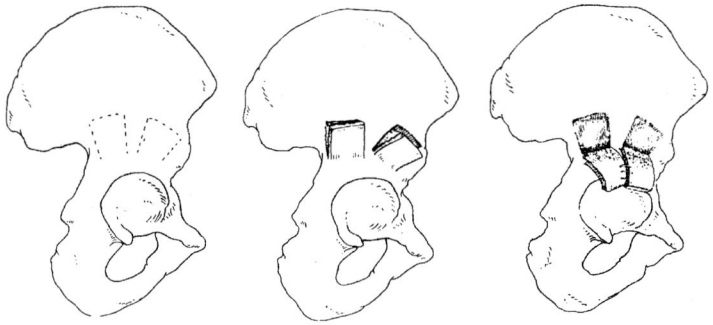

Hey Groves was one of many to build up the acetabulum. Br J Surg 1926, 14, 486.

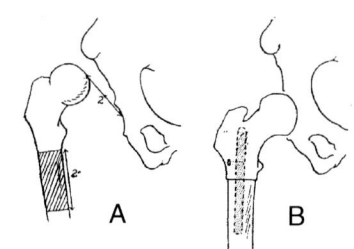

The Hey Groves shortening osteotomy of 1926 facilitated reduction of DDH. He removed 2 inches. From Br J Surg 1926, 14, 486.

> **RESULTS**
>
> 1847 After Pravaz published a book on the treatment of DDH, the Academy of Medicine appointed Nélaton to check the results, and he confirmed Pravaz' results.
> 1923 American Commission organized by Goldthwait
> 1941 Severin classification of the results of treatment of hip dislocation

OPEN REDUCTION OF CONGENITAL DISLOCATION OF THE HIP
ALFONSO POGGI
1890

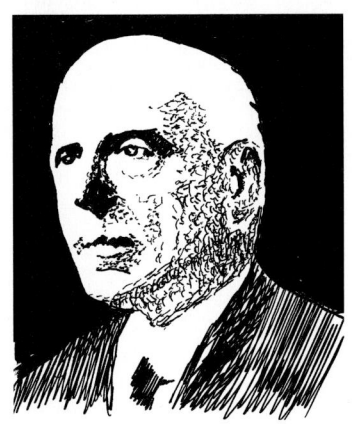

◆ Alfonso Poggi

"Olga La Forni, aged 12, was a student in Bologna. When she first began to walk, a defective gait was noticed by her parents. However, nothing was done. During the following years the defective gait became more severe until it became an obvious limp. Recently she could no longer stand or walk because of pain in her left hip. Therefore she was admitted to the Clinic on August 11, 1888.

"The nature and extent of the dislocation offered little hope for significant improvement by conservative orthopedic measures. Having tried in vain the method of closed reduction recommended by Professor Paci on January 29, 1888, I prepared to operate in the surgical amphitheater in the presence of the students instead of the late lamented Professor Loreta. I had decided in my own mind to hold myself to the most rational method, to replace the femoral head in its natural position, deepening or reconstructing the acetabulum, even adjusting the femoral head if it were altered in shape. The operation was performed under chloroform anesthesia and with meticulous attention to asepsis and antisepsis.

"I preferred to open the articulation with the semi-circular incision of Anthony White rather than the currently more popular incision of Langenbeck, because it seemed to me that in this specific case the transverse division of the muscular fibers would lead more easily to the femoral head. Having cut the fibrous capsule, which was rather thick, the bare head appeared within the large capsular sac covered with synovia, but without any signs of a new acetabulum, with the inner capsule interposed between the articular head and the outer surface of the ilium, though not too adherent to it. A little effort in forced adduction and internal rotation of the limb caused the head to come out. The head was small and deformed, did not have the shape of a spherical segment, but that of an irregular oval with the surface in contact with the slightly altered ilium. The rest of it was covered with cartilage and at its apex was topped by a small protuberance, the remains of the insertion of the round ligament, which was absent. The head was attached to a slender and short neck at a greatly obtuse angle to the greater trochanter. The capsular sac already referred to disclosed a foramen in the antero-inferior part through which I passed my index finger with some difficulty, and reached the acetabulum. I enlarged

the pathway of communication with longitudinal incisions and discovered the boundaries of the acetabulum although they were of small circumference. The cavity was filled and I noted a small swelling of cartilaginous consistency which may have been a remnant of the insertion of the round ligament.

"Because of these observations it seemed possible to me to reconstruct the articulation to its normal form. I deepened the acetabulum, reshaped the deformed head giving it its proper contour, and by means of well directed traction and incisions in the capsular ligaments, I was able with only little difficulty to replace the head into the newly deepened acetabulum. I then detached the capsular edge from the iliac bone, removing the exuberant parts, and with three layers of sutures in the capsule, the muscles and the skin, with drainage tubes inserted, I closed the large incision.

"With the reduction of the dislocation the disappearance of the marked deformity was noted in the supine position and therefore the disappearance of the protrusion of the greater trochanter, the lumbosacral curve, and the feeling of emptiness on palpation of the inguinal region. The shortening of the limb was notably less, being only 2 cms, this the result of atrophy of the limb as was noted in the physical examination; and to the shortening of the neck and femoral head, both incompletely developed. Finally one might add that proof of a good reduction was the fact that the limb could be raised without difficulty.

"The dressing was applied and the patient returned to her bed in the supine position with one pillow under the buttocks to keep the pelvis elevated and with traction (extension and counter extension on the operated limb by means of Volkmann's apparatus).

"The postoperative course was uneventful. After 50 days, the patient began to be about with crutches, the use of which was advised for a time to spare the articulation while walking. The joint was mobilized by massage and manipulation. The wound had healed and the patient enjoyed a good result for the duration of her stay in the hospital.

"Now nothing of importance remains except to add that the correction was maintained and that the present condition of Olga was satisfactory 13 months after the operation. In truth none of the deformities returned, the shortening has remained 2 cms; but the joint has regained its principal movements, not at all painful. Because of this the patient can sit comfortably and can walk at length without discomfort. There remains only an insignificant degree of limp which would be corrected with a proper shoe."

OSTEOTOMY, VIENNA
KARL CHIARI
1950

"The basic concept underlying the procedure consists in constructing a congruent shelf above the intact hip joint without bone grafting and its inherent risks, and in optimally correcting

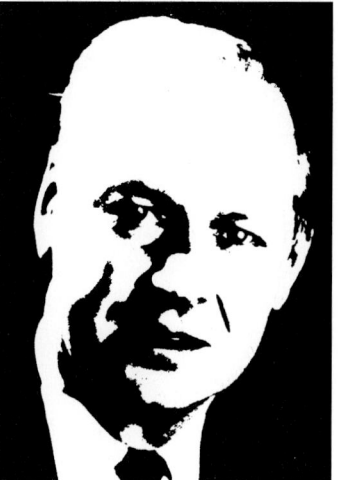

◆ **Karl Chiari**
Professor of Orthopaedics in Vienna.

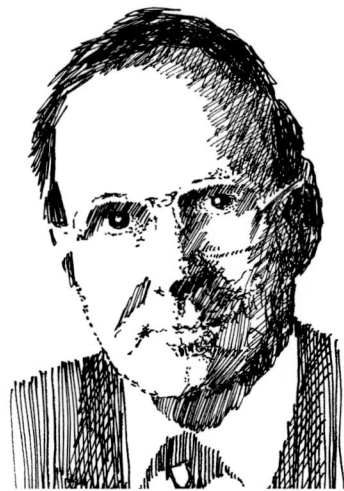

◆ Robert Bruce Salter

Orthopaedic surgeon-scientist in Toronto. The results of treatment of DDH by the methods of the fifties were seldom good, and this stimulated him to develop better methods. Well-focused benchwork in the laboratory has been the jumping-off point for his clinical innovations: innominate osteotomy, a classification of growth plate injuries, and continuous passive motion. He spends much time teaching, and there can be few orthopaedic surgeons in the world who have not met him in person.

the pathologic position of the femoral head. Lateralisation of the head is corrected by pushing it medially."

INNOMINATE OSTEOTOMY
ROBERT B. SALTER
1961

"There is much more than a defect in the roof of the acetabulum. Indeed, the entire acetabulum, rather than facing downwards, is directed antero-laterally more than is normal, so that the femoral head is inadequately covered when the hip is extended and laterally when the hip is adducted. This observation explains why the reduced hip is stable in a position of abduction and flexion and why it redislocates or resubluxates. . . . The basic abnormality responsible for instability of the reduced congenital dislocation is the abnormal direction in which the acetabulum faces. If the entire acetabulum could be made to face in a normal direction the reduced hip would be stable in the position of function. Consequently, an operation has been designed to redirect the acetabulum as one piece."

Perthes' Disease

Infarction of the Femoral Head

A century ago, when a child began to limp and had hip pain, this used to mean only one thing—tuberculosis. With the advent of X-rays, a small number of children who did well were found to show a different radiologic appearance. Some time passed before the concept of avascular necrosis (AVN) was introduced. And we are still stuck with empirical treatment because the basic cause is still a mystery

Perthes' disease produces such a characteristic deformity of the head of the femur that it seems unusual that it was not discovered in bone specimens. Bone is very durable, and all kinds of collections of pathologic material provided learning material before X-rays. The only picture of Perthes' disease I found was in Benjamin Bell's collection, though he didn't know what it was.

First pictures were in Alban Kohler's *Atlas* of 1905, and Fragenheim had provided a pathologic description in 1909. Today we call it Perthes' disease or even Legg-Calvé-Perthes-Waldenström disease because he/they popularized it. This is the tradition. Diseases are named for the original describer only by mistake. Too much confusion and revisionism would arise if diseases had to be named for the original describer.

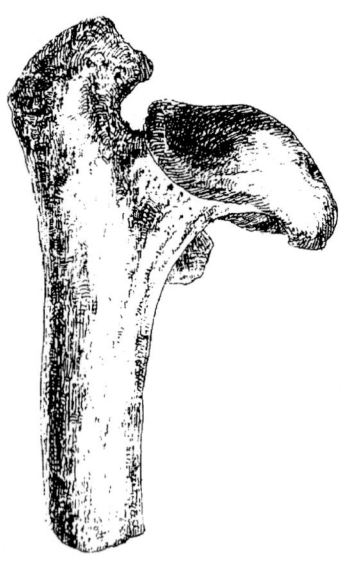

The earliest picture of Perthes disease that I have been able to find. Benjamin Bell calls it "interstitial absorption." A treatise on disease of bone, Edinburgh, 1828.

AN OBSCURE AFFECTION OF THE HIP JOINT

ARTHUR T. LEGG, 1910

"We are at times painfully aware of the fact that there are many symptoms which we readily recognise in our clinical observations to which we can assign no cause, and it is also an undoubted fact that there are many conditions which exist today of which we are ignorant.

"The cases which I bring to your attention today seem to me illustrative of the fact that we, in the past, have not observed certain conditions which truly exist, and that now, having observed, we naturally must ask ourselves, are our observations faulty or are they correct? and, assuming them to be correct, what is the cause of the condition?

"The first case, a well-developed girl of eight, was brought to the Children's Hospital in October, 1907, with a history of a fall nine months before, immediately followed by a limp on the right which had persisted. There had been no pain or constitutional symptoms.

"Examination showed normal flexion of the right hip with other motions much limited. There was very slight spasm, slight atrophy of the thigh and calf, but no shortening. There was a slight amount of thickening anterior to the neck. The motions of the left hip were normal.

"A traction hip splint was applied, which she has worn since. She has had no acute symptoms, nor pain, and has remained in excellent general condition. The very slight spasm present at the first examination disappeared in about a month.

"Examination of the right hip at the present time shows motion in flexion to 100 degrees, abduction to 50 degrees, adduction normal. Internal and external rotation is possible to about 45 degrees. The thickening about the joint has remained the same, and the right leg now measures one quarter of an inch longer than the left.

"There has been no pain or limp on the left, and the motions of this hip are normal. A slight amount of thickening, however, is felt about this hip.

"The Von Pirquet test was negative. Roentgenological examination shows the head of the right femur to be flattened and apparently spread out. The neck appears thickened and shorter than normal. An area of increased radiability appears in the upper part of the head and neck. The left or apparently normal side shows the same condition with the exception of the area of increased radiability."

[He describes four further cases.]

"In reviewing the cases, the following facts in a general way are observed: (1) Age, five to eight years. (2) History of injury. (3) Limp. (4) Thickening about the neck of the femur. (5) Absence of pain. (6) Absence of constitutional symptoms. (7) Little or no spasm. (8) Absence of shortening.

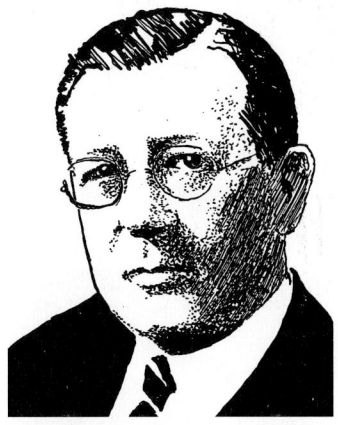

◆ **Arthur T. Legg (1874–1939)**
Legg studied at Harvard, trained in Harvard, worked at Harvard, and died in the Harvard Club of a heart attack. You could say he was a Harvard man. He pioneered the first adult orthopaedic clinic with Goldthwait.

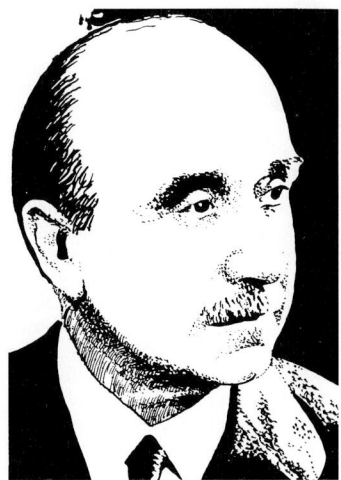

◆ **Jacques Calvé (1875–1954)**
After studying in Paris he went to Berck-Plage on the coast. There were 1100 beds serving Paris for the cases of bone and joint tuberculosis. An X-ray machine was purchased about the time of his arrival, and he found 10 children out of 500 with hip disease who had something different—he called it "coxa plana." He also described vertebra plana. He married an American.

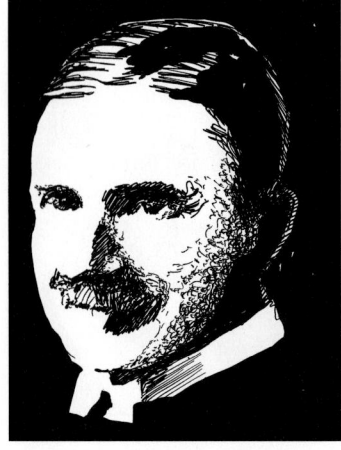

◆ Georg Clemens Perthes (1896–1927)

◆ Georg Clemens Perthes (1896–1927)

Perthes was born the son of a teacher in the Rhineland. His mother died of tuberculosis. A relative introduced him to Trendelenburg, who suggested he take up medicine. He became Trendelenburg's assistant and took the photos for the article on the Trendelenburg sign. He went to China with the German army and wrote a study of Chinese bound feet. He was a pioneer of radiotherapy; he wrote on jaw injuries and nerve repair. His assistant Schwarz had taken an X-ray of Perthes' disease in 1898, soon after the first machine was working, but nothing was published until 1910.

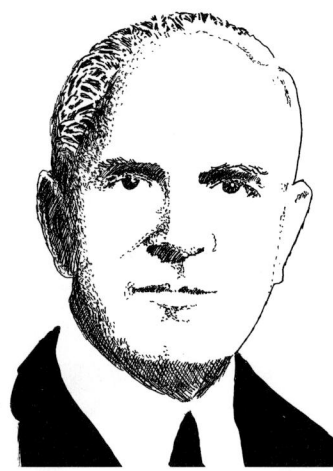

◆ Dallas B. Phemister (1882–1951)

Phemister graduated from Chicago and left only to study in Vienna for a time. He was a general surgeon with a special interest in bones and joints. He coined the magic phrase "creeping substitution" to describe bone healing in Perthes' disease in 1921. It may have been more helpful if he had seen it as a pathologic fracture complicated by delayed union. He was an advocate of bone grafting—the Phemister graft—and an originator of epiphyseodesis.

◆ James Gordon Petrie (1905–1982)

From New Brunswick in Canada, Petrie separated orthopaedics from general surgery in Montreal. He was an early advocate for stabilizing fractures of the spine. He is remembered for abduction casts and the principle of containment for Perthes' disease.

"It is worthy of note that all these cases sought advice solely on account of the limp. It is also of interest that in two of the cases (the first and the fourth) the condition of flattening of the head of the femur exists on both sides; and it is of the greatest interest that in both cases there was entire absence of symptoms in one of the hips.

"Direct injury, if severe enough, might cause a flattening of the head of the femur, and in children of this age the head is certainly impressionable. Should this be the cause in these cases, the thickening and shortening of the neck without evidence of fracture remains unexplained. We all know that the history of injury, especially in children, should be given much latitude, but in this group of cases, with a history of distinct injury in all of them, it seems to me that it must be considered, and at this time it seems to me that a possible explanation of the condition is that the injury may directly cause this condition by causing injury or displacement at the epiphyseal line, whereby the nutrition of the head, coming mostly through the neck, is impaired, and by the poorly nourished epiphysis bearing on the acetabulum, it becomes flattened. From such an injury a hyperemia of the neck of the femur would occur, and by this to stimulate bone growth the thickening of the neck may be explained.

"Of the occurrence of a similar condition appearing in the apparently normal hip, I shall not, at this time, attempt to offer any explanation. Contrecoup and sympathetic inflammation may be considered, but these are, to my mind, very remote possibilities."

Three authors published in 1910: Legg in February, Calvé in July, and Perthes in October. They were magnanimous to each other in subsequent papers. Perthes pointed out that Legg had lectured on the subject a year before, and Legg wrote that it was largely due to Perthes that the disease was widely recognized.

Slip of the Capital Femoral Epiphysis

In the days before X-ray, slip was just another cause of limp. And rather a benign cause. Today we make a great fuss about early diagnosis, because delay increases the risk of a catastrophic slip, avascular necrosis, and other complications. Earlier in the 20th century, the main interest in slips was the invention of osteotomies for the late case. Most slips today are internally fixed in an outpatient setting without complications.

ACUTE SLIPPED EPIPHYSIS
AMBROISE PARÉ, 1564

Ambroise Paré is often said to have described a slipped epiphysis, but the following description was the closest thing I could find. It seems to refer to growth plate injuries in general, but it would do for an acute slipped epiphysis.

Paré describes several types of dislocations, including the changes due to people having been tortured and put on the rack and those who have suffered the strappado on their arm. And then he goes on to say:

"There is also a fourth one added to these, as when the epiphyses and heads of the bones are plucked from the bone whereon they were placed or fastened: which unproperly called kind of luxation, hath place chiefly in the bones of young people, and it is known by the impotencie of the part, and by the noise and grating together of the crackling bones when they are handled."

JEAN-LOUIS PETIT, 1723

"Décollement—separation of the head from the neck—in the sense that one says a criminal has been beheaded; or else one may understand this word, the separation of the epiphysis from the neck, looking upon the cartilage that is found between them as a cement that joins both parts."

ON THE DEFLECTION OF THE FEMORAL NECK IN CHILDHOOD: A NEW SYNDROME
ERNST MULLER, 1888

"In this paper I describe an affection of the upper end of the femur of which I have found no notice in the literature. In past years in the Surgical Clinic at Tübingen I have seen and carefully examined increasing numbers of cases, including one autopsy, and besides in individual cases found so closely conforming characteristic features that it seemed proper to describe a special pathologic process.

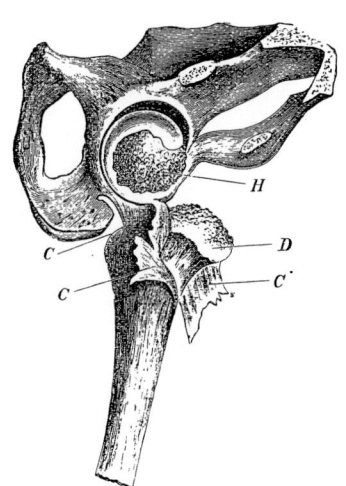

The pathology of a traumatic separation of the proximal femoral epiphysis. *H*, head of the femur; *D*, end of diaphysis; *C*, detached periosteum and capsule. From Poland, 1898.

"The course of the affection is as follows: In young individuals from 14 to 18 years there occurs without special cause or the result of any preceding painful trauma of the hip a limp, a weariness and a gradual shortening of the affected limb.

"The symptoms develop quite gradually and attain no special intensity that might confine the individual to extended bed rest. The patients are in other respects, except for fortuitous affections, healthy, specifically without evidence of other joint or bone disease.

"On objective investigation there is found an absolute shortening of the diseased limb in a manner that shows equal measurements from the trochanter to the external malleolus with the trochanter moved 2 to 3 cm. higher. There is no swelling; instead, with further progress, atrophy sets in. The limb lies outwardly rotated to a limited degree with some contraction at the hip; movement at the hip, especially flexion, is but little diminished; rotation and abduction is somewhat more restricted. The mobility at any rate is so good that one must assume that the head will be found in its socket (observing that the whole appearance of the limb was not that found in a dislocation) and that no serious changes would be found in the joint itself such as a wandering acetabulum due to destruction from caries. In one case an examination was made under anesthesia, and thereby one was convinced that the flexion and the extension which had previously appeared to be somewhat restricted had disappeared and that these movements were completely free and without crepitus, so that the femoral head must be in a healthy joint. Abduction and rotation remained somewhat limited even under anesthesia.

"The shortening of the limb depends on the fact that the diaphysis is shifted on the epiphysis so that the angle between the shaft and the neck of the femur is lessened. That no separation of the epiphyseal line exists is demonstrated by the rotatory restriction of the arc of motion of the greater trochanter. Based on the evidence in the living subject, one must conclude that the symptom complex must lie in the femoral head. A more exact insight into the changes is gained by a specimen of femoral neck and head prepared from a case of resection of the hip joint (S. W. Hauber). The changes in this specimen are quite remarkable on the sawed cross section of the head and the neck. The femoral neck gives the impression of being molded by pressure from above downward. In accordance with this is the circumstance of the neck's being strongly extended in the longitudinal direction. The cartilaginous joint surface is entirely healthy. The epiphyseal line is clearly seen as a narrow band. The epiphysis a distinctly crescent shape, and lies like a cap over the diaphysis; if one draws a line from both end points of the epiphysis in a frontal plane, the greatest distance of this from the epiphyseal line is 1.2 cm. The diaphysis simulates an impacted fracture driven into the epiphysis.

"With this changed direction of the femoral neck, the femoral head by its constant relationship to the extremity must accommodate itself to an extreme position of abduction, or rather in a *position of abduction that it could not attain in a normal relationship; one can only think that a larger part of the upper extent of the femoral neck was being drawn into the socket.*

"Therefore, it is easily understood that abduction was restricted even under narcosis.

"If we ask about the process which has taken place in the bone and has led to its deformity, we have a group of bone affections to choose from which could lead to the bending of the femoral neck. The diseases that come to mind are rickets, osteomalacia, osteitis deformans and deformity of the neck following inflammatory softening from an adjacent osseous focus.

"That it is rickets which gives rise to the described typical softening and bending of the femoral neck allows no direct proof, but it appears to me that it represents the most plausible explanation with no known facts in contradiction."

CHONDROLYSIS

HENNING WALDENSTRÖM, 1930

"I have treated three cases of necrosis in the joint cartilage after epiphysiolysis. All of these cases got repositioned under anaesthetics and were plastered in abduction and inward rotations. For two months they remained in plaster bandages, whereupon they walked about for one month on crutches. These three patients acquired a satisfactory mobility in their hip joint, though it did not become normal. After some months the joints began to grow more and more stiff and finally all mobility ceased. During the anaesthetic the fixation loosened very easily with a creaking sound, as if the surfaces of the joints had been cemented together. Immediately after this the joint showed a fine mobility, but the next day it already began to get stiff again. After a time it was evident that nothing could be done.

"If one studies the X-ray films, only five months after the reposition one discovers, in case three, a thinning of the joint cartilage. In the other two cases it was not visible quite so soon.

"I have seen no necrosis of the cartilage among the patients that have not been repositioned. For this reason I have not repositioned during the last few years, but have put the patient to bed with permanent extension. Rotatory bandages are applied. The patient has to remain like this for two months. During the last few years I have used this method in 24 cases and have not seen any cartilage necrosis."

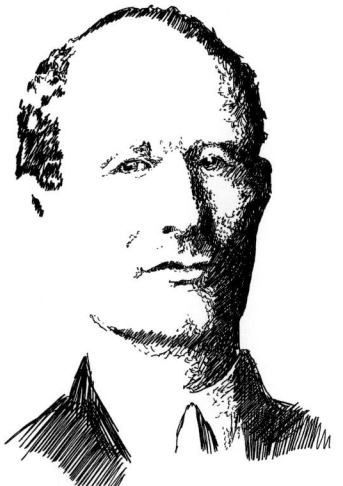

◆ **Johan Henning Waldenström (1877–1972)**
Waldenström was a surgeon in Stockholm, Sweden. He thought that Perthes' disease was a form of tuberculosis when he first described it in 1909.

Sickle Cell Disease

Sickle cell disease had been known for years. In 1949, Linus Pauling and others demonstrated the abnormal hemoglobin. This was one of the early studies of the bone problems.

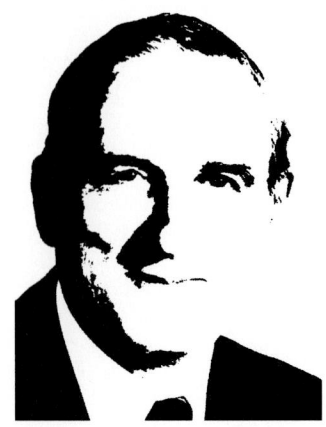

◆ **Sir John Golding**
After working with Phillip Wiles, Golding started orthopaedics in Jamaica at the new medical school. With the support of the community he built up rehabilitation, schools, and surgical care, using a mixture of enthusiasm, charm, and brains.

JOHN GOLDING, 1959

"The bone changes can be conveniently divided into four groups:

(1) Bone changes due to marrow hyperplasia.

(2) Bone changes due to thrombosis and infarction may cause severe and crippling disability. The femoral head is most often affected.

(3) Growth effects—a chronic anaemia will cause retardation of growth.

(4) The crises and secondary osteomyelitis. If a bone is affected the part becomes hot and swollen. This quite often occurs in the metacarpals, metatarsals and phalanges of small children. If a joint is affected it becomes acutely tender and a large effusion develops: the fluid is deep yellow and glairy, and it contains a few red cells, some of which are sickle shaped. Organisms of the salmonella group have often been found in these cases."

Paralytic Hip Dislocation

As more children with DDH are treated in the newborn period, PDH (paralytic dislocation of the hip) has become the commonest cause of hip dislocation in older children.

It was first described in 1866:

A. VERNEUIL, 1866

"A certain number of displacements of the femur are due to more or less complete paralysis of the muscles that surround the hip, in other words the pelvi-trochanteric and especially the buttock muscles; we will call it paralytic dislocation of the hip."

◆ **William Mustard**
Mustard was a general, orthopaedic, and cardiovascular surgeon at the Hospital for Sick Children, Toronto.

He was a man with a great sense of fun in public—he wore his tuxedo inside out at his retirement party and was reputed to scoop fish out of an aquarium and swallow them live. Behind this was the man who repaired arteries with glass tubes in the war, invented an operation for blue babies, and, while caring for polio epidemics, invented his psoas transfer. The chief surgeon of the day finally told him that he would have to decide what kind of specialist he wanted to be and stick at that. He chose cardiovascular surgery, saying that it would take no more than 6 months to teach anyone the necessary carpentry to be an orthopaedic surgeon.

PAUL RECLUS, 1878

"Two conditions are necessary for dislocation—atrophy of one group of muscles while their antagonists retain their integrity. If all the muscles are paralysed, very great laxity and an increased range of movement will be produced but no dislocation.

"At the hip an iliac dislocation is the most frequent. It is due to the pull of the adductors which is not counterbalanced by the atrophied extensors and abductors."

SPONTANEOUS DISLOCATION OF THE HIP

REGINALD WATSON JONES, 1926

He studied 157 cases of polio affecting the hip. There are 9 with severe adduction flexion contractures and *"Of these 9 cases there were 6 with paralytic dislocation of the hip, and these were the only dislocated hips in the whole series of 157 cases.*

"It would appear clear that unopposed activity of the flexors and adductors of the hip is the cause of paralytic dislocation."

He includes in spontaneous dislocation those children with cerebral diplegia and septic arthritis.

"I believe that spontaneous dislocation is rarely inevitable, and that in the great majority of cases it is an entirely preventable condition. The cause of spontaneous dislocation is a derangement of the normal muscle balance with the production of a flexion-adduction deformity; it is clear that the prevention of dislocation resolves itself into the prevention or early correction of that deformity, with re-establishment of muscle balance.

"Unfortunately, however, that Utopian state in which there is no treatment apart from prophylaxis is yet unrealised, and, whatever the future may hold, the demand for corrective measures still exists."

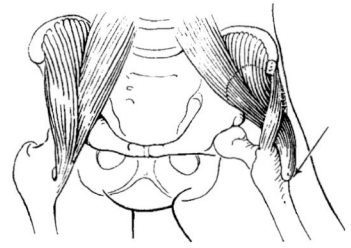

Mustard's psoas transfer for paralysis of the gluteus medius. From Mustard WT: Iliopsoas transfer for weakness of the hip abductors. J Bone Jt Surg 1959, 41B, 289. Used with permission.

Rebalancing muscle forces is an essential part of treatment. Various muscles were used, such as the tensor and sacrospinalis, but these did not work. Mustard and later Sharrard used the psoas, which had the power needed.

Iliopsoas transfer was reported by William Mustard in 1951 to replace the hip abductors. The muscle had the necessary bulk to equal the hip abductors, the iliac muscle fired electromyographically when taking weight on the leg, and the distance of the lesser trochanter from the crest was the same as the distance to the greater trochanter.

W. J. W. Sharrard moved the muscle posteriorly to replace both the abductors and the extensor in 1958, and this operation enjoyed some popularity for spina bifida children.

◆ **John Sharrard**

Orthopaedic surgeon in Sheffield, England.

After he identified the sites of the anterior horn cells in the spinal cord for each muscle with a view to understanding the pattern of paralysis in polio, the disease began to disappear due to immunization. He transferred his enviable enthusiasm to spina bifida and made Sheffield a mecca for patients with this disease. Many children had progressive hip dislocation. He modified Mustard's transfer to take a more posterior course so that it would substitute for both abductors and extensors.

He is a musician and a linguist and has done much both to create pediatric orthopaedics as a subspecialty in Europe and to bring kindred spirits together.

Snapping Hip

This was described by Maurice Perrin (1826–1889) in France in 1866 and redescribed by Louis Ferraton in 1905.

References

Chapter references are located in Chapter 26.

◆ Chapter Four

The Foot

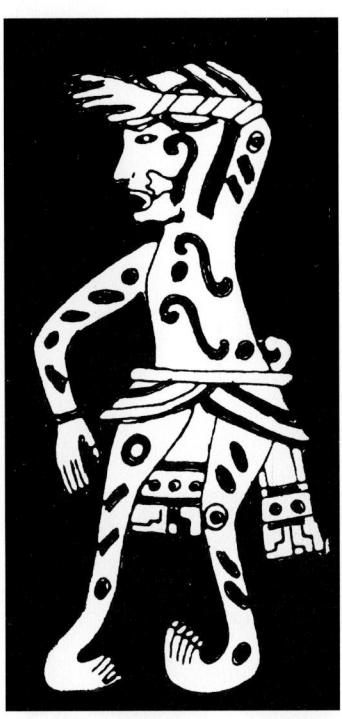

The foot does not have the glamor of the hip, spine, or knee. It is not 'scoped, instrumented, or replaced. There are few orthopaedists who puzzle more than a minute or two over the diagnosis. Patients self-diagnose and think of podiatrists when they have trouble with their feet.

Toward the end of the 19th century, the disease of *flat foot* was invented, and insoles and special shoes became a commercial success. In addition, there were many people with abnormal feet due to polio, rickets, uncorrected clubfeet, and malunited fractures. People walked more. Shoe stores were few. There were shoemakers who carved a last—a wooden copy of the foot—and made the shoes on this.

The foot is a complex machine, and better understanding of it has not resulted in major advances yet. Oddly enough, it was attempts to make a better lower limb prosthesis that ignited studies of foot mechanics by Verne Inman in California in the 1950s.

As the population ages, more and more people cannot reach their feet to take care of the calluses, nails, and ischemic lesions. Chiropodists provide these services.

Pre-conquest Mexican depiction of a clubfoot.

History of Podiatry

Doctors used to have little to offer for foot diseases and disguised their uselessness by pretending that the subject was beneath them.

Today chiropodists in the United Kingdom and podiatrists in the United States provide a lot of services. The word *chiropody* goes back to 1785 when David Low published a book called *Chiropologica*. Several books followed, and gradually chiropodists have gained professional status. In the United States, there was a New York Pedic Society in 1895, which became the National Asssociation of Chiropodists. They were confused with chiropractors and started to call themselves podiatrists in 1918. Only in 1958 did this become official. Today members of the American Podiatric Medical Association carry out about three fourths of the bunion operations in the United States and provide large numbers of orthotics.

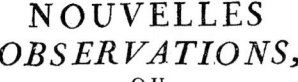

The first book of podiatry, 1762, *The Treatment of Corns.*

THE ART OF PRESERVING THE FEET BY AN EXPERIENCED CHIROPODIST
ANONYMOUS, 1818

"It has been too much the fashion, ever since the commencement of the modern school of medicine and surgery, to consider certain ailments of the human body as beneath the dignity of science; in consequence of which the neglected extremities of the system have been either consigned to the case of ignorant quackery or to the absurd and often dangerous remedies of vulgar prejudice and tradition."

The writer suggested the name podology and the need for examinations to qualify a person.

Clubfoot

Clubfoot is not a proud story in orthopaedics. The cause of clubfoot remains unknown. The treatment remains the same in principle as it was hundreds of years ago, and it is unsatisfactory because the finest result always shows some giveaway signs. Clubfoot still has an impact on the course of a whole life.

Famous Patients

Somerset Maugham, better known as a novelist than a physician, was born with a foot deformity and made the hero of his story in *Of Human Bondage* a person with a clubfoot.

Chinese ladies with bound feet. For a thousand years Chinese girls had their feet bound to make them look sexy. Today as I listen to the crying in our clubfoot clinic and think of all the troubles a tight cast will inflict, I am amazed that such a habit was widespread. Children did die of binding. The idea was to prevent the foot from growing—like a bonsai tree—and approximate the metatarsals to the calcaneus and telescope the toes. These women walked with difficulty, contributing to the chauvinist myth of female helplessness. The practice was banned in the 20th century.

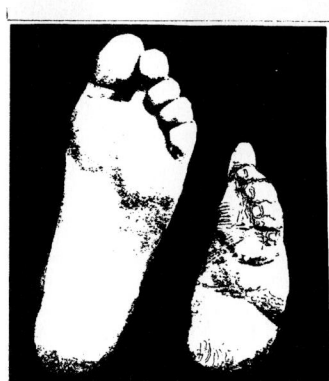

Chinese women's bound feet in the last century. When Perthes was working in China, he took this photograph of the foot and the shoe it had to fit.

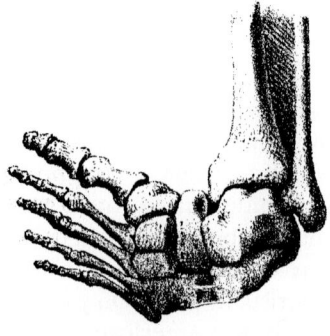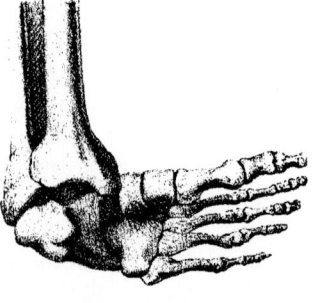

Clubfoot. The medial deviation of the head of the talus is clear, as is the joint between the medial malleolus and the navicular. From Lionel Beale, 1833.

Lord Byron was a poet, protagonist of Greek nationalism, and scandalous figure of the 19th century. He was born with a clubfoot, which was cared for by one of a family of bracemakers. This was a time when gentlemen wore knee breeches and hose. Byron concealed his thin calf and twisted foot with a padded shoe insert that has been preserved. An engraving of his foot deformity was made after his death and published. He wrote a play entitled "The Deformed Transformed"; the climax was a fairy going around touching deformities and making them go away. He was said to have the form and features of an Apollo with the feet and legs of a satyr. Denis Browne photographed his prosthesis.

Madame Bovary. In this French novel, the author, Gustave Flaubert, tells the story of an operation for clubfoot. Flaubert's father, a surgeon in Rouen, died with gangrene of his leg, and Flaubert describes an operation for Hippolyte, an adult with a clubfoot, that ended with gangrene and amputation.

In the novel, Monsieur Bovary, a village doctor, persuades Hippolyte that an operation would improve his walk and help his chances with the women. He reads a book and makes a splint.

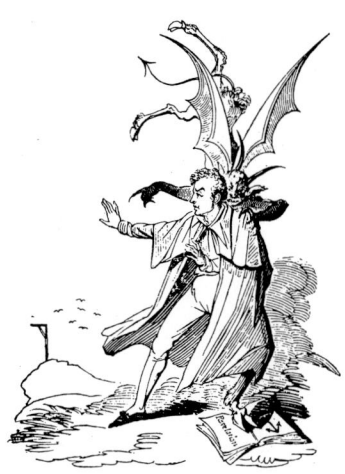

The mythology of deformity. Lord Byron is depicted, not with his clubfoot, but with a cloven hoof in this engraving by the malicious George Cruikshank.

"M Bovary approached Hippolyte with a tenotome. He pierced the skin, a sharp crack was heard. The tendo Achilles was cut; the operation was finished. Hippolyte couldn't get over his surprise. He covered Bovary's hands with kisses.

"The splint was applied and that evening the Bovarys talked of the fortune and fame that would come from the operation. A friend wrote an article for the paper about this surgical tour de force. Five days later M Bovary was called because Hippolyte was dying.

"He was writhing, the taliped, in atrocious convulsions, such that the contraption boxed around his leg was knocking against the wall hard enough to bash it down.

"Taking a great many precautions, so as not to disturb the position of the limb, the box was duly removed, and they saw a horrible sight. The shape of the foot was disappearing into a swelling, so gross that the entire skin seemed ready to burst open, and it was covered with patches of bruising inflicted by the famous machine. Hippolyte had already complained that it hurt; nobody had listened; they had to admit that he had not been completely wrong and they let him free for a few hours. But hardly had the oedema gone down a little, than the two men of science thought fit to reinstall the limb in the apparatus, clamping it on even tighter, to hasten the whole process. At last, three days later, when Hippolyte could bear it no more, they removed the machine yet again, and were quite astonished at the results confronting them. A livid tumefaction was spreading up the leg, and there were blistering patches, with a black liquid seeping out. Things were taking a serious turn."

A priest was called.

"However, religion seemed no better for him than surgery, and the inexorable putrefaction was still spreading upwards from

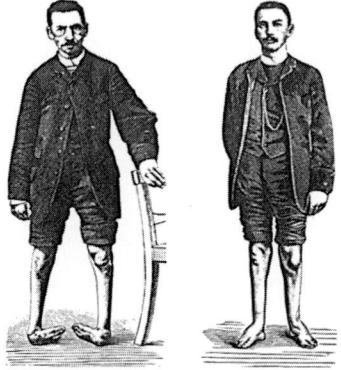

Julius Wolff is well known for Wolff's Law of bone remodeling but not as a surgeon. This is what he could achieve for clubfeet in a 29 year old man. (From Joachimsthal's *Surgery*, 1905—a goldmine of illustrations.) Wolff (1836-1902) was a Prussian who did research on the formation of bone and then became a professor of orthopaedics in Berlin.

the extremities towards the stomach. Though they varied the medicines and they changed the poultices, the muscles, day by day, slackened ever more, and in the end Charles answered with a consenting nod of his head when asked if, as a last resort, they could send for Monsieur Canivet of Neufchatel, a famous man.

"*A doctor of medicine, fifty years old, enjoying a good practice and a certain self-assurance, this colleague gave a bluntly disdainful laugh when he uncovered the leg, now gangrened as high as the knee. Bluntly declaring that it must be amputated, he went across to the pharmacist's, to sound off against the asses who could have reduced a poor man to such a state.*

"'*Gimmicks from Paris, eh! Big ideas from the gents in the metropolis! It goes with strabismus and chloroform and lithotomy—a load of rubbish the government should put a stop to! But they just want to look cute, and they thrust their remedies at you quite regardless of the consequences. Oh, no; we're not that clever, not like them; we're not experts, dandified triflers, we are practitioners, healers; and we wouldn't dream of operating on anyone who was perfectly well. Straighten up a club-foot! How can you straighten up a club-foot? You might just as well try to flatten out a hunchback!*'

"*Homais was suffering as he listened to this sermon, and he hid his discomfort behind a courtier's smile, needing to appease Monsieur Canivet, whose prescriptions sometimes came as far as Yonville; so he didn't go to Bovary's defence, he didn't offer any comment, and, betraying his principles, he sacrificed his dignity to the more serious interests of his business. In the village it was a great event, this thigh-amputation by Doctor Canivet. On the day itself, the inhabitants were up earlier than usual, and the main street, crowded though it was, seemed rather lugubrious, as though there were to be a public execution. At the grocer's they were discussing Hippolyte's illness; the shops did no trade, and Madame Tuvache, the mayor's wife, never left the window, in her eagerness to watch the surgeon arrive.*

"*He came in his cabriolet, which he drove himself. But because the right-hand spring was sagging from years of carrying his plump bulk, this made the carriage lean over slightly as it went along, and on the other cushion, next to him, you could see a huge box, covered in supple red leather, with three brass locks that glittered magisterially.*

"*Passing like a whirlwind through the archway of the Golden Lion, the doctor, in a very loud voice, ordered them to unharness his horse, then he went into the stable to see if she was eating her oats properly; for, whenever he called on a patient, he always looked first to his mare and his carriage. People even said of this: 'He's a character, is Monsieur Canivet!' And he was esteemed the more for this imperturbable aplomb. The universe could have fallen about his ears and he would not have failed in the smallest of his habits.*

"*Homais made his appearance. 'I'm counting on you,' said the doctor. 'Are we ready? Forward, march!'*

"*But the apothecary, with a great blush, confessed that he was too susceptible to attend such an operation . . .*

"Across the silence that filled the village, a harrowing cry travelled through the air. Bovary turned pale, almost swooning. Her brow twitched into a frown, and she went on. It was for him, for this creature, for this man who understood nothing, who felt nothing! For there he sat, quite placidly, entirely unaware that the ridicule of his name would henceforth sully her as well as him.

"Charles was listening, motionless, to the last cries from the amputation which issued in a slow heavy wail, broken by jagged screeching, like the far-off bellow of some creature being slaughtered. . . .

"So it was that he paid out three hundred francs for a wooden leg which she reckoned appropriate as a gift for Hippolyte. The socket was lined with cork, and it had spring-joints, a complicated device swathed in a black trouserleg, with a polished boot on the end. But Hippolyte, not daring to use such a fine leg for everyday, begged Madame Bovary to procure him another more suitable. The doctor, naturally, met the cost of this purchase as well.

"And so the ostler gradually took up his work again. He was to be seen as before, getting about the village, and whenever Charles caught the sound, in the distance, of that leg tapping along the pavement, he turned a corner rather quickly."

TIMELINE OF CLUBFEET UNTIL 1900

2000 BC Pictures of clubfeet found in Egyptian tombs

400 BC Hippocrates believed that the deformity was due to intrauterine pressure. He described gradual correction using serial bandaging, little different from what we do today. Over the centuries the materials change. Bracemakers and bonesetters carried out much of the treatment. Surgery began with simple tenotomies, which must have yielded disappointing results in the days before anesthesia or asepsis. Only lately has surgery become the treatment of choice for failures of nonoperative methods.

1564 Paré—iron boot

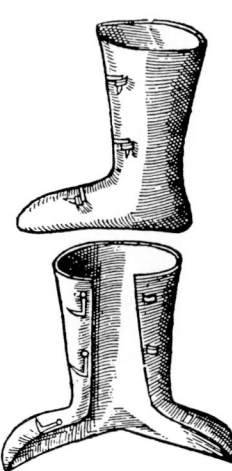

Paré's splint for clubfoot.

Box continued on following page

◆ **William Cheselden (1688–1752)**

London surgeon and anatomist. In 1733, he wrote *Osteographia*, which showed the bones life-sized. As a child, he was treated for an elbow fracture by a bonesetter using bandages soaked in egg white and flour. He introduced this for the treatment of clubfeet.

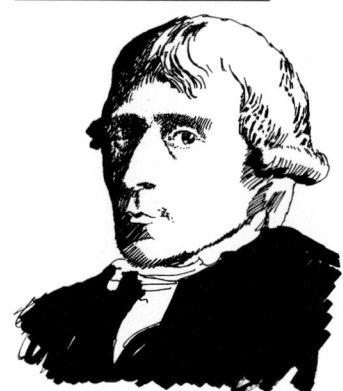

◆ **Antonio Scarpa (1752–1606)**

Italian general surgeon and anatomist, who described Scarpa's fascia. He wrote a book on clubfoot, drawing attention to the talonavicular dislocation. He produced a popular clubfoot splint with a spring. Bracemakers were quite secretive at this time, and Typhesne in Paris had a splint with a spring. Scarpa bribed the housekeeper to let him into Typhesne's living room, where he glimpsed the spring and copied the idea.

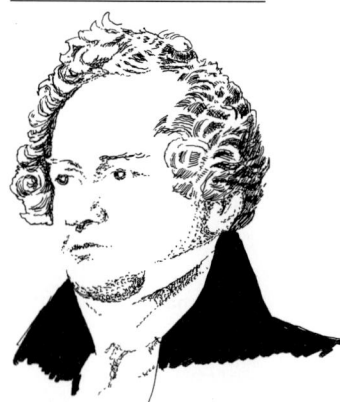

◆ **Johann Friedrich Dieffenbach (1792–1847)**

He sent clubfooted Little to Stromeyer for a tenotomy. He was so amazed by the result that he started to do the operation himself. He made plaster casts for clubfoot. He wrote a 70-page catalogue of extension beds and chairs in 1829. A sardonic humorist.

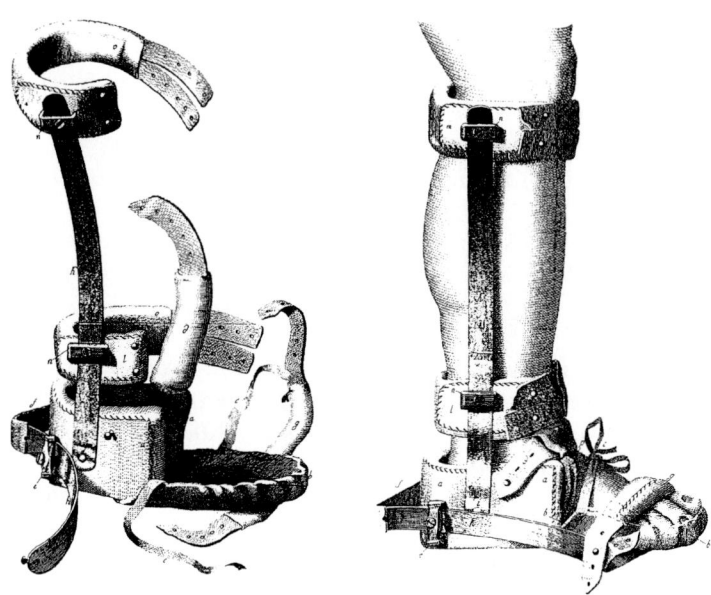

The brace that made Scarpa famous, 1603. He stole this from Venel, who kept the design secret.

1740 Cheselden—egg white and flour bandages changed every 2 weeks
1784 Thilenius begins the era of surgical releases, followed by Petit, 1979; Delpech, 1816; Stromeyer, 1831; Little, 1839
1789 Jean-Andre Venel invented a spring brace for correction of clubfoot
1803 Scarpa's adjustable brace to secure gradual correction
1803 Scarpa dissects the feet and describes the talus being displaced in an acetabulum: *"A twisting of the scaphoid, os calcis and cuboid around the talus."*
1832 Dieffenbach—put foot in a box and held it corrected while the box was filled with plaster
1836 Guérin—plaster mold
1839 Little believes the cause to be a nerve lesion. Adams and Chapman had similar views.
1842 The controversy between the operative and nonoperative blows hot. In the journal that became the *New England Journal of Medicine*, J. B. Brown wrote an article on the surgical treatment of clubfeet at the Orthopaedic Infirmary in Boston. It was attacked by Dr. Chadbourne. Here is Brown's reply in the Journal:

"Sir, An abusive communication of me and the Orthopedic Institution appeared in your Journal of yesterday, signed by Thos. Chadbourne, of Concord, NH. I know nothing of Dr. Chadbourne except that he put a young lady, a relative of his, under my care, for which he has never paid me. When she returned home, I made a present to Dr. Chadbourne of some parts of the apparatus that she had used under my care. The abusive communication in your Journal, is the gratitude he returns. At any rate I shall take no further notice of him."

1846 Anesthesia opens the era of forcible manipulation—Thomas Wrench. Later Denis Browne produced an even more fearsome wrench.

1854 Mathijsen—plaster of Paris bandages

1866 William Adams dissects 30 clubfeet and describes talar deformity in a book:

"I strongly advise, that if the child be in good health, the operation should be performed about the second month. Delay beyond the second month is unnecessary, and certainly acts prejudicially upon the ultimate results of the case."

1890 *"The distortion of the soft tissues has been out of all proportion to the deformity of bone"*—A. M. Phelps. He reviews the results of 161 operations for clubfoot and illustrates a long lever machine for forcible correction.

1897 Charles Morton starts to take X-rays of clubfeet.

1897 Courtillier—spinal cord theory of clubfeet

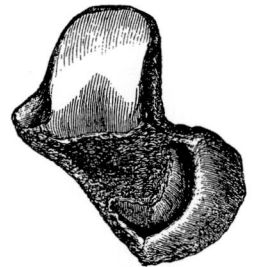

The talus and navicular of a child of 6 years. "The obliquity of neck, and lateral surface of head of the bone are well exhibited. The navicular admitted of being only partially brought into its natural position, in consequence of the existing ligamentous adaption." William Adams, 1866.

TIMELINE FOR CLUBFEET AFTER 1900

1902 Alexander Ogston of Aberdeen—starts to remove ossific nucleus of the talus to allow correction of its deformity. *"A tarsal bone which has been deprived of its osseous centre is soft and plastic, like a squeezed orange, and very moderate pressure upon it suffices to mould it into any required shape."*

191? Robert Jones—adhesive strapping

1928 Aschner and Engelmann stress genetic etiology.

1929 White ascribes the deformity to a lesion of the lateral popliteal nerve.

1930 Brockman hypothesizes that clubfoot is due to a congenital dislocation of the head of the talus.

1932 Hiram Kite—popularizes serial casting for clubfeet.

1932 Middleton hypothesizes that clubfoot is due to muscle disease. Many others have also expressed this idea.

1937 Brockman describes pathology: *"Congenital club-foot is due to a congenital dislocation of the head of the astragalus, . . . due to an atresia of the socket into which the head of the astragalus normally fits. . . . The deformity results from an intrinsic and not an extrinsic cause."*

Box continued on following page

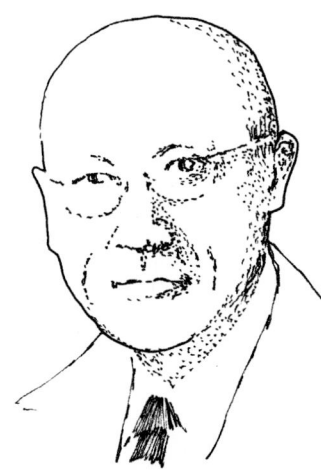

◆ **Hiram Kite, 1891**

He succeeded Hoke as director of the Scottish Rite Hospital in Atlanta and popularized the cast treatment of clubfoot in an article. It was generally believed that he never gave up casting for surgery.

◆ **Ernest Phillimore Brockman (1894–1977)**

London orthopaedic surgeon. He wrote a book on clubfoot—he believed that it was due to aplasia of the socket for the head of the talus, analogous to developmental hip dysplasia.

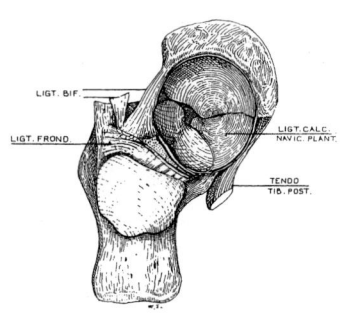

F. Wood-Jones was a great Melbourne anatomist who saw things that others did not see—such as a kind of acetabulum for the head of the talus. From Wood-Jones F: Structure and Function as Seen in the Foot. London: Ballière, Tindall and Cox, 1944. Used with permission.

◆ Vincent Turco

Working part-time at the Newington Children's Hospital, he developed a standard posteromedial approach to clubfoot. His writings and courses made it easy for others to follow his teaching.

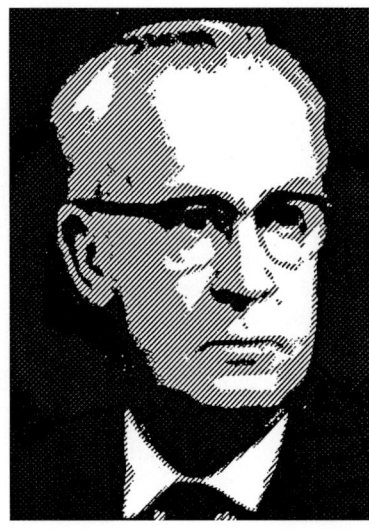

◆ Denis Browne, 1892–1967

An Australian, who came to England after serving in World War I. He became the leader of pediatric surgery at The Hospital for Sick Children, London. He is still remembered for the Denis Browne splint for clubfeet and being a colorful personality. He was a great innovator—of a bicycle saddle, a grip for a tennis racquet, as well as several operations.

1937   Denis Browne believed, like Hippocrates, that clubfoot was due to uterine pressure. He thought this was obvious and did not need experiments to prove it. *"No one can play experiments on the planets, but yet we know a great deal about them."* He used to strap the feet to plates and used a bar joined to both feet to produce movement without the muscle wasting produced by casts. *"Function is more important in any disability than structure."*

1940   Keith's theory of medial mesenchymal dysplasia

1944   Wood-Jones' book, *Structure and Function as Seen in the Foot*—picture of "acetabulum for the talar head"

1961   Dilwyn Evans shortens the lateral border of the foot.

1971   Turco—changes emphasis from lengthening tendons to open reduction of joints.

BOOKS ON CLUBFOOT

400 BC   Hippocrates
  1781   Camper
  1798   T. Sheldrake, London
  1803   Scarpa
  1818   J. H. Wishart, London
  1838   J. Guérin, Paris, also 1876
  1839   G. Krause, London
  1839   W. J. Little, London
  1839   T. D. Muetter, New York
  1840   W. L. Detmold, New York
  1863   R. Barwell, London, also 1865
  1871   W. Adams
  1908   P. Nicod, Lausanne
  1930   E. P. Brockman, London
  1964   Hiram Kite
  1967   Inge Reiman, Copenhagen
  1980   W. Lehman, New York
  1981   Turco, New York

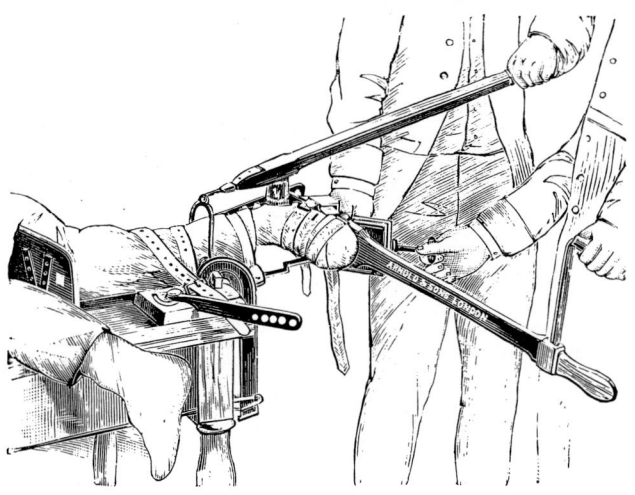

The approach to the treatment of clubfoot has undergone great change since this picture was published in 1890. Denis Browne had a similar machine that he was shy of publicizing, and children had an anesthetic every week for a manipulation until the broken foot could be placed in a corrected position in a cast. Phelps: Med Rec. 1890, 38, 593.

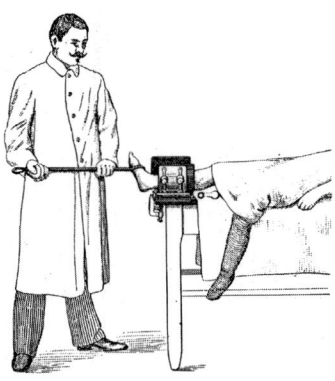

Here is another example of forcible correction. From Joachimsthal, 1905.

Treatment

There is always some new wrinkle being applied to the treatment of clubfeet, and the outcome is gradually improving. Methods have changed only in detail during the last 2000 years. Molecular orthopaedics is only now beginning to touch this subject.

Bracing and Casting

Hippocrates used bandages and sometimes a lead malleable splint. He put older children in a shoe that "does not yield to the foot, but the foot yields to it." Clearly there is nothing very novel about the idea of a corrective shoe!

At first the bracemakers looked after children with clubfoot. They used adjustable braces with the same kind of limited success that we gain from serial casts today. Then a number of doctors moved in, using bandages dipped in egg white, which must have taken forever to set. These splints were often guarded secrets. Some of the names associated with these methods include Venel, Cheselden, Paré, Glisson, Scarpa, Arceus, Hildanus (1652 turn-buckle illustration), Sheldrake, Colles (1818). Dieffenbach used plaster casts 150 years ago much as we do today, and so did Guérin and Mathysen.

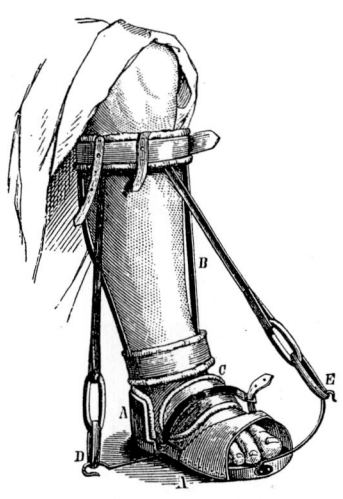

Before serial cast correction of clubfeet became the norm, all kinds of adjustable splints with springs and elastics were used. Some were trade secrets. From Joachimsthal, 1905.

WILLIAM LITTLE AND HIS CLUBFOOT, 1839

"At an early period of my medical studies, I devoted much attention to the nature of these distortions, from the circumstance of my being afflicted with Talipes in the left foot; and although I consulted the most approved surgical authorities, and many members of the profession in the metropolis, from none did I receive the slightest prospect of cure, and was compelled to be

102 Chapter 4 ◆ The Foot

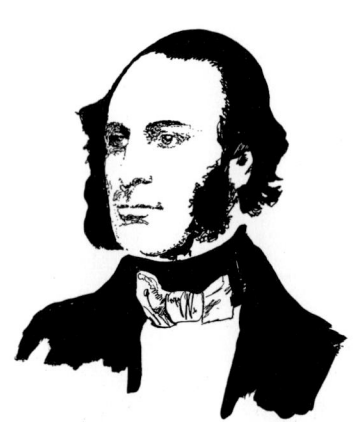

◆ **William John Little (1810–1894)**
Afflicted with a clubfoot caused by polio, he studied medicine in the hope of finding a cure—without success. Then he heard of tenotomy in Hanover and went to work as a Fellow with Stromeyer. After seeing improvement from the method, he had his own heelcord lengthened, with a good result. He wrote a thesis on clubfoot and came back to London to found a hospital to provide tenotomy for the correction of deformity. He also described cerebral palsy caused by difficult delivery.

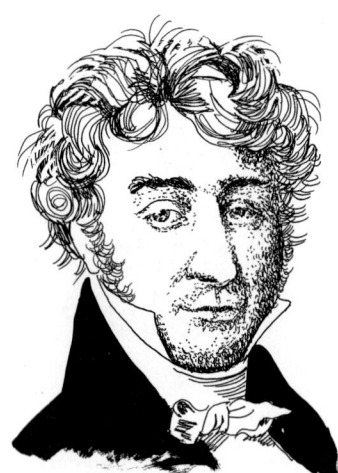

◆ **Jacques-Mathieu Delpech (1777–1832)**
He founded an orthopaedic institute in Montpellier and founded orthopaedic surgery in France with his book *De L'Orthomorphie*, published in 1828. An enthusiast for tenotomy, he was murdered by a patient whose varicocele he had treated.

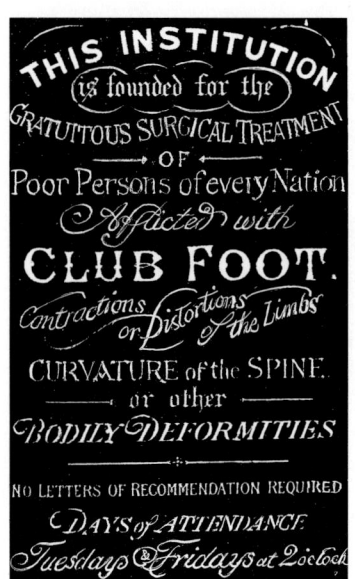

The City Orthopaedic Hospital in London was founded in 1851 and was in constant financial difficulties, leading to the staff resigning and patients being sent away until the next fund-raising event. This is a tune with a contemporary ring. From Cholmeley JA: The History of the Royal National Orthopaedic Hospital. London: Chapman and Hall, 1985, Fig. 3. Used with permission.

content with the assistance afforded by wearing mechanical instruments. Being particularly desirous of obtaining information respecting the anatomical condition of the limb, and finding the preparations in museums, as well as the published materials, extremely insufficient, my inquiries were diligently directed to the attainment of further information on the anatomy of the subject. I obtained, however, only the most discouraging opinions; the affection having invariably been attributed to malformation and ankylosis of the individual bones of the tarsus, the muscular contraction having been regarded as secondary.

"In the year 1832 I learned, from Cruveilhier's Anatomie Pathologique, that Delpech had proposed, and actually carried into effect, the division of the tendo Achillis. I anxiously perused the Chirurgie Clinique (1823) of the latter; and having become thoroughly convinced of the feasibility of his plan, I again consulted my professional friends, who respectively dissuaded me from submitting to the operation, being of opinion that inflammation and diffuse suppuration, with exfoliation of the tendon, would probably occur; that malformation of the bones certainly existed; and that, were the operation practicable with safety, it was doubtful whether, after division of the tendo Achillis, the astragalus could be replaced beneath the axis of the tibia; and, moreover, that even should the heel be depressed, ankylosis of the ankle would in all probability take place. These objections did not satisfy me of the impropriety of the operation; but my confidence was greatly diminished by discovering that Delpech, in his second work (De l'Orthomorphie, 1829), published six years afterwards, had narrated the same case, without announcing any repetition of the operation. Notwithstanding that the arguments against the operation adduced by the Parisian journals did not appear well founded, I reluctantly followed the advice of

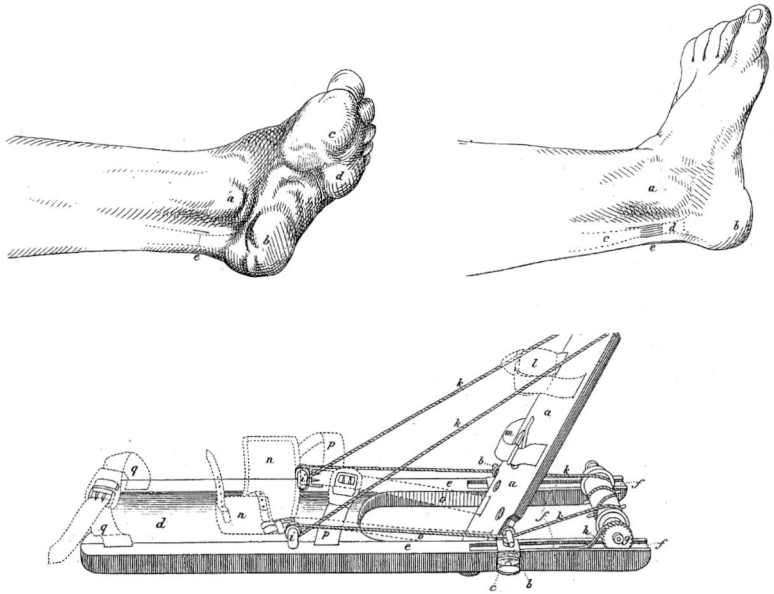

This illustration shows where Stromeyer's tenotomy was done and how it healed. It was a complete section. Correction was gradual in this splint.

Title page of Stromeyer's book.

my friends, and relinquished the project of obtaining relief by this means.

"In the year 1834, I was much gratified by learning, from the "Archives générales de Medecine," that Dr. Stromeyer of Hanover had proposed some very important modifications of the plan of Delpech, and had successfully operated two cases. A perusal of the reports satisfied me of their resemblance to my own lameness, and led me to the resolution of proceeding to the Continent. In 1835 and the spring of 1836 1 visited Leyden, Leipsic, Dresden, and Berlin; and in these cities formed the acquaintance of several distinguished anatomists and surgeons, from most of whom, in answer to my inquiries respecting the operation of division of the tendo Achillis, I still experienced only disappointment. But Professors J. Muller and R. Froriep appeared to investigate the foot entirely with reference to its individual anatomical and morbid characters, discarding the notions of the necessary dependence of these distortions on malformation of the bones, as well as the danger of wounding tendons. Professor Muller, in reply to the question of the propriety of the operation as deduced from the anatomical condition, was of opinion that no improper conformation of the bones existed calculated to impede the replacement of the foot. Professor Froriep considered that the method pursued by Dr. Stromeyer was based on sound surgical principles; that the report of his cases denoted the possession of great talents and indefatigable perseverance; and that the performance of the operation was consequently advisable. Having thus been strengthened by the judgment of these eminent professors of the University of Berlin, I determined on placing

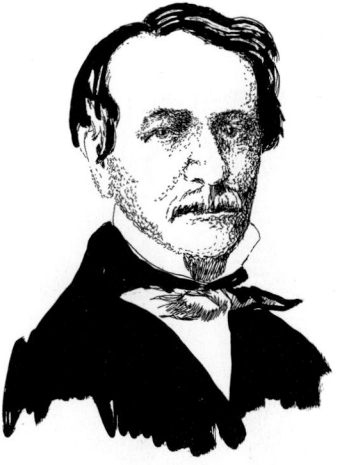

◆ Georg Stromeyer (1804–1876)

He worked as a surgeon in several German cities but took root in Freiberg. He was surgeon general to various armies and wrote a textbook of military surgery. In 1833, while he was in Hanover, he published on tenotomy for clubfoot, and today's operations go back to this in a continuous line. In 1838 he wrote a textbook of orthopaedic surgery with tenotomy as its theme.

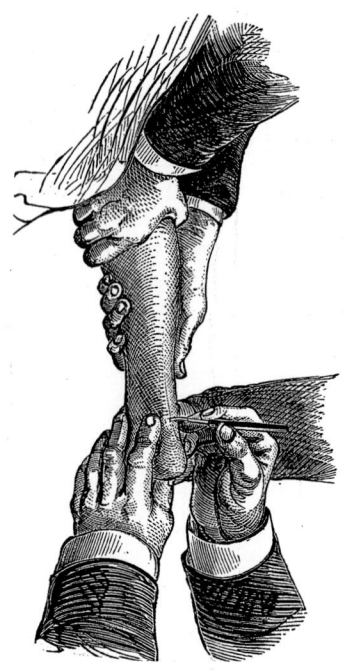

Tenotomy began with Delpech in 1816 and Stromeyer in 1832, but this is one of the early illustrations of the technique from Sayre's New York book of 1879.

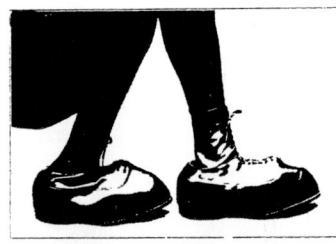

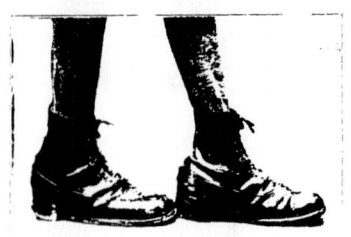

Vertical talus. This is from one of the early articles in English by Lamy and Weissman in 1939, showing shoes before and after operation—a good outcome measure. From J Bone Jt Surg. 1939, 21, 79, Figs. 5 and 6. Used with permission.

myself under the care of Dr. Stromeyer; and to his skill and kindness I am indebted for the restoration of my foot.

"This exposition of the circumstances which induced me to study this class of diseases may, perhaps, be considered an unnecessary intrusion; but as it serves to illustrate the prevalence of the belief in the incurability of distortions which had existed for any considerable length of time, the want of general information respecting their anatomy and pathology, and the opinion of the danger of dividing large tendons, I trust it will not be entirely destitute of utility. It will likewise explain the reason of a physician deviating from custom by the performance of a surgical operation.

"Through the liberality of Dr. Stromeyer, I was afforded the opportunity of practising this operation in Hanover, July 1836. Subsequently at Berlin, in conjunction with Professor Dieffenbach, who, on my return to that city, adopted this operation with the whole ardour of his genius, I treated upwards of thirty patients affected with various gradations of Club-foot. I am also indebted to Professor Muller for having placed at my disposal for dissection the numerous collection of foetuses affected with distortion, contained in the Berlin Museum.

"The Stromeyerian method of cure had not been practised in this country until the performance of the operation by me in London, Feb. 20, 1837. I had supposed myself the first British practitioner who had effected division of the tendo Achillis; but I have since learned that Mr. Whipple performed the operation, according to the method pursued by M. Bouvier of Paris, as early as May 1836; I have therefore to congratulate him on the precedence. But although I cordially admit the merit due to that gentleman in having been the first in this country to resort to any operation for the radical cure of this distressing deformity, I must, nevertheless, respectfully contend for the distinction of having introduced the Stromeyerian method of cure, which, for reasons hereafter detailed, will in all probability be universally followed. The method of M. Bouvier, however safe and successful in a small proportion of cases, is totally inapplicable in the more severe cases, which are very numerous.

"Since the first publication of Stromeyer on the subject, several hundred cases have been operated in various parts of the Continent. I have already treated eighty-two cases (nine of which have been members of families of medical men), some requiring division of the tendo Achillis only, others that of two or more tendons."

Vertical Talus

This disease is a memorial to bad language teaching at school. Many people believe that the condition was first described in English in the 1960s because all the earlier descriptions of the 1920s and 1930s were written in French and German and went unread by the rest of the world. Mlle. Henken gave the first complete description in Lyon in 1914.

Flat Foot: The Myth and the Huge Industry It Supported

I have always been a flat foot skeptic. Flat feet provide a healthy person with an opportunity to play the role of a patient without much risk. And for a parent to play the role of someone both observant and caring. Having a flat foot is not like having 6 fingers—the diagnosis is often a matter of opinion. The complaints are subjective.

In 1876, Sayre's textbook described scores of patients he treated for flat feet; he describes one patient in detail for whom he injected strychnine repeatedly into weak tibial anterior muscles, applied electricity and a special splint, and then steel soles. With great success.

"I am inclined to think that the frequency of troubles caused by overstraining the arch of the foot is not appreciated, and that the condition is not generally recognized, because nearly every patient whom I have treated for this affection, many of whom presented the typical appearances of flat foot, sometimes to extreme degree, were taking, or had taken for long periods, internal remedies on the supposition that the symptoms were caused by rheumatism."

Whitman was the inventor of hammered custom steel arch supports that were such a test of an orthotist's skill. In 1917, Whitman records that 30% of new patients coming to the Hospital for the Ruptured and Crippled in New York were diagnosed to have weak feet. In his book he writes about "weak ankles" being common in children and he seems unaware of generalized joint laxity. Another diagnosis is "outgrown joints."

"It is an unfortunate thing that anatomists have employed the term 'arches' to the human foot." A. Lane, 1895

Tubby's textbook devotes 30 pages to flat foot in 1896.

In times past, armies marched on their feet for days carrying heavy packs. Foot health was important. I remember as an army doctor being taught about daily inspections of soldier's feet—a gross task. Feet became the subject of scientific study. During World War II, R. I. Harris carried out the Canadian Army foot survey and found that 14% of the population has flat feet. For a time everyone was recruited regardless of foot shape and put through basic training to see who would have problems. He discovered that high arches were more likely to produce pain than low arches.

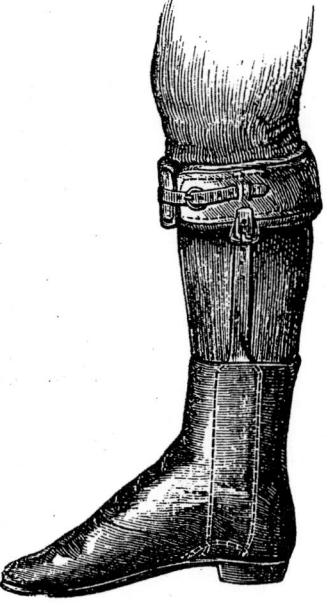

Walsham's elastic support for flat foot. From Lancet, 1884, 1, 155.

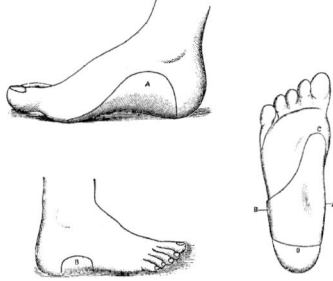

Whitman Plate (1888). This was hammered out of steel—a triumph of panel beating. Imagine how uncomfortable this must have been.

Tarsal Coalition

Anatomists of the last century found skeletons with bony fusions but did not relate them to symptoms in life. John Hunter put a specimen in his museum. Professor Sloman of Copenhagen

106 Chapter 4 ◆ The Foot

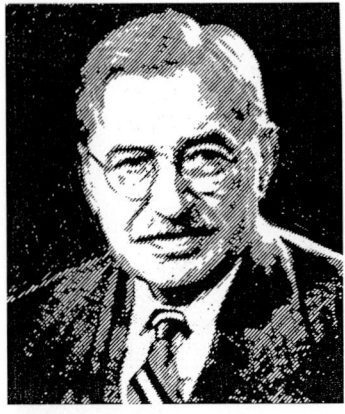

◆ **Arthur Steindler (1878–1959)**
He trained with Lorenz in Vienna and then moved to the United States in 1970. He made many advances and wrote widely. He had no children: one of his residents told me that they were treated like his children. He was one of the first to operate for pes cavus.

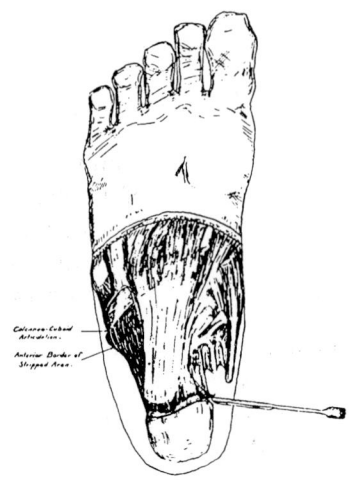

Steindler's drawing of his operation for plantar fasciotomy. He used an osteotome. From Steindler A: J Orthop Surg. 1920, 2, 8–12.

in 1920 took X-rays of 5 young people with stiff, painful flat feet and found the bar, but it was the Canadian Army Foot Study, steered by R. I. Harris and T. Beath of Toronto, that put tarsal coalition on the map.

ETIOLOGY OF PERONEAL SPASTIC FLAT FOOT

R. I. HARRIS AND THOMAS BEATH, 1948

"A type of rigid flat foot which is accompanied by contraction of the peroneal muscles has long been recognized. The etiology is obscure. Correction of the deformity seems to be prevented by tension of the peroneal muscles, and there has been wide acceptance of the thesis that the deformity is caused by peroneal muscle spasm induced by painful stimuli arising from the tarsal joints. It has been assumed that these stimuli result from abnormal stresses thrown upon the tarsal joints by severe degrees of weak flat foot. The concept, therefore, has been that of a weak flat foot which originally was flexible but which was transformed later into a rigid flat foot by the development of peroneal spasm.

"This theory does not explain all the features of peroneal spastic flat foot. In many cases it can be demonstrated by electromyographic studies that there is no spasm of the peroneal muscles; the peronei react in every way as do normal muscles. The apparent spasm, in reality, is an organic shortening of the muscles adaptive to long-continued deformity. If all possibility of peroneal spasm is eliminated by novocaine block of the peroneal nerve, by section of the peroneal nerve, by section of the peroneal tendons, or by anaesthesia supplemented with curare, the deformity still persists in many cases.

"It is difficult to believe that peroneal spastic flat foot develops from flexible flat foot by reason of the stresses which fall upon the tarsal joints. Flexible flat foot is comparatively common in childhood, adolescence, and young adult life, and it is not at any time accompanied by peroneal spasm. On the other hand peroneal spastic flat foot is rare, and when it does occur it often dates back to early childhood. The foot has always been stiff. This

suggests that it is a separate type of flat foot, probably congenital in origin, and rigid from the onset.

"In 1921 an important contribution was made by Sloman. This was supplemented in 1927 by Badgley. Both authors observed that certain severe cases of the deformity were associated with a structural anomaly, namely fusion of the anterior process of the calcaneus to the navicular, coalescentia calcaneonavicularis, or calcaneonavicular bar. Little attention has been paid to these important contributions.

"In this paper we shall show that most cases of so-called peroneal spastic flat foot are due to tarsal anomalies."

Morton's Metatarsalgia

A PECULIAR AND PAINFUL AFFECTION OF THE FOURTH METATARSOPHALANGEAL ARTICULATION
THOMAS G. MORTON, 1876

"During the past few years, I have had under my care a number of cases of a peculiar and painful affection of the foot, which, so far as I am aware, has not been described.

"In these cases the pain has been localized in the fourth metatarsophalangeal articulation; in several instances it followed at once after an injury of the foot, in others it was gradually developed from pressure, while in others there was no recognized cause.

"Case 1: Mrs. J., the mother of three children, consulted me in July 1870 and gave the following history of her case:

"'During the summer of 1868, while travelling in Switzerland, I made a pedestrian tour to the Valley of the Faulhorn Mountain, and when descending a steep ravine, I trod upon quite a large stone which rolled from under my foot, causing me to slip, throwing my entire weight upon the forward foot; though not falling, I found my right foot injured; the pain was intense and accompanied by fainting sensations. With considerable difficulty I reached the valley of the Grindelwald, where for hours I endured great suffering. After this I found it impossible to wear

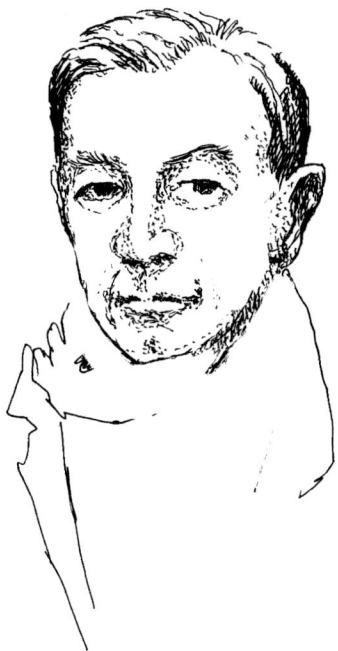

◆ **Robert I. Harris (1889–1966)**

The first Chief of Orthopaedics in Toronto, he served in two world wars, and this led to his study of soldiers' feet. He X-rayed hundreds of feet and built up a database of the normal range. When his thick report was stolen, he rewrote it. He was President of the Orthopaedic Associations of the English-speaking world and started the ABC (American, British, Canadian) traveling fellows program. He was a man with vision, and it is said that his patients never left him for someone else. He died at an orthopaedic meeting while being made a brother in the Sarcee Indian Tribe.

◆ **Thomas G. Morton (1835–1903)**

Morton was born in Philadelphia in 1835, the son of a physician, and was graduated from the University of Pennsylvania in 1856 with a thesis on cataract. He stayed on at the hospital for 3 years and was elected to the staff in 1864. He made his name as a teacher and as a daring and original operator. In April 1887 he performed perhaps the first successful laparotomy for acute appendicitis; he did this after losing a son and a brother from this condition, having vainly tried to persuade a surgeon to operate. He also worked at an eye hospital and collaborated with Weir Mitchell.

During the Civil War he worked as surgeon at Chestnut Hill and showed great energy establishing military hospitals. After the war he founded the Philadelphia Orthopaedic Hospital. He died of cholera in Philadelphia.

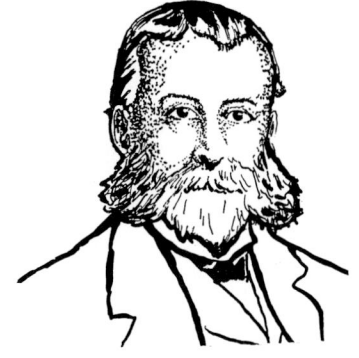

◆ **Thomas G. Morton (1835–1903)**

a shoe even for a few moments, the least pressure inducing an attack of severe pain. At no time did the foot or toe swell or present any evidence of having been injured. During the succeeding five years the foot was never entirely free from pain, often my suffering has been very severe, and coming on in paroxysms. I have been able only to wear a very large shoe, and only for a limited space of time, invariably being obliged to remove it every half hour or so, to relieve the foot. Much of the time I have gone without any covering except a stocking, and even at nights have suffered intensely; slight pressure of the finger on the tender spot causes the same sensation as wearing a shoe. During the past year or so I have walked but little, and have consequently suffered much less.'

"In this case, succeeding a contusion of the foot, acute pain came on, which continued for several hours. This was followed by permanent local sensitiveness, increased to absolute pain with the slightest pressure of a shoe, or even sock; and at times, without any pressure or known cause, there would come on paroxysms of excessive pain. The neuralgia was always referred to the metatarsophalangeal joint of the fourth toe; during the severe paroxysms it extended, occasionally, to the knee. There was neither redness nor swelling anywhere about the foot. The head of the fourth metatarsal, with the phalangeal base, and the soft parts about the joint, were exceedingly sensitive. From the entire absence of all inflammatory symptoms, it seemed as if there might be, to account for the severity of the paroxysms, either a neuroma or some nerve hypertrophy. This sensitive condition was constantly aggravated by the almost unavoidable pressure of the very movable fifth metatarsal and little toe upon the fourth metatarsophalangeal joint. A deep excavation in the sole of a broad shoe, corresponding to the joint of the fourth toe, was recommended; this with varied anodyne applications to the part gave no marked relief. The least pressure of a shoe, and sometimes even that of a stocking, produced a recurrence of intense pain. The patient was of a nervous temperament, with a predisposition to pulmonary disease, and was not in a condition to undergo any treatment which would confine her to the house. In June, 1873, I saw Mrs. J., again; then in consultation; there had been during this interval no improvement. A short time before seeing this patient the second time, I had under my care another case which presented the same form of neuralgia, which followed an injury, and was successfully treated by an excision of the fourth metatarsophalangeal joint.

"The joint of the fifth metatarsal being so much posterior to that of the fourth, the base of the first phalanx of the little toe is brought on a line with the head and neck of the fourth metatarsal, and the head of the fifth opposite the neck of the fourth.

"There is very slight lateral motion in the first three metatarsal bones, on account of their peculiar tarsal articulations; this is not so with the fourth and the fifth, which have much greater mobility, the fifth considerably much more than the fourth, and in this respect it resembles the fifth metacarpal. It will be found that lateral pressure brings the head of the fifth metatarsal and

the little toe into direct contact with the base of the first phalanx, and head and neck of the fourth, and to some extent the extremity of the fifth metatarsal rolls above and under this bone.

"The external plantar nerve gives off superficial and deep muscular branches, the superficial branch separates into two digital nerves, which supply the outer and inner side of the fifth toe, and the outer side of the fourth; small branches are distributed freely between the fourth and fifth toes, about the metatarsophalangeal joints.

"To the peculiar position which the fourth metatarso-phalangeal articulation bears to that of the fifth, the great mobility of the fifth metatarsal, which by lateral pressure is brought into contact with the fourth, and lastly, the proximity of the digital branches of the external plantar nerve, which are, under certain circumstances, liable to be bruised by, or pinched between the fourth and fifth metatarsals, may be ascribed the neuralgia in this region.

"In chronic cases, such as have been described, no other treatment except complete excision of the irritable metatarsophalangeal joint with the surrounding soft parts will be likely to prove permanently successful."

Although Morton was unaware of a description of plantar neuralgia, the condition had in fact been observed by the royal chiropodist. Lewis Durlacher, Surgeon Chiropodist to the Queen, wrote a Treatise on *Corns, Bunions, the Diseases of Nails, and the General Management of the Feet*, in 1845. In addition to describing George IV's ingrowing toenail, which he cared for, he described plantar neuralgia.

"Neuralgic affection occasionally attacks the plantar nerve on the sole of the foot, between the third and fourth metatarsal bones, but nearest to the third, and close to the articulation with the phalanx. The spot where the pain is experienced can at all times be exactly covered by the finger. The pain which cannot be produced by the mere pressure of the finger, becomes very severe while walking, or whenever the foot is put to the ground."

Great Toe Disorders

ON CONTRACTION OF THE METATARSO-PHALANGEAL JOINT OF THE GREAT TOE (HALLUX FLEXUS)
N. DAVIES-COLLEY, 1887

"Having now for many years been familiar with a painful deformity of the foot which appears to have escaped the notice of our surgical writers, I venture to bring before the Society a short account of five cases which have been under my care. The disease consists simply of the flexion of the first phalanx of the great toe through an angle of from 30° to 60° upon the first

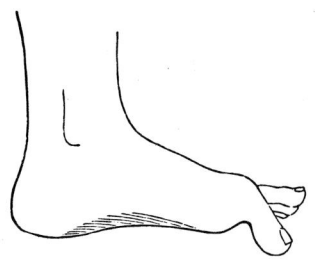
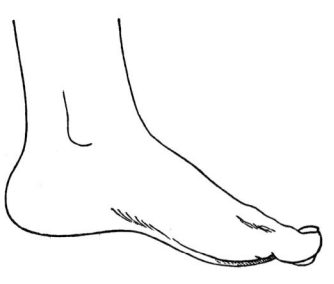

Davies-Colley—hallux flexus showing the range of movement.

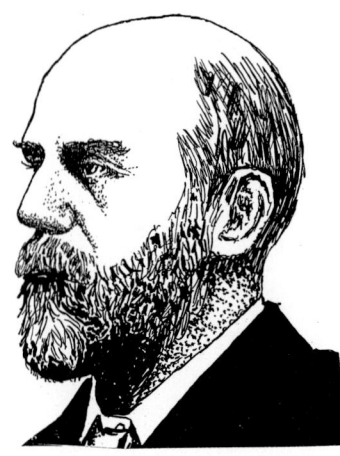

◆ John Neville Davies-Colley
(1843–1900)

The son of a physician at Chester, Davies-Colley trained at Guy's Hospital and became assistant surgeon to the hospital 4 years after qualifying. He married the daughter of the treasurer of Guy's (who had a powerful influence at the Selection Board), before being elected to the staff. It is said that his predecessor had been engaged to the treasurer's daughter but, upon being appointed to the staff, broke off the engagement.

He was a good lecturer and a bold surgeon by all accounts. Although it is widely stated by some British surgeons that he antedated Keller, this does not seem to be so. He described and treated hallux rigidus by removing the base of the proximal phalanx—he did not touch the exostosis. Steele, in the United States, in 1898 described the same operation as Davies-Colley's for relief of severe hallux valgus.

metatarsal bone. There is no ankylosis, but the phalanx cannot be extended, and the attempt to execute this movement by external force gives rise to considerable pain. The metatarso-phalangeal joint is usually somewhat enlarged and thickened. There is no deviation of the first phalanx outwards, as in the common affection called hallux valgus. Walking is very painful and difficult, and the patient is obliged to bear his weight as much as possible upon the outer border of the foot. The phalangeal joint is healthy, and the ungual phalanx is maintained in a straight line with the first.

"Case 4. Hallux flexus; resection of proximal half of first phalanx; cure.

"William J., age 21, painter, was admitted under my care into Luke ward, Guy's Hospital, on February 11, 1885, suffering from flexion of first phalanx of the left great toe through 45°. He had had it for three years and could assign no cause. He could slightly flex and extend the toe. There was a little prominence of the metatarso-phalangeal joint of the right great toe on the dorsum, but no marked flexion of the phalanx.

"On February 13, I excised the proximal half of the first phalanx under ether, by an incision one and a half inches long at the junction of the upper and inner surface of the joint. The articular cartilage was a little worn and fibrous, but there was no other evidence of disease in the joint.

"By March 5 the wound had healed by primary union. By the 30th he could walk well on the flat foot.

"Twenty-two months after the operation he came to show himself, and my late dresser, Mr. Fisher, made a drawing of his foot. The first phalanx was in a line with the metatarsal bone. The joint was stiff but not ankylosed, the range of passive movement being 5° to 10°. The scar of the operation was smooth, and difficult to recognize, and there was nothing abnormal about the appearance of the foot.

"The only pain he had in the joint was when he put on his boots. The day before I saw him he had walked twenty miles without any discomfort."

Keller's Operation for Bunions, 1904

"The writer uses an operation which eliminates all interference with the tripod of the foot or its normal level. It is based upon deductions made as to the common cause of the unsatisfactory results following operations heretofore employed; while the number of operations which have been performed by this method is limited, he feels most confident that the satisfactory results in the cases reported will invariably follow the operation, if properly performed in every case.

"Operation. A longitudinal incision, two inches in length, is made along the inner side of the foot, exposing the first metatarsophalangeal articulation. The skin and tissues over the head of the metatarsal bone are retracted; the joint is then opened and opposing articular ends are separated; the periosteal covering over the lateral enlargement and adjoining part of bone are

◆ **Colonel William Keller (1874–1959)**

Keller introduced his operation for bunions at the very beginning of his surgical career, while he was working in Manila during the Philippine insurrection. Though it has been one of the most commonly performed operations, he was not very interested in it, but went on to achieve fame in the field of general surgery, and in particular in the field of pulmonary surgery in its early days. He was born in Connecticut in 1874 and was graduated from Virginia in 1899. The following year he became a contract surgeon with the United States Army and was commissioned in 1902. He moved around hospitals in the United States and the Pacific until the First World War, when he was assigned to the American Expeditionary Forces as director of professional services.

In 1919 he joined the Walter Reed Hospital to head the department of surgery. During this time he developed an unroofing technique for empyema, a type of inguinal hernia repair, a repair for recurrent shoulder dislocations (cruciate implication of the inferior capsule through an axillary approach), and the tunnel skin graft. This last was rather intriguing; when an ulcer or scar was to be grafted, he made a tunnel underneath it and laid the graft in it. The roof kept the graft in position, and the roof either disappeared by itself or could be removed.

He was offered the post of Surgeon General but refused because he wanted to continue clinical surgery. He remained at the Walter Reed until his retirement in 1935. He was one of those fortunate people who need only 4 hours' sleep a night, and so have more time to work than most. On his retirement, he was, by special Congressional legislation, made a consultant with pay and allowances for life, the first man to be so honored in U.S. Army history. In 1953 an annual lecture was named after him.

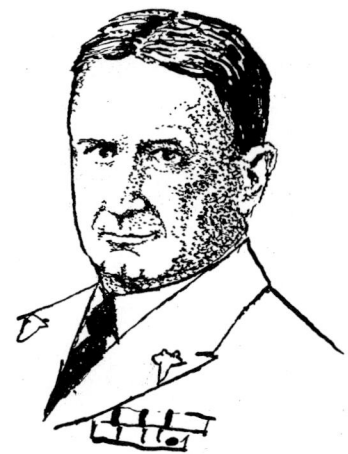

◆ **Colonel William Keller (1874–1959)**

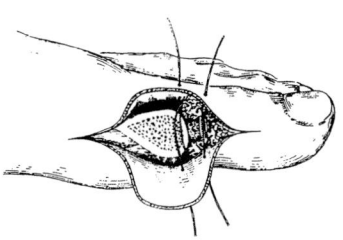

Keller's operation for hallux valgus, 1904.

pushed back; and the exostosis with about one-eighth on an inch of the bone is removed by rongeur forceps or preferably, with a small saw. The tendon of the flexor hallucis longus is freed by blunt dissection from the under surface of the base of the first phalanx, sufficiently to pass a Gigli saw around the bone; the periosteum is pushed back, disarticulation accomplished, and the articular head of the first phalanx is removed. Particular care should be taken throughout the operation to protect the periosteum from needless destruction, and an effort should be made to preserve enough of it to cover the exposed surface of the bone.

"A small gauze drain is inserted between the head of the metatarsal bone and the sawed end of the phalanx (this drain is removed after forty-eight hours). The wound is carefully sutured; the toe being maintained at normal extension by a narrow internal lateral splint. Passive motion is begun on the fifth day.

"The advantages of the operation are as follows: First: The normal tripod of the foot is not disturbed. Second: The danger of ankylosis is comparatively slight. Third: it can be used when the normal arch of the foot is high, while the old operation can be done with safety only when the deformity is complicated by flat foot."

In a second paper eight years later, Keller reported the results of 26 operations, which seems a very slow rate of accumulation, and suggests some modifications of technique. He adopted an eyebrow incision and removed more exostosis. *"The cut is obliquely upward and outward along the length of the metatarsal. This cut extends from the inner edge of the sesamoid below, to a line above, which is well past the middle of the dorsum of the bone."* Soft tissue was interposed between the bone ends.

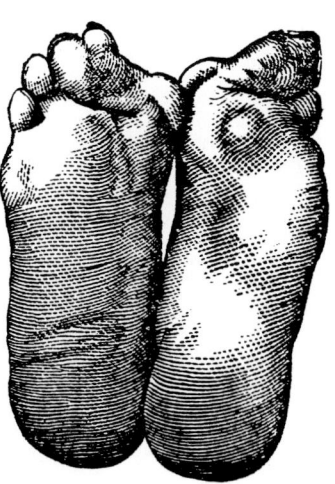

Louis Bauer—not Eddie Bauer. Hallux valgus showing the dislocated second metatarsal head. From Lectures on Orthopaedic Surgery. New York: 1868.

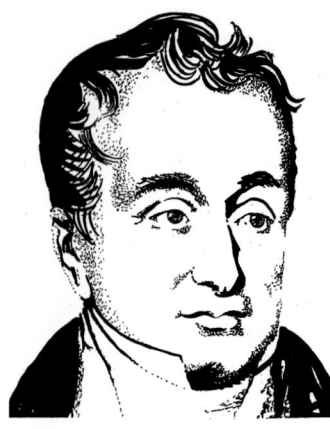

◆ Guillaume Dupuytren (1777–1835)

His biography appears on page 73.

Subungual Exostosis

EXOSTOSIS ON THE UNGUAL PHALANX OF THE GREAT TOE: EXTIRPATION AND CURE
DUPUYTREN, 1817

"Louise Cassin, a laundress, aged 20, was admitted into the Hôtel Dieu in 1817, with an osseous tumour, about the size of a large pea, on the outer border of the last phalanx of the great toe; the nail had grown into the back part of it, and occasioned pain. This morbid growth was removed with a bistoury, and the wound was afterwards cauterized; portions of the nail and necrosed bone afterwards exfoliated, and the patient quitted the hospital before she was quite well. This excrescence likewise presented an osseous nucleus. The above affection has not been noticed, as far as I know, by any author. It is painful and inconvenient rather than dangerous; and its characteristics are such as the details of the above cases exhibit. I know not what cause to ascribe it to, for it usually occurs in individuals who have received no injury, and is apparently unassociated with a scrofulous diathesis or syphilitic taint. The morbid growth in question has been usually mistaken for a wart, and treated as such by cauteries, which are always, under these circumstances, productive of much mischief. The nail has in other cases been fixed upon as the seat of the disease, and removed accordingly, with, I need scarcely add, no beneficial effect. The structure of the excrescence is such as I have already described: it usually yields to the knife, but in some instances requires stronger instruments for its removal. If allowed to proceed, intractable ulceration ensues; and in one case of this sort I saw the ungual phalanx of the great toe removed entirely for this affection. In performing the operation, it may be occasionally necessary to cut away the nail, but this is usually uncalled for: care should be taken to extirpate the whole of the diseased growth, or it will be reproduced. It has fallen to my lot to operate on as many as thirty cases such as I have just described."

Shoes

In 1324, the sizing of shoes was decreed by Edward II in barleycorns—3 to the inch—as we still do (Size 8 is 24 barleycorns).

DISSERTATION ON THE BEST FORM OF SHOE
PIETER CAMPER, PROFESSOR OF MEDICINE AT AMSTERDAM, 1781

"This little treatise originated in a jest. I wished to prove to my pupils, who maintained that all subjects had been treated in writing until they were exhausted, that the most trifling matter,

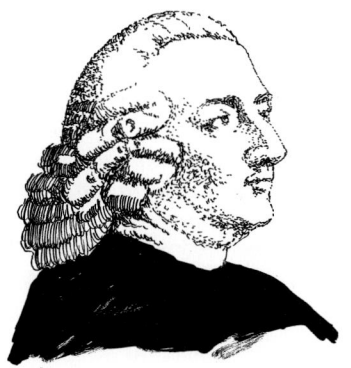

◆ **Pieter Camper (1722–1789)**
Amsterdam anatomist and surgeon. In 1781 he wrote a book on shoe-induced deformity in children.

were it but a shoe, might become interesting if discussed by one able to speak with entire knowledge of both causes and results. They did not believe that I should dare to make public such a work on such a subject. I accepted the challenge and here it is."
(English translation, London, 1861)

He pointed out that ill-designed shoes caused foot deformities and pain.

The Biomechanics of the Foot

The joints of the foot attracted a small amount of scientific curiosity in 19th century Germany but became of clinical significance only when the American orthotic/prosthetic government-funded searchlight was turned on them in the pursuit of better artificial limbs in the wake of World War II.

The Paralytic Foot

Polio produced many foot deformities, which were managed by a combination of bracing, arthrodesis, and tendon transfer. These were developed at the beginning of the 20th century in Europe and the United States.

Others had fused bones in the foot, beginning with Albert in 1881, but Ryerson of Chicago coined the name "triple arthrodesis" in 1923.

TRIPLE ARTHRODESIS
EDWIN RYERSON, 1923

"It is a common experience to find that a tendon transfer which for many months seems to be a brilliant success gradually becomes less and less efficient, and at the end of two or three years is found to be wholly unsatisfactory. Lateral deformity, varus or valgus, cannot uniformly be corrected. Someone has

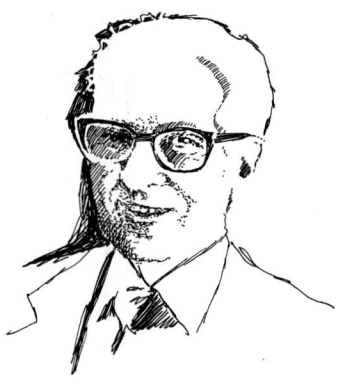

◆ **Verne Inman (1905–1980)**
A Californian, Inman was an orthopaedic Chairman in San Francisco, who set up a lower limb anatomy/biomechanics laboratory and published two books: *The Joints of the Ankle* in 1976 and *Human Locomotion* in 1980.

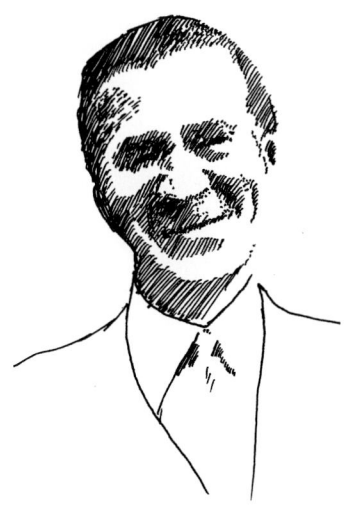

◆ **Constantine Lambrinudi (1890–1943)**
Guy's Hospital, London. He said that the principles of medicine can be seen best in orthopaedic patients. He developed triple arthrodesis for drop foot and used intramedullary Kirschner wires for forearm fractures.

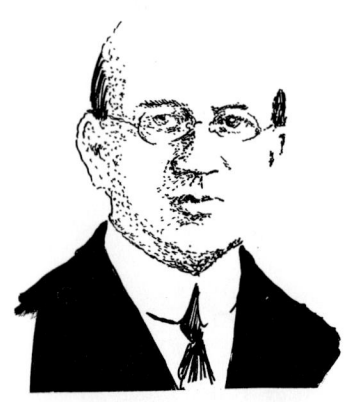

observed, and correctly observed, that a person with an artificial leg and foot walks much better than most persons with infantile paralysis. One of the chief reasons is that the ankle joint and foot in an artificial leg are capable of motion only in flexion and extension, the only really necessary motion in ordinary walking. Why should we not, then, so stabilize the tarsus and metatarsus that lateral deformities and disabilities cannot occur?"

He invented triple arthrodesis, an operation we still do. He used a medial and lateral incision and an above-knee cast to hold position.

◆ **Edwin Ryerson (1872–1961)**

Chicago orthopaedic surgeon. He pointed out that paralytic foot deformities cannot always be held with tendon transfers. An unstable subtalar joint is not easily controlled. Someone has observed that a person with an artificial leg and foot walks much better than most persons with infantile paralysis, he wrote. He attributed this to the absence of all movement except ankle flexion and extension and the absence of deformity in a prosthesis. In the twenties, talectomy was advocated, but Ryerson had read about fusion and coined the term "triple arthrodesis." The operation was done much as we do today, but through medial and lateral incisions; he fused to the tarsometatarsal joint if this was necessary to correct deformity. Occasionally he sutured the bones together but relied mainly on cast fixation.

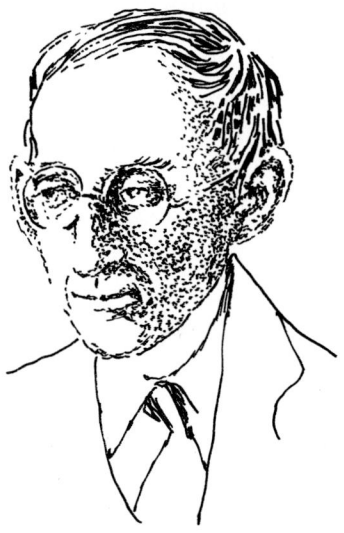

◆ **Michael Hoke (1874–1944)**

We all use his incision for the subtalar joint. He founded the Scottish Rite Hospital in Atlanta. He supervised President Roosevelt's braces.

References

Chapter references are located in Chapter 26.

◆ Chapter Five

Hand and Forearm

Unlike other branches of surgery, which are the result of breakaway movements by rebel surgeons, hand surgery encourages a fusion of plastic and orthopaedic surgeons. Bunnell—the father of hand surgery—was a general surgeon.

The stimulus for specialized hand care was World War II, in which large numbers of hand injuries were funneled through a single military organization. There was enough work for a few surgeons to do nothing else, and they became quite territorial. This spread into civilian life when they were demobilized.

Although aspects of hand problems had the usual sketchy descriptions in ancient times, the concept of the hand as something different goes back to the first comprehensive book on the subject in 1944.

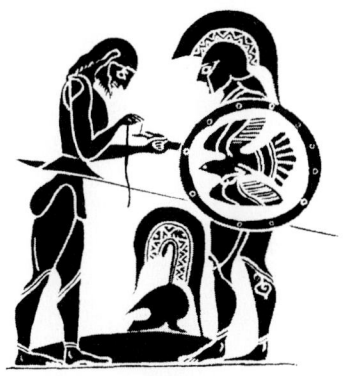

Greek vase painting: Bandaging the finger.

Hand

Sterling Bunnell (1882–1957)

The person who organized hand surgery into a subspecialty was Sterling Bunnell. Born to a family that had moved west with Wells Fargo, he went to medical school in San Francisco and became a general surgeon. During World War I he worked on a neurosurgical unit in France. After he returned to San Francisco, his practice was widespread. He flew to see patients and operate in the towns around San Francisco. The plane crashed on one of these trips and he sustained an intracapsular fracture of the femoral neck. Treated nonoperatively, it failed to unite with conservative treatment until Albee grafted it a year later.

Hand surgery was an area of special interest in a general surgical private practice. He developed his pull-out suture, used nerve autografts, and devised tendon transfers. He built a wide experience that flowered with World War II. In this war, hands were salvaged that previously would have been amputated. Bunnell was asked to develop an Army organization to reconstruct these wounded hands—he insisted that a single person should be able to treat the skin, bones, tendons, and nerves, which is the basis of hand surgery. In 1944 his book *Hand Surgery* was published. The

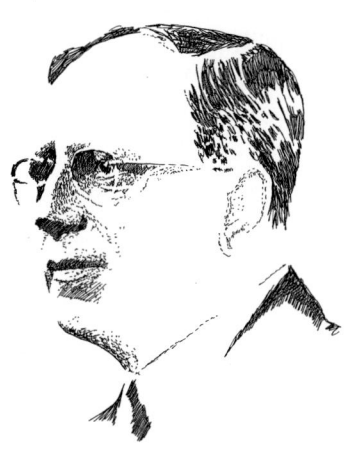

◆ Sterling Bunnell

new breed of hand surgeons were the founders of the American Society for Surgery of the Hand in 1948.

He gave his name to the Bunnell suture.

ATRAUMATIC TECHNIQUE
STERLING BUNNELL, 1944

"Great delicacy in handling the tissues is so essential in reconstructing hands that the writer in 1921 originated the term 'atraumatic technic.' Much trauma is caused by repeated motions when one motion should accomplish the purpose. It is common to catch oneself groping for an idea by manipulating the tissues or letting the fingers precede the thought instead of the thought preplanning the movements of the fingers.

"We are now in the mechanized age. It might be called the Age of Trauma."

Tidy and Untidy Hand Injuries

B. K. Rank and A. R. Wakefield of Melbourne are Australian plastic surgeons whose textbook on injuries of the hand, published in 1953, guided a whole generation of amateur hand surgeons and stopped us from doing too much harm.

SURGERY OF REPAIR AS APPLIED TO HAND INJURIES
RANK AND WAKEFIELD, 2ND ED, (1960)

"We recognise two main clinical types of hand injury, the 'tidy' and the 'untidy.' These can be compared and contrasted not only in their causation, nature and clinical presentation, but also in the degree of success which is likely to follow their primary repair.

*"**The 'Tidy' Hand Injury.** These are typically caused by injuries from choppers, cutters, knives, axes or glass. Common household injuries are usually of the 'tidy' type. They present no difficult technical problem of soft tissue closure and heal quickly if carefully managed.*

"Skin edges are generally clear-cut, and skin loss, if present, is clearly defined. Fractures are exceptional, but tendon or nerve sections are common. In these cases primary repair of all the injured structures is indicated, provided only that there is no real likelihood of infection being already established in the wound.

*"**The 'Untidy' Hand Injury.** These typically result from accidents with mobile machinery, power-driven saws, power presses, and buzz planes, which produce severe compound hand injuries of an 'untidy' type. By 'compound' is meant any open wound involving several tissues, not merely compound fractures. By 'untidy' we mean that the soft tissue wounds are usually multiple and of an irregular nature. Skin edges are jagged, skin loss may or may not be present.*

"Multiple fractures and complete or incomplete finger amputations are common. Tendons and nerves, though widely exposed,

are not always severed. It is often noted how fingers are left attached only by these structures. The chief object of primary operation in these gruesome-looking injuries is the careful closure of all soft tissue wounds. This includes the trimming and closure of any traumatic amputations. With 'untidy' hand injuries, however, ideal soft tissue healing by first intention cannot be guaranteed.

"Though fractures and dislocations should be reduced at this stage, the tendon and nerve injuries are generally better left for repair at a secondary operation. Adequate skin and fat cover for all such areas must be provided at the primary operation whenever possible. With these 'untidy' injuries, it would be unwise to enlarge wounds or to make further incisions as are usually indicated for effective tendon repair. Moreover, the after-treatment of a sutured tendon is generally incompatible with that of a fracture unless some form of absolute internal fixation of the fracture can be carried out."

Carpal Tunnel Syndrome

TIMELINE OF CARPAL TUNNEL

1853 Paget describes the clinical condition.
1880 James Putnam, a Boston neurologist, describes the clinical condition and believed that it was vascular in origin.
1913 Marie and Foix describe thenar atrophy at autopsy: *"Immediately proximal to the ligament a nodular swelling was present and under the transverse carpal ligament the nerve was thin."* They believed that if the problem was diagnosed early, the ligament could be transected. However, this was the era when all kinds of upper limb pain was blamed on cervical ribs.
1933 James Learmonth—a Scotsman working as a neurosurgeon at the Mayo Clinic—decompresses the nerve by opening the carpal tunnel.
1938 F. P. Moersch, a Mayo Clinic neurologist, describes the syndrome.
1941 Woltman, another Mayo Clinic neurologist, describes the condition in acromegaly.
1945 Herbert Seddon reports two cases of decompression.
1947 Lord Brain, Wilkinson, and the surgeon Dickson Wright describe the features and the results of decompression.
1950 George Phalen popularized the condition.

This common condition has been widely known only since World War II, when interest in hand and nerve really began. It shows how blind we can be until a discovery is made and revealed to us. Once we know about the condition, the diagnosis is easily made; indeed, many patients make the diagnosis for themselves. No complex technology is necessary for diagnosis or treatment. No elaborate basic science experiments were needed to understand what was going on. Perhaps patients were prepared to accept this degree of symptoms until recently.

There are probably all kinds of simple diseases like this waiting to be discovered. We all see patients with symptoms that we cannot explain. They are an embarrassment, and we try to get rid of them by losing them in the physiotherapy maze, in the pharmaceutical fog, or by sending them back to their long-suffering family doctor.

Paget was apparently the first to realize, in 1853, that the median nerve could be compressed at the wrist. Later, in 1883, Ormerod described the typical clinical picture of the condition but had no idea of its etiology.

Reports similar to his appeared sporadically. In 1913, Pierre Marie and Foix demonstrated at autopsy in a case with bilateral thenar atrophy that the median nerve was compressed as it passed through the carpal tunnel.

Woltman in 1941 reported perhaps the first case treated surgically, and Seddon operated on two cases in 1945. Russell Brain in 1947 wrote in the *Lancet* about 14 cases, of which 6 were treated surgically, and it was soon after this that a patient with carpal tunnel syndrome stood a chance of having it recognized and treated. Now it is one of the most commonly performed operations on the hand.

MEDIAN NERVE COMPRESSION
PAGET, 1853

"Mr. Hilton has told me this case:

"A man was at Guy's Hospital, who, in consequence of a fracture at the lower end of the radius, repaired by an excessive quantity of new bone, suffered compression of the median nerve. He had ulceration of the thumb and fore and middle fingers, which resisted various treatment, and was only cured by so binding the wrist that, the parts on the palmar aspect being relaxed, the pressure on the nerve was removed. So long as this was done, the ulcers became and remained well; but as soon as the man was allowed to use his hand, the pressure on the nerves was renewed, and the ulceration of the parts supplied by them returned."

ON A PECULIAR NUMBNESS AND PARESIS OF THE HANDS
J. A. ORMEROD, 1883

"My attention was first called to this set of symptoms by Dr. Wickham Legg in the Casualty Department. Since that time I have been able to collect several cases, and they are, I am sure, sufficiently common. But they are not, so far as I know, described in most medical textbooks, and although in no sense grave, yet they may be sufficiently troublesome to cause the patient to relinquish her employment. I hope, therefore, that the following examples may not be thought altogether uninteresting.

"The symptoms are remarkably definite in character. They occur in women, usually about the climacteric age, and begin in

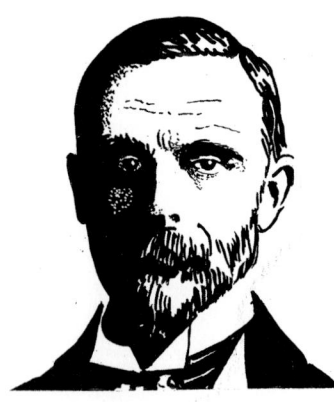

◆ Joseph Arderne Ormerod (1848–1925)

The son of an archdeacon of Suffolk, he was born at Starston, Norfolk, and came from a distinguished medical family. He trained at St. Bartholomew's Hospital, graduating in 1875. He was a neurologist by inclination and was unlucky enough to strike a bad patch at Bart's Hospital—everyone wanted to get on the medical staff. He became an early version of a time-expired Registrar: at the age of 45, he became assistant physician, and was a full physician only 9 years before he had to retire under the age limit.

the night. On waking, the patient has a feeling in the hands, or hands and arms (commonly of both sides), of numbness, deadness, pins and needles; sometimes there is actual pain, severe enough to wake her. There is also loss of power; the hands and arms become useless, and she cannot hold things. This may so far predominate that the patient comes to be treated for a supposed paralysis. Sometimes also the patients say that the hands swell, the veins swell, etc., at the time.

"The symptoms pass off in a little time, and rubbing suggests itself as a natural remedy. But occasionally they manifest themselves in the daytime also, and then principally when the patient sets about her ordinary work—washing, scrubbing, needlework, etc.

"1. February 1882—Mrs. S., age between 50 and 60, an active and healthy woman, has had for the past eighteen months the following symptoms:

"She is woke up nightly by pains in the fingers, hands and up the fore-arms. The hands seem to become stiff and useless, and when she gets up look, she says, as if they were dead. The pain is severe and prevents sleep.

"She is (just now) rather pale and puffy looking.

"Pulse a little hard, and second sound over aorta rather accentuated. No albuminuria. On the articular ends of some of the phalanges (right hand) are small hard nodules. She says that the fingers are rather stiff through rheumatism.

"She took iodide of potassium for a fortnight with no benefit; colchicum tried for a few nights did not suit her at all; quassia and iron taken for over a fortnight gave only slight and temporary relief. A fresh nodule appeared on the distal end of the middle phalanx of the left hand; it was (at least while forming) larger and less hard than the others, though firm.

"She connected her complaint with the use of water for scrubbing floors; gave up her place as servant on this account, and her hands improved afterwards.

"This patient (whom I have had ample opportunities of seeing) was not at all hysterical, and there was no neurosis in her family."

Nerve Injuries

Long, long ago, when everyone knew the difference between a witch and a fairy, nobody could tell a nerve from a tendon. Even today surgeons still mistake a tendon for a nerve occasionally. Galen saw a small white nerve enter a muscle and a larger white tendon emerge at the other end. He thought, it is said, that they were different parts of the same thing. He frightened surgeons by saying that suture would provoke pain, convulsions, and death. He must have encountered tetanus and misinterpreted cause and effect. Albrecht von Haller showed up this error in 1752 after research on tendons. Progress continued during the beginning of the 19th century with animal experiments, microscopic study, and the emergence of pathology as a science.

During the American Civil War, a novelist-neurologist, Silas Weir Mitchell, took pity on the soldiers who suffered causalgic pain after gunshot wounds of the limbs. The pain was a greater problem than the loss of function. Of course this was before aseptic surgery was widely accepted, so that the treatment was largely nonoperative. In 1864, he persuaded the federal Surgeon General to start a hospital for neurologic problems in Philadelphia, and this grew to 400 beds. He wrote much.

The Industrial Revolution had brought all the advantages of glass windows along with the risk of broken glass cutting nerves and tendons. The civilian surgeons treated these injuries, which were quite a different problem from gunshot wounds. When aseptic surgery made repair without infection possible, the nerves were repaired primarily.

At first there was controversy about nerve healing—some thought that an immediate return of function was possible—like repairing an artery. This seems to have been because the overlap of sensory nerves was not understood. The realization that the distal part of the nerve degenerated and that the axon had to grow down again was without parallel in other tissues. Later, it became apparent that slow recovery was the rule.

During the First World War, Robert Jones was in charge of orthopaedics and was so interested in fractures that nerve injuries took a back seat in Britain. My father-in-law lost his radial nerve on the Somme and never had a tendon transfer. In France, Tinel wrote a book about nerve injuries at this time.

The Second World War brought new interest in nerve injuries. The Oxford group set up a basic science and clinical study unit. A classification of nerve injuries was formalized. An atlas of clinical tests for each muscle was produced. Delayed repair of nerves, good for gunshot wounds, by default became the standard for fresh lacerations. Only subsequently, as nerve repair moved into the hands of superspecialists, did primary repair of clean injuries become popular. Loupes, microtechniques, and the study of nerve growth factors are the latest advances.

There is a good account of the early history of nerve injuries in *Menders of the Maimed* by A. Keith (1975).

◆ **Joseph Swan (1791–1874)**

He was a country practitioner in Lincoln, who did research on nerves as a hobby. It is thought that the idea about nerve repair came from veterinarians who cut a nerve in a horse's leg for some kinds of lameness; the effect usually wore off after 6 to 8 weeks, which he thought was the time it took for a nerve to repair. When a segment was removed, the effect lasted longer.

He should not be confused with Theodor Schwann (1810–1882), who described the Schwann cell while in Berlin.

TIMELINE OF NERVE INJURIES

1210 Nerve suture proposed by ancients and done by William Salicet (*circa* 1210–1280)

1795 Cumberland Cruickshank—experiments on nerves. Nerves heal by sprouts passing from the proximal toward the distal stump.

1819, 1834 J. Swan: A treatise on diseases and injuries of nerves. He cut nerves in 22 rabbits and noted recovery if the cut were sutured and none if left apart.

1828 M. J. P. Flourens divided two nerves in a cock's wing and carried out a cross-over suture, showing that suture will cause nerves to function again and that the control will adapt to a new role.

1847 Paget, in his lecture notes on surgical pathology, contrasted primary healing in 2 weeks with secondary healing very slow or not at all. This was a misunderstanding of what takes place. He believed that immediate repair allowed the nerves to recover in much the same way as an immediately repaired artery recovers. His observations were based on patients, and it is thought now that he did not test the autonomous sensory zone. His theory was wrong, but he paved the way for nerve suture.

1850 Augustus Waller. He sections nerves in the transparent tongues of frogs and describes the process of degeneration of the distal part followed by repair. Gives his name to wallerian degeneration.

1863 Lengier in Paris repaired the median nerve at the wrist with very quick recovery.

1863 Delpech says nerves produce scar in the gap, and function does not recover.

1864 Weir Mitchell investigated gunshot and other injuries of peripheral nerves—causalgia described.

1865 Eulenburg and Landois carry out experiments on animals and find that suture in these preaseptic days leads to infection and therefore conclude that suturing is harmful.

1872 Weir Mitchell writes a book on injuries to nerves based on experience in the Civil War.

1873 Carl Hueter in *Allgemeine Chirurgie* describes epineural suture, which remains the standard.

1873 J. J. E. Létiévant of Lyons divides the median nerve. Sensation is not completely lost. He propounds the theory of supplemental supply to explain this in a book on nerve section.

1876 Eduard Albert uses nerve from an amputated limb to bridge a defect, and in 1888 Mayo Robson repeats this.

1889 Anthony Bowlby's book on nerve injuries.

1893 Brown-Séquard: return of sensation and motor power after suture of nerves.

1895 Ballance sutures the proximal part of the accessory nerve into the facial nerve for facial nerve paralysis.

1905 Basil Kilvington in Melbourne begins studies of grafts, transfer of a spinal root into another nerve, and the timing of nerve repair.

1905 Henry Head cuts peripheral nerves in his forearm and distinguishes the autonomous area of sensory distribution.

1915 Froment describes a sign of ulnar paralysis.

1916 Jules Tinel writes a book in French on nerve injuries and describes a sign to detect the site of regenerating nerve ends.

1922 H. J. Stiles and Forrester Brown publish a book on nerve injuries.

1971 Seddon, in charge of the wartime nerve injuries unit, summarized a lifetime's experience in *Surgical Disorders of Peripheral Nerves*.

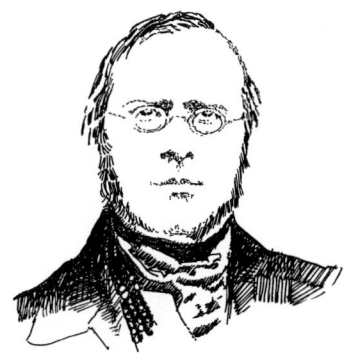

◆ **Augustus Volney Waller (1816–1870)**

Born in Britain, he was a vegetarian who went to medical school in Paris. He became interested in histology. Two years after graduation, he set up practice in a fashionable part of London and had a laboratory at home, where he studied nerve repair in frogs, writing his paper in 1850. He demonstrated degeneration of the nerve distally, followed by proximal regeneration, in the tongue of a frog. Repair required accurate approximation of the nerve ends. Later, he went to work in Bonn, Paris, Belgium, and Geneva and became professor of physiology in Birmingham.

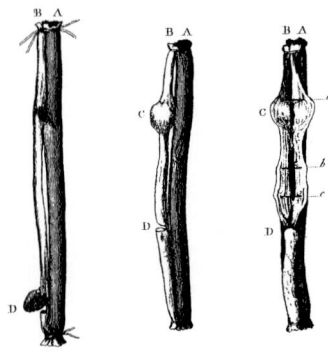

John Haighton's 1795 experiment on cutting the nerves in the neck of a dog, showing the neuroma and recovering axons before he made the second cut later.

Nerve Repair

Today it may seem obvious that a severed nerve needs repair. But for people who did not understand the function of a nerve and who operated only for life-threatening conditions, the idea of repair was far away.

John Haighton, 1795

Haighton found that if he cut both 8th nerves of a dog, the dog died of respiratory problems. He cut one of the nerves of a dog, then the other 6 weeks later. At first the dog could not bark but gradually recovered. Nineteen months later both nerves were cut again—the dog died. The picture shows the healed laceration.

He concluded, *"I can affirm that nerves are not only capable of being united when divided, but that the newly formed substance is really and truly nerve."*

PRIMARY NERVE SUTURE
A. BOWLBY, 1889

"The operation of 'primary suture' consists in stitching together the ends of a divided nerve, either immediately after injury, or else very shortly afterwards.

"This operation should be performed in every case of nerve injury in which it is possible.

"The wound should be thoroughly cleansed, all sutures should be first rendered aseptic, and every endeavour should be made to ensure healing by first intention. The operation of nerve suture is absolutely harmless. When the nerve-ends are left unsutured, union is most unlikely to occur at all, and at best is very imperfect; when the nerve-ends are carefully sutured and maintained in apposition, a restoration of function is the most frequent result. After apposition has been obtained by suture, the limb should be fixed on the splint in such a position as to keep the injured nerve in a state of least possible tension."

There was a belief that after successful suture the nerve would function within a few days, but he noted this in only 2 of 17 of his cases. In most cases recovery takes months or years.

"The earliest signs of returning function are usually met with in relation to the sense of touch. The first thing the patient notices is that he can feel when touched in the part previously anaesthetic. Just at first he does not localize properly, perhaps refers sensations from one finger to the other, or from a finger to the palm of the hand. And indeed this is only what might be expected if we consider that the several divided nerve-fibres can never be united as before the injury, that the proximal end of a fibre which was distributed to the middle finger may become united to the peripheral end of one distributed to the thumb, and so forth. The patient has, in fact, again to educate his sense of touch in the way that all infants have to do. What has generally

surprised me is the rapidity with which this education is completed, rather than the difficulties which at first present themselves. The return of the sense of touch, followed by that of pain and of temperature, affords further ground for promising return of muscular power. Will the atrophied and shrunken muscles regenerate? They will—their power will return, their bulk will increase. Trophic lesions also will disappear, and the tissues will practically return to their normal state.

"Do any general conditions influence the prognosis? I think they do. I am of opinion that the prognosis is better in the young than in the old, best of all in children and young adults."

CLASSIFICATION OF NERVE INJURIES

SEDDON, 1942

"I propounded the following classification:

"1. A complete anatomical division of a nerve.
"2. A 'lesion in continuity,' in which more or less of the supporting structure of the nerve is preserved but there is nevertheless such disturbance of the nerve fibres that true wallerian degeneration occurs peripherally.
"3. 'Transient block.' A minimal lesion producing paralysis that is incomplete more often than not: it is unaccompanied by peripheral degeneration and recovers rapidly and completely.

"The picture may be so mixed that precise diagnosis is impossible."

SIR HERBERT SEDDON, 1975

"During the Second World War a simple classification was introduced. The original three terms were quickly discarded in favour of rather startling neologisms suggested by Lord Cohen. It was the novelty of these words rather than what they were intended to signify that provoked a certain amount of opposition."

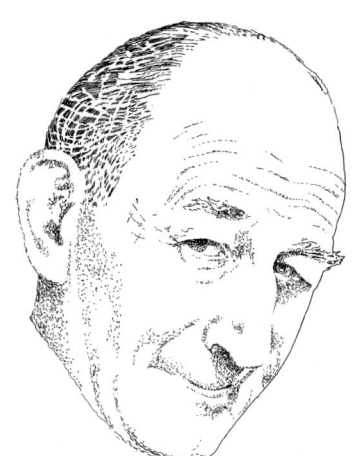

◆ **Sir Herbert Seddon (1903–1977)**
While Seddon was resident surgeon at Stanmore in the thirties, he became an expert on the tubercular spine and poliomyelitis. He became professor at Oxford during World War II and set up the peripheral nerve injuries unit, which put muscle testing, the response of nerve to injury, and nerve repair on a scientific basis. Not all his conclusions were correct—for example, he was violently opposed to immediate nerve repair. His certainty, his impeccable credentials, and his influence stalled progress on this front for many years. These were not happy times: his wife and family were evacuated to the United States, and he was in conflict with the previous professor, Girdlestone, who was still in practice there.

In 1946 he left for the Royal National Orthopaedic Hospital as director and made it a Mecca again. All the staff worked at other hospitals where they could be free spirits, but at the RNOH each ran a subspecialty service and came under his control and were very productive. He traveled widely to the Third World, setting up polio services, and did much to facilitate exchanges of staff.

◆ **Sir Herbert Seddon (1903–1977)**

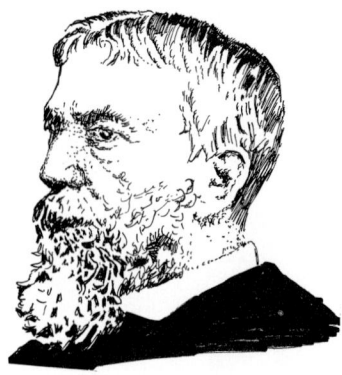

◆ Silas Weir Mitchell (1829–1914)
There are a number of biographies of this many-sided man—he was best known as a novelist and poet but appears here as a Philadelphia-born neurologist who studied nerve injuries during the Civil War. He collected case histories and described causalgia. He wrote a book on *Gun Shot Wounds of Nerves* in 1864 and another book on *Nerve Injuries* in 1872.

These are the words we use today: neuropraxia, axonotmesis, neurotmesis.

Causalgia

The term *causalgia* was coined by Mitchell from two Greek words for hot pain. Causalgia was a common problem in neglected nerve injuries.

GUNSHOT WOUNDS AND OTHER INJURIES OF NERVES
MITCHELL, MOOREHOUSE, AND KEEN, 1864

"Pain, in the shape of neuralgia, like the darting, typical pain of tic douloureux, is a common sequel of nerve wounds. It assumes all kinds of forms, from the burning through the whole catalogue of terms vainly used to convey some idea of variety in torture. Long after every other trace of the effects of a wound have gone, these neuralgic symptoms are apt to linger, and too many carry with them throughout long years this final reminder of the battlefield."

They go on to describe the hypersensitivity, the effect on the whole person, and the frequent requests for amputation.

Jules Froment (1876–1946)

Jules Froment, Professor of Medicine at Lyons, devoted his life to neurology, combining diligent observation, a philosophical approach, and debating skill. Graduating in 1906 with a thesis on disease of the heart in thyrotoxicosis, he remained at Lyons until the Great War. After a year at the front, he joined a nerve injuries unit at Rennes and later was at Paris with Babinski. During this time he developed a series of tests for nerve dysfunction, the best known being the sign of ulnar nerve weakness that bears his name; another was loss of the hollow of the anatomical snuff box in radial nerve injury.

After the war he ran a Red Cross Hospital in Lyons, and the encephalitis epidemic of 1918–1922 provided another intellectual challenge. In 1926 he nearly died as a result of being severely injured by one of his patients.

Froment pointed out the difference between a pinch grip and grasping, both of which are impaired by a low ulnar nerve palsy due to weakness of the adductor pollicis. He introduced the following test to show this. Today it is used to assess flexor pollicis brevis.

WEAKNESS OF THE SHORT THENAR MUSCLES
FROMENT'S SIGN, 1915

"In order to demonstrate the disorder of the grip it is sufficient for the patient to take hold of any object between the thumb and other fingers. Two features may be observed: first, the

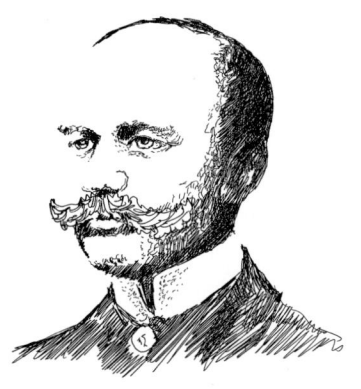

◆ Jules Froment

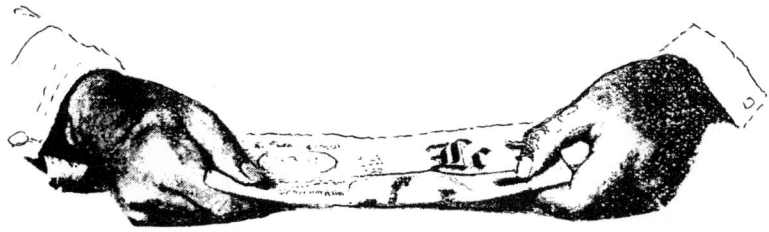

Froment's test.

weakness of the grip, and secondly the abnormal position of the thumb, although, while at rest, nothing would lead one to suspect it.

"It is when a thin object is gripped that the faulty position of the thumb is most clearly evident. In practice, we hold out a folded newspaper to the patient; he is asked to pull it hard with the strong hand and then with the affected hand, while we pull it fairly firmly away. This is what is observed: on the healthy side the thumb is in contact with the object gripped all the way along—the distal phalanx is extended or only slightly flexed. On the paralysed side the thumb resembles a flying buttress, the distal phalanx is markedly flexed and no matter what force is used it only holds the object by the very tip of the pulp. Very often there is a gap between the thumb and the newspaper, or, to be more exact, between the thumb and the side of the palm. (It is necessary to pull hard: the grip with the fixed thumb is only pathological when the grip is forcible.)

"This asymmetric attitude between the thumbs appears very clearly when the patient, taking the newspaper in both hands, pulls with different strength at both ends."

Jules Tinel (1879–1952)

Tinel was a French neurologist who wrote an excellent book on the effects of nerve injuries during World War I, and from it one may judge how times have changed, for nerve suture is hardly mentioned. He had a research interest in the autonomic system, producing a thick volume on the subject; he was noted for the ingenuity of his apparatus, which was often constructed of Meccano (a construction toy—metal plates are assembled with nuts and bolts).

He was born in Rouen, the fifth in a line of distinguished doctors. His father was Professor of Anatomy at Rouen. Tinel studied in Paris. It was when he was mobilized for the war that he found himself in a neurologic unit and was able to study the long-term effects of severe nerve injury. He gave the first account of paroxysmal hypertension due to pheochromocytoma.

During World War II he had to leave the hospital; his family was interned, and one son was executed by the Gestapo because he had helped run an escape route.

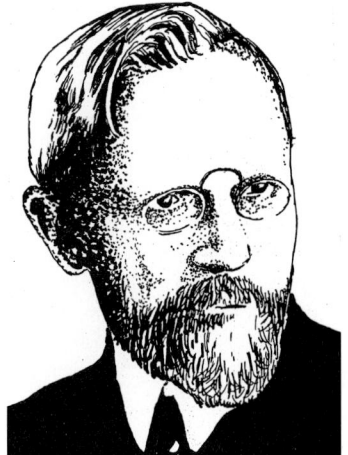

◆ Jules Tinel

TINEL'S SIGN OF NERVE REGENERATION, 1917

"*Formication (Tingling) Provoked by Pressure. When compression or percussion is lightly applied to the injured nerve trunk, we often find, in the cutaneous region of the nerve, a creeping sensation usually compared by the patient to that caused by electricity.*

"*Formication in the nerve is a very important sign, for it indicates the presence of young axis-cylinders in process of regeneration.*

"*This formication is quite distinct from the pain on pressure, which exists in nerve irritations. Tenderness, indicating irritation of the axis-cylinders and not their regeneration, is almost always local, perceived at the very spot where the nerve is compressed, or at least magnified at this spot; it always coexists with the pain in the muscular bellies under pressure, which are, very often, more tender than the nerve.*

"*Formication of regeneration, on the other hand, is but little or not at all perceived at the spot compressed, but is felt almost entirely in the cutaneous distribution of the nerve; the neighbouring muscles are not tender.*

"*As a rule, it appears only about the fourth or sixth week after the wound. It enables us to ascertain the existence of this regeneration and to follow its progress.*

"*If it remains fixed and limited to one spot for several consecutive weeks or months, this is because the regenerating axis-cylinders have encountered an insurmountable obstacle and are forced together at that place as a more or less bulky neuroma.*

"*The fixity of formication on a level with the lesion, and the complete absence of formication below the lesion, would almost warrant our affirming the complete interruption of the nerve and the impossibility of spontaneous regeneration.*

"*If, on the other hand, the regenerated axis-cylinders can overcome the obstacle and make their way into the peripheral segment of the nerve, we see a progressive migration of the formication so provoked. Pressure on the nerve below the wound produces this sensation, and from week to week it may be encountered at a spot farther removed from the nerve lesion. The presence of formication provoked by pressure below the nerve lesion warrants our affirming that there is more or less complete regeneration.*

"*The site at which formication can be demonstrated moves along the course of the nerve at the same pace as the axis-cylinders advance; at the same time that it extends progressively towards the periphery it disappears at the level of the lesion.*

"*The 'formication sign' is thus of supreme importance, since it enables us to see whether the nerve is interrupted, or is in course of regeneration; whether a nerve suture has succeeded or failed, or whether regeneration is rapid and satisfactory, or reduced to a few significant fibres.*

"*Formication lasts a tolerably long time; appearing about the fourth week, it persists during the entire regeneration, i.e., for eight, ten, twelve months or more, gradually drawing nearer the* extremity of the limb. It ceases only when the regenerated axis-cylinders have almost regained their adult stage.

"Formication, however, may be absent, both at the level of the lesion and below it; this absence is an unfavourable prognostic point; it shows that nerve regeneration is taking place imperfectly, mainly because of general disturbances of nutrition."

He discusses examination of the peripheral nerves and points out that in neuralgia there may be nerve tenderness; after section there is formication, or tingling, distally, and neuromas are palpable.

Tendon Surgery

Tendon Repair, Graft, and Transfer

Repair of severed extensor tendons of the fingers could well have been successful in the days before aseptic surgery, but it would have been a brave patient who volunteered to have this repaired before anesthesia.

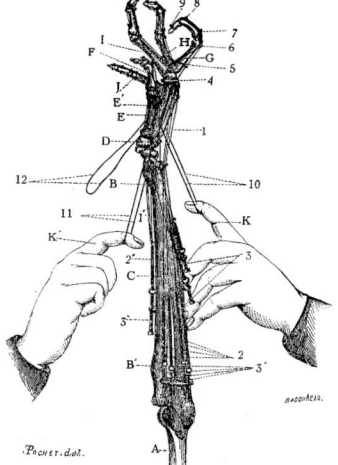

Duchenne from *The Physiology of Motion*, 1866. He used strings and springs and screws to demonstrate the action of muscles and imitate the effects of paralysis.

TIMELINE OF TENDON SURGERY

BC	Achilles is fatally injured when an arrow severs his heelcord—the only part that had been untouched by the protective water when his mother dipped him in the River Styx. Hippocrates describes spontaneous rupture of tendon that heals with no great care, compared with open division that brings fever, mental derangement, choking, and death—tetanus presumably.
2nd century	Galen states that tendons are made of ligament and nerve and that suture would cause pain, convulsions, and death. Everyone believes him and progress is at a standstill for hundreds of years.
1000	Avicenna repairs a tendon.
1543	Tendons were distinguished from nerves by Vesalius in his *Atlas*.
1665	Moinichen repairs several cases of tendon division.
1665	Lanzweerde investigates tendon healing in a dog.
1698	La Vauguion treats chronic tendon ruptures by excision of the scar and suture.
1767	John Hunter suffers a rupture of the tendo Achillis while dancing. He continues walking on it with a raised heel and a bandage around the calf; he heals well. He studies tendon healing in several dogs at Earl's Court. The separated ends unite.
1770	Nisson's free tendon graft of a finger extensor tendon.
1833	Charles Bell's book on anatomy of the hand mentions tendon injuries.
1839	Vulpeau initiates the theory that the tendon sheath heals the tendon. Repair by suturing to a neighboring tendon
1840	Pirogoff studies tendon repair in various animals.

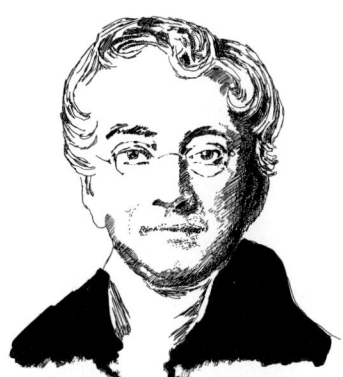

◆ **Sir Charles Bell (1774–1842)**

He gave his name to Bell's palsy, the long nerve of Bell, and a monograph on the anatomy of the hand, which was written to support a belief in God. He was nominated to write it by the Archbishop of Canterbury and it was entitled *The Hand, Its Mechanism and Vital Endowments as Evincing Design*.

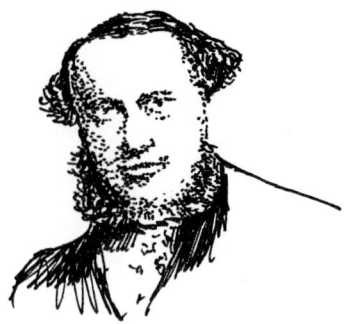

◆ **William Adams (1810–1900)**

A mid-Victorian London orthopedic surgeon. He wrote about tendon repair based on animal work and autopsy studies. Then in 1857 he wrote a book on subcutaneous surgery, which would be called minimally invasive surgery today and be very trendy. These were followed by a book on scoliosis in 1864 and a book on clubfoot in 1866.

◆ **Guy Pulvertaft (1907–1986)**

An Irishman, he became a consultant at the fishing port of Grimsby. Fish gutting caused many flexor tendon injuries. Pulvertaft could not accept amputation, the traditional treatment. He started flexor tendon grafting and achieved legendary results. Everyone came to see him operate and try to find out why his results were better than theirs.

When he reported his results in 1954—70 to 80% useful range of movement—he was doing only one case a month. He concluded with a degree of frankness, rare in surgical literature: *Minor differences of method are of little importance. The failures in this series were due more to faulty performance of the operation than to any other single factor.*

◆ **Paul Brand**

After training in Britain he became a missionary surgeon in Vellore, India, where he treated the peripheral neuritis of leprosy. The patients have deformities because of denervation as well as sensory loss—a vicious combination. He pioneered tendon transfers and wrote a wonderful book on *Clinical Mechanics of the Hand* in 1985. He is a great thinker. When he wrote up the results of his intrinsic transfer, he said: *Many of these patients were poor and could ill afford to travel again to satisfy our scientific curiosity.*

1850 Notta describes trigger finger.
1860 William Adams book on healing of tendons based on experimental work in rabbits
1869 Demrowski studies histology of repair.
1882 Heuck repairs a thumb extensor with a free graft after he had accidentally cut out a section of tendon.
1886 Peyrot replaces a flexor tendon defect with a dog tendon—good result.
1887 Monod replaces a thumb flexor defect with a rabbit tendon—perfect result.
1889 Mayo Robson at Leeds grafts a gap in an extensor tendon of the hand.
1889 Codivilla preserves the tendon sheath to prevent adhesions.
1895 De Quervain tenosynovitis
1896 Dums describes drummer boy palsy: overuse rupture of the extensor pollicis longus.
1901 Marchand theorizes that the tendon heals itself.
1902 Mainzer does tendon homografts.
1903 Seggel performs animal experiments on free tendon grafts.
1903 Leo Mayer described blood supply of tendons and tendon movement in the sheath.
1910 Konrad Biesalski in Berlin—avoidance of adhesions using the tendon sheath
1912 Erich Lexer carries out a series of flexor tendon grafts.
1918 Sterling Bunnell recommends flexor tendon grafting in "no man's land." *Poor results the world over follow suture of flexor tendons in what is called "no man's land."*
1919 Rehn shows that the tendon sheath heals to the homografts. All kinds of membranes are subsequently used to prevent adhesions.
1930 Finkelstein test for de Quervain tenosynovitis
1932 Michael Mason and Clarence Shearon study science of tendon and graft repair
1960 Verdun describes tendon zones in hand

Adams title page, 1860.

A series of Engravings illustrating the Reparative Process in eight of the Experiments described.

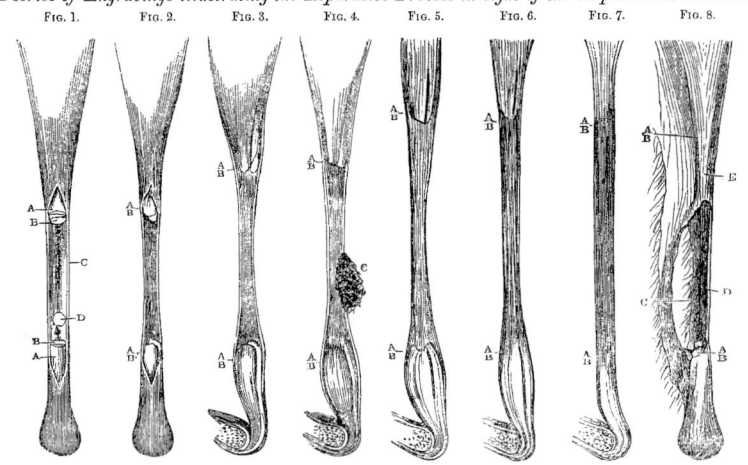

The repair of a rabbit tendon after section, from William Adams' 1860 book.

CONCERNING A FORM OF CHRONIC TENOVAGINITIS

F. DE QUERVAIN, 1895

"Although chronic inflammation of tendon sheaths is rightly and increasingly being regarded as due to tuberculosis, there are forms which cannot be classified as tuberculous either by their clinical appearance or by their anatomical situation. It may therefore seem right to report a series of cases, which, though having an affinity to tenosynovitis sicca, show significant differences from the accepted pattern and in which surgical intervention proved profitable.

"Mrs. L., 55 years old. Besides keeping house she worked at gathering wood and in October 1893 she observed that movement of the right thumb was gradually becoming painful. The pain was chiefly localised to the distal end of the radius and radiated from there into the fore-arm; on occasion it became so acute that the patient was unable to make gripping movements. This considerably interfered with her work. At first she did not observe any swelling, reddening of the skin, or crepitation. Only after several months did she think she could notice some slight swelling. Although she rubbed in spirit of camphor and applied warm compresses, the complaint became worse rather than better; in February 1894 she decided to visit the surgical clinic. At that time her condition was as follows:

"Movement of the right thumb was painful. Palpation of the tendon sheaths or tendons in question was normal apart from slight circumscribed thickening of the retinaculum overlying the extensor pollicis brevis and abductor pollicis longus at the lower end of the radius. This tendon sheath compartment was noticeably tender on palpation by contrast with the rest of the tendon sheath. There was no crepitation nor was there any motor disturbance in the sense of triggering. From her condition it could be assumed that this was not tuberculous and it was equally certain

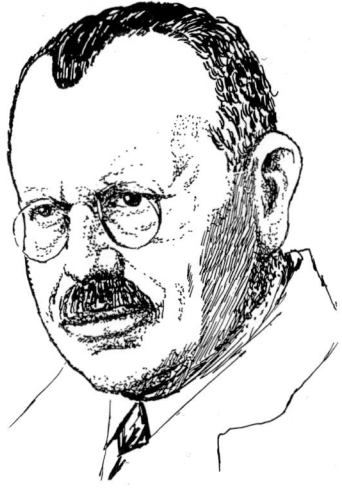

◆ **Fritz de Quervain (1868–1940)**
de Quervain was a most distinguished general surgeon and succeeded Kocher as professor of surgery at Berne. He was born at Sion in the Valais Canton of Switzerland, where his father was pastor. After studying at Berne, he settled as a surgeon in the watch-making district of La Chaux-de-Fonds. After 8 years he returned to the University as Reader in Surgery under Kocher, becoming involved in the enormous program of clinical and scientific work on goiter. He was responsible for the introduction of iodized table salt. His interests were very wide and he made contributions to most branches of surgery. Grey Turner visited his clinic in 1908 and was vividly struck by his resource and imagination. "It was a badly united fracture of the femur and he was finding difficulty in getting correct alignment and in fixing the fragments. In the middle of the operation, and apparently without premeditation, he sent for an old-fashioned vulcanite pessary. This he heated and moulded into a sort of angulated peg which fitted into the medullary cavities of the bone ends and served to give stability to the fragments while the wound was closed and the limb put up in a fixation apparatus."

that it was not a form of gouty arthritis. It seemed most likely that it was a thickening of the tendon sheath at a specific point, i.e., at the fibrous extensor tunnel roofed by the extensor retinaculum. The functional disturbance was produced by an increase of friction at this point.

"On 7 March 1894, setting out with the idea that stenosis was the cause of the condition, I excised (under cocaine anaesthesia) the common tunnel of extensor pollicis brevis and abductor pollicis longus over a length of one centimeter, laying the tendons open to the subcutaneous tissue. The outer surface of the synovium showed not the slightest change; there was no effusion of fibrin, etc., and the underlying bone was sound. Only the excised tunnel of the tendon sheath seemed to show a certain thickening which was hard to define.

"After the operation the pain which the patient had previously felt disappeared, and, after the incision had healed per primam, she began to use her thumb again without trouble. A report on 7 March 1895 shows that the patient remained perfectly well and the lack of the tendon sheath tunnel caused her no disturbance."

He operated on a further case and describes three others seen by a colleague. On the basis of these cases he draws a clinical picture of the disorder.

"The patients feel more or less acute pain when moving the thumb; this radiates from the wrist to the thumb and the forearm and is of such degree that often they cannot continue to hold an object that they have picked up. Palpation shows either nothing or slight thickening of the tendon sheath tunnel at the distal end of the radius, which is in every case definitely tender to touch, whereas the rest of the tendon sheath is either less tender or not tender at all. This affection is always chronic."

De Quervain wondered why this should occur. Perhaps it is because the thumb is the most used digit and the radial styloid area is liable to injury. Kocher wrote to him about the condition and took the view that it began as an occupational hypertrophy of the tunnel. He compared it with Nelaton's description of trigger finger but observed that for no very obvious reason the secondary nodule in the tendon was absent. De Quervain, too, thought that the thickening of the tendon sheath or of its synovial lining was responsible for the condition and that the friction generated by the stenosis aggravated it.

He advocated surgery as the most rewarding method of treatment. He suggested a 4-cm incision in the line of the tendons, taking care to avoid the radial nerve. The roof of the tunnel should then be removed.

Trigger Finger in the German Army, 1897

Schulte described nine cases. He did some experiments and found that the tendon sheath checked movement. And when the arch at the entrance was divided, motion was easy.

Hand Infection

In 1912, A. B. Kanavel published a book, *Infections of the Hand.* In experiments, he demonstrated the tendon sheaths and fascial spaces in the hand, which are the clue to recognizing the spread of advanced infection.

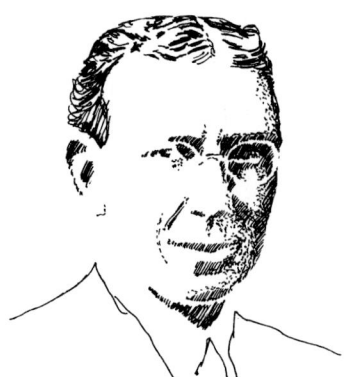

◆ A. B. Kanavel

Replantation

> **TIMELINE OF MICROSURGERY**
>
> 1906 Alexis Carrell: macrotechnique for experimental replantation
> 1917 Esser: island flaps
> 1921 Nylen of Sweden uses a microscope to dissect the inner ear of a rabbit.
> 1923 Holmgren introduces the Carl Zeiss binocular operating microscope for ear surgery.
> 1950s Kidney grafts begin.
> 1960 Jacobsen works on small vessel anastomosis.
> 1962 May 23: Ronald Malt replants a severed limb at the midarm level in Boston. Fifteen years later the patient is working as a truck driver delivering beef carcasses.
> 1962 November: Harold Kleinert reanastomosed a digital artery for a partially amputated thumb.
> 1964 J. W. Smith uses the microscope for nerve repair.
> 1968 July: first complete thumb replant by Komatsu and Tamai in Japan.
> 1970s Many replant services are organized, laboratories develop for training, and elective free transfers become frequent.

REPLANTATION
R. A. MALT, BOSTON, 1962

"Everett Knowles knew a severed arm lay within his sleeve and innocently assumed we could restore it. The idea didn't seem so far-fetched to the residents of the West Surgical Service either."   R. A. Malt and C. F. McKahn

◆ CASE 1

"A 12-year-old boy was brought to the Massachusetts General Hospital on May 23, 1962, 30 minutes after his right arm below the shoulder had been sheared from his body between the side of a freight train and a stone abutment.

"His blood pressure was 120/80 mm Hg and his pulse was 120 beats per minute. The end of the axillary artery, sealed with thrombus, was seen within the stump of the right shoulder. The dismembered arm was unblemished below the level of injury. There were no signs of damage to the central

nervous system, chest, or abdomen, but the tips of his left thumb and index and middle fingers were crushed.

"The severed arm was immersed in a mixture of ice and sodium chloride solution as blood transfusions were begun and tetanus toxoid and antitoxin given. When the vital signs became stable and no systemic injury was apparent, replantation was considered.

"To free the vascular system of altered blood and to detect covert damage the limb was removed to an operating room. There, intra-arterial perfusion was carried out, first with Ringer's solution containing sodium heparin, bacitracin, and neomycin sulfate, and then with 25% sodium diatrizoate for arteriography. As the X-ray picture of the arterial system was apparently normal and the boy's condition good, we decided to attempt reunion.

"Preparation of the stump was restricted to irrigation with Ringer's solution and removal of a few comminuted fragments of bone. Circulation was restored by an anastomosis of two brachial venae comites and then of the artery itself with No. 000000 polyester thread inserted by a modified Carrel technique. The bone was fixed by driving a Kuntscher intramedullary nail from the fracture site through the head of the humerus and by subsequently impacting the distal bone on the exposed length of nail. Corresponding ends of each of the four major nerves were joined with a marking stitch.

"By this time the extent of permanently devitalized tissue was obvious, so judicious debridement was possible. Healthy muscle was coapted with mattress sutures of chromic catgut, the remaining skin closed with silk, a spica cast applied and the injured fingers of the left hand repaired. A large denuded area over the deltoid muscle and a smaller one in the axilla were covered with split-thickness skin grafts five days later.

"No anticoagulants were used at any time during surgery or the postoperative period. Penicillin G and streptomycin sulfate were given intramuscularly for eight days and phenoxymethyl penicillin orally, for an additional five. The body temperature varied from 99° F (37.2° C) to 101° F (38.3° C) for six days, from 99° F to 100° F (37.8° C) for four more, and was thereafter normal until the boy was discharged from the hospital three weeks after entry. Intensive physiotherapy involving passive movements of all joints below the elbow and galvanic stimulation of accessible denervated muscles, begun early in the hospital stay, was continued daily until neurolysis on Sept. 11, 1962. (Plans for an earlier operation were deferred because of a paronychia.)

"Each of the four nerves in the upper arm was involved in a neuroma, 5 to 10 cm long. In addition, the distal end of the musculocutaneous nerve was severely scarred throughout its entire length, and the diameter of the distal radial nerve was uniformly only a fifth that of the proximal

segment. (Long gaps in these two nerves were bridged by free autogenous nerve grafts.) Lysis of the median and ulnar nerves well into the forearm and flexion of the elbow permitted generous resection and an end-to-end anastomosis of these structures, but a neuroma remained in each proximal segment as far proximal as could be discerned. A spica cast was again applied. Chloramphenicol and erythromycin readily controlled a postoperative staphylococcal cellulitis, and the patient left 11 days after surgery.

"Four months later, active contraction appeared in the flexor muscles of the forearm. Strength grew slowly for three months, then quite rapidly for three more. Movement of the opponens pollicis was detected 11 months after neurolysis, and by that time two-point discrimination and the sensations of temperature and light touch were present in all digits; contraction of the biceps was unequivocal. Bulk began to return to the hypothenar eminence after 14 months. Twenty months after neurolysis strength in the biceps, pronator, and the opponens pollicis was about 30% to 40% of normal and in the deep and superficial flexors of the fingers and wrist, over 80% of normal. Sensation had returned to the extent that a 200-mg hair, pain, and temperature could be appreciated in all fingers. Abduction of the shoulder was limited to 75' because of the nail impinging on the acromion, but was otherwise full. The elbow had normal flexion but lacked 10' of full extension. The boy could lift 10-lb weights and write his name. His interest and performance in school have improved.

"At 15 years post injury the patient has done extraordinarily well physically and psychologically. He works full time as a truck driver, moving heavy carcasses of beef."

Dupuytren's Contracture

It is strange that a disease that occurs nowadays in about one in five of the population over the age of 60 years, and is so obvious to all, did not attract attention until the last century. Surgeons, artists, and writers did not notice the condition, but players of bagpipes apparently called it the Curse of the MacCrimmons for centuries (D. Elliot). Not being a fan of the pipes, I had always assumed that every player had this condition, but in fact the contracture makes playing the pipes impossible.

Dupuytren certainly gave the best account of this contracture in a lecture at Hôtel Dieu, Paris, in 1833. This was published in the *Lancet* the following year, in accordance with Thomas Wakeley's plan to give publicity to the teachings of the men at the forefront of the profession. Apart from giving the condition the name of Dupuytren and acquainting doctors with the contracture, it encouraged one man, John Windsor, to look through lecture notes he had made as a student 25 years before. He had heard **Henry Cline** lecture on this in 1808 at St. Thomas' Hospital, London:

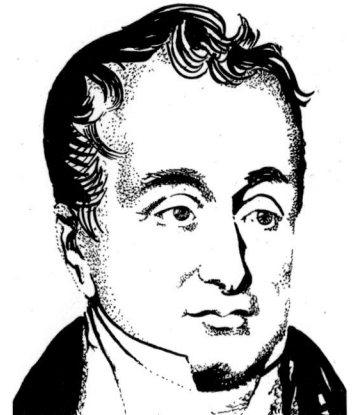

◆ Guillaume Dupuytren

"One or more of these tendinous columns of the aponeurosis palmaris sometimes becomes contracted and thickened; most generally only one is affected, but sometimes more and proportionably so many fingers are bent into the palm of the hand. The treatment is easy and efficacious; it consists in cutting through the aponeurosis with a common knife. In performing the operation, in order to avoid the blood vessels and nerves underneath, the fingers or finger may be kept extended afterwards by a splint, for the flexor muscle has in some degree become shortened and without this the disease might be reproduced."

In 1777 Cline wrote in his notebook:

"The contraction of the fingers which so frequently happens in laborious people, arises from a thickening of the fascia of the palm of the hand, without any alteration in the muscles and tendons. This has been seen in dissecting two subjects, in one all the fingers were contracted, but upon cutting through the fascia, they were immediately extended."

Astley Cooper, too, recognized the condition, writing about it in his treatise on dislocations and fractures of the joints in 1822:

"The fingers are sometimes contracted in a similar manner, by a chronic inflammation of the thecae, and the aponeurosis of the palm of the hand, from excessive action of the hand in the use of the hammer, the oar, ploughing, etc., etc. When the thecae is contracted, nothing should be attempted for the patient's relief, as no operation or other means will succeed; but when the aponeurosis is the cause of the contraction and the contracted band is narrow, it may be with advantage divided by a pointed history, introduced through a very small wound in the integument. The finger is then extended and a splint is applied to preserve it in the straight position."

PERMANENT RETRACTION OF THE FINGERS, PRODUCED BY AN AFFECTION OF THE PALMAR FASCIA
DUPUYTREN, 1833

"Retraction of the fingers, Gentlemen, and particularly that of the ring-finger, has been observed for many years, but it is only very lately that the cause of this deformity has been investigated with success.

"The greater number of individuals affected by this disease have been obliged to make efforts with the palm of the hand, or frequently to handle hard bodies. Thus the wine-merchant and coachman of whom we shall presently speak were obliged, the one to perforate continually the casks with a gimlet, the other to ply his whip unceasingly on the backs of his jaded horses; it is also seen in masons who lift stones with the extremities of the fingers, in ploughmen, etc.; hence we see that the disease occurs most frequently in those who are forced in working to make the palm of the hand a point d'appui. *Individuals who are predisposed to the disease of which we speak, perceive that they extend*

the fingers of the injured hand with less facility than usual; the ring-finger soon begins to contract; the deformity first attacks the proximal phalanx, and the others follow its movement: as the disease advances, the finger becomes more contracted, and the flexion of the two neighbouring fingers begins to be remarked. We do not feel any nodosity in front of the chord which runs along the palmar surface of the ring-finger; the two last phalanges are straight and movable at this period; and the proximal one is bent nearly at a right angle on the metacarpal bone, but still retains some motion; in this state it cannot be brought to its original position by the most violent effort. A person attacked by this infirmity attached to his finger a weight amounting to 150 pounds, without influencing in the least the degree of flexion. When the ring-finger is flexed to a great degree, the skin presents various folds, the convexity of which looks towards the articulation of the wrist.

"But you may ask, what are the inconveniences of this affection? As the ring-finger cannot be extended, the motion of the two neighbouring fingers is much limited; the patient can only seize a very small body; if he attempts to grasp it strongly, he feels great pain; the very act of catching any body is painful. A man, who had been for a long time affected with this disease, happened to die. I had kept my eye on him for some years, and was determined not to lose this opportunity of investigation. Accordingly I possessed myself of the arm of this man, had the state of parts accurately drawn by an artist, and then proceeded to dissect them. When the skin was removed from the palmar surface of the hand and fingers, the folds which I have before noticed, disappeared altogether. It was evident then that the folded arrangement of the skin during life depended on some other affection; but what was this? The dissection was continued by exposing the palmar fascia, and I was astonished to perceive that this fascia was tense, retracted, and shortened. From its lower portion were given off kinds of chords, which passed to the diseased finger. In flexing and extending the fingers, I could clearly see that the fascia underwent a sort of tension, or crackling; this was a trace of light, and made me suspect that the aponeurosis had some connexion with the complaint. But the precise point affected remained to be discovered. I cut through the prolongations extending from the fascia to the fingers; the state of contraction immediately ceased, and the slightest effort was sufficient to bring them to complete extension; the tendons were all sound, and the sheaths had not been opened; but in order to leave no doubt on the subject, I examined the tendons with care. Their surfaces were smooth, and they enjoyed their usual degree of motion. The joints also were in a healthy state, the bones were neither swollen nor changed in any degree. I could distinguish no alteration of the articular surfaces or ligaments. The synovial membranes, the synovial cartilages, all were sound. It was, therefore, natural to conclude that the disease commenced in an exaggerated tension of the palmar fascia, which depended on the violent or long-continued action of some hard body on the palm of the hand.

"Cases of Contraction of the Ring and Little Fingers Completely Cured by Division of the Palmar Aponeurosis

◆ CASE 1

In 1811, M. L., wine-merchant, having received from the South a great deal of wine, was desirous to assist his workmen in arranging the casks in the store. While endeavouring to raise one of the casks, which was very heavy, by placing his hand under the edge of the stave, he felt a sensation of cracking and a slight pain in the palm of his hand. For some time the part remained stiff and sensible, but these symptoms soon went off, and he paid little attention to the state of his hand. The accident was nearly forgotten, when he perceived that the ring-finger commenced to contract towards the palm of his hand, and could not be extended as much as the other fingers. As there was no pain, he neglected this slight deformity. By degrees the disease advanced, and made a sensible progress each year, so that in 1831 the little and ring fingers were completely flexed, and applied to the palm of the hand; the second phalanx was folded on the first and the extremity of the third applied to the middle of the ulnar edge of the palmar surface. The small finger was firmly flexed on the palm of the hand; and the skin of this part was folded, and dragged towards the retracted fingers.

"The patient, annoyed by seeing this deformity getting daily worse, consulted several surgeons, who all said that the disease existed in the flexor tendons, and advised their section as the only remedy; but some would cut both tendons, whilst others proposed to divide only one.

"The moment I saw the man's hand I recognized the affection of the palmar fascia, declared the disease was not situated in the tendons, and that a few incisions practised in the aponeurosis would be sufficient to restore entire freedom of motion to the finger.

"**Operation.** The hand of the patient being firmly fixed, I commenced the operation by making a transverse incision nearly an inch long, opposite the metacarpophalangeal articulation of the ring finger; the bistoury divided first the skin and then the palmar fascia, with a crackling sound perceptible to the ear; after this incision the ring-finger recovered its position and could be extended nearly as completely as ever. As I was desirous to spare the patient the pain of a new incision, I attempted to prolong the division of the fascia by gliding the bistoury deeply under the skin towards the ulnar edge of the hand, in order to free, if possible, the little finger; but this attempt failed. I was in consequence obliged to make another transverse incision opposite the articulation of the first and second phalanx of the little finger, which enabled me to detach it from the palm of the hand, but the rest of the finger remained obstinately fixed towards this part. A new incision, however, divided the skin and fascia opposite the metacarpal joint of the finger, to give it some slight liberty; finally, a third transverse cut was made opposite the *middle of the first phalanx, and immediately extension of the finger was easily accomplished; this proved clearly that the last incision had divided the point of insertion of the fascial process. The wounds were simply dressed with dry lint, and the fingers kept in a state of extension by a suitable apparatus.*

"***Progress of the Case.*** *Next day, little pain; merely some uneasiness from the continued extension. On the following day the back of the hand was slightly oedematous from the pressure of the apparatus, which was clumsily made; another was applied, but the state of irritation continued, great pain set in, and the hand became much swollen. Not wishing to remove the machine applied to extend the fingers, I ordered the hand to be bathed continually with Goulard's solution, which gave considerable relief. On the 15th we found some suppuration had set in; the hand was still swollen and painful. Extension was continued to the same degree as formerly, and the cold lotion applied. On the 16th the swelling had abated considerably, the fingers remained stiff, and suppuration was fully established. 17th: The symptoms were more favourable, and the extension could be increased somewhat without determining any pain. Finally, in the course of some days the swelling of the hand disappeared, and the wounds were healed on the 2nd of July.*

"*The cause of this slowness in the cicatrization depended, without doubt, on the forced extension in which the fingers were constantly kept. The patient continued to carry the apparatus for another month, in order to oppose the reunion of the edges of the divided fascia; and when at length this was removed, we had the satisfaction of seeing that he could flex his fingers with facility, and that the stiffness which remained was only due to the forced extension in which the articulations were held for so long a time; but this rigidity disappeared when the patient had, for a short time, resumed his accustomed exercises.*

"***Remarks.*** *This case can leave no doubt of the nature of the disease but we may be inclined to ask, how can the palmar fascia determine similar effects? To answer this question, we must recall to your memory a few anatomical particulars concerning this fibrous envelope. The superficial palmar fascia is partly formed by the expansion of the tendon of the palmaris longus, and of the anterior portion of the annular ligament of the wrist. Though very strong in its origin, it thins by degrees, and sends off from its inferior margin four fibrous slips, which pass towards the inferior extremity of the four last metacarpal bones; here each of these slips bifurcates for the passage of the flexor tendons, and each branch of the bifurcated slip passes on to be attached to the side, and not to the front, of the phalanx, as most anatomists have thought. These are the slips of fascia which should be cut, whenever the operation becomes necessary. When we dissect off the skin from the fascia beneath, we find a certain difficulty in separating it, because the* *cellular tissue is dense, and because various fibrous filaments pass from the fascia into the integument; these adhesions explain readily the wrinkled state of the skin, and its motion. At first sight we might be inclined to dread cutting the nerves and vessels of the finger, but these parts are well protected by a kind of bridge formed by the contracted fibres, and run no risk of being divided."*

William Heberden (1710–1801)

He was born in London and studied medicine, partly at Cambridge and partly in London. Having taken his degree of Doctor of Physic, he practiced in the University for about ten years, and then settled in London and was elected into the Royal Society. He very soon ran a big practice.

In 1766 he recommended to the College of Physicians the first design of the *Medical Transactions*, one of the first medical journals. He declined all professional business several years before his death, which was mercifully postponed until the year 1801, when he had advanced to the age of 91.

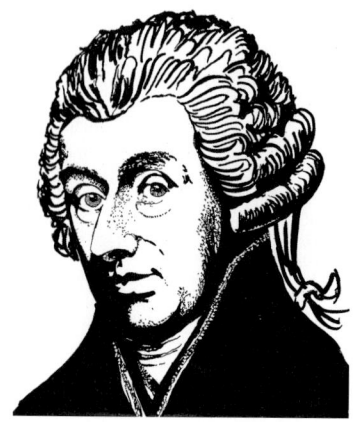

◆ William Heberden

HEBERDEN'S NODES, 1802

*"**Digitorum Nodi.** What are those little hard knobs, about the size of a small pea, which are frequently seen upon the fingers, particularly a little below the top, near the joint? They have no connection with the gout, being found in persons who never had it: they continue for life and being hardly ever attended with pain, or disposed to become sores, are rather unsightly than inconvenient, though they must be some little hindrance to the free use of the fingers."*

Robert Kienbock (1871–1953)

He studied in Vienna and after travel, started a medical clinic with radiology as a sideline. Soon it became his main occupation. He wrote on both diagnostic and therapeutic radiology, with a particular interest in bone. He wrote about avascular necrosis of the lunate in 1910. Although much handicapped after being thrown from a horse in midcareer, he continued to be productive.

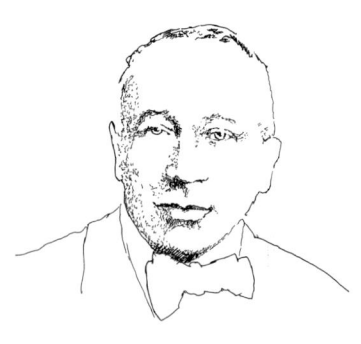

◆ Robert Kienbock

CONCERNING TRAUMATIC MALACIA OF THE LUNATE AND ITS CONSEQUENCES: DEGENERATION AND COMPRESSION FRACTURES

ROBERT KIENBOCK, 1910

"There is a characteristic traumatic lesion of the lunate which occurs alone, or in association with analogous changes in the navicular, or with fractures of the navicular, triquetrum, epiphysis of the radius, and styloid process of the ulna. It apparently arises as a result of a contusion or sprain of the wrist, especially in the case of a dorsal perilunar dislocation in association with tears of the interosseous ligaments and blood vessels. The disturbance of nutrition which follows leads to a weakening

and progressive porosis evidenced by sclerosis and gradual wearing away of the proximal portion of the lunate, and finally in the decay of the bone.

"The diagnosis can be made only on the basis of the X-ray findings. On the anteroposterior view of the wrist one can find changes in the form and structure of the bone, beginning in the proximal portion. This shows itself as a spotty irregularity with areas of increased and decreased density corresponding to the weakening and atrophy of the bone. Later on, one finds occasionally defects and sclerosis in the remaining portion of the bone. The bone is often abnormally flattened, the proximal portion appears to disappear, showing only as a thin shadow, as the bone wears away. In the oblique views of the wrist, the flattening of the bone is more obvious. Here one can see the results of compression and wearing away. One may also see small pieces of bone debris.

"The diagnosis cannot be made on clinical grounds as a rule. In acute cases, only swelling of the wrist is noted. In other cases the following factors point toward the diagnosis. There is often diffuse swelling of the wrist with pain on motion and limitation of motion in all directions. Occasionally crepitus can be elicited on dorsiflexion of the wrist. With the wrist in volar flexion there may be a pressure-sensitive prominence on the dorsum of the wrist over the lunate. Rarely, distinct moveable fragments can be palpated. Sometimes percussion over the head of the third metacarpal (the hand held in a fist) may produce pain over the lunate. Occasionally the wrist bone may be shortened as measured from the distal radius to the base of the third metacarpal.

"Over a period of months and years, the surface of the proximal portion of the lunate will be worn away, becoming generally smaller. The joint surface of the adjacent radius will be damaged and the cartilage destroyed. Finally, the lunate can become fragmented into two or more small pieces. Arthritis deformans, however, does not spread to the other neighboring carpal bones.

"In the beginning, treatment consists of the usual measures; massage, hot packs, hot air, etc. Similar treatments are used later on for recurrent swelling, but in the fact of progressing bone destruction, they are, on the whole, worthless. In cases with severe difficulty, considerable pain and disability, the lunate can be excised.

"At operation, the proximal portion of the lunate is found to be fragmented. The fragments are held, loosely bound, in connective tissue. The radiocarpal joint is covered with thick, yellow connective tissue. After decades, at post mortem examination, the anatomic findings are the same. The proximal portion of the lunate has been destroyed for the most part. The major portions of the articulating surfaces for the navicular, capitate, hamate, and triquetrum are reasonably well preserved. Usually the lunate is found in two equal-sized fragments, one volar and one dorsal.

"This traumatic lesion of the lunate is quite common, occurring perhaps as frequently as the similar lesion in the navicu-

lar. It is treated, since it initially was considered to be only a contusion or sprain, only when it causes increasing difficulty. The patient usually does not complain of the minor episode of injury, but considers an earlier, more severe injury as causing the condition. This should be considered in rendering a medical legal opinion."

Otto Madelung (1846–1926)

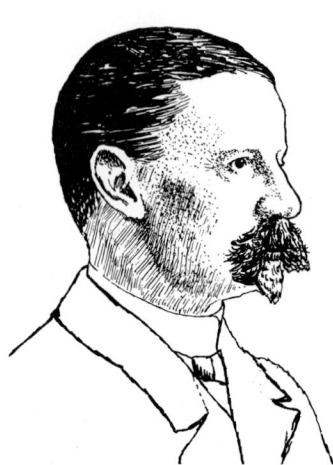

◆ Otto Madelung

Madelung was an abdominal surgeon—he flourished during the time that surgery was beginning to have something to offer the patient with abdominal disease. His orthopaedic contributions, though they caused his name to decorate textbooks, were slight.

He was born in Gotha, the son of a merchant, and he studied at Bonn and Tübingen. After serving in the Franco-Prussian war of 1871 he settled in Bonn, and during this time he wrote his paper on wrist deformity. He became assistant professor of surgery at Bonn in 1881, then at Rostock before becoming professor at Strasbourg in 1894, where he was the youngest member of the medical faculty. He built up the hospital at Strasbourg along German lines and continued to work there until the city was recovered by the French at the end of the First World War. Then all the German professors were replaced by French, and after a period under house arrest, he retired to Göttingen.

Apart from his work on intestinal resections, intestinal typhoid, obstruction, and so on, he was one of the first advocates of early laparotomy for abdominal injuries. In 1909 he described arthrotomy of the shoulder from behind. His description of deformity at the wrist was not original, and only a little more complete than descriptions by Dupuytren and R. W. Smith which had appeared many years previously.

It is difficult to give much impression of his personality—someone described him as a "serious and conscientious man with a powerful will," and this rather stern picture is supported by one of his sayings: "*Every clinical lesson must be prepared and conducted in such a way that every student who contemplates missing the class must feel that he would miss something important.*"

SPONTANEOUS ANTERIOR SUBLUXATION OF THE HAND
OTTO MADELUNG, 1878

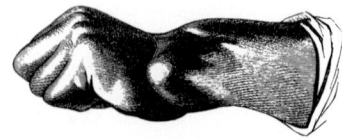

Madelung's deformity.

"The deformity is most noticeable looking at the subluxation from the ulnar side. The forearm is apparently normally formed. The distal end of the ulna is distinct under the normal though rather tense skin and the styloid process and articular surface can be recognised with the eye and encircled by the finger. The hand viewed on its own is normal but has dropped forwards. The diameter of the wrist is almost twice the normal.

"The hand, viewed from the radial side, is less obviously displaced forwards. The extensor tendons, which pass over the radius towards the dorsum of the hand, bridge and obscure the step that was so noticeable on the ulnar side. The antero-posterior diameter appears to be almost doubled. When the distal end of the radius is palpated with the hand dorsiflexed, i.e., with the extensor tendons relaxed, a large portion of the articular surface of the radius may be palpated. At the same time it is noticeable that the posterior lip of the lower end of the radius, which is normally rather sharp, has become more obtuse. If it is compared with the radius of the healthy side it is noticed that the whole distal epiphysis of the radius is angulated volarwards. In some cases, when the hand is inspected in the neutral position between flexion and extension, there is slight deviation of the hand radially and sometimes laterally. Viewed anteriorly, the bridge-like prominence of the flexor tendons, particularly flexor carpi radialis, flexor carpi ulnaris, and palmaris longus, becomes noticeable."

Madelung regarded the condition as a defect of growth of the wrist joint. It was not due to trauma or infection. Heavy work by young people produced more pressure on the anterior part of the distal radial epiphysis than on the posterior part. In those with "primary weakness of bone," this degree of pressure may cause the anterior part of the epiphysis to stop growing. As a result the lower end of the radius comes to be angulated forward. The carpal bones are also compressed and show changes.

Today, this deformity is regarded as a frequent feature of dyschondrosteosis.

Treatment was not successful. Surgically replaced hands relapsed. However, Madelung noted that the pain disappeared after a time even when the subluxation was gross, and that the capacity for work was not impaired.

PARTIAL EXCISION OF LOWER SHAFT OF ULNA FOR DEFORMITY FOLLOWING COLLES' FRACTURE
WILLIAM DARRACH, 1913

The patient had a malunited fracture with pain, limitation of motion, and radial shortening only 7 weeks after fracture.

"It was decided to shorten the ulna, preserving the ulnar articular surface.

"Through a small posterior incision the lower end of the ulna was exposed, its periosteum carefully reflected and about half an inch of shaft removed. The bone was cut through with cutting forceps, resulting in a good deal of splintering, an effort thus being made to obtain a more rapid regeneration."

The range of movement improved, but the ulnar osteotomy was un-united at the time of the report. This is interesting, because many people believe that he shortened the ulna by removing the articular end.

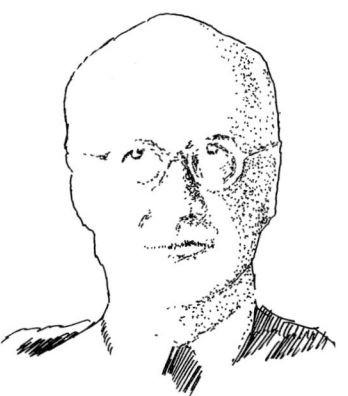

◆ **William Darrach (1876–1948)**
He was a Yale graduate who worked in New York. He became dean of medicine at Columbia and played a big part in building up the Columbia–Presbyterian Medical Center before resigning and running the fracture service. He was a negotiator and teacher.

References

Chapter references are located in Chapter 26.

◆ Chapter Six

Deformity of the Spine

Scoliosis

Scoliosis has been a major concern since the beginning of recorded time. Although it is much less frequent than back pain, all the early interest was on visible deformity rather than on hidden suffering. So there were many scoliosis institutes and publications during the last 300 years; however, we are still no nearer understanding the cause of idiopathic scoliosis. There is still contention as to whether bracing makes any difference. Arthrodesis, which has been given up for most conditions, is still used; indeed, we are still devising implants to create a more secure arthrodesis of the crooked spine.

Early on, scoliosis was distinguished from tuberculosis of the spine. Scoliosis was a benign condition, whereas tuberculosis produced a gibbus, wasting, paraplegia, and death.

Title page of Pravaz's book, 1827.

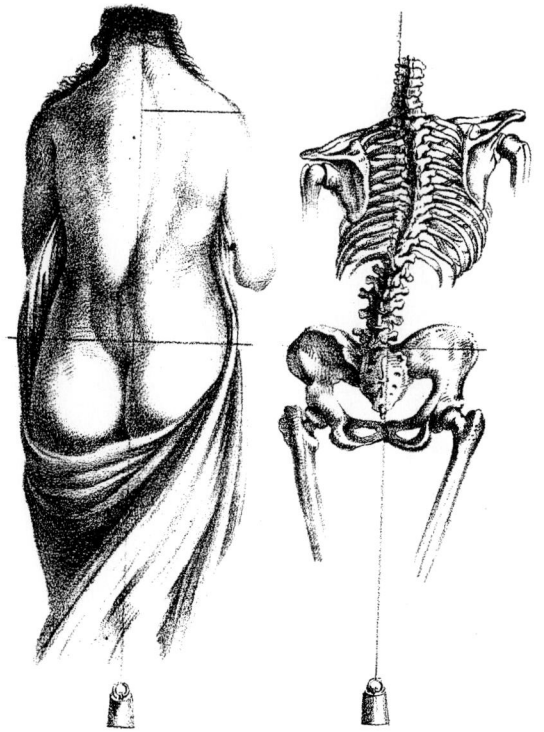

From Pravaz, 1827.

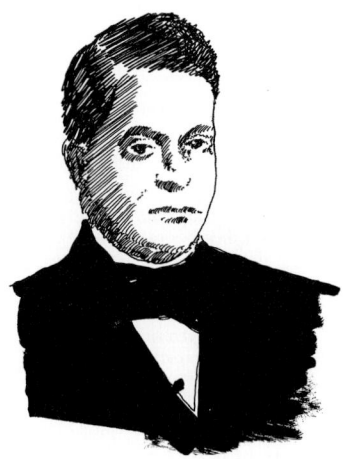

◆ **Charles Gabriel Pravaz (1791–1853)**

He founded an orthopaedic institute in Paris and took Guérin into partnership. He used traction for scoliosis. He is known for his *Balançoire Orthopaedique*. In 1834 he moved to Lyon and started to reduce developmental dysplasia of the hip.

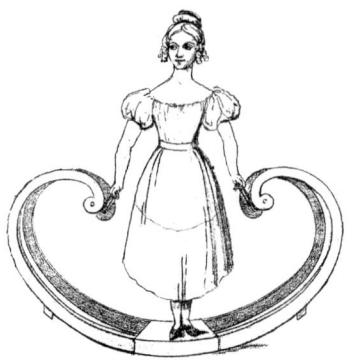

Rocker exerciser for scoliosis. From Edward Duffin: Lateral Deformity of the Spine, 2nd ed. London: 1835.

Famous People with Scoliosis

The Mysterious Scoliosis of Catherine the Great (1729–1796). About 18 months after Catherine was born, her mother gave birth to a crippled son, Wilhelm. Mother loved him idolatrously, whereas Catherine was ill treated. The son died at age 12 and at autopsy was found to have congenital dislocation of the hip.

At the age of 7 years, Catherine was kneeling at prayer when cough and delirium struck. For three weeks she lay on her left side. When she was able to sit up, her body had taken the form of

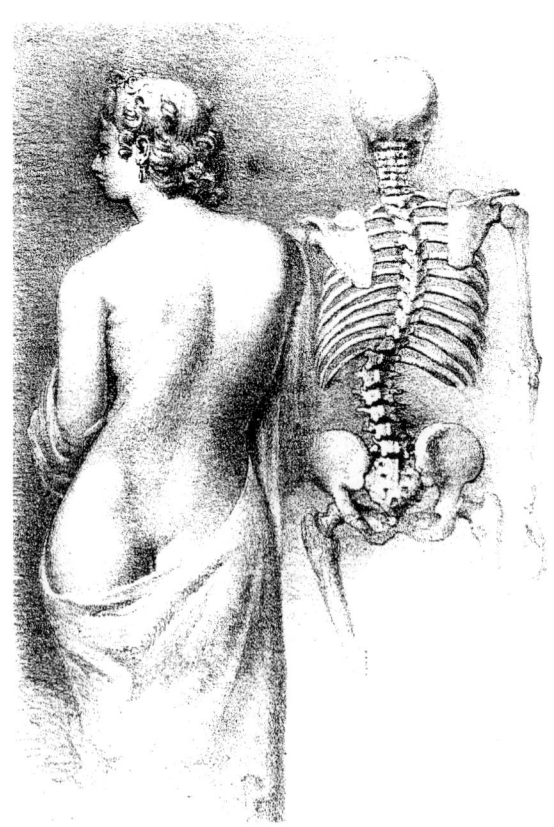

Title page of Beale's book, 1833.

Lionel J. Beale used this as the frontispiece for his book on deformity in 1833.

a Z. *The right shoulder was higher than the left, the backbone had a zigzag form, and the left shoulder was hollow.*

The local executioner was summoned to treat this. He advised daily massage with the saliva of a girl who had not eaten breakfast. He made a brace and checked it every other day for three years. Then she was straight.

Catherine became one of the great leaders of Europe and was generally believed to be a nymphomaniac. However, she had a great fear of venereal disease and had her Scottish doctor, Dr. Rogerson, examine her lovers first. He did well, because she lived to the age of 66 years.

What was this mysterious disease that was so successfully treated? Perhaps it was a chest infection; old books on scoliosis show deformities due to pleurisy and empyema. Although this may have been a common cause of scoliosis in the past, it is rare today.

Quasimodo. The Hunchback of Notre Dame was driven deaf by the church bells; he was a foundling with one eye and knock-knee who roared around the cathedral. What is the diagnosis here? Proteus syndrome.

Alexander Pope (1688–1744). This leading English poet was a lifelong cripple, standing only 4′6″ tall, with a hunchback. It was difficult for him to stand up without a corset. His legs were so thin that he wore 3 pairs of stockings. I imagine that he had a congenital scoliosis.

He wrote these well-known lines:

That long disease my life

♦

To err is human, to forgive divine.

♦

Hope springs eternal in the human breast.

Title page of Delpech's book, 1828.

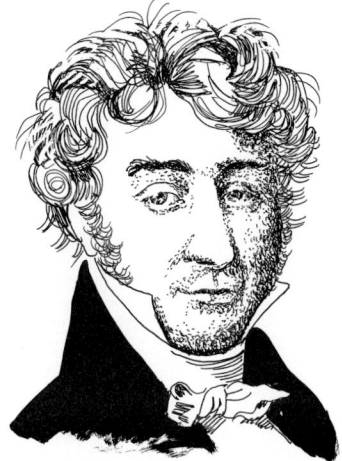

◆ **Jacques-Mathieu Delpech (1777–1832)**

A surgeon in Montpellier who pioneered tenotomy on 6 May 1816, but then stopped because of problems with infection. He founded an Orthopaedic Institute in 1825, where girls with idiopathic scoliosis were treated by continuous correction, using exercises, traction in bed at night, and suspension by day. In 1828 he wrote his classic book, *De L'Orthomorphie*, with an atlas. He was murdered by a patient he had operated on for varicocele.

146 *Chapter 6* ♦ Deformity of the Spine

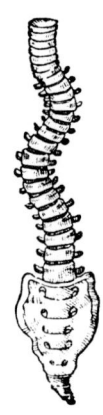

This is perhaps the earliest picture of scoliosis. Guilhelmus F. Hildanus, 1652.

♦ **Robert Chessher of Hinckley (1750–1831)**

The stepson of a surgeon, he never wrote a paper or a book and had no followers and is known only from references to his work by others. He lived in the nonoperative days of orthopaedics; he invented the double inclined plane, a splint for leg fractures, and a spinal brace bearing similarities to the Milwaukee brace. The idea was to take the weight of the head off the spine.

It was said of him, *"He appears more anxious to do good than to make money."* He was featured in George Eliot's novel *Middlemarch*: *"I remember Mr Cheshire and his irons, trying to make people straight when the Almighty had made them crooked."* In those Victorian days some people regarded treatment as fighting God's Will.

TIMELINE OF SCOLIOSIS
Pre-19th Century

300 BC Hippocrates   Lateral curves due to "the positions in which patients lie"
1575   Paré's metal jacket for scoliosis
1641   Ulhoorn in Holland—overhead traction in a chair
1652   Claes and Peter Schot are running a scoliosis clinic in Utrecht.
1652   Hildanus—first picture of a scoliotic spine
1666   Johannes Scultetus: pictures of straightening the spine on a scannum—Hippocrates' Traction Table.
1671   Francis Glisson believes that rickets is the cause of scoliosis and devises swing suspension by head and armpits, "The English Swing."
1719   Lorenz Heister, iron cross splint for scoliosis
1742   Andry: *"The shoulder that carries the burthen rises always higher than that which is not loaded."* He had pictures of poor sitting posture and advised carrying books on the high shoulder side.
1772   Antoine Portal, axillary crutches in a chair
1778   Robert Chessher, scoliosis clinic in Hinckley, England
1783   Timothy Sheldrake's book, an essay on the various causes and effects of the distorted spine. He and his brother made braces for scoliosis patients.
1789   J. A. Venel has a traction bed for sleep.
1792   David van Gesscher—metal vertical brace with pressure on prominences
1796   Erasmus Darwin, neck swing

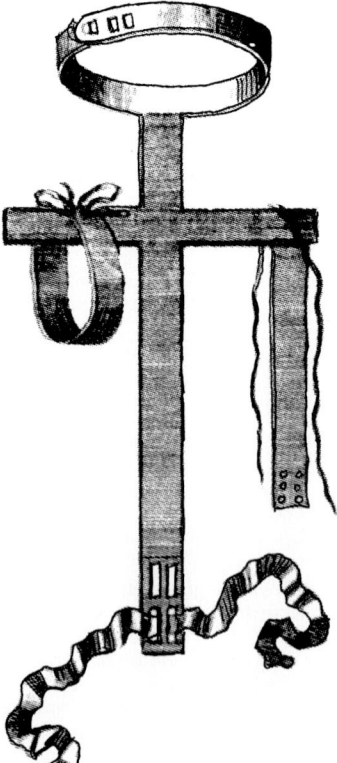

The iron cross scoliosis brace. From Heister, 1719.

◆ Jean Andre Venel (1740–1791)

Born in Switzerland, he studied in Geneva and started work as a surgeon in 1763 in Orbe. He went on to study obstetrics in Paris and Strasburg and in 1770 went to work for a Polish count. In 1775 he settled in Yverdon; the following year he wrote a book on health and medicine for women about to get married. In 1778 he wrote a book and started a school for midwives. He developed an interest in clubfeet and studied in Montpellier before returning to Orbe, where he bought an old abbey and started an orthopedic hospital in 1780. It was staffed with orthotists and teachers. He kept plaster casts and drawings of the patients to document change. Venel had a mechanical turn of mind and built machines for correction of deformity. He developed a day brace for scoliosis, and when it came off the child went into an orthopedic bed to relax with traction at night. The idea of an orthopedic bed became very popular, and his successors, such as Heine and Delpech, developed their own. His clubfoot brace became famous though the design went with him to his grave. He achieved a lot in 51 years and rivals Andry for the title "Father of Orthopaedics." He died of tuberculosis.

The 19th Century

- 1821 Borella, screw plate compression of the hump
- 1827 Jalade-Lafond, oscillating bed
- 1827 Pravaz, *Balançoire Orthopédique*
- 1828 J. M. Delpech writes *Orthomorphie*. This is illustrated with many pictures of before and after plaster casts of scoliosis. He used traction and exercises and no braces. His results were dramatic.
- 1829 Dieffenbach catalogues the various special beds and chairs—it takes 70 pages. It would seem that every parent concerned about their child's posture was likely to be taken in by these gadgeteers.
- 1831 Stromeyer: "*It is so easy and important to make the spine straight momentarily, while nothing is more difficult than to make the causes disappear which cause irregular nutrition of the bone.*"
- 1835 J. Hossard, surgical mechanic in Paris. A three-point pressure brace with girdle used muscles to correct curve. He showed an excellent result. Guérin thought this was fraudulent and said so, provoking a legal action. Guérin paid out damages.
- 1839 J. Guérin uses traction and then subcutaneous tenotomy. The publication of his results led to criticism and a retaliatory legal case which Guérin lost.
- 1840 Guérin: "*Lateral curvature of the vertebral column is the clubfoot of the back—that is, a contracture of the muscles of the spine.*"
- 1858 S. H. V. Bouvier wrote a book on chronic disorders of the locomotor system, with beautiful engravings depicting scoliotic spines and the effect of spinal deformity on the lungs, heart, and abdomen. He used traction for treatment.

◆ Jean Andre Venel (1740–1791)

Title page of Bouvier's book, 1858.

◆ Sauveur-Henri Victor Bouvier 1799–1877

Born and educated in Paris, he took over an orthopaedic institute started by a patient, and joined the Children's Hospital in 1831. He published his lecture series on disorders of the locomotor system in 1858. It included an atlas illustrating the pathology, equipment, and results of care. For scoliosis he used traction rather than braces. Almost blind, he died when he fell into the cold waters of the Tuileries Gardens.

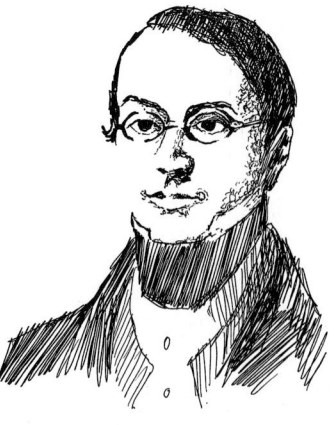

◆ Sauveur-Henri Victor Bouvier 1799–1877

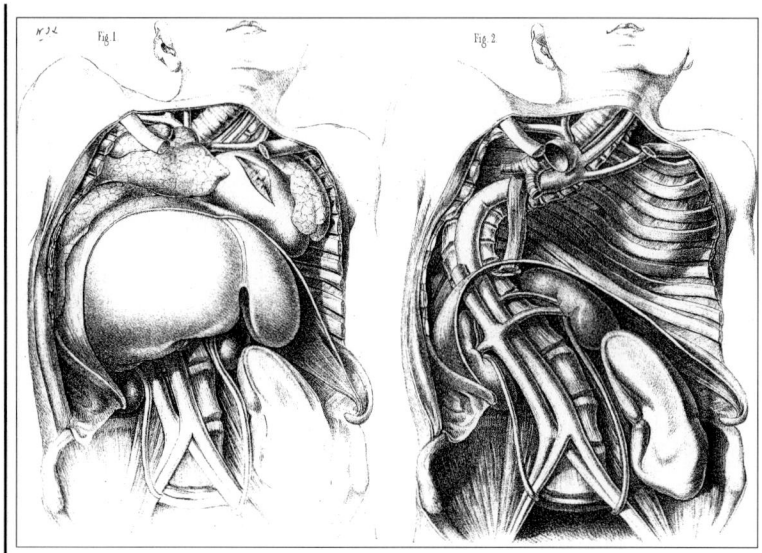

Bouvier was well aware that crowding of the viscera was produced by scoliosis.

◆ **Edward Harrison (1766–1838)**

He founded an Institute for Diseases of Curvature of the Spine in Lincolnshire. He wrote a book about scoliosis, a tract on Sarah Hawkes, and gave his name to Harrison's sulcus.

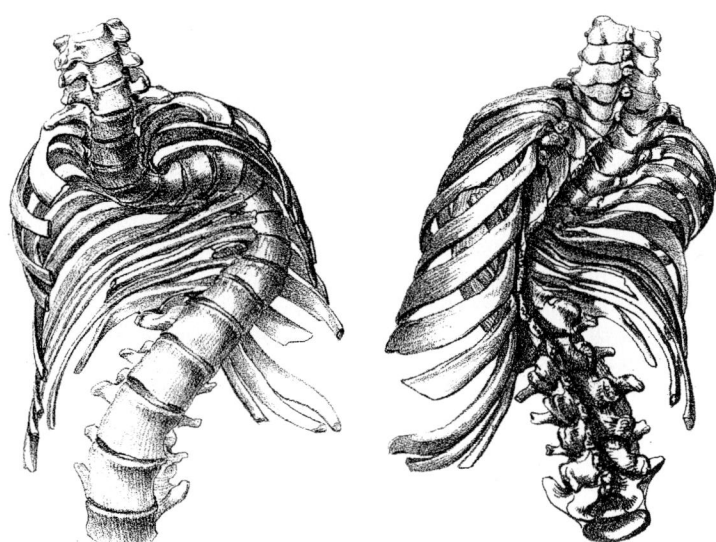

Bouvier illustrated many scoliotic spines.

◆ **James Knight (1810–1887)**

Baltimore graduate and New York City surgeon from 1835. A "surgico-mechanic," he used his home as a hospital for the New York Society for the Relief of the Ruptured and Crippled. He refused to have an operating room because he did not believe in operations or plaster—he used bandages and splints. Only after he died were these introduced. He was an autocrat. When one of his staff, Gibney, wrote a book on the hip in 1884 mentioning traction and operation, Gibney had to resign.

In 1868 Knight wrote *The Improvement of the Health of Children and Adults by Natural Means* and, with Gibney's help, *Orthopaedia* in 1874.

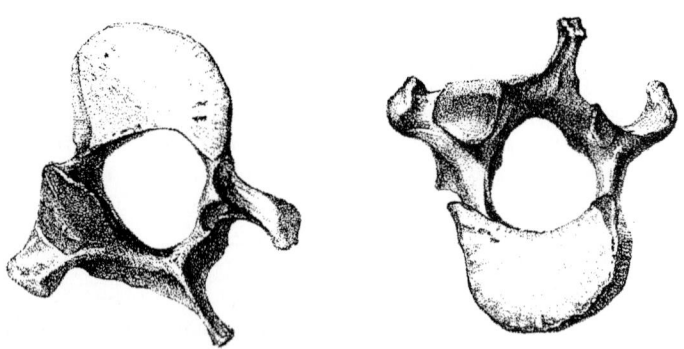

Bouvier showed the deformity of the individual vertebrae. As we struggle today to straighten the spine and restore symmetry to the chest, we should remember this picture.

◆ Charles Fayette Taylor (1827–1899)

A Vermonter, he studied the Swedish exercises and thought these were the answer. He wrote a book in 1861: *Theory and Practice of the Movement Cure.* He invented a back brace that he used on Theodore Roosevelt's sister. In 1867 he wrote on polio. A nonsurgeon. He resigned when a New York orthopedic clinic built by Teddy Roosevelt was turned into New York Orthopaedic Hospital.

Bauer had views on the patented Taylor brace. He said it should be freely available. *"Dr. Taylor need not have gone to the expense of patenting this, because it is not likely to be employed by anyone else."*

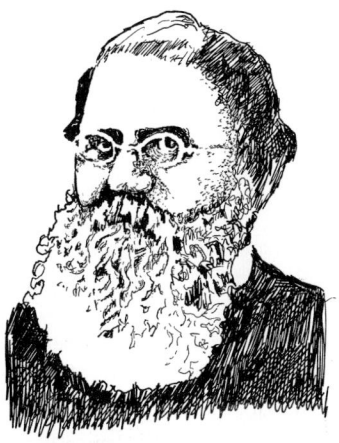

◆ Charles Fayette Taylor (1827–1899)

1861 Charles Fayette Taylor in the United States advocates exercises.
1864 Adams' forward bend test
1865 Heather Bigg, an engineer, writes *Orthopraxy; The Mechanical Treatment of Deformities, Debilities and Deficiencies of the Human Frame.*
1877 Lewis Sayre's book about serial plaster casts applied with the patient in vertical traction
1883 Wilhelm Schulthess opens a clinic in Zurich, using a machine for measuring the 3-D deformity.

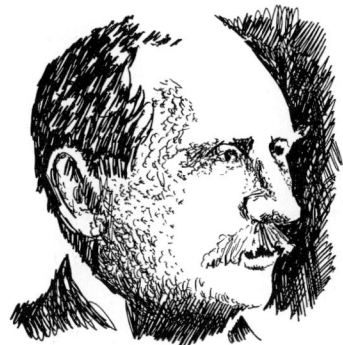

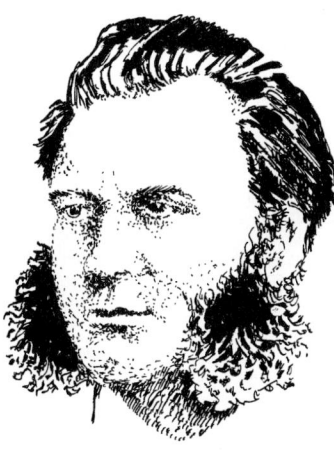

◆ Lewis Albert Sayre (1820–1900)

Born in New Jersey and worked in New York City. First American professor at Bellevue. Lister visited him and was impressed. He wrote a book on spinal disease and spinal curvature in 1877, describing his methods of suspension and casting—a forerunner of the Boston brace treatment of scoliosis. Also known for bone lengthening, tenotomies, immediate closure of myelomengocele, an inflatable tourniquet, and a book on clubfoot; he maintained fractures as a part of orthopaedics.

He was President of the American Medical Association in 1880 and a founder of the *Journal of the American Medical Association.* He initiated several public health measures in New York. A strong, high-profile person.

◆ Louis Bauer (1814–1898)

Born in Stettin, he studied with Stromyer and was jailed for his political views. He was a refugee with Little in London and translated Bishop's book on deformities into German. He went to the United States in 1853, aged 39, and founded the Orthopaedic Institution of Brooklyn in 1854. He wrote the second textbook of orthopaedics in the United States in 1864. He was a member of the rest school: immobilization must be absolute and unconditional. He was critical of his colleagues and left under duress for St. Louis in 1869. His writing was polemic.

He wrote one of the first American textbooks in 1868. The review! *"The term Orthopaedia applied to surgery—literally the rectifying by education—is defined to be the prevention and treatment of deformities. Once but little known, it has now grown into a great specialty.*

"We regret that the author cannot avoid the besetting sins of the class he espouses—that of criticizing all brother specialists. We can also readily pardon the errors in style and finish on account of the foreign origin of the writer; but we do think he . . . uses too many long words—Spondylitis, Kyphosis. . . ."

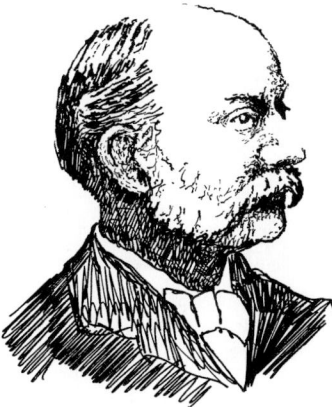

◆ Newton Melman Shaffer (1846–1928)

A New Yorker and a nonsurgeon—he referred cases that needed an operation to the general surgeons. He was second President of American Orthopaedic Association and active in the New York City scene. He wrote a book on the *Hysterical Element in Orthopaedics* in 1880.

Box continued on following page

◆ John Ridlon (1852–1936)

A New Yorker who visited Hugh Owen Thomas in 1888. On his return he made a Thomas splint and put it on a patient at St. Luke's Hospital. Shaffer ordered it off and Ridlon lost his job. Thomas wrote a vituperative book in Ridlon's defense, *An Argument with the Censor of St. Luke's Hospital,* and sent a copy to every orthopaedic surgeon in the world. Ridlon moved to Chicago but fell on hard times. In response to a letter, Robert Jones sent him a thousand dollars to keep him going. Later Ridlon became President of the American Orthopaedic Association.

◆ Pehr Henrik Ling (1776–1839)

A Swedish fencing teacher who started the application of exercises to medicine.

◆ Jonas Zander (1835–1920)

Stockholm. He invented powered machines to exercise patients passively or using resisted exercises. They were popular during World War I.

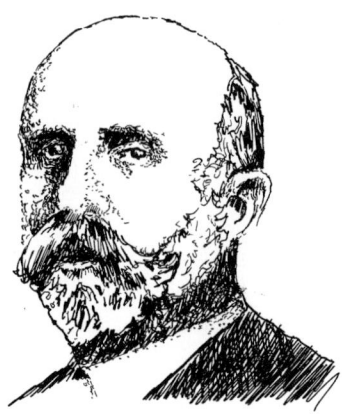

◆ Virgil Gibney (1847–1927)

Kentucky-born. Worked at Bellevue in New York City. He worked with the nonsurgeon Knight at the Ruptured and Crippled Hospital, resigned, and then after Knight died he was reappointed and turned it into a real hospital. However, another 50 years elapsed before it became the Hospital for Special Surgery. Gibney was the first President of the American Orthopaedic Association.

He wrote 176 papers. He was a surgeon at a time when many orthopaedists were not. Just suppose that the antisurgeon wing had won—where would we all be now?

1889 Volkmann operates on the rib prominence, improving appearance, and he allowed some correction of the deformity by traction.
1890 Alfred Schanz: traction, manipulation under anesthesia, and serial plaster casts
1891 Hadra rods
1893 Bradford and Brackett in Boston use recumbent traction, local pressure, and a plaster jacket. Many others do this and add derotation forces.
1897 Calot in France—forcible correction under anesthesia

The 20th Century

1900 Robert Lovett starts writing on lateral curvature.
1910 Lange rods
1911 Russell Hibbs fuses the spine for tuberculosis and suggests it for scoliosis. He does an in situ fusion in 1914 and later corrects the curve with a cast and then fuses; he reports increasing series in 1917, 1924, and 1931. He advocates a long fusion undertaken before the deformity becomes severe.
1924 Lovett and Brewster—turnbuckle cast

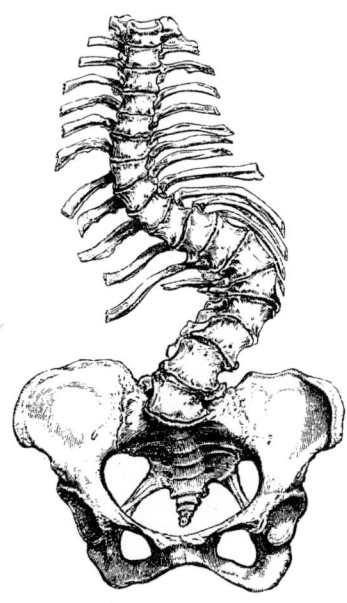

Thoracolumbar scoliosis. Many of the old books pictured skeletons. There were no X-rays to depict the condition, and people died young and poor. From Bernard Brodhurst: The Deformities of the Human Body. London, 1871.

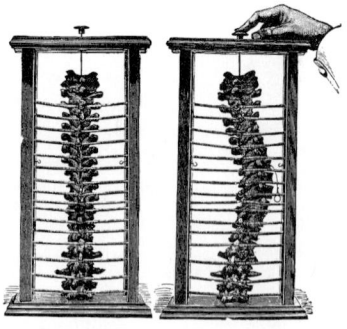

Explaining the rotation that accompanies a lateral curve. Judson's experiment illustrated in Young JK: Orthopaedic Surgery. Philadelphia, 1894.

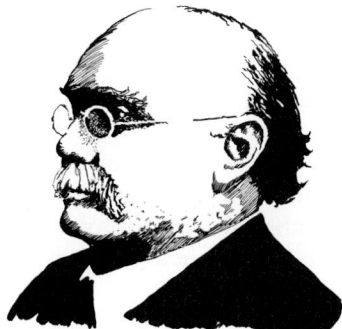

◆ **De Forest Willard (1846–1910)**
Like Little, he had a polio foot deformity that was treated by tenotomy. He became a pediatric surgeon and wrote a book in 1910. He is known for costotransversectomy and nerve grafting.

1929 Arthur Steindler in Iowa—nonoperative methods of increasing the compensatory curves to achieve "shoulders square over the pelvis, pelvis square over the ankles"
1931 Risser: hinged correction cast with turnbuckles
1936 Fergusson method of measuring the curve
1948 Cobb angle described
1954 Paul Harrington in Houston, Texas, is awarded a grant to develop his rods and starts the intraoperative correction of deformity in polio curves and then in idiopathic scoliosis. After he published a paper in 1962, the method quickly spread to other centers.
1954 Bount and Schmidt introduce the Milwaukee brace
1958 Risser sign
1966 John Moe—first President of the Scoliosis Research Society
1969 Allan Dwyer in Australia—anterior instrumentation
1970s Boston brace
1984 Cotrel Dubousset derotation system

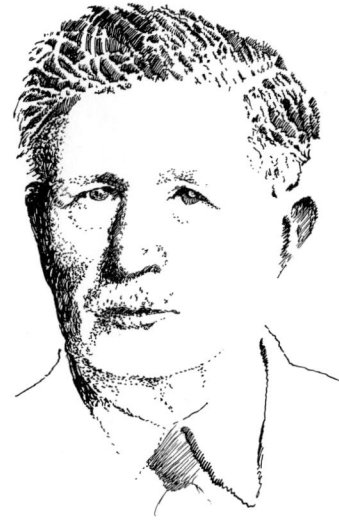

◆ **Rudolf Klapp (1873–1949)**
He studied in Wurzburg and worked in Berlin. Like many before him, he invented scoliosis exercises—the crawling method—and I am sure this delighted many parents.

Title page of Duffin's book, 1835.

Pathology

People used to die young, so that opportunities to study the skeleton in scoliosis were greater then than now. Bouvier's engravings of the bones are among the best, but there were many others. The rotation that accompanies lateral curvature was appreciated and demonstrated in models. The extension deformity was not noticed until Edgar Sommerville in Oxford made a point in recent times.

The etiology of most curvatures is still unsolved. It has been attributed to poor posture causing a fixed deformity since the beginning of time. Rickets and subclinical polio have been blamed. Apart from the cucumber experiments you will read about, experimental studies on animals are recent. Lovett did some gross studies on a cadaver at the beginning of the century.

The shape of the back was recorded with plaster casts and the benefits of treatment in the early 19th century were based on the very dramatic improvements obtained. Though it is hard for us

◆ **Robert Lovett (1859–1924)**

He was a Harvard graduate who studied orthopedics with the New York group. He worked both in Boston and New York. He wrote a textbook with E. H. Bradford in 1890, which taught a generation, and then collaborated with Robert Jones on a new version that was published in the year of his death. He organized crippled children services and made a special study of the biomechanics of scoliosis.

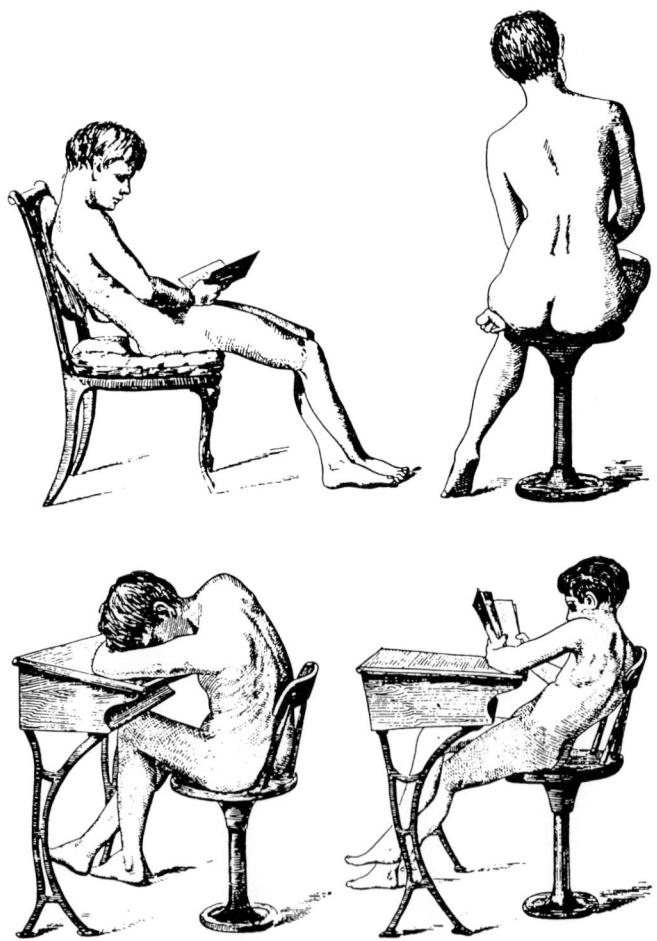

The faulty posture theme. All Boston school desks were redesigned as a result of acceptance of this theory. From Bradford and Lovett, 1899.

today to believe that traction can produce longlasting results, there is no doubt that recording the shape is a better outcome measure than recording the Cobb angle.

Detection

Adams' Forward Bend Test, 1864

"The stooping position is diagnostic of lateral curvature in the early stages. When rotation of the bodies of the vertebrae has taken place, in however slight a degree, the patient cannot stoop in a direct line, and at the same time preserve the symmetrical form of the back. If rotation of the bodies of the vertebrae has occurred, the patient will always stoop in the oblique direction, and the angles of the ribs will be observed to project posteriorly, and give a general prominence, or a fulness on the corresponding side: whilst on the opposite side a flattening—in slight cases not amounting to a depression—will be observed.

"The spine will also bend or curve forwards, with less regularity through the region affected, so that it appears less flexible at this part, and remains straighter."

Paget, 1891

"Among the fears of disease for which one is consulted none is more frequent than that of lateral curvature of the spine. These fears are felt, especially, by mothers among the richer classes; and usually the fear is only for their daughters' spines. It is thought essential to the welfare of a young lady that her spine should be straight...."

He describes the forward bend test.

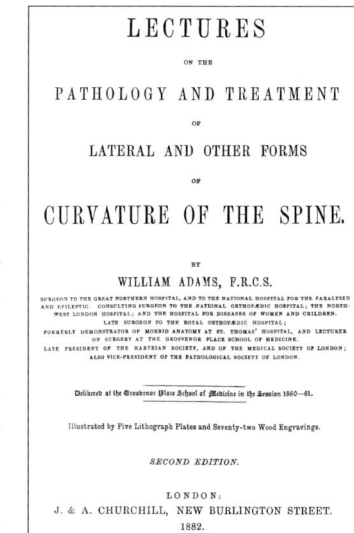

Title page of Adams' book on curvature of the spine, 1882. In this book he describes the forward bend test.

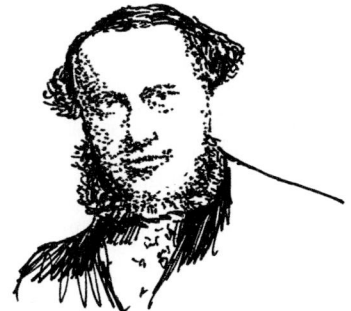

◆ William Adams (1820–1900)

◆ **William Adams (1820–1900)**

Apprenticed to his father, a general surgeon, he studied at St. Thomas' Hospital in London. While waiting for a surgical appointment, he was curator of pathology at St. Thomas'. Adams went on staff at the Orthopaedic Hospital (1851 to 1872) and was a protégé of Little. He did some research on tendon healing in rabbits and looked at patients who died after tenotomy. Because he started work in the era before aseptic surgery, he was a proponent of subcutaneous surgery—tendon, bone, and fascia.

Among the rules of the hospital, one stated, "No serious or new operation is to be carried out without a consultation having been previously held with the whole of the medical staff." Adams was reported for breaking this rule. In the end, he was forced to resign and subsequently the *British Medical Journal* advised surgeons not to apply for his job because of poor labor relations. He worked at other places. He was known for original work on clubfoot, writing that much of the deformity was in the talus in his book *Clubfoot: Its Causes, Pathology and Treatment*. In 1866, this book won a prize at the Royal College of Surgeons. Other book topics included subcutaneous fasciotomy for Dupuytrens in 1879, the principles and practice of subcutaneous surgery in 1857, and scoliosis in 1864. Subcutaneous osteotomy of the neck of the femur to correct deformity was introduced in 1871. In 1876 he visited the United States with Lister to watch Sayre and was made a fellow of the American Orthopaedic Association in 1898. He should not be confused with Robert Adams.

Measurement

How was scoliosis measured before X-rays?

Delpech made plaster molds of the patients, much as we still do for the fabrication of a spinal brace.

Schulthess modified the tools that a sculptor uses to transfer a design in clay to a block of marble. He made a three-dimensional representation on paper of the deformity from all directions. We lost something when the two-dimensional thinking engendered by X-ray dominated thought.

Moire photography and laser systems show the shape of the trunk with greater ease than does the Schulthess system. Today all kinds of computed surface topography methods are possible.

The early X-ray machines did not produce clear spinal images. It was not until the 1920s that long X-ray images were taken that allowed measurement. Lippman described the Cobb method in 1935, and it was used for the multicenter end result study done in 1941. Cobb popularized it in an instructional course in 1948. Perhaps the lesson to you, dear Reader, is that you should never miss the opportunity to give an instructional course at the Academy. The Ferguson method dates to the early 1920s. He was a radiologist at New York Orthopaedic Hospital.

Today computed tomography and 3-D computer-generated images are giving us a clearer idea of the deformity and its correction.

Risser believed that the iliac apophysis develops at the same time as the vertebral growth plates. He decided that vertebral growth could be judged by observation of the development of the iliac apophysis.

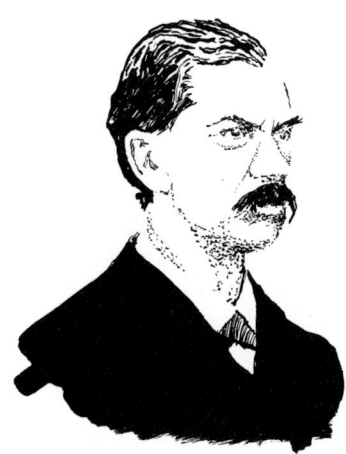

◆ **Wilhelm Schulthess (1855–1917)**

Son of a farmer, he was graduated in medicine in 1880 at Zurich and specialized in pediatrics and internal medicine. He opened the first orthopaedic clinic in Zurich with a surgeon from the University Hospital, A. Lunning. It is still in operation today, with the multidisciplinary approach much alive. Scoliosis was a major focus, and Schulthess had to be able to chart the progress of spinal deformity. In 1885 he constructed a measuring machine, and this led to many presentations until X-rays took over as the measure of severity at the turn of the 20th century.

He invented stereotactic machines to produce calibrated corrections and a machine to measure rotation. In 1906 he wrote a thick book on spinal deformities, which was the standard work in the German-speaking world for many years. His other interests were muscle balance and principles of tendon transfers. He was active in the social integration of handicapped children into society.

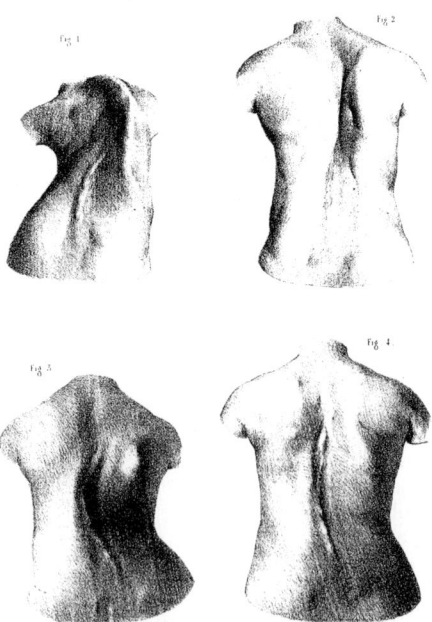

Delpech recorded scoliosis by making plaster casts of his patients. These before and after pictures would be hard to beat today. Both patients were treated with traction and casts for long periods, and both kept the correction for at least a year.

Chapter 6 ◆ Deformity of the Spine 155

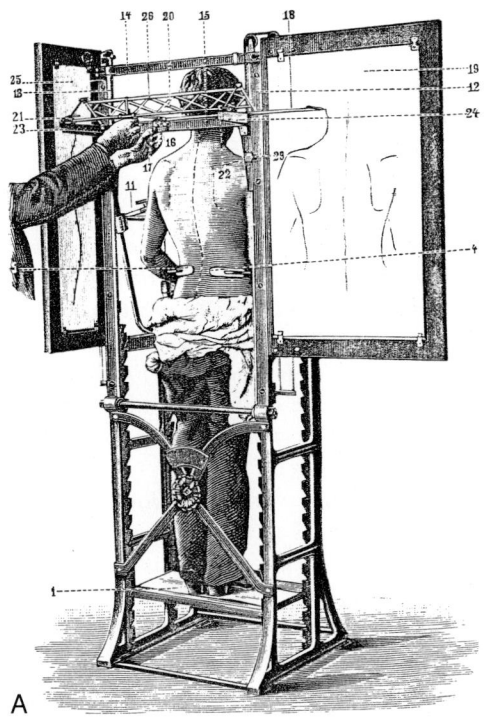

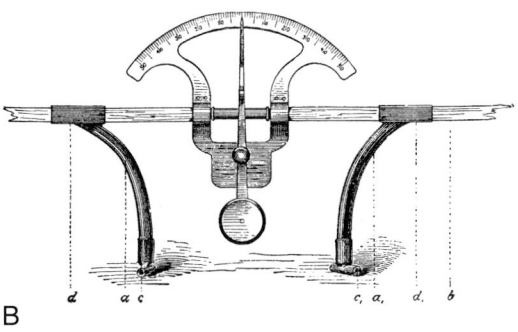

(A) Recording scoliosis, 1885. Schulthess used a machine modeled on one used by sculptors to carve marble from a clay original. (Joachimthal). (B) This is Schulthess' 1885 version of a scoliometer.

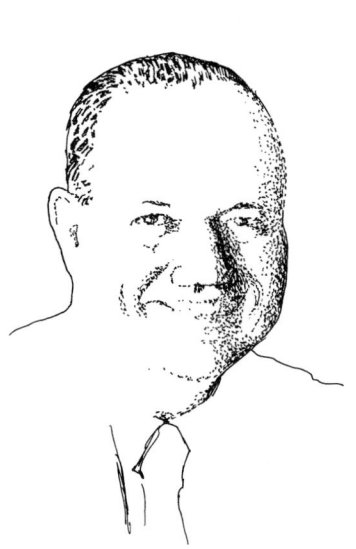

◆ John Cobb

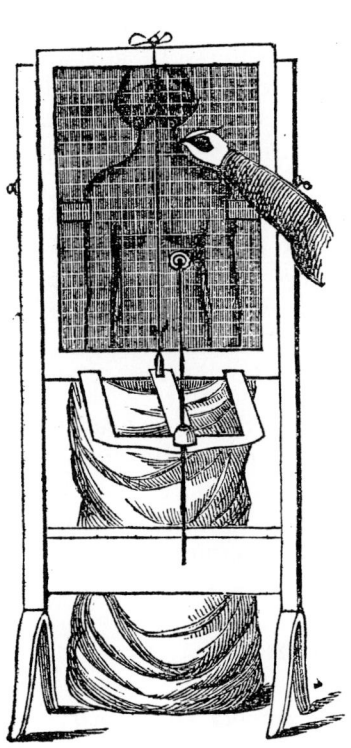

Recording deformity in scoliosis. From Louis Bauer, 1868.

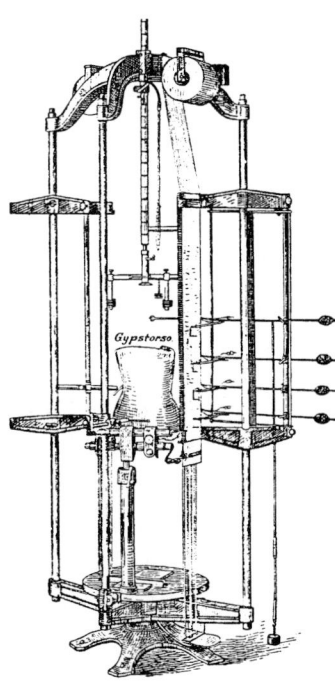

The concept of CAD-CAM is not new. From Joachimsthal.

Risser Sign, 1958

"In the anteroposterior roentgenographic view of the pelvis, the iliac apophysis appears laterally and anteriorly on the crest of the ilium as an ossification center. This is termed capping. With continued growth it develops posteriorly in its excursion of ossification across the iliac crest to dip down to contact the ilium medially at its junction near the sacrum. This is considered to be attached or completed. When this completed ossification occurs, vertebral growth can be considered to be complete. Closure of the line between the apophysis and the ilium has no vertebral growth significance. Two or three years may be required for its closure.

"The average time for completion of the iliac apophysis to its medial and posterior attachment is about 1 year. The shortest time was 7 months; the longest, 3 years.

"The average chronological age when the iliac apophysis is completed is 14 years in girls and 16 years in boys.

"In the occasional use of the localizer cast without surgery to prevent an increase in the lateral curve, it is important to know when the cast can be safely discarded. The attachment of the iliac apophysis is used as a criterion. If the growth center has completed its excursion of ossification, then it is safe to conclude that cast treatment ... can be stopped. But if the cast is removed before the iliac apophysis has attached, then we may expect a return of the deformity and an increase in proportion to the anticipated spinal growth."

This paper is a fine example of the effect of ill-chosen words. Risser uses the word "attached" to describe complete medial extension of the apophysis—now known as Risser 4. Most people understand "attached" to mean that the apophysis has fused to the iliac crest—Risser 5—and feel guilty if the brace is removed before this. Not what Risser meant!

More and more studies suggest that the Risser sign is well suited to a historical book—it is so misleading that it should be given up. But even though we know it is discredited, most people cannot resist looking for it. Strange!

Prognosis

"During this (adolescent) growth period, the average yearly increase in curvature was 5.9 degrees in males and 8.2 degrees in females.

"Increase in curvature ceases when vertebral growth stops."
Risser and Fergusson, 1936

Treatment

Why Correct Deformity?

"Deformity is a chronic source of discontent and unhappiness, and too commonly it gives occasion to petty insult, annoyance, and neglect. To relieve deformity is to promote the welfare

of a community to a very appreciable and not unimportant extent. I have little hesitation in saying, so great is the remedial power which science now has at its command, that the time will come when deformity will be a rare evil among civilised nations."
HH Bigg, *Orthopraxy*, London, 1865

Methods of Treatment

You may think it extraordinary that so many useless methods of treatment have been thrown at scoliosis. One reason may be that about 40% of scoliosis stops progressing before growth ends and the rest certainly slows or stops with the completion of growth. Any kind of treatment to halt progression will seem effective if it is offered to this 40% during growth, or to 100% after growth ends.

Until 150 years ago, surgical treatment was impossible. We can hope that in a few years' time, folks will be laughing at our pride in exchanging a crooked spine for an ankylosed one—trading one problem for another.

Look at the various approaches that have been tried:

1. **Short acute stretches**
   First there was the strong pull of Hippocrates on his prototype of a traction table; then there was the idea of Vidus Vidius in the 16th century. He tied the patient upside down to a ladder by the ankles and then dropped the ladder to give the patient a jerk. It sounds like the kind of thing that could only be done once.

2. **Special apparatus to exert a prolonged pull and push**
   Scoliosis straightens with traction and with the application of three-point pressure. This is easily done with the hands. All kinds of equipment was invented to work on the same principles. Despite so much ingenuity, putting the spine back in place has not proved to be of any value. When the pressure is released the scoliosis is back to where it was. This approach is useless. Vertical suspension was used by

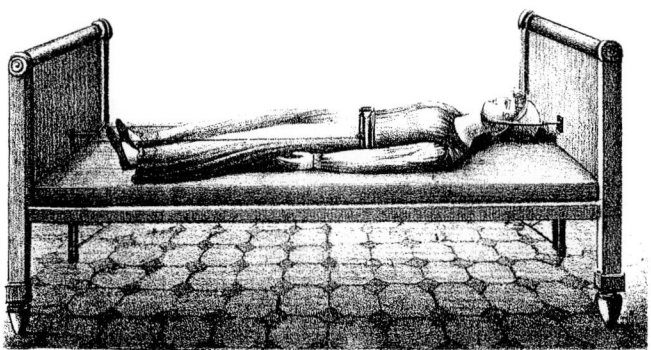

Lit à Extension Progressive.

Pravaz traction in 1827. We still use halo femoral traction occasionally—where is the progress since then?

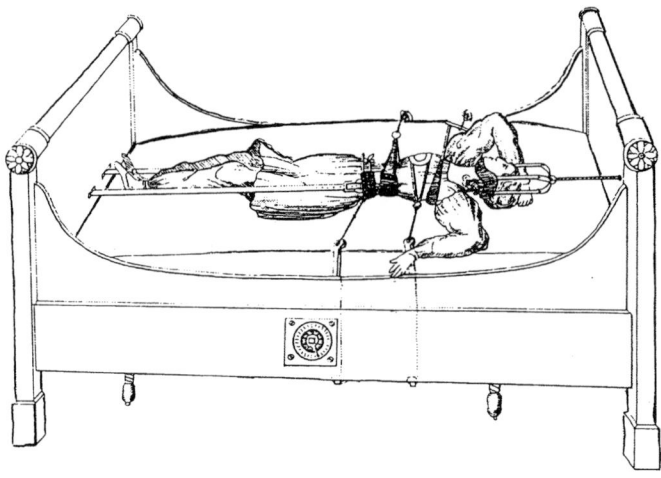

Traction plus lateral pull for scoliosis. From Delpech, 1828.

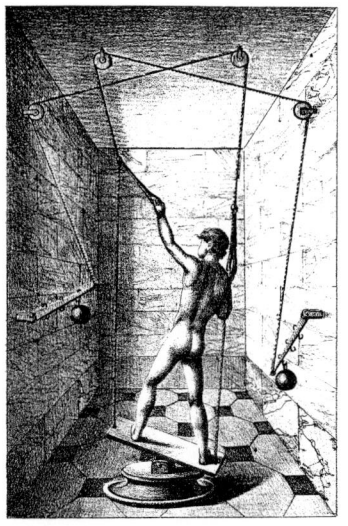

The orthopaedic balancing machine to exercise scoliosis away. From Pravaz, 1827.

Deventer in 1739, by Levacher in 1772, by Darwin, and in 1796 by Snow. Horizontal traction in special beds was used at night in conjunction with braces by day in 19th century Europe. For horrible curves, halo-femoral traction still has a small place as a prelude to instrumentation.

3. Exercises

The notion that the spine curves because the muscles are weak is pervasive. After all, each of us can stand a little straighter if we try. By strengthening the muscles, the condition should improve. If only diseases responded to common sense treatment, we would have solved disease years ago. Despite the large and lucrative orthopaedic gymnasiums of the 19th century in France and Germany, which were filled with as much equipment as a modern-day health club, this was another useless approach. Yet even today, no parent can leave a scoliosis clinic without wanting exercises.

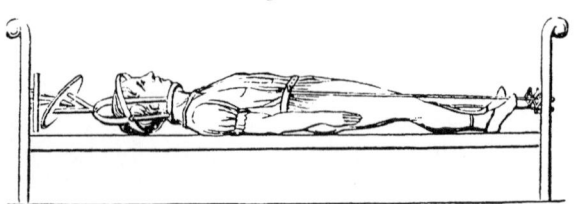

Spring traction for scoliosis. Paris, 1825. From John Bishop: Deformities of the Human Body. London, 1852.

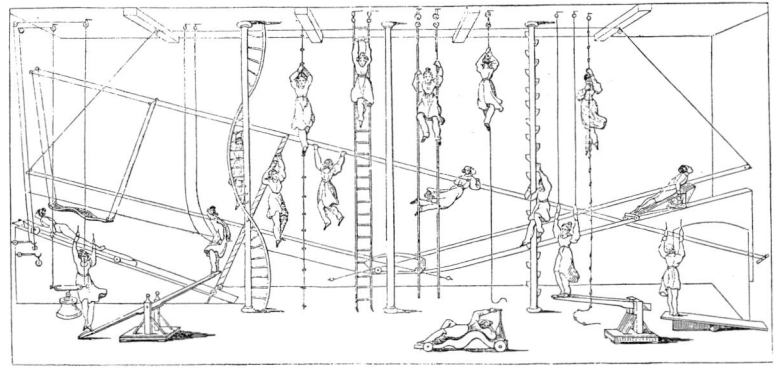

The exercise room for scoliosis in 1837. This represents a considerable financial outlay and suggests that the exercise cure was as popular in the past as fitness is now. From Jules Guérin.

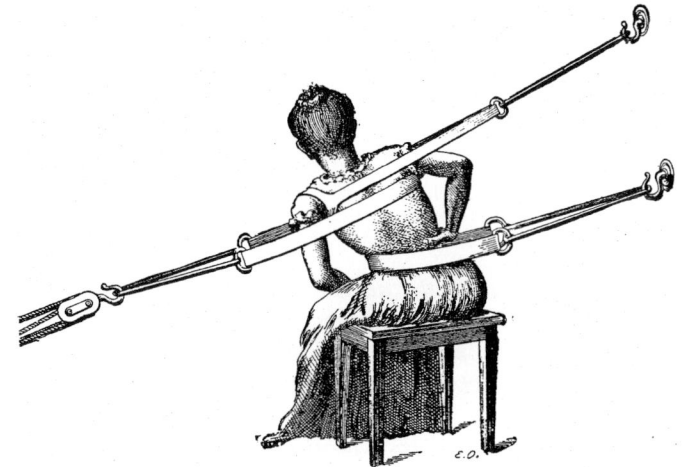

Elastics to correct scoliosis. (Barwell in Joachimsthal.)

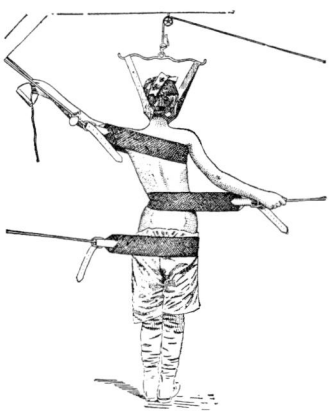

Bradford's self-correction apparatus for scoliosis. From J. K. Young: Orthopaedic Surgery. Philadelphia, 1894.

INFIRMARY FOR THE CURE OF DISTORTIONS OF THE SPINE AND LIMBS

ANONYMOUS, 1841

"I have been much gratified by a visit to the Orthopedic Infirmary in this city, under the care of Dr. Brown.

"The remedies formerly applied to the cure of spinal distortions, have generally been such as, whether successful or otherwise, have produced a vast amount of suffering to the patient. Thus, some have been required to pass months and years, lying, almost in one position. Others have been subjected to instruments of torture, not unlike those formerly applied to criminals. Racks have been used with great mechanical power to extend the spine forcibly, and violent pressure applied to reduce the vertebrae to their proper places. The body has been encased in steel collars and corsets, to force it into the straight shape, and many other equally violent methods made use of.

"By the progress of scientific improvement, these violent applications have been superseded, and more moderate and gentle

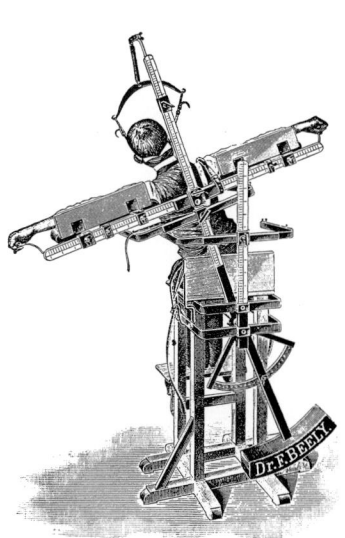

Dr. Beely's machine to improve posture. From Joachimsthal.

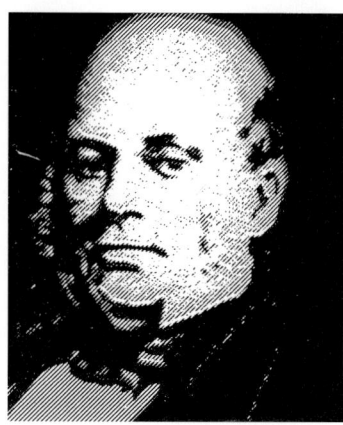

◆ Jules Guérin (1801–1886)

◆ **Jules Guérin (1801–1886)**

He was a contentious original thinker and one of the first to operate for scoliosis. He was born in French-occupied Belgium and was a graduate in medicine from Paris. In 1828 he became editor of the oldest medical journal in France. Interested in deformities, he founded an excellent Orthopaedic Institute just outside Paris in 1834. He and Bouvier won a prize for an essay on orthopaedics in 1837. In 1839 the hospital council for Paris started an orthopaedic service at the Children's Hospital and appointed Guérin chief. After Delpech introduced tenotomy in 1818, Guérin became an enthusiast for the method and applied it to scoliosis. Some thought he carried this to excess. A debate on this controversial technique took place at the Academy of Medicine in 1842. Malgaigne carried a report of the debate between Bouvier and Guérin in the first issue of a surgical journal he founded. Tempers flared. Guérin published results in his journal; he reported on 740 patients with various deformities treated by tenotomy: 358 were completely cured, 287 were benefited, 77 were not benefited, and 18 died. Malgaigne wrote an editorial on orthopaedic illusions, and Guérin took him to court for defamation and damages. Malgaigne argued that freedom to discuss scientific matters and results is a basic right. Repudiation of false claims and valueless treatment is essential for the health of the public. Charges against Malgaigne were dismissed. Myotomy fell into disrepute, and Guérin lost some of his appointments.

Guérin was also involved in other cases. Hossard, a Parisian brace maker, patented a spinal orthotic and was asked to demonstrate this to the Institut de France; Guérin and Bouvier were appointed assessors. They were shown a very deformed patient who was seen not long afterward with a straight back. Guérin thought that it was not the same patient. Hossard sued Guérin and won.

In 1848 he was the subject of another commission of enquiry by the Faculty of Paris, which tried to decide the line of demarcation between orthopaedics and general surgery.

---

means adopted, suited to the nature of each particular case. Most distortions arise from a weakness of some of the muscles intended to support the spine. Muscles acquire size and strength by use; and become enfeebled, diminished in size, and waste away, by disuse.

"An essential part of every plan of cure must be to contrive some mode of giving a moderate and regular exercise to the enfeebled muscles. The wearing of any machine that supports those parts which need support, relieves these enfeebled muscles from their duty still more, and they consequently continue to grow weaker, and the disease is further than ever from a cure."

4. Corrective Posture

Posture is how we stand and sit when we are not thinking about it—something under the control of involuntary reflexes. For a long time it was believed that various stimuli,

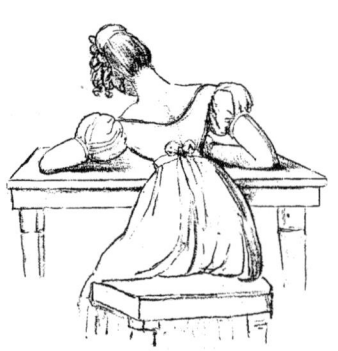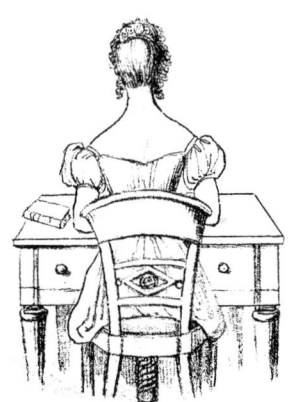

Poor sitting posture is blamed for scoliosis by mothers. Poor and recommended posture. Edward Duffin: 1835

such as school bags, provoke a scoliotic postural reflex. Doctors falsely believed that avoiding these provocative stimuli would prevent or cure scoliosis. Even today most mothers of scoliotic daughters ask about school bags.

At one time all Boston schoolchildren used desks designed by an orthopaedic surgeon with the aim of preventing scoliosis.

5. **Braces**

Scoliosis braces are one of the few forms of medical treatment that have remained relatively unchanged for more than 500 years, starting with Paré's brace modeled on armor. Bracing has survived comparisons with medieval instruments of torture, suggestions that it is ineffective, and the loathing of everyone who wears one. If there is anything constant in orthopaedic life, it is that someone somewhere is adding a new wrinkle to a scoliosis brace.

Scoliosis was regarded initially by doctors as "a disease not to treat," to use the words of the doctor to the Pharoahs, because treatment is ineffective. For centuries doctors left scoliosis entirely to the bracemakers. Only in the past 150 years have doctors taken charge and tried to tell the bracemakers what to do.

Casts applied in combination with traction have enjoyed popularity. This began as a spin-off from the treatment of the tuberculous spine by Sayre. We still use an Abbott frame to apply casts for juvenile scoliosis.

Bracing in the 17th Century. The Schott brothers ran a spinal deformities clinic in Utrecht with 2000 international patients attending at one time in the middle of the 17th century. A diary has been preserved about Mun Verney, who developed a scoliosis between the ages of 11 and 16 years, when he went for treatment. The diary for January 1652 records:

"I would never have thought he could have been so crooked if I had not seen it. The backbone is quite awry and his right shoulder is half a handful lower at least than his left. Herr Schott has undertaken the cure, if your son will stay here three quarters of a year: and already he is about to make harnessing for him for which your son is very willing to undergo.

"If he cannot cure, he takes nothing, accounts his labour lost, and if he do cure, then he takes so reasonable that they who receive benefit by him are willing oftentimes to give more than he is willing to take . . .

"He hath been in harness two weeks, so finely fitted for his crookedness. It is perfect massive iron all along (excepting some holes here and there) back and breast, lined with quilted fustiane and all so light . . .

"Then he felt his harness somewhat loose upon him, whereupon we went the second time to let him see; he straighted it, by pinning some iron buttons closer, and drawing some strings . . .

"Mr. V. wears his harness under his doublet very patiently.

"July 1653   Mun's harness is very irksome, especially in hot weather. [The iron front and back shell were fastened by Herr

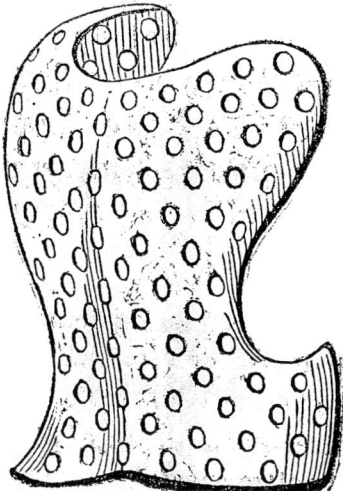

Scoliosis brace, 1564. Metal with leather padding. From Paré.

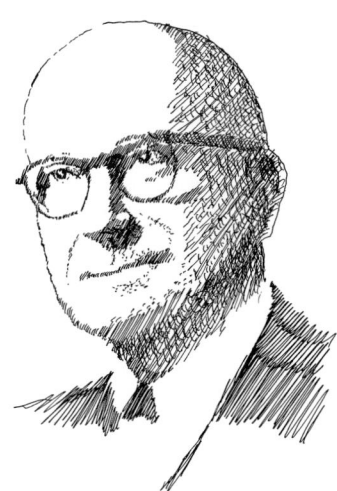

◆ **E. G. Abbott (1870–1938)**

Orthopaedic surgeon in Portland, Maine, who used lateral pressure pads to correct scoliosis—either with a hammock or using a horizontal frame.

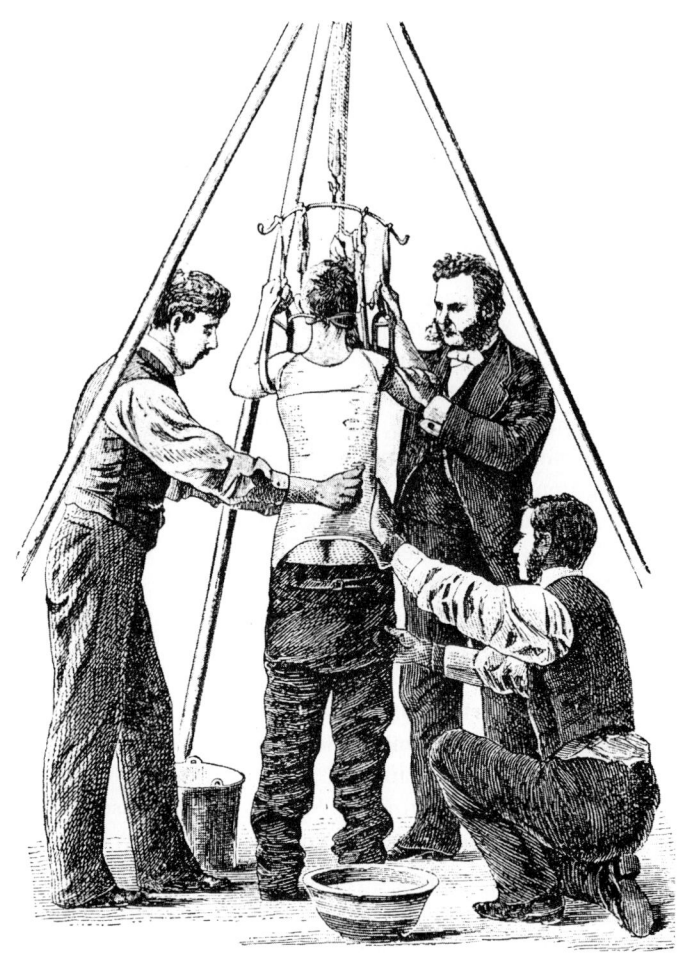

Not a drop of plaster messes their clothes as Sayre supervises the application of a traction cast for scoliosis. 1877.

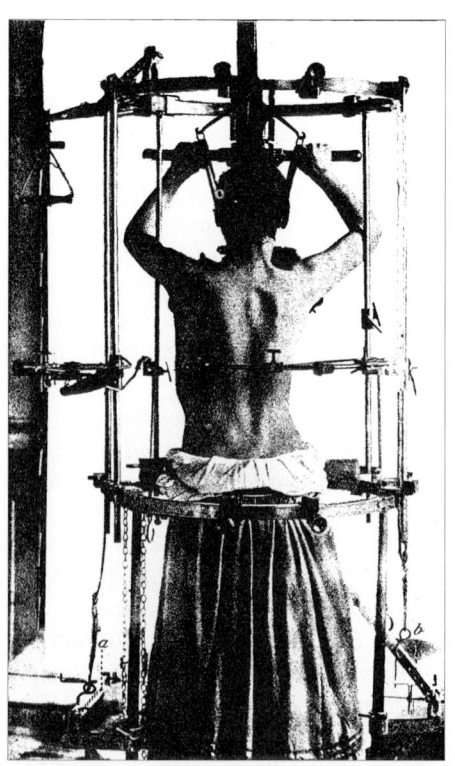

Detorsioning apparatus. Schulthess, 1905. From Joachimsthal.

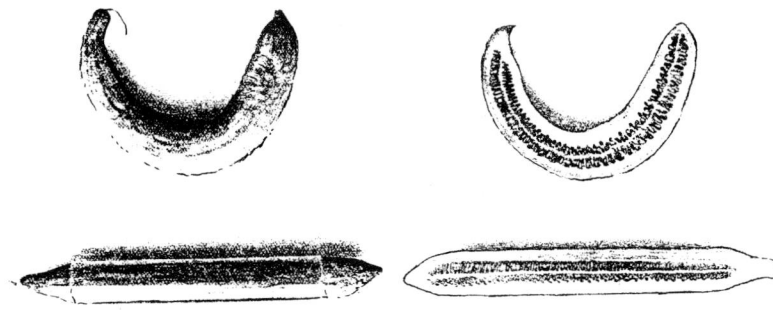

Top, two cucumbers of the curly kind grown into unrestrained curvature. Bottom, two cucumbers on the same plant persuaded into straightness by growth in glass tubes. This is the cucumber experiment. When a naturally curly cucumber is grown in a glass tube, it grows straight. Bigg developed the principle of "Advenience" from this experiment: "*The human body, when unsymmetrical, will gradually come to the shape of an appliance.*" From Heather Bigg: An Essay on the General Principles of the Treatment of Spinal Curves. London, 1905.

Schott over a shirt and could not be removed by the patient. Mun went every week to have the harness removed so that he could put on a clean shirt underneath.]

"*Jan 1654 Herr Schott's bill is a heavy one—he is at great charges in maintaining 16 or 17 servants daily and 3 sons that do nothing but work in iron and steel and brace and unbrace crooked limbs. He has done a notable cure on Mr. Verney.*

"*March 1654 Mun manages to dance in his armor.*

"*Feb 1657 Herr Schott came to London and provided new apparatus at a cost of 30 pounds sterling.*"

[1688   Mun died at the age of 51 years.]

Heather Bigg, Designer of Spinal Braces, 1905

"*I purchased crooked saplings, and when they were established in the soil tried various methods of straightening them ... I subjected them to treatment ... A tolerably crooked sapling could readily be straightened during one season.*"

He also did experiments on cucumbers.

Much ingenuity has gone into bracing from the days when manufacturers of armor solved the problem of peacetime employment by making scoliosis braces, such as Paré's quilted iron corset in 1582. In the years that followed, every kind of pad and strut, buckle and spring, turnscrew and belt has been tried—some not all that different from those in use today.

6. **Surgery—myotomy**

   Before anesthesia, deformities were treated by subcutaneous tenotomy. Tenotomy/myotomy was used for severe scoliosis because the paraspinal muscles stand out like cords. It is interesting that myotomy for scoliosis was one of the first reasons for doctors criticizing each other in print and attacking each other in court.

   Guérin, Malgaigne, and Velpeau were involved in legal cases in 1842 about myotomy. Guérin was a myotomy enthusiast. He published the results of treating 1349 patients. In an editorial, Malgaigne called this an orthopaedic illusion. Malgaigne was sued for defamation but won the case, and the principle of free scientific criticism was accepted.

   "*Division of the Muscles of the Back. A delicate lady, who had the misfortune to have a distorted spine, submitted to the*

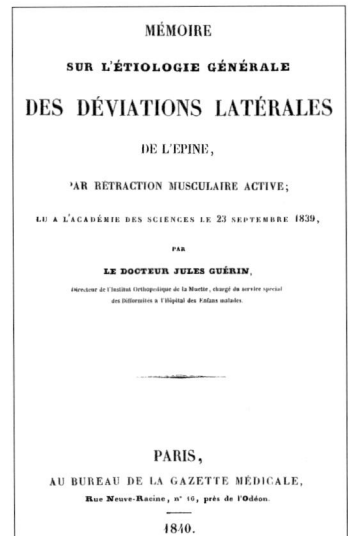

Guérin's book on Scoliosis, 1840. He saw it as a problem of muscle contracture and carried out myotomies. He lost his job after adverse comment.

apparently severe operation one day last week, of having the muscles, at certain points on the broad surface of the back, severed in twain with a knife, in order that the bones might be brought into their original condition. Dr. Brown, of this city, well known of late in this new branch of surgery, was the operator. Although a most formidable matter to think about, it is not very terrible in reality. The patient never sighed nor moved, till the last thread to cut and the operator satisfied that he had overcome the cause of the distortion. Any one in a similar condition might probably be made straight very soon—and it will no longer, therefore, be necessary for so many to remain cripples, when there is really, balm in Gilead. Dr. Brown, we believe, has the honor of being the first to divide the great muscles and tendons of the back, for curvatures of the spine, in this country. We hope for a more extended notice of this important matter, whenever Dr. Brown has leisure for reporting the particulars of the case."
Boston, 1841

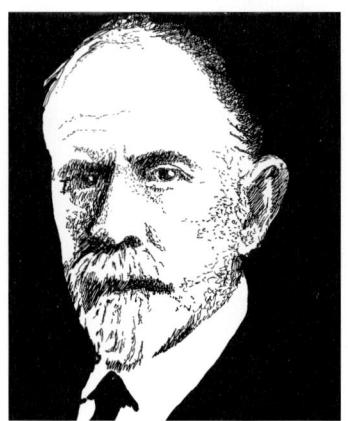

◆ **Russell A. Hibbs (1869–1933)**
Born in Kentucky, he was the last of 10 children. After studying at Vanderbilt he went into general practice for a time before going to New York, training in orthopedics, and becoming the chief at what was to become the New York Orthopaedic Hospital.

7. Fusion

Fusion proved to be helpful for tuberculous spinal deformity and was tried for scoliosis. The deformity was corrected with plaster casts and then the spine was fused through a window in the cast. This was the standard treatment until the early 1960s. Scoliosis was seldom touched by general orthopaedists because these casts were difficult to apply and produced pressure sores that wrecked everything.

Albee used cortical grafts to strut the concavity, and Hibbs started joint excision plus cancellous graft, as early as 1911.

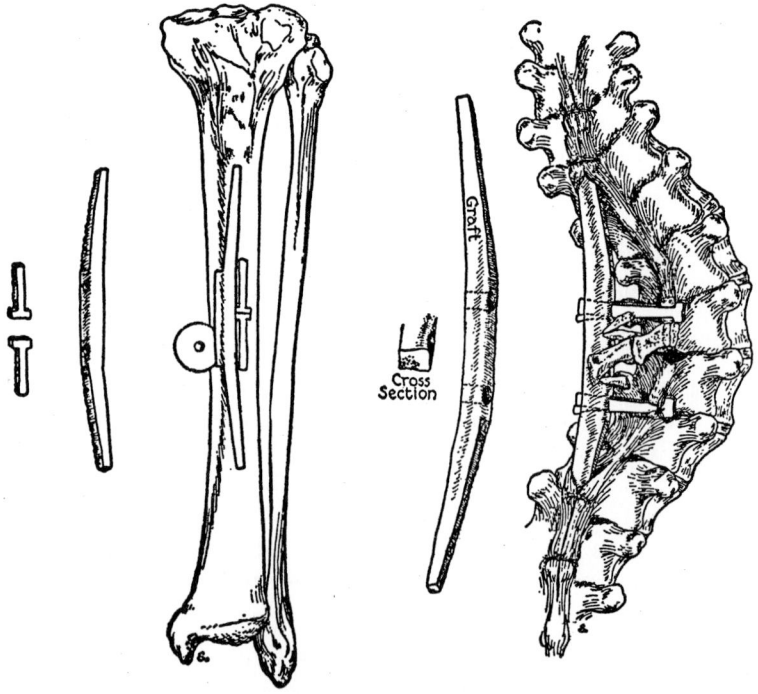

At the left is shown the source of bone graft material and the method of obtaining it. At the right is illustrated use of this bone graft material in the correction and control of most extreme cases of curvature. The two vertebrae at the apex of the curvature are immobilized by bone keys joining the graft to the vertebrae. From Albee FH: Bone Graft Surgery in Disease, Injury and Deformity. D. Appleton-Century Company. New York: 1940.

A REPORT OF 59 CASES OF SCOLIOSIS TREATED BY THE FUSION OPERATION
RUSSELL A. HIBBS, 1917

In the period of 1914 to 1919, inclusive, 59 patients with scoliosis were treated by the fusion operation at the New York Orthopaedic Dispensary and Hospital. These were mostly polio patients, and most were treated in head-pelvic traction preoperatively to reduce deformity.

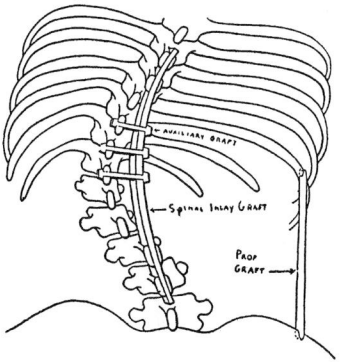

THE PROP GRAFT

Albee used a bone-distracting rod and bone segmental graft to pull like a Luque wire in 1936. He even propped up the ribs. From Albee FH and Kuscher R: The Albee spine fusion operation in the treatment of scoliosis. Surg Gynecol Obstet, 66:797–803, 1938. Reproduced with permission.

"An incision is made through the skin and subcutaneous tissues, from above downward, exposing the spinous processes of the vertebrae to be fused. The periosteum over the tips of these processes is split longitudinally, and, with a periosteal elevator, pushed to either side, leaving them bare. The periosteum and interspinous ligaments in turn are still farther split and pushed forward a short distance from each spinous process, as two lateral halves, gauze packs being inserted to prevent oozing. The dissection is carried farther and farther forward upon each vertebra in turn, until the spinous processes, the posterior surfaces of the laminae, and the base of the transverse processes are based, thereby exposing the ligamentum subflavum attached to the margins of the laminae and the articulations of the lateral processes.

"The ligament is removed from the laminae with a curette, and the articulation of the lateral processes is destroyed in order to establish bone contact at this point. With a bone gouge, a substantial piece of bone is elevated from the adjacent edges of each lamina, of half its thickness and of half its width. The free end of the piece from above is turned down to make contact with the lamina below, and the free end of the piece from the lamina below is turned up to make contact with the lamina above. In transposing these pieces of bone from the laminae, it is better to avoid severing their continuity.

"Each spinous process is then partially divided with bone forceps and broken down, forcing the tip to come into contact with the bare bone of the vertebra below. The spinous process of the last vertebra below should be turned up to bring about contact with the next above. As the spinous processes of the lumbar region are wide, it is sometimes practicable to split them, turning one half up and the other half down. Thus is established contact of abundant cancellous bone at the articulations of the lateral processes, laminae, and spinous processes. The periosteum and ligament, which together have been pushed to either side and lie practically as an unbroken sheet, are brought together in the middle with interrupted sutures of ten-day chromic catgut. The subcutaneous tissue is then closed with sutures of plain catgut, the skin wound is closed with sutures of silk, and dressings are applied.

"The dissection may be made in a practically dry field, without injury to the muscles, if it is subperiosteal and if a free use is made of gauze packs. Only in an operative wound that is free from hemorrhage can the operator see to exercise the care

necessary for thorough work. Not only the baring of the bones may be complete, but the periosteum may be separated from them in a practically unbroken sheet and without disturbance of its relation to the surrounding tissues and blood supply. The greatest care should be exercised in the dissection, as by its extent and thoroughness the area of fusion is measured. After the bones are bared, they may be treated as indicated above or in any manner which establishes their contact and stimulates bone formation. With the closure of the periosteum, practically a tube of periosteum is formed, with its abundant blood supply undisturbed, filled with healthy, living cancellous bone, lying in continuous contact. This situation is entirely consistent with the physiologic laws of bone growth; it furnishes a great stimulus to their operation, and insures a fusion of the lateral processes, the laminae and the spinous processes.

"Usually no immediate postoperative support is applied, the patient being placed in a bed without springs. At the end of two weeks, when the wound is healed, the final traction jacket is applied. The greatest amount of correction is, as a rule, obtained at this time, because the deformed area of the spine is temporarily much more mobile from the operative dissection. This jacket is worn for another six weeks, the patient being confined to bed, after which a removable jacket is applied and worn during the day for the next six to twelve months. At the end of this period all support is removed.

"The extent of fusion in each case varies with the extent of the curve, and, as a general statement, should extend from the neutral vertebra above to the neutral vertebra below the apex. In the series of 45 cases a cervicodorsal curve was present in 3, a dorsal curve in 17, a dorsolumbar curve in 19, and a dorsosacral, or total, curve in 6 cases. Six vertebrae were fused in 3 cases, seven vertebrae in 5 cases, eight vertebrae in 7 cases, nine vertebrae in 8 cases, ten vertebrae in 7 cases, eleven vertebrae in 5 cases, twelve vertebrae in 6 cases, and fourteen vertebrae in 2 cases; fifteen and sixteen vertebrae were fused in 1 case each. In the last instance, the fusion of the sixteen vertebrae was performed in two operations.

"In five of the cases, secondary operations were done to extend the area of fusion. One patient had a pseudo-arthrosis at one point in the operative area and had to have a secondary operation."

[Operative mortality was 2 in 59 patients.]

"Conclusions

"1. The study of these cases gives evidence that we have in fusion a means of preventing the progress of deformity of scoliosis in cases in which it is caused by muscle imbalance.

"2. That the operation should be done before gross deformity has developed, it being easier to prevent than to correct deformity.

"3. That after fusion the upright posture is maintained with greater ease and trunk movement exercised with less fatigue."

The report is interesting in that there is no mention of the severity in terms of angles. The results are related to outcome—walking, sitting, and posture in these polio patients. Although prevention of progression is claimed, there is no evidence for this.

8. **Instrumentation**

The systems of plates and screws used for fractures at the end of the 19th century were not readily applicable to the spine, and there was a gap of about 60 years before internal fixation was developed for the spine. Why was this—was it just a lack of imagination or was it that people had tried and failed? Or was it that the spine was sacrosanct?

Fritz Lange (1864-1952) was Professor of Orthopaedics in Munich. He lived at a time when there were two competing ideas in orthopaedics. On the one hand there was tissue transplantation achieving remarkable, but transient, success; it looked as if the future lay in replacing diseased tissue with healthy tissue. On the other hand there was plaster of Paris and prolonged immobilization. Lange struck out in a third direction, looking to *"replace certain parts of living organs, which serve exclusively mechanical purposes, such as movement or support, by inorganic material. We always have inorganic material at hand in any quantity."*

In 1902 he tried to create *"an artificial spinal column of steel"* but had metal problems. He was working before the invention and use of stainless steel. He carried on with different designs and metals.

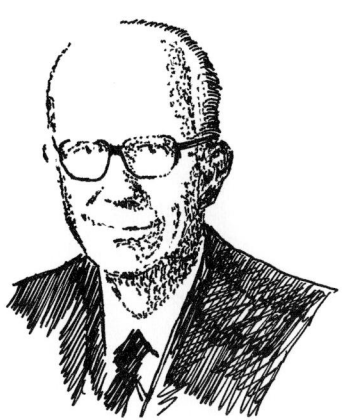

◆ **John Moe in 1958**

He compared different fusion techniques in un-instrumented patients and concluded, *"A meticulous fusion with wide exposure, with all soft tissue removed from the posterior surfaces of the spine, with decortication carefully and completely done, and with articular facets carefully fused, is productive of the best overall results."*

INSTRUMENTATION FOR TUBERCULOUS SPINAL DRFORMITY

FRITZ LANGE, 1910

"Incisions are made in the skin from 3 to 4 cm long, corresponding to the lower and upper ends of the rod, and the fascia is opened on both sides, close to the spinous processes, with incisions 1 cm long. The steel rods are then inserted in an incision through the muscles as deep as possible and close to the bone to the right and the left of the spinal column. The attachment to the spinal column is made with a double sling of Turner silk No. 12 above or below the spinal process. The incision in the skin is then sewed up and drained at the upper corner of the wound for forty-eight hours by a wick of sublimate gauze. A plaster-of-Paris jacket is then applied. The jacket is not removed until 6 weeks after operation.

"My first operation was two years ago. This patient was in the acute stage and had very much pain. I operated because I thought that the exact fixation of the diseased spinal column would stop the pains and heal the spondylitis quicker than would be possible in a simple plaster-of-Paris jacket. This supposition was fulfilled, the patient not having pain again after the operation, though he has not been careful at all; for instance, he worked with the anvil in his father's smithy. Now, the spinal

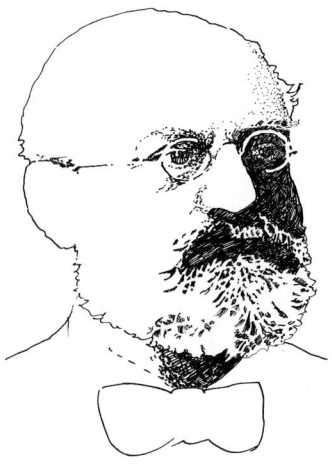

◆ Berthold Ernst Hadra (1842–1903)

column has such an excellent mobility in the healthy parts that the stiffness of the operated portion is not apparent when the patient is moving, the steel wires have been healed in without any reaction for two years. The number of my operations on the spinal column is not yet large enough to judge finally, but I believe that this new operation offers the best chances of curing spondylitis without long treatment in plaster-of-Paris and without having great deformity."

Hadra, Lange, and Meurig Williams had used internal fixation for short segments. But it was not until Harrington that a workable system was developed.

TIMELINE FOR INSTRUMENTATION
- 1891 Hadra—spinous process wiring
- 1910 Lange rods. Metal rods were attached to the spinous processes to prevent tuberculous spinal deformity and promote healing.
- 195? Meurig Williams plates bolted to the spinous processes to prevent fracture deformities
- 1962 Harrington rods—posterior distraction hooks
- 1969 Dwyer—anterior compression system
- 1973 Luque—posterior segmental fixation
- 1978 Zielke—anterior rigid instrumentation
- 1984 Cotrel Dubousset posterior derotation system

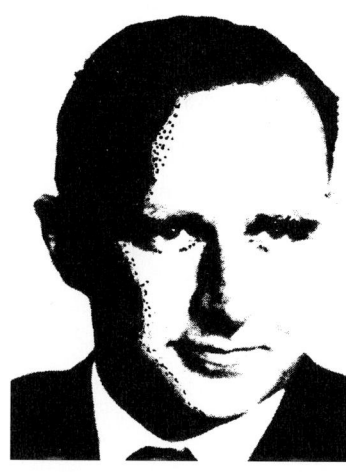

◆ Alan Dwyer (1920–1975)

Not a scoliosis surgeon, Dwyer was an Australian surgeon who went to New Guinea to look after some of the orthopedic problems in this Third World country. Scoliosis was big and in the fifties there were no good answers. Anterior approaches to the spine had been pioneered in Hong Kong for tuberculosis by Hodgson and Stock. Dwyer built his system of instrumentation on this approach.

TREATMENT OF SCOLIOSIS; CORRECTION AND INTERNAL FIXATION BY SPINE INSTRUMENTATION

PAUL HARRINGTON, (PRESENTED 1960 AND PRINTED 1962)

"The development of the treatment of scoliosis to be described began in 1947 with the study of the anatomy of the spine and the problem of scoliosis as seen in approximately 3,000 patients with poliomyelitis. It was thought that a metal device for the correction of the scoliotic curve and for the maintenance of the correction could be implanted, and in the period between 1949 and 1954 such a device was used in nineteen patients. Thirty-five modifications in the device were made in this five year period."

Harrington gave the details in table form of every one of 129 patients treated over 8 years. At first the spine was instrumented without fusion or immobilization, but he learned that both were necessary.

9. Immunization

Immunization against scoliosis! Must be a dream. Yet in the past, polio produced as much scoliosis as the idiopathic gene does today in the developed world. Polio causes scoliosis still in large parts of the world. In the Third World, communities would do more toward eradicating scoliosis by setting up an immunization program than a scoliosis service.

Results

In 1941 the American Orthopaedic Association put together an end result study based on 425 patients with idiopathic scoliosis treated at 16 orthopaedic centers across North America.

TREATMENT OF IDIOPATHIC SCOLIOSIS
AMERICAN ORTHOPAEDIC ASSOCIATION, 1941

"Excellent rating was reserved for those in whom residual deformity was slight and roentgenograms revealed the curve to be of minor degree. Good rating included those patients who had a moderate curvature, but were well balanced and concealed the deformity satisfactorily. Results were rated fair when the curvature was moderately severe and the patient displayed obvious cosmetic defects, while a poor rating was given for those with severe curvature and marked body asymmetry.

"Of 425 cases reviewed, 12, or 3 per cent, were rated excellent; 119, or 28 per cent, good; 191, or 45 per cent, fair; and 103, or 24 per cent, poor.

"If the clinical appearance of the back at end result is compared with what it was when the patient was first seen, it will be noted that the best cosmetic results were obtained in the group treated by correction in the Risser jacket and spine fusion.

"Fifty per cent (214) of the patients reviewed had fusions done either immediately or after conservative treatment had been abandoned in favor of surgery. Correction was by means of the turnbuckle jacket in 80 per cent of those corrected and fused. The average percentage of correction obtained was 65 and the average percentage of correction at end result was 27. . . . There was complete loss of correction in 29 per cent.

". . . The incidence of pseudarthrosis for the entire operative group amounted to 28 per cent.

"The results in 69 per cent of the cases at end result were rated fair or poor, and 31 per cent, good or excellent.

"Conclusions

"1. Practically none of the patients with scoliosis are cured, if correction of lateral deviation is a criterion.
"2. In approximately 60 per cent of those treated by exercises the deformity increased and in 40 per cent, it remained unchanged.
"3. Correction without fusion resulted in complete loss of correction after support was discontinued in the majority of instances.
"4. Correction by the turnbuckle jacket and subsequent fusion has yielded better results in this series than have other types of treatment."

Eduardo Luque looked after poor children at the Shriner's Hospital in Mexico City. Harrington instrumentation was too expensive, and so he developed his system of segmental fixation on the priority of cheapness. The ability to get more correction and a stronger purchase so that there was no need for postoperative immobilization became evident later. Sagittal curve could be preserved. The risk of neurologic damage led to the principle of segmental fixation being applied through various hook systems instead of the sublaminar wires.

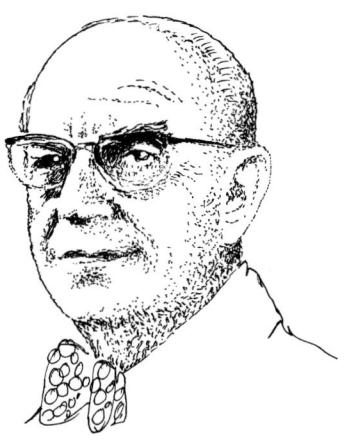

◆ **Paul Harrington (1911–1980)**

He was not a spinal surgeon when he invented his rods. He returned from the war to Houston at a time when opportunities were scarce. He was given the least prestigious job available—surgeon to the polio clinic. Scoliosis was a big problem and with his brace maker he made the hooks. His memoirs are at the University of Kansas.

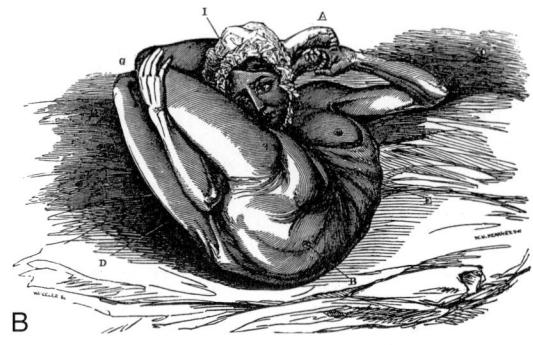

Title page (A) and illustrations (B and C) from Harrison's book, The Extraordinary Case of Sarah Hawkes, 1832. Pillows and positioning were used to produce the cure. Probably hysteria on a grand scale.

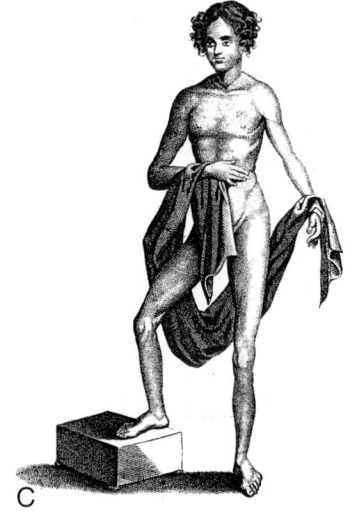

This careful study, done about 50 years ago, shows in conclusion what would now be regarded as the natural history of scoliosis. The study shows that our success in gaining correction today is not much better than it was—65% correction, but that internal fixation prevents us losing correction and securing fusion.

Kyphosis

Stamford Raffles, founder of Singapore, had a kyphosis.

THE STOOP OR SEMICIRCULAR CURVE FORWARD

R. A. STAFFORD, 1832

"Nothing is more common than to see a weakly, over-grown boy, about fourteen or fifteen years of age, stooping forwards, as if he would fall at every step he takes. The poor lad is blamed, both by his parents and school master, and is laughed at by his companions, for so careless a habit. The fact, however, is, that the muscles of his back are so weak that they have not sufficient strength to support him. In spite, therefore, of all remonstrances, he still stoops, and, vexed at constant reproofs, he seeks, by lolling in all directions, to relieve himself, till at length he falls into bad habits, and the deformity becomes confirmed."

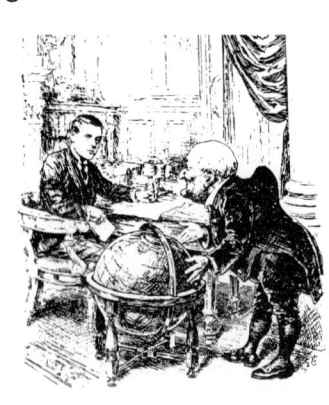

Mr. Punch—a hunchback—gave his name to a satirical magazine that has lasted more than 100 years. A whole psychologic thesis could be based on changing attitudes to deformities.

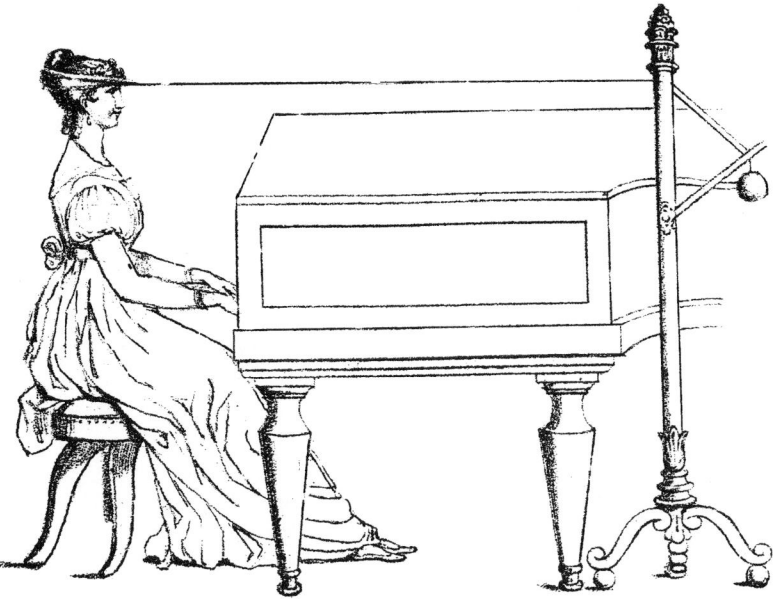

Exercise for round back, keeping the extensors active during hours of piano practice. This would not make young ladies into enthusiastic piano players. From Edward Duffin, 1835.

KYPHOSIS DORSALIS JUVENILIS

H. SCHEUERMANN, 1921

"It is possible to distinguish a group of cases amongst the curvatures of the spine which begin during puberty that are morphologically different from the rest and have other features in common which command interest.

"The type to be discussed below is the dorsal kyphosis—a genuine sagittal curve due to a fixed curvature of the vertebral column and distinct from a round back, an error of posture, which can be actively corrected in whole or in part."

Scheuermann describes a series of 105 such patients in whom the curvature was purely sagittal in 60 and accompanied by slight lateral deviation in 45. The peak incidence was at the age of 16, and 88% of the cases were males.

"At first sight it seems that puberty, a period of rapid growth culminating at about the age of 16, must be an important factor. The case histories of most of these patients reveal that the deformity of the back followed manual work of some kind. The agricultural workers are in the absolute majority and most of them state that the curvature of the spine developed slowly over the course of six months or a year, often accompanied by pain in the back which radiated to the sides, and all the patients stated that the pain definitely disappeared on lying down.

"An X-ray picture in a recent case (i.e., during the first six months) of a typical dorsal kyphosis shows that the vertebrae

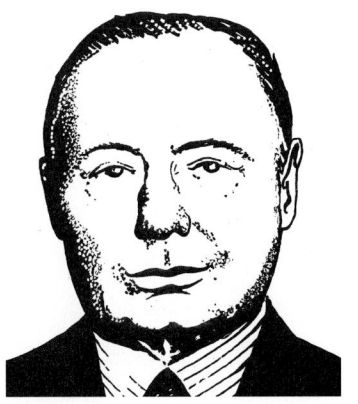

◆ **Holger Werfel Scheuermann (1877–1960)**

The son of a Danish doctor, Scheuermann trained in orthopaedics and radiology. In 1935 he became chief radiologist at the Cripple's Hospital and was the best-known radiologist in Denmark. He described juvenile kyphosis in 1921 and presented a thesis on this subject to the university for his doctorate. They would not accept it. Finally at the age of 80 he was granted an honorary doctorate in recognition of his work. Clearly Scheuerman was not the first to recognize this condition, as a description written in 1826 shows. He did, however, recognize the cause of the deformity.

which lie at the most concave portion of the curvature are considerably narrower anteriorly than posteriorly. The vertebrae become wedge-shaped. The epiphysis is no longer triangular but becomes broad and irregular; the vertebrae are also irregular, which points to abnormal conditions in the line of growth."

The deformity will remain despite any treatment known, he wrote. He had not reckoned with the power of spinal instrumentation.

MYOSITIS OSSIFICANS PROGRESSIVA
JOHN FREKE, 1740

Extract from a letter to the Royal Society:

♦ **John Freke (1688–1756)**
Born in London, apprenticed to a surgeon, and in 1729 he joined the staff of St. Bartholomew's Hospital and became a Fellow of the Royal Society. He suffered from gout, which forced him to retire. He was a man of wide culture, well known in literary circles—a friend of Fielding, who mentioned him in *Tom Jones*.

"Yesterday there came a boy of healthy look, and about fourteen years old, to ask of us at the Hospital, what should be done to cure him of many large Swellings on the Back, which began about Three Years since, and have continued to grow as large on many Parts as a Penny-loaf, particularly on the Left Side: they arise from all the vertebrae of the Neck, and reach down to the os sacrum; they likewise arise from every Rib of his body, and joining together in all Parts of his Back, as the Ramifications of Coral do, they made, as it were, a fixed Bony Pair of Bodices.

"If this be found worthy of your Thoughts it will afford a Pleasure to, Gentlemen,

"Your Most Humble Servant, John Freke

"It is to be observed that he had no other symptoms of rickets in any joint of his limbs."

References

Chapter references are located in Chapter 26.

◆ Chapter Seven

Spinal Pain

Old books have little information about back ache. There was a lot about tuberculous spine, and I suppose that if the patients were lucky enough not to be dying of tuberculosis they were regarded as having so much to celebrate that their back ache was ignored. For example, Sayre wrote a textbook of orthopaedics in 1876. In 471 pages there is not a word on back ache. There is much on spinal tuberculosis and scoliosis, but nothing on back ache.

In 1915 Bradford and Lovett's book had 2 pages on back ache out of 406. The subject was included in the section on emotional and excitable and temperamental patients with hysteria!

By 1926 Cochrane has 24 pages on back ache out of 500 and writes about posture, asymmetrical articulations, muscle tears, and sacroiliac displacements as responsible for back pain. He starts off by writing about industrial back pain.

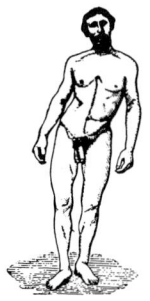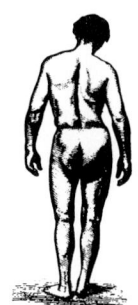

Sciatic scoliosis. Lewis Sayre in 1876 used this illustration to depict that disease of the imagination: sacroiliac joint disease, a misinterpretation or false trail that led many patients to sacroiliac fusion.

Important people had weird ideas about focal infection and kissing spines, which retarded progress. In the 1930s the disc was rediscovered as the cause of sciatica. Schmorl's book, based on spinal autopsies, did much to put the subject on a scientific basis. In 1925 he began to examine the spine at every autopsy and wrote a book on the first 10,000 in 1932. It was translated into English in 1959. For anyone with lectures to give, his 400 illustrations of vertebral pathology are a gold mine. Today, our understanding of spinal pain still leaves much to be desired.

Pain is a common complaint. The relationship between the complaints and the pathology is not as close as we would like. The relationship between treatment and outcome is often unclear because so many attacks of back ache improve with time.

When Did the Average Patient Stand a Chance of His Problem Being Recognized and Treated?

Disc protrusion, 1930s
Spondylolisthesis, 1950s
Stenosis, 1960s

Until back ache was auditioned and allowed to play a role in the orthopaedic theater, there was no treatment. Bottles of liniment and patent medicines provided self-treatment. The osteopathy school of practitioners was first interested in the spine because they believed that spinal manipulation cured deafness and other problems. They were not interested in spinal pain.

Manipulators of the spine for spinal pain were the chiropractors and a few doctors.

The discovery of the disc brought about a "disc rush"—a Klondike at every surgeon's back door. The early indications for operating were disc prolapse, instability and spondylolisthesis, and then stenosis. Operating started in the late 1930s and reached a crescendo in the 1960s.

More recently, the back school movement has helped patients understand how they can help themselves.

Famous People with Back Ache

President John F. Kennedy

Kennedy suffered a football injury to his back at Harvard and was turned down for the Army because of a bad back. He was accepted by the Navy; his boat was sunk under him, and he emerged a hero with sciatica. On June 23, 1944, he had a disc removed at the Lahey Clinic but was no better. He had many other health problems. When he ran for the Senate in 1952 he traveled with crutches hidden in the car and had pain on walking. He continued to use crutches but concealed this. On October 21, 1954, a spinal fusion was carried out at the Hospital for Special Surgery in New York. A plate and graft was used, and he almost died of postoperative infection. The plate was removed a few months later, in 1955, because of continuing infection. His pain continued and, while he was depressed and being treated by bed rest, he wrote *Profiles in Courage*. In the fall of 1957 a lumbar abscess was drained and he improved after this for a time. He was on vapocoolant therapy, procaine injections, swimming, calisthenics, a shoe lift, a back brace, and his mother's mustard plasters at various times.

In addition, he was diagnosed with adrenal insufficiency in 1947 and was treated with steroids from this time. He was written up in the AMA *Archives of Surgery* as Case 3, 1955, Vol. 71. Attempts were made to steal his medical records, and his physician's office was vandalized. Kennedy denied that he had Addison's disease—a tuberculous destruction of the adrenals, a play on words.

MANAGEMENT OF ADRENOCORTICAL INSUFFICIENCY DURING SURGERY

◆ CASE 3

A man 37 years of age had Addison's disease for seven years. He had been managed fairly successfully for several years on a program of desoxycorticosterone acetate pellets implanted every three months and cortisone daily. Owing to a back injury, he had a great deal of pain, which interfered with his daily routine. Orthopaedic consultation suggested he might be helped by a lumbo-sacral fusion together with a sacro-iliac fusion. The operation was accomplished on Oct. 21, 1954. This patient had a smooth postoperative course insofar as no Addisonian crisis ever developed.

TIMELINE OF INVESTIGATIONS

1895 X-rays helped with diagnosis but they were of much less help than in other fields of orthopaedics. Knowledge about back ache did not take the same great leap forward as did other diseases at the time of the invention of X-rays. The quality of spinal films was abysmal at first.

1918 Dandy: Air myelography, but it was poor for the spine.

1921 Sicard and Forestier: Lipiodol myelography. Sicard, a Parisian neurosurgeon, was using injections of Lipiodol for low back pain. An assistant injected some and then aspirated with the syringe. Back came cerebrospinal fluid. Horror. Would the patient die? "Fluoroscope the patient." Surprise. The first myelogram. Fame. Later the arachnoiditis was discovered to be a problem. Water-soluble media were used widely in the 1970s.

1931 Burman myeloscopy

1948 Lindblum discography

1973 Minnesota Multiphasic Personality Inventory applied to low back pain patients

1973 Prototype computed tomography

1977 First primitive magnetic resonance imaging

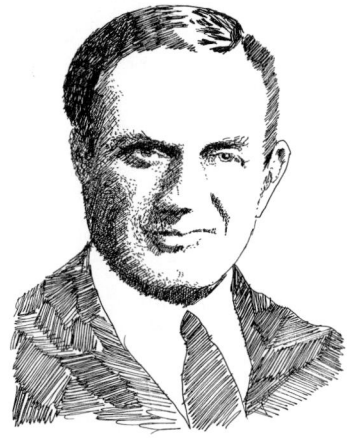

◆ **Walter C. Dandy (1886–1946)**
While a general surgical resident, he was struck by the intraperitoneal gas seen on the radiograph of a patient with a perforation. He injected air into the cerebrospinal fluid space and invented ventriculography—the first way in which the brain and cord were visualized. Later he pioneered disc surgery while a neurosurgeon at Johns Hopkins.

Spinal Stenosis

The spinal canal and foramina become too small for the lumbar roots, resulting in pain and intermittent claudication. Usually due to arthritis in the elderly, it can occur in the young owing to diseases such as achondroplasia.

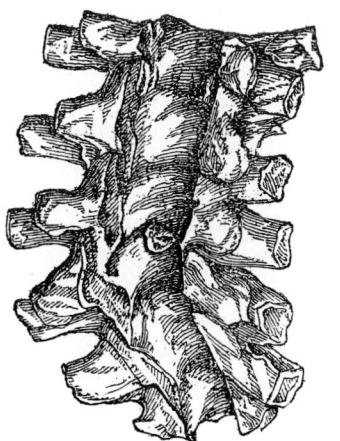

Angular deformity with an exostosis projecting from the posterior surface of a thoracic vertebral body. The patient did not recount an injury and had a partial cord lesion. From Marshall Hall, 1838.

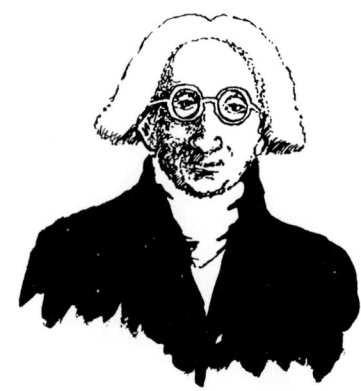

◆ **Antoine Portal (1742–1832)**

Parisian surgeon who wrote a major anatomy text. He was President of the Academy of Science for much of his life.

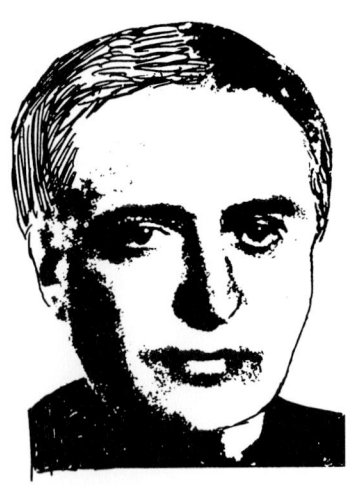

◆ **Vittorio Putti (1880–1940)**

He was the dynamo of European orthopaedics from the time he became Director of the Rizzoli Institute in Bologna in 1911. He brought people together—not easy in this egotistic specialty. He made the Rizzoli famous for education and excellence. He is mentioned here for his leg-lengthening equipment, a report of 3600 cases of closed reduction of developmental dysplasia of the hip, arthroplasty, and sciatica.

TIMELINE OF SPINAL STENOSIS

1000 BC   Stenosis found in Egyptian mummies

1803   Antoine Portal found that the spinal canal varied in size and described cases in which the spinal cord was slowly compressed, resulting in wasting and varying degrees of motor loss.

1864   S. Jacqoud noted spinal stenosis in a book on paraplegia: *"Paraplegia which results from compression of the spinal cord by a spinal canal which is too narrow."*

1893   Arbuthnot Lane decompresses a degenerative spondylolisthesis with relief.

1893   von Bechterew describes a syndrome which has been interpreted elsewhere as ankylosing spondylitis.

1896   Sottac invented the expression "intermittent claudication of the spinal cord."

1899   Sachs and Fraenckel describe a patient who had pain in the legs, paresthesia, and a forward stoop, which was relieved by two-level laminectomy.

1910   Sumita describes the narrow canal in achondroplasia.

1911   Bailey and Casamajor of New York describe the weakness, stoop, and claudication due to arthritis of the spine causing pressure on the cord and roots. It was relieved by laminectomy. They note the thickened lamina, bony overgrowth from arthritis, and the thickened ligamentum flavum. Multiple other reports are published of small series during the next few years.

1925   Parker and Adson describe cord compression by hypertrophic joints relieved by laminectomy.

1927   Putti tries to popularize root compression by hypertrophic joints, but he is ignored.

1945   Sarpyener in Istanbul describes the congenital stricture of the spinal canal.

1949   Henk Verbeist, a neurosurgeon in Utrecht, finally popularizes the subject; Brodsky, Ehni, and Kirkaldy-Willis add more information.

PATHOGENESIS OF SCIATIC PAIN

VITTORIO PUTTI, 1927

Sciatica may be due to disease of the nerve, he writes. *"In other cases the cause is local, and the pain is due to compression or irritation of the nerve at some point or other along its course.... The idea is not new that a nerve may be irritated in the canal or foramen which it traverses ... The study shows one constant factor—the association of pain with anatomical alterations of the lumbar spine.... The anomalies may have a two-fold effect on the intervertebral foramen; Firstly, they may alter its shape and reduce its capacity; secondarily, by altering the mechanics of the spinal column, they may induce a localised arthritis. The diseased joint, by its swelling and deformity, changes the shape and capacity of the foramen, thus irritating and compressing the nerve within."*

He mentions that Sicard had advised lumbar laminectomy to decompress the roots, but he had found immobilization in a plaster jacket sufficient.

SPINAL STENOSIS
HENK VERBEIST, 1954

"My English paper was repeatedly rejected by editorial boards of important English and American neuro-surgical and neurological journals. The reasons given for rejection varied from disbelief to irrelevant comments. It was ironic to me, a neurosurgeon, that the paper was not published by a neurosurgical or neurological journal, but rather by the British volume of JBJS [Journal of Bone and Joint Surgery].

"The clinical symptoms described were disturbances of walking or standing which included pain, paraesthesias, and loss of power or sensation or both. The walking disturbance was called 'intermittent claudication' and was considered pathognomonic of stenosis of the lumbar vertebral canal."

Discogenic Back Pain

Sciatica

The best early description of sciatica comes from a monograph by Cotugno written in 1764. About 90 years later pathologists found necropsy evidence of disc profusion. Another 90 years passed before it was realized that there was any connection between these two observations.

Virchow gave a brief account of protruded disc and shortly afterward, in 1858, von Luschka described it more fully. At autopsy Luschka found a soft, grayish knob of tissue on the surface of the posterior longitudinal ligament between L2 and L3; on sectioning the disc horizontally, he found that this tissue had arisen from the nucleus pulposus that had burst through the annulus. He postulated that if this mass continued to expand, it could burst through the ligament and cause cord compression. In 1896 Kocher found a high disc protrusion in the course of an autopsy on a man who had fallen 100 feet.

In 1911 two classic papers appeared, one from Glasgow and the other from Boston. The Glasgow paper describes a man who died from a traumatic paraplegia and was found to have a massive disc prolapse. Goldthwait's paper from Boston discusses a man who developed a paraplegia after a spinal manipulation for back pain (a warning to all). He theorizes on the basis of this and produces a speculative description of lumbosacral instability as a cause of lumbago and sciatica. Among other ideas, he thought that a disc prolapse could cause cord and root pressure. He includes a drawing of this notion, which is so accurate that it could be used in a textbook today.

These papers did not attract much attention. Surgeons had by this time started to operate on the spinal cord with increasing

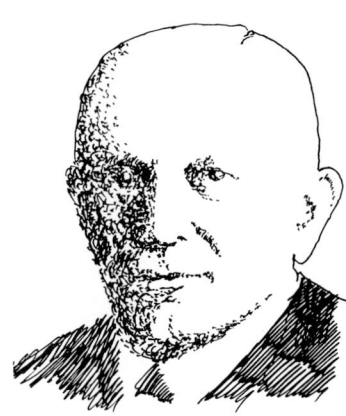

◆ **Christian George Schmorl (1861–1932)**

He was the director of the Pathological Institute in Dresden for his working life. He had a photographic memory and wrote many papers. Best known for his work on bone, he always examined the spine at autopsies. After examining 10,000 spines, he wrote a book, *The Human Spine,* in 1932. An edition co-authored with Herbert Junghanns was published in English in 1959.

Schmorl died of septicemia after scratching his finger on a bandsaw while cutting a specimen.

frequency, but regarded disc protrusions as sessile chondromata or fibromata.

In the 1920s, Schmorl and his school were studying the spinal column as a routine during autopsies and found disc protrusions in about 15%. In the later twenties, "chondromata" were a fairly commonplace finding for the neurosurgeon. However, it was not until 1934 that Mixter and Barr established, first, the fact that these chondromata were in fact disc prolapses and, second, the connection between sciatica and disc profusion. These two surgeons from Massachusetts General Hospital described 19 cases they had operated on: 4 cervical discs, 4 thoracic, 10 lumbar, and 1 sacral. The paper ended with these words, "I think fusion should be combined with operation where there is any question of an unstable spine, and I believe that a ruptured disc may be unstable."

At first the prolapse was removed by full transdural laminectomy, but within a few years, in 1939, Love had evolved the interlaminar approach, which did not require the removal of any bone. After World War II, disc surgery was very popular but did not prove to be a panacea for sciatica, and today a more conservative mood prevails.

TIMELINE OF DISCOGENIC PAIN

1764 Cotugno describes sciatica.
1841 Valliex describes a fractured disc at autopsy after an injury.
1857 Virchow describes a disc prolapse briefly.
1858 Von Luschka describes disc prolapse at autopsy.
     Brissaud describes sciatic scoliosis.
1881 Forst describes the Lasègue sign.
1896 Kocher describes disc prolapse at autopsy.
1909 Oppenheim and Krause operate on disc prolapse but think it is an osteochondroma.
1911 Middleton and Teacher described a patient who died of paraplegia due to disc prolapse and experimented to show that longitudinal vertebral compression made the disc bulge.
1911 Goldthwait develops a hypothesis about disc prolapse after an unfortunate experience. His armchair drawing is a good forecast of what will be found. But he does not connect this with sciatica.
1917 Bertolotti in Italy attributes sciatica to an enlarged transverse process—a wrong turning.
1926 Smith-Petersen popularizes sacroiliac fusion for low back pain and sciatica. A wrong turn?
1927 V. Putti tries to popularize the disc but without success.
1929 Walter E. Dandy (Baltimore) entitles a paper "Loose cartilage from the intervertebral disk simulating tumor of the spinal cord." He describes two cases: *"The early symptoms are those of localized vertebral pain plus bilateral sciatica—one side being affected more than the other. Later, the symptoms are rapidly increasing paralysis, sensory and motor paralysis*

> and loss of urinary and vesical control and of reflexes—all due to compression of the cauda equina.... This lesion offers a pathological basis for cases of so-called sciatica, especially bilateral sciatica.... The lesion is cured by operative removal of the cartilage."

1932 Georg Schmorl in Dresden studies 5000 spines at autopsy and writes a wonderful book on pathology.

1932 Mixter and Barr—the first laminectomy for disc. Joe Barr gives an off-the-cuff account of the events surrounding this. *"We had a very difficult time getting the neurologists to accept the possibility that a tumor pressing on a nerve root could be present without producing objective neurological changes. It just seemed to them incredible that such a thing could be true."* No one believed him, but the irony was that he realized that he had discovered nothing new. *"We rediscovered something that had been known."* The dynasty of the disc—Farfan's phrase—begins.

1936 Shordania—the pyriformis syndrome. Another wrong turn in the explanation of sciatica.

1939 Love at the Mayo Clinic introduces keyhole laminotomy.

1944 Magnuson decompresses the intervertebral foramen for sciatica.

1963 Lyman Smith and Joe E. Brown: papain is used to break down the disc with enzymes but, despite a lot of success, the risks (anaphylaxis or neurologic damage) take it off the market after a few years.

1970 Harry Crock: isolated disc resorption

1974 Robert Williams of Las Vegas: microdiscectomy

False Trails

Before root compression by disc and bone was accepted, many imaginary diseases were invented, such as sacroiliac disease piriformis syndrome, and visceroproptosis. And operations were done for them. For example:

END-RESULT STUDY OF ARTHRODESIS OF THE SACROILIAC JOINT FOR ARTHRITIS—TRAUMATIC AND NONTRAUMATIC

M. N. SMITH-PETERSEN AND WILLIAM A. ROGERS, 1926

"It is the purpose of this paper to offer evidence justifying the diagnosis of traumatic arthritis of the sacroiliac joint. This evidence will be offered in such a way that surgeons of the opposite viewpoint in order to refute it will have to do more than simply state 'There is no such condition as traumatic sacroiliac arthritis.' There are a great many orthopaedic surgeons who hold this latter point of view in a passive, non-aggressive way."

Results: Complete recovery, 85%; failures, 8%.

Spondylolisthesis

This condition was known well before X-rays were invented, from pathologic specimens that were obtained from women who had died in obstructed labor. It was not important as a cause of back ache. Neugebauer's article was written in a gynecologic journal to show obstetricians how to recognize the condition from the posture and gait of the patient. He collected cases from the literature, added some of his own, and described a number of bony specimens.

A 14-year-old girl had a fall when carrying a bucket of water on her head in 1861. She could not stand or walk for three months because of sacral pain. Subsequently she had attacks of back pain and after a stillbirth came under the care of gynecologist Hegar (of dilator fame). He could feel the 5th lumbar vertebra prolapsed in front of the sacrum on rectal examination. Neugebauer believed that she had a fracture followed by spondylolisthesis.

"My investigations at present have led me to take the following view of the etiology of the so-called spondylolisthesis: a congenital spondylolisthesis interarticularis may exist in the arch of the fifth lumbar vertebra on one or both sides ... (But) in by far the greater number of cases the anamnesis gives evidence that the spondylolisthesis commenced in a fracture."

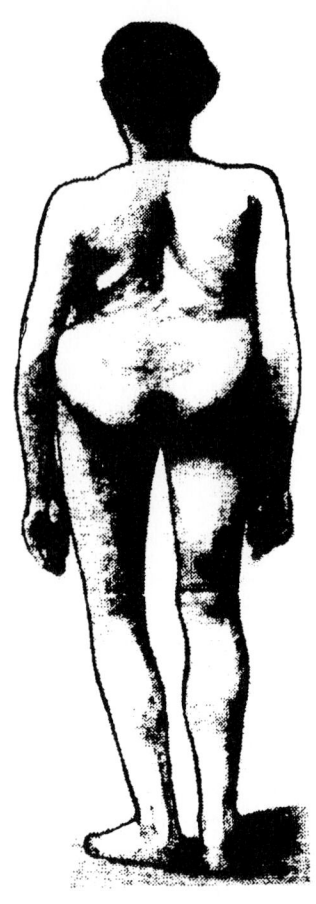

Spondylolisthesis, 1868. From Franz Ludwig Neugebauer (1856–1914), who was an obstetrician in Warsaw, Poland, when he noted the striking appearance of women with severe spondylolisthesis. The trunk appears short, and the pelvis is extended. Transverse abdominal creases are common. This, he wrote, should warn obstetricians about a narrow birth canal. He was writing in the days before spinal surgeons existed.

◆ **Ernest Adolph Gustav Gottfried Strumpell (1853–1925)**

Leipzig internist and pathologist. His textbooks went through 30 editions and were translated into several languages. He wrote a classic on ankylosing spondylitis.

TIMELINE OF SPONDYLOLISTHESIS

18th C Herbineaux describes the condition.
1839 Rokitansky described it in a textbook of pathology.
1854 Kilian's description
1882 Neugebauer describes the clinical features in a 70-page monograph republished in English by the New Sydenham Society.
1936 Jenkins tries to reduce the slip with traction and fusion.
1953 Watkins introduces posterolateral fusion.
1970 Scott wiring to secure healing of the pseudarthrosis
1976 Harrington is the first to instrument reduction of a slip. Many others have followed in his footsteps.
1976 Classifications by Wiltse, Newman, and Macnab: dysplastic, isthmic, degenerative, traumatic, and pathologic types of spondylolisthesis

---

Spinal Osteoporosis and Senile Kyphosis

Wedge compression fractures and stenosis are such a common cause of misery in older women that I thought that there would be a lot written. I could find nothing—perhaps because old age is a modern phenomenon.

Original Papers on Sciatica

SCIATICA: TREATISE ON THE NERVOUS SCIATICA OR NERVOUS HIP GOUT
DOMINICUS COTUGNO (COTUNNIUS), 1775

"1. *It is a thing very well known amongst physicians, that the name Sciatica is given to that species of pain which seizes the hips about those parts where the thighbones form the joints; a pain seldom felt in both, but often in one, so as to render the patient lame on that side which it invests. This name is of Greek origin, and is derived from the seat of the disorder; for the hip in Greek is called ischios but I much doubt whether it was adopted by the Latins before the time of Pliny the Elder. For altho' Cato has the word Ischiacos, yet Celsus, who was very accurate in his knowledge of the Latin names, which were affixed in his time to diseases, when he has occasion to mention this pain, chuses to call it Dolor Coxae.*

"2. *The species of the Sciatica are various, according to the various parts in which the pain is felt; and altho', as hitherto, physicians have not discriminated between them so accurately as they ought; yet every one is separately to be distinguished and marked out by its characteristic symptoms, as each demands its proper treatment in the cure. The principal species of Sciatica that deserve our attention are two; one, where the pain is fixed in the hip, and extends no further; the other, where it runs along, as it were, in a track, and is propagated even down the foot, on the same side. Altho', in the former, it is not only one part of the hip that is always affected, nor the pain produced always by the same cause; yet because it is generally felt about the joint, I think it would be properly termed the arthritic Sciatica. The latter, because it has its situation in the nerves which run along the hip (notwithstanding it is by some called the true, as by Prosperus Martianus and by others the bastard Sciatica, as by Riolanus) I am of opinion ought to be called the Nervous Sciatica.*

"3. *At present, I shall leave the Arthritic Sciatica out of the question. I shall take upon me to speak only of the Nervous Sciatica, the principal causes of which lie as yet buried in obscurity. But I shall divide this Sciatica into two species. The one is a fixed pain in the hip, situated chiefly behind the great trochanter of the thigh, and extends itself upwards to the Os sacrum, and downwards by the exterior side of the thigh even to the knee; this pain seldom stops at the knee, but often runs on the exterior part of the head of the Fibula, and descends to the fore part of the leg, where it pursues its course along the outside of the anterior spine of the Tibia, before the exterior ancle, and so ends on the Dorsum Pedis. The other is fixed pain in the groin, which runs along inside of the thigh and leg. The former, as it is situated in the posterior part of the hip, and arises from an affection of the Ischiadic Nerve, I shall call the Posterior Nervous Sciatica: the latter, which invests the fore part of the hip, and is propagated*

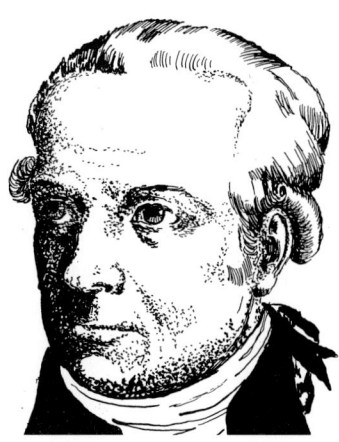

◆ **Domenico Cotugno (Cotunnius) (1736–1822)**

Cotugno was born in Ruvo, Italy; his father, not rich, spared nothing to give his son a good education. This decision was rewarded. At the age of 9 years Domenico could speak the Latin tongue with fluency: at the age of 18 he was elected to the position of Physician at the Hospital for Incurables in Naples, perhaps considered a safe appointment for a teenager. By the age of 20 he was Professor of Surgery and occupied the chair for 66 years until his death at age 86.

He is remembered for his discovery of cerebrospinal fluid, his discovery of the aqueducts of the inner ear, descriptions of sciatica, typhoid ulcers, and the presence of a substance that coagulated on heating the urine of patients with nephritis.

On his deathbed he left 100,000 ducats to the hospital he had served so long.

along the Crural Nerve, I shall term the Anterior Nervous Sciatica. I shall now, as briefly as I can, relate what discoveries and observations I have made, and what judgment I have formed on these two species of the disease.

"4. To begin with the Posterior Sciatica Nervosa, I have observed that it is either continual or intermitting: sometimes it tortures the patient day and night, without any intermission; but more commonly remits now and then, and returns again at stated intervals.

"5. As I observed all the symptoms accurately, I concluded the judgment I had formed was right; and that it consisted in an affection of the Ischiadic Nerve. Though chance has never thrown an opportunity in my way to prove this by the dissection of any person who died in this disorder, I do not in the least imagine that I am assuming a dubious state of the case, in pointing out its seat. For in this particular I am very well satisfied both by my own diligent observations of the symptoms, as well as by the happy and absolute cures I have performed in consequence of them. If I am here deceived, I am happily deceived, and I am not very solicitous to be delivered from the infatuation, since in it I have such success with my patients.

"6. Not only the situation and track of the pain demonstrate that the seat of the disorder is in the Ischiadic Nerve, but likewise the various affections which follow prove it clearly. For the insuperable lameness that is sometimes the consequence of it, shews, that the powers of the muscles in moving the thigh and leg are weakened: but the power of those muscles that maintain the free motion of the nerves, are not commonly weakened for a long time. For a Semi-palsy coming on, gives us a striking proof that the nerves are affected. It is usually accompanied with an emaciation, which distinguishes the torpor of the limbs arising from long inactivity, from that impotence which is brought on by wounding the nerves. Therefore, if the nerves of the hip in this Sciatica are affected, I do not see how it can be doubted that the Ischiadic, of all the nerves traversing the hips, as the pain is fixed there, is not the cause and seat of the disorder. In this nerve the pain is felt, in this nerve we are to search for the cause of lameness, and from its affection the origin of the Semiparalysis and Tabes."

[He drew attention to the cerebrospinal fluid circulating in the dural sacs. He thought this could be present in excessive amounts, diffusing into the peripheral nerves.]

"Since, therefore, an abundant, or acrid fluid, abiding in the outer Vaginae of the Ischiadic Nerve, may cause the Posterior Nervous Sciatica, let us now see how it generates all the symptoms and effects of it. In the first place, if it arises from too great an abundance of fluid, the Vaginae of the nerves will consequently be strained, and the enclosed nervous filaments compressed, so that the leg will be rather benumbed than painful. On the other hand, if the fluid be acrid, then the pain will be sharp and permanent. But from whichsoever of these causes it arises, the

pains will be exacerbated towards the evening; for at that time a man's body grows warm, and the pain is increased, either by the more rapid circulation of the blood's causing a greater quantity of fluid to be thrown into the Vaginae; or by the increased heat's exciting or adding a greater stimulus to the acrid matter. The pain that the patient suffers in this exacerbation, can hardly be expressed."

[Cotunnius goes on to compare sciatica with brachial neuralgia.]

"I now flatter myself that I have produced some probable reasons, and causes, of the generation of pain in the Ischiadic Nerve; and why its trunk and branch, which descends to the leg, feel the track of the pain and are more adapted to receive the causes, than the other nerves of the body, except the Cubital. Nor is there here any room to cavil at me, because the Cubital Nerve has almost the same disposition, and yet is seldomer affected with pain. For, although this may be owing to the Cubital Nerve's having but a small track uncovered with muscles, the pain is not so rare to be met with as is imagined. Indeed, I have often known the Cubital affected at the same time with the Ischiadic Nerve; and especially when the cause of the pain was internal, and might be communicated to both nerves. This consent, and agreement of pain in the elbow and hip, have been observed by me more than once, in curing those who were harrassed with a rheumatic or venereal Virus; and I do not doubt, but that, if anyone would attend to it, we should frequently observe an alliance between these two pains. Nay, as I have often observed, the pain of the hips descends by degrees to the foot, or rises from the foot to the hip, I have in like manner found the pain of the elbow ascend to the shoulder, and reach to the extremities of the fingers. There is so great a similarity and consent between these pains, whether we regard the disposition of the affected parts, or the nature of the pain, that I think Celsus, in judging these two pains, has done right to couple them together, and even put them upon a par. Indeed, if the name of the Sciatica had not taken its origin from the seat of the pain, but from its appearance, I myself should not hesitate to call that pain of the arm, the Nervous Cubital Sciatica; for it agrees with the Posterior Nervous Sciatica, in appearance, situation, symptoms, and cure."

The Lasègue Sign

The remarkable feature of this sign is that it was never described by Lasègue—the "universal specialist." In 1864 Lasègue wrote *Thoughts of Sciatica* and since then most authors have been happy to imagine that this includes a description of the sign. This error has been copied from one learned book to another. Lasègue in fact described two cases of sciatica, observing that weight bearing and flexing both hip and knee together aggravated the pain.

His pupil Forst described the sign in a doctoral thesis in 1881, and wrote that his attention was attracted to it by Lasègue—his teacher, sponsor, and President of the University examiners. Forst

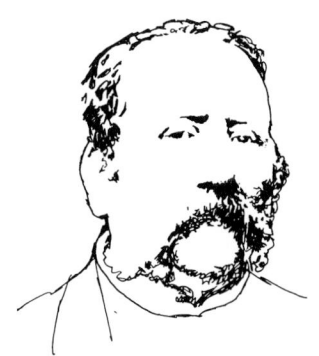

◆ **Ernest Charles Lasègue (1816–1893)**

considered that the sign depended on the sciatic nerve becoming compressed by the hamstrings.

However, in the year before Forst went into print a Yugoslavian physician, Laza K. Lazarevic, had described the sign in the *Serbian Archives*. Lazarevic based his observations on six patients and realized that the sciatic nerve could be stretched by straight leg raising. He mentioned two other ways of eliciting the sign: by attempted toe touching or by instructing the patient to sit up in bed with the knees extended. Due to the lack of popularity of this last technique, it is a useful way to separate a malingerer from the genuine article.

In 1884 de Beurmann studied the mechanism of the sign; he removed the sciatic nerve from a cadaver, replacing it by a piece of rubber tubing. On straight leg raising the tube elongated by 8 cm.

There seems little point in immortalizing the name of Lasègue in this connection. Lazarevic or Forst would prove no more popular with medical secretaries—perhaps it should be called the sciatic stretch test.

SCIATIC STRETCH TEST
J. J. FORST, 1881

"*We do not intend to make a complete study of sciatica but will limit ourselves to study, in particular, one clinical sign of very great value from the point of view of diagnosis. In spite of all that has been written on sciatica, we have been unable to find any mention of the symptom that we are about to discuss. Professor Lasègue attracted my attention to this sign.*

"*What then is this sign?*

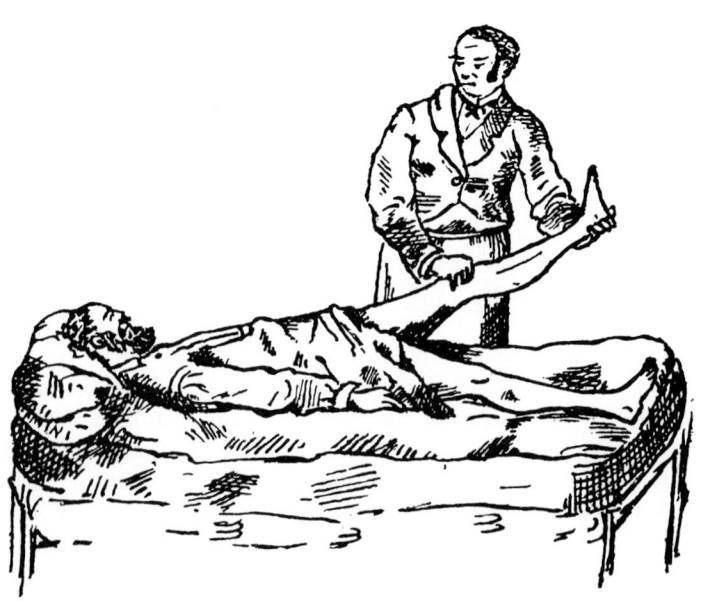

The Lasègue sign. From J. J. Forst, 1881.

"We place the patient on the bed lying on his back; in this position we take the foot of the affected leg in one hand as shown in the Figure, and place the other hand on the knee of the same leg; having done this, we flex the thigh on the pelvis, keeping the leg extended. It is only necessary to lift the limb a few inches for the patient to experience acute pain at the level of the sciatic notch just at the emergence of the nerve. We replace the limb on the bed, and proceed with another manoeuvre, which gives further verification of the sign that we have mentioned.

"We have just seen that the patient experiences acute pain when the thigh is flexed on the pelvis while the leg is held in extension. If we now flex the leg at the knee, we are able to flex the thigh at the hip without causing the patient any painful feeling."

Forst reasons that the pain is produced by the muscles at the back of the thigh becoming tense when the straight leg raising test is performed. These muscles compress the sciatic nerve. When the knee is flexed, the relaxed muscles do not compress the nerve and the maneuver is painless.

INJURY OF THE SPINAL CORD DUE TO RUPTURE OF AN INTERVERTEBRAL DISC DURING MUSCULAR EFFORT

GEORGE S. MIDDLETON AND JOHN H. TEACHER, 1911

"The following case is of interest, because it seems to throw light upon certain cases of spinal myelitis and haemorrhage into the spinal cord arising out of strains and racks of the back in men engaged upon heavy work. So far as we are aware, the lesion is one which has not hitherto been observed, as we have been unable, after considerable search in literature and enquiry among pathologists and surgeons, to find any record of an exactly similar case.

"A man was lifting a heavy plate from the floor to a bench, when he felt a "crack" in the small of his back. He suffered intense pain, and was unable to straighten himself. Paraplegia soon developed, and the patient died sixteen days later, principally from the effects of bedsores and septic cystitis. The cause of the paraplegia was haemorrhage and softening in the lumbar enlargement of the spinal cord, and the cause of this was found in a mass of the pulp of an intervertebral disc which had been displaced into the vertebral canal.

"With regard to the mechanism of the injury, it can be inferred from the history of the case that the man, at the moment at which he felt the "crack" in his back must have had his back more or less bent forward, with the lumbar and abdominal muscles in full action.

"This would cause powerful compression of the intervertebral discs, with the anterior margins of the vertebrae approximated to one another, and, therefore, in a favourable position for displacement of the pulp of the intervertebral disc backwards, if that were possible.

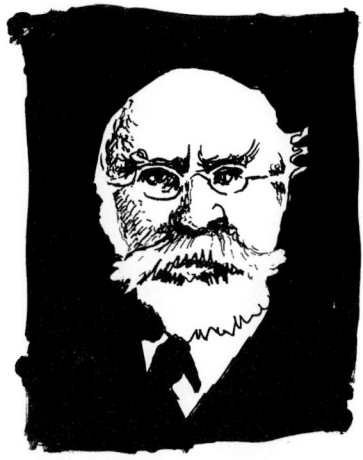

◆ George Stevenson Middleton (1853–1928)

He was born in Aberdeen and graduated from Glasgow University. As a physician he joined the teaching staff and instituted a postgraduate class on Sundays, probably initiating postgraduate education in Glasgow. His writings were mainly descriptions of unusual and interesting cases.

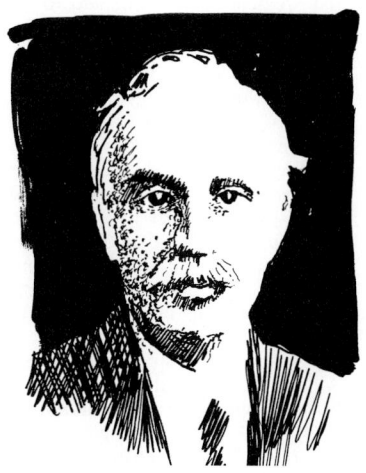

◆ John Hammond Teacher (1869–1930)

A graduate of Glasgow University who became Professor of Pathology. His main interest was in gynecological pathology, and he achieved fame for describing a very early fetus.

"To test this theory of the injury experiments were made to see whether the pulp of the intervertebral disc could be squeezed out through the strong surrounding ligaments, and the direction which it would take.

"In one a successful result was obtained. The first three lumbar vertebrae from the body of a well-developed man with no disease of the column were placed in a carpenter's wooden vise, and pressure made rather more to the front than to the back. The cord and the nerves had been cut out, leaving the dura in situ. It was noted before pressure that the position of the intervertebral discs was shown by a slight bulging inwards. After pressure had been applied a definite rounded prominence could be seen opposite the disc between the first and second lumbar vertebrae, close to the side of the posterior longitudinal ligament.

"The pressure had not been very powerful—certainly not enough to crush the bones at all. Repeating the experiment with more powerful pressure, the swelling was seen to increase slightly.

"The arches were then cut out and the dura mater raised. The rounded swelling was found with the fibrous outer layer of the disc intact. Pressure with an iron vise to crushing of the bone failed to produce any further swelling.

"On cutting through the disc with a sharp knife it was found that the swelling actually was due to displacement of the soft pulp, which had forced its way through the inner fibrous layers of the disc as far as the outer sheath. The corresponding area on the other side was unchanged. The pulp of the disc had, therefore, been displaced, and it had travelled in the direction which it must have followed in the victim of the accident."

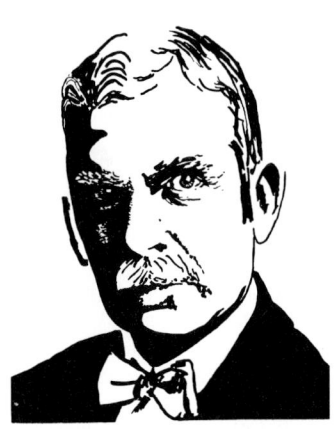

◆ Joel Goldthwait (1866–1961)

Goldthwait was born in Marblehead, Massachusetts. He planned to work in scientific agriculture and graduated, but after one unhappy day in business, he decided to try something else. He graduated again in medicine from Harvard in 1890. He worked for an orthopaedic surgeon and made this his specialty. At the turn of the 19th century there were no hospital facilities in Boston for the crippled and disabled over the age of 12. As a result of agitation he acquired a third floor room to work from, and the success of this led to an orthopaedic outpatient clinic being formed at Massachusetts General Hospital. He raised funds to build a ward that was opened in 1909, and he became its first head. A little later he published his article on the importance of the lumbosacral joint. Later he organized a school of physical education and another for occupational therapy students, in addition to his great activity in writing and teaching. During his life he was at the forefront of the American orthopaedic scene and played a major role in the development of the Boston school of orthopaedics.

THE LUMBOSACRAL ARTICULATION; AN EXPLANATION OF MANY CASES OF "LUMBAGO," "SCIATICA," AND "PARAPLEGIA"

JOEL E. GOLDTHWAIT, 1911

"An experience of the writer within the past year in connection with the treatment of a patient with a spinal lesion was so disastrous to the patient and so distressing to the writer that a series of investigations were started in the hope of bringing some relief to the patient and at the same time of preventing such happenings in the future. It is this study which represents the basis of this communication, and in order that it may be fully understood the case that led to it is first reported."

Goldthwait described a 39 year old man who strained his back. A displacement of the right sacroiliac joint was diagnosed, and it was replaced under anesthesia. He made a normal recovery, but three months later his pain recurred and a strain of both sacroiliacs was diagnosed. The following day he felt something "slip" in his back as he leaned forward to get out of a bath. It produced sudden severe pain; his body was drawn forward and to one side, and the pain radiated into the legs. Goldthwait manipulated his sacroiliac joint under anesthesia but without relief, so later in the day he started to apply a plaster jacket in hypertension. While he was doing so the patient had another severe pain and within a few minutes developed a motor and sensory paraplegia with paralysis of the sphincters. When he was put on his side this disappeared but returned when he turned over in bed. By the following morning the paraplegia was complete and remained so.

After six weeks Harvey Cushing explored the spinal canal from L1 to S3 but found no abnormality. The patient improved somewhat and eight months later was able to move with canes.

Goldthwait's powers of reasoning were stimulated. He thought that this cauda equina lesion had occurred at the lumbosacral level because of clicks from this region, tenderness, and the pattern of paralysis. He studied the anatomy and abnormalities of the region, and suggested that the lumbosacral joint could become subluxated by the transverse process of L5 striking the sacral ala and prising the joint open. He mentions that Dr. A. H. Crosbie had seen, but not published, a case of paraplegia due to proven disc prolapse. The illustration gives his impression of what it would look like.

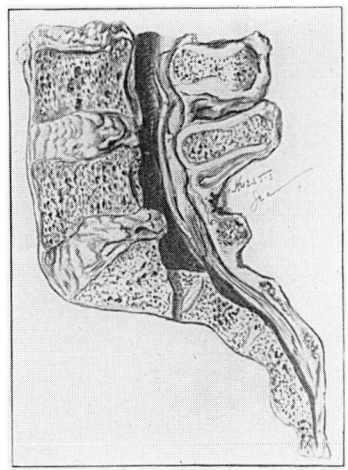

Goldthwait's concept of a disc compressing the cauda equina.

It is a paper that covers possibilities, because in view of the negative laminectomy, he had no evidence to incriminate a massive disc prolapse, which would today seem the most likely cause of his patient's troubles.

Here are his final conclusions.

"The lumbosacral articulation varies very greatly in its stability, depending upon peculiarities in the formation of the articular processes and of the transverse processes; that these peculiarities not only result in less than the normal strength of the joint, but may represent mechanical elements which not only produce strain and cause pain but may lead to such great instability that actual displacement of the bones may result, with at the same time the separation of the posterior portion of the intervertebral disk.

"In such displacement, if the fifth lumbar slides forward upon the sacrum, spondylolisthesis, the condition is usually compensated for, and pressure upon the cauda equina or the nerve roots does not occur.

"If the displacement be upon one side, the spine must be rotated and the articular process of the fifth is drawn into the spinal canal with such narrowing that paraplegia may result, or the crowding backward of the intervertebral disk alone may be so great as to cause paraplegia, but of more gradual development.

"Weakness of the joints or the partial displacements may cause irritation of the nerves inside or outside of the canal and produce the bilateral leg pains often called sciatica."

JOE BARR REMEMBERS DIAGNOSING A DISC IN 1932

"My first concept with regard to lumbar disk lesions as causing clinical symptoms dates back to 1932. At that time I was just a little over 30 years old, and was in private practice. Those of you who are old enough to know about 1932 know that there wasn't much private practice at that time. It was scratch as

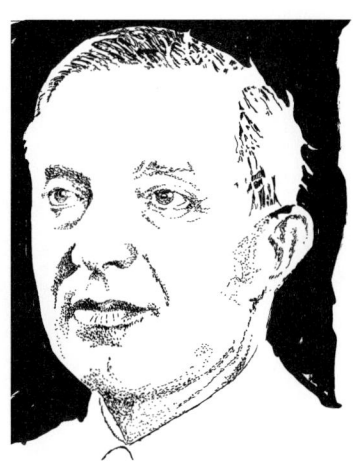

◆ Joe Barr

scratch can. There wasn't a great deal of work and the work there was went to much older and much wiser doctors than I was at that time and perhaps ever will be.

"I worked with Dr. Ober.

"In any case, in 1932 a young fellow came down to see Dr. Ober. I examined this fellow. His name was Kenneth Newton. He was in his 30s.

"Kenneth Newton had what we now recognize as a classical disk syndrome. He had hellish pain down his leg. He had a list in his back and he was miserable. Plain X-rays were negative. We put him in a little hospital to cool off. He stayed uncomfortable. Well, in those days we thought the cause of this syndrome was either sacroiliac strain, as exemplified by Smith-Petersen, or perhaps lumbosacral strain. Phil Wilson was a great person to defend the sacroiliac region as the cause of low back and sciatic pain. We knew that spondylolisthesis caused pain in the legs sometimes. We knew that infectious arthritis did also. We knew that tumors did and then we sort of stopped and we didn't know much more about it than that.

"Anyway, Kenneth Newton didn't do very well under conservative treatment so we considered manipulating his back. This was a standard form of treatment. I couldn't understand, if it was strained, why it failed to be relieved by complete bed rest. It seemed to me very odd that this could be true. Any other strain of ligaments that I had ever heard of would be relieved by rest. It was also hard to understand why strain of any ligament could produce what appeared to be typical nerve pain, deep seated and agonizing.

"So I said to Dr. Ober, 'Before we manipulate his back, isn't it possible that we are missing something?' Dr. Ober said, 'Yes, he might have a tumor. Let's get Jason Mixter to see him.' Jason Mixter was a neurosurgeon, of course, and the man in New England who knew most about the spine. So Jason saw the patient and said, 'Well, it could be a tumor all right.' He had operated on a few chondromas of the spine and he advised that we do a Lipiodol myelographic examination. We put in 2 cc of Lipiodol to fill a big broad spinal sac and those 2 cc ran a little pencil line up and down the back. We didn't even know enough to do fluoroscopy. We just took a couple of films. These were negative as far as this was concerned. The patient was no better.

"Jason said he would be willing to explore the spine. So he did. Here I missed an excellent opportunity because I wasn't present at the exploration. I was busy doing some orthopedic examination or other and didn't see the surgery. But I was told the patient had a chondroma of the spine. I saw the operative note and in the clinical records at the M.G.H. is a very lovely pen-and-ink sketch that Mixter had made. He found the tumor by opening the dura, doing a rather radical laminectomy, removing the 2 laminae and removing the tumor through the opening in the dura. He found the first sacral nerve root under compression and removed it transdurally. The patient was much better, in fact was completely relieved of his back and leg pain.

"I wasn't so busy in those days and so on the next Sunday morning after the report had come back from pathology, 'chondroma of the spine,' I went over to the Pathology Department, got the slides out and asked to see them. Here was this tumor but I couldn't see any cells. That seemed to me very odd. I asked Tracy, the pathologist, about this chondroma that didn't have any cells. He said, 'Well, that is a characteristic of chondromas of the spine. They don't have cells.'

"Just about that time something happened which gave us a clue. I was sent a book by Schmorl and Junghanns. I won't give the German title of it but it was a book on the spine in disease and health and, as you all know, Schmorl was a German pathologist who spent his life, especially his later years, studying spines which had been removed at autopsy. He described these little posterior protrusions which he saw which he thought were of no clinical significance. 'Nicht wichtig,' they were called. I had been asked to review this book. My German was very bad. It took me about 3 or 4 weeks of hard slogging before I could make out just what this was all about. I asked Tracy Mallory if this could be a disk protrusion because from Dr. Mixter's description this had arisen from an intervertebral disk. Tracy said he didn't know. It might be. I went to the medical school and asked to see some slides of disk tissue and there were no pathological histological slides of normal intervertebral disk tissue at Harvard Medical School. This was extraordinary, but it was a fact. It was a tissue of no importance.

"So we made some disk tissue slides and compared them with this 'tumor.' Of course, it was the same sort of material. Fortunately, the Pathology Department had a very lovely index of all material they had ever examined at the M.G.H. since it was opened in 1812 or so.

"We were able to find about 20 or 30 cases of chondromas of the spine. They ranged from the cervical spine on down to the lumbar spine with 1 or 2 in the dorsal spine. And of these 'chondromas' of the spine, there were 3 or 4 of them that anybody, even a fourth year medical student, could tell were chondromas. They had cartilage cells in them. The rest of them all looked like normal disk tissue.

"So we were on the hunt then for other clinical cases with this same type of thing. Our first case in which we made the diagnosis preoperatively was a fellow by the name of John Andrade who was a Portuguese chap from down on Cape Cod.

"Phil Wilson and I operated on him. He had a severe forward and lateral list of his spine so he was cocked off to the side. Phil Wilson was sure that strain had a lot to do with this. So we took a massive tibial graft and did a fusion on him after the disk had been removed. He fused solidly but he fused with the list still present. John Andrade is living today with his spine bent off to the side about 30° and listed forward about 30°.

"Then the struggle was on. We had a very difficult time getting the neurologists to accept the possibility that a tumor pressing on a nerve root could be present without producing *objective neurological changes. It just seemed to them incredible that such a thing could be true."*

MYELOSCOPY, OR THE DIRECT VISUALIZATION OF THE SPINAL CANAL AND ITS CONTENTS
MICHAEL BURMAN, NEW YORK, 1931

Burman examined 11 cadaver spines. His arthroscope was too big for most spines. *"In cases where the canal was wider, we were able to see the spinal cord, the dura mater, and some of the nerve constituents of the cauda equina."*

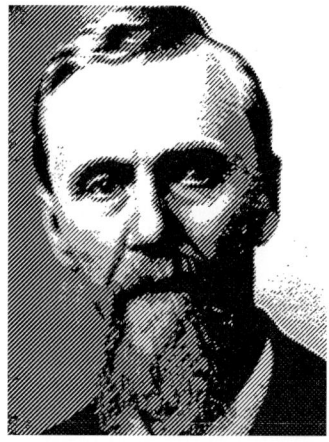

◆ **Andrew Taylor Still (1828–1917)**

Osteopathic medicine was founded by Still after he had served as a surgeon in the Civil War and after his three children died of meningitis in 1874. He lost his faith in the medicine of the day and started a school based on the idea that diseases were caused by musculoskeletal derangements and could be corrected by manipulation.

TIMELINE FOR THE TREATMENT OF BACK PAIN

Nonoperative Treatment

- 1813 Royal Central Gymnastic Institute founded in Sweden—Ling's exercises
- 1825 Delpech runs a Back School, but mostly for spinal deformities.
- 1874 Andrew Still—osteopathy founded
- 1874 Back braces. James Knight publishes *Orthopaedia*. He describes many orthotics since he was a champion of nonsurgical treatment. The only brace he is known for—the chairback brace—is not in the book. Women had been wearing corsets for centuries. Braces had been widely used for spinal deformity and tuberculosis for many years.
- 1895 D. D. Palmer: Chiropractic founded
- 1914-18 War sees the beginning of medically supervised physiotherapy.
- 1929 Evans: epidural blocks
- 1937 Williams' famous back exercises.
- 1946 John Bonica, an anesthetist, organizes a multidisciplinary Pain Clinic in Tacoma, Washington. This employed operant conditioning and reducing drug dependence.
- 1979 Zacrisson—back school—the aim is to educate patients about back pain and empower them.

Anterior Fusion

- 1880s Anterior approach begins to be used for draining tuberculous abscesses. The pus did all the tricky dissection.
- 1933 Burns of Britain fuses a spondylolisthesis from in front.
- 1934 Ito in Japan uses an anterior approach for tuberculous spine.
- 1960 Paul Harmon introduces the retroperitoneal approach.
- 1960 Hodgson and Stock in Hong Kong revolutionize spinal surgery with their anterior approaches for tuberculosis—these are used later for disc disease.
- 1969 Dwyer anterior instrumentation.
- 1971 Freebody of Croydon uses the transperitoneal approach for a large series of spondylolisthesis patients.

Posterolateral Interbody Fusion (PLIF)

1944 Briggs and Milligan used spinous process to stuff into the discotomy.
1946 Jaslow uses the same technique.
1957 Wiltberger uses plug cutters.

Many other systems are used today.

Posterior Fusion

1887 W. F. Wilkins in Kansas sutures the pedicles of a dislocated spine in a newborn baby.
1891 Berthold Hadra in Texas does an interspinous wiring.
1909 Fritz Lange uses steel bars wired to the spine to stabilize a fracture.
1911 Fred Albee uses a tibial cortical graft to stabilize the spine.
1911 Russell Hibbs fuses spines—interlaminar fusion.
1933 Ghormley introduces iliac graft.
1944 Don King—screw fusion of facets
1952 Wilson plate
1959 Boucher of Vancouver—screw fusion of facets, with the screws going down pedicles
1962 Harrington rods
1963 Roy Camille, pedicle screws and plates
1964 Knodt rods
1982 Luque rod and sublaminar wire
1984 Cotrel-Dubousset pedicle screws and rods

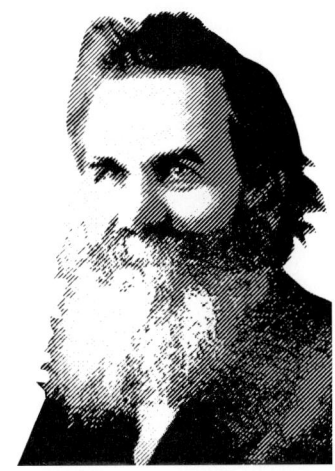

◆ **Daniel Palmer (1845–1913)**

In 1895, a janitor was bending over when he heard a pop in his back and became deaf. Palmer repositioned the vertebra where the janitor had heard the pop and his hearing returned. Palmer, a Canadian, became famous and founded the chiropractic school in Davenport, Iowa in 1898. *Cheir* is the Greek word for hand, and *praktikos* is Greek for action. Chiropractors believe that disease is due to nerve malfunction brought on by spinal malalignment, which can be corrected by spinal manipulation.

Vertebra Plana, 1925

A LOCALIZED AFFECTION OF THE SPINE SUGGESTING OSTEOCHONDRITIS OF THE VERTEBRAL BODY, WITH THE CLINICAL ASPECT OF POTT'S DISEASE
JACQUES CALVÉ, M.D., CHIRURGIEN EN CHEF DE LA FONDATION FRANCO-AMÉRICAINE DE BERCK PLAGE, FRANCE

"In this paper are submitted two observations, one of a case of my own, and one a case of my friend, Dr. Brackett, of Boston, who has been good enough to allow me to use the notes and illustrations of his case. They both occurred in patients in private practice and were observed carefully from the time of their first symptoms until their evident cure. Both cases were believed, during their entire evolution, to be Pott's disease, and were treated as such.

"Observation 1. P. F., 2½ years of age. Onset: November, 1921, insidious, gradual, accompanied by pain in the back, and stiffness, with the appearance of a small knuckle in the dorsal region which rapidly increased. Parents consulted a specialist, who made the diagnosis of Pott's disease and sent the child to the Riviera. The case came under my observation for the first time in May, 1922, six months after the onset. At this time there were the usual symptoms of Pott's disease with a sharp knuckle. The child was difficult to manage and, the diagnosis appearing evident, it did not seem necessary to have an X-ray picture taken at that time, and the case was treated at Berck by hyperextension in a recumbent position until January, 1924. The knuckle disappeared progressively, no abscess threatened at any time, nor were there any symptoms, at any time, suggesting compression of the spinal cord. The child made a recovery without deformity and now walks like a normal child, and is wearing, at present, a celluloid jacket as a matter of protection."

[Observation 2 was similar.]

"As seen from a clinical point of view, these were cases of dorsal Pott's disease. Neither developed an abscess or symptoms of spinal cord compression, the evolution was rapid, and the disease was, perhaps, cured in a shorter period than usual. Nevertheless, at the time this did not seem a sufficient reason for doubting the diagnosis of the tubercular nature of the affection, nor was there any doubt of the diagnosis until the evidence of the first roentgenograms was considered. As has already been stated, my patient was extremely difficult to manage, which prevented a roentgenogram being taken at the beginning of the treatment. When, from a clinical point of view, it was considered that the disease was cured, a roentgenogram was taken to confirm this clinical diagnosis of cure, and at once the abnormal aspect of the picture was apparent and raised a doubt of the original diagnosis. As there had appeared in an American journal at the same period a roentgenogram of the case treated by Dr. Brackett, which bore a striking resemblance to that of my own case, I obtained a picture of this case.

"A study of the two roentgenograms shows, in my opinion, the difference between them and pictures taken of a case of true Pott's disease.

"1. In these two cases the lesion attacks only one vertebra (there is but one pedicle).
2. In striking contrast here is the absolutely intact condition of the adjacent discs above and below the diseased vertebra.
3. The cartilage is thicker and there is a neoformation of this tissue. The transparent part above and below the lamellar osseous nucleus is at least a third higher than it is normally. (This is never seen in tuberculosis, which is markedly destructive of cartilage tissue.)
4. Greater opacity is to be remarked, which indicates that the bone density has increased. We are, therefore, justified in ruling out a diagnosis of tubercular infection in either of these two cases, and this observation, combined with the similarity of the roentgenograms, justifies the consideration of these two cases in the same category. It might seem presumptuous on my part to suggest a pathologic entity from the observation of two cases only, but one may advance a suppositional diagnosis while waiting for

other observations to corroborate these findings, and it is hoped that other observations will be stimulated by this short paper.

"In what type of disease can these two cases be catalogued? The affection which I have just submitted to you is, I believe, to the spinal column what coxa plana is to the hip, and what Koehler's disease is to the foot."

References

Chapter references are located in Chapter 26.

◆ Chapter Eight

Cervical Spine and Whiplash

At one time in Britain, more than 200 crimes were punishable by hanging, and only in 1868 was public execution abolished. About this time, interest in more minor degrees of neck pathology surfaced. The railways had been built, and trains were involved in all kinds of crashes, resulting in many cases of what is known now as whiplash injury. The first Model T Ford rolled off the assembly line in 1908 and made this injury commonplace.

Whiplash

Head and neck pain after a car accident is common and is still a bit of a mystery. This is nothing new. Before car insurance companies, there were railways with deep pockets, and in the early days, injury claims were common after a collision.

RAILWAY SPINE
JOHN ERICHSEN, 1866

"Concussions of the spine and of the spinal cord not infrequently occur in the ordinary accidents of civil life, but none more frequently or with greater severity than in those which are sustained by Passengers who have been subjected to the violent shock of a Railway Collision.

"The absence often of evidence of outward and direct physical injury, the obscurity of their early symptoms, their very insidious character, the slowly progressive development of the secondary organic lesions, and the functional disarrangements entailed by them, and the very uncertain nature of the ultimate issue of the case, they constitute a class of injuries that often tax the diagnostic skill of the surgeon to the very utmost. He must separate that which is real from that which is exaggerated."

It became the most common reason for a doctor going to court, and there were frequent differences of opinion.

The next year came a rejoinder:

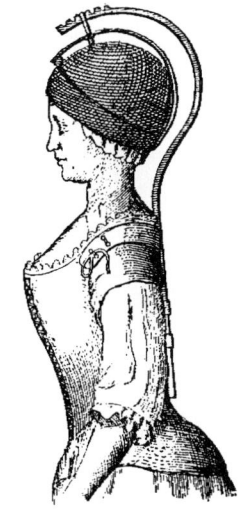

The jury mast for tuberculosis of the cervical spine—1768 (Joachimsthal). This was invented by François-Guillaume Le Vacher (1732-1816); his younger brother developed scoliosis braces.

ON COMPENSATION FOR RAILWAY INJURIES
JAMES SYME, 1867

"Since the passing of Lord Campbell's Act—a most unjust piece of legislation as it has always seemed to me, which established the principle of regulating the amount of damages for personal injuries in accordance with the value of individuals to society and to their families . . . For instance at this time last year a trial took place . . . on the part of a commercial traveller, who prosecuted the Great Northern Railway Company for compensation on account of an injury alleged to have been sustained from a collision on their line."

[Then he names nine doctors who gave evidence on one side or the other: Erichsen's side predicted death and Symes' side said there was no organic disease and good health was expected.]

"The jury, instead of the 12,000 pounds asked, gave 4700 pounds of damages; and before many months, the plaintiff, who had been rapidly recovering, admitted that he was quite well, as he still continues to be.

"The truth is, that when juries find medical evidence so conflicting, not being able to judge for themselves as to the merits of the case, they almost always decide in favour of the claimant, so that there is thus the greatest encouragement afforded to unfounded or exaggerated demands for redress."

Symes says that a patient only has to read Erichsen's book in order to learn how he should behave to win. He then gives a case of exaggeration he encountered and how he dealt with it. He hoped that publishing these cases would discourage them.

Contemporary Whiplash

Harold Crowe of Los Angeles used the word "whiplash" at a meeting in 1928.

INJURIES OF THE CERVICAL SPINE
A. G. DAVIS, 1945

This was one of the first articles to use the word "whiplash."

"Starting with the fact that the great majority of injuries to the cervical spine are in the nature of 'whiplash,' and accepting the meaning of the term "whiplash" as a hyperflexion followed by spontaneous extensor recoil, the nature of a great variety of injuries of this section of the spinal column becomes understandable.

"Two types of injury are immediately separated by the severity of the accident. For convenience these will be referred to as 'obvious' and 'obscure.'

"The 'obscure' lesions are those confronting the physician, with pain and spasm in the neck, variable pain radiation with graduations from those of trivial annoyance to those exhibiting intractable neuralgia. The question of injury is frequently slurred over by the patient for the reason that the painful symptoms do not develop until some time after the injury occurs."

Experiments on monkeys by Ian McNab in the 1960s showed that hyperextension of the neck did produce widespread damage to disc, muscle, and ligament.

COMPENSATION
J. G. JOHNSON, NEW YORK, 1883

"In 1866 an able and rising surgeon of England published a book of his triumphs in a new specialty he had worked up for himself, as a personal damage surgeon against railroad corporations, in a new disease he had discovered, resulting from the mighty power of steam in railway concussions upon the nervous system of human beings. The ingenuity and plausibility with which his book was written spoke more for his skill as a partisan than did the contents appear as that of a searcher after truth."

The English railways paid out 2.2 million pounds in compensation in 5 years for cases of concussion of the spine. In 1863 there were 35 killed and 401 injured in railway accidents in the United Kingdom.

MALINGERING AND FEIGNED SICKNESS
SIR J. COLLIE, 1913

"The many provisions made by the Legislature in recent years for securing benefits to injured workpeople have, undoubtedly, given rise to a large number of cases of malingering. Not many years ago it was practically only in naval and military circles that one heard the term used, where the ingenious Jack or Tommy feigned all sorts of ailments in order to avoid an unpleasant duty or get discharged from the Services. Chewing cordite or running gunpowder into self-inflicted wounds were among their more drastic means....

"As long as medical men who attend the working-classes are dependent on the working-men themselves and the club officials for their tenure of office, so long will gross exaggeration and malingering be rampant."

Cervical Spondylosis and Myelopathy

Nontraumatic neck pain due to disc degeneration has taken a century or more to be accepted. Beginning in 1824, Wenzel, Rokitansky, Luschka, and Lane appreciated that the discs degenerate with age and described the changes of cervical spondylosis. Olliver in 1824, Key in 1838, Jaccoud in 1864, and Leyden in 1874 discussed spondylosis causing paraplegia. Gowers in 1886 described spondylosis causing both root and cord compression. Also in 1886, Horsley removed an acute disc protrusion. From 1909, disc protrusions were thought to be chondromas, and several papers were written about neurologic defects due to them. In the 1920s, Schmorl started examining the spine at every autopsy and observed disc protrusions but stated (wrongly) that they did not produce neurologic deficits. Only after Joe Barr's paper (reproduced in Chapter 7) in the early 1930s did people accept that these so-called chondromas were really disc protrusions and could damage roots and cord.

Suprisingly, for a condition so common, it was not until the landmark paper by Brain in 1952 that disc protrusion, cervical spondylosis, radiculopathy, and myelopathy were put together. Decompression, foraminotomy, and fusion have become areas of rapid evolution.

THE NEUROLOGIC MANIFESTATIONS OF CERVICAL SPONDYLOSIS

W. R. BRAIN, D. NORTHFIELD, M. WILKINSON, 1952

"Forty-five cases of cervical spondylosis have been investigated. In 38 cases the spinal cord was compressed: in the remaining seven cases the nerve roots only. The primary lesion is a degeneration of the cervical discs, to which the changes in the bodies of the vertebrae and the neurocentral joints are secondary. The intervertebral disc is the site of a degeneration which evokes an osteophytic reaction in the bodies of adjacent vertebrae. The pathological lesion responsible for radicular symptoms is described as a root-sleeve fibrosis."

The paper is long and pictures the spinal cord indented by transverse bars.

SURGERY FOR THE CERVICAL SPINE

1864	Boudof drains an abscess from the front.
1891	Hadra in Texas fuses C6–C7 for a dislocation in a child.
1900	Louis Pilcher in New York tries to reduce a C1–C2 dislocation.
1910	Mixter and Osgood write about C1–C2 instability and reduction.
1928	Stookey reports difficulty in removing "chondromas" through a posterior transdural approach. They were bulging discs.
1937	Gallie in Toronto popularizes C1–C2 fusion with wire and ilium.
1942	William Rogers of Boston uses traction, fracture reduction, and interspinous wiring.

1951	Scoville and others write up 115 operative cases of posterior cervical discotomies.
1953	Mason: osteotomy of the cervical spine for ankylosing spondylitis
1955	Robinson and Smith in Baltimore report anterior discotomy and fusion.
1957	Perry and Nickel in Los Angeles—halo cast
1958	Ralph Cloward of Honolulu uses a circular graft for anterior body fusion.
1960	Bailey and Badgley in Ann Arbor describe anterior fusions at multiple levels.
1960	Anterior discotomy without fusion by Hirsch in Sweden
1960s on	There have been new approaches and many kinds of plates and screw methods developed—this book is about history, not current events, so I will stop here.
1961	Garrett—halo vest
1971	Hattori laminoplasty for ossification of the posterior longitudinal ligament
1978	Brooks and Jenkins improve the Gallie technique.

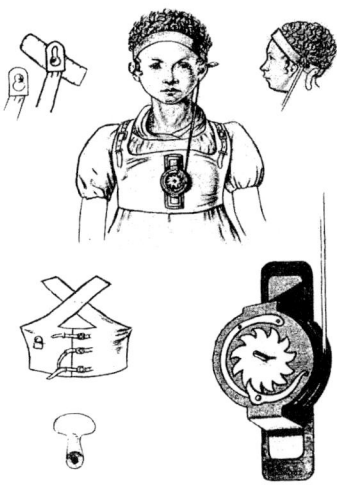

Jorg's brace for torticollis. Leipzig, 1810.

Torticollis

Congenital muscular torticollis is common, and one of the first patients is said to have been Alexander the Great (354 BC) because statues of him show head tilt—but this was a popular classical pose. A Dutch surgeon, Isaac Minnius, in 1652 carried out one of the first tenotomies for this condition. It would not be a place I would choose to start to do a tenotomy. Soon afterward Daniel Florianus tied a 14 year old boy to a chair and divided the tendon, which gave way "with such a snap as if one had plucked the string of a musical instrument." Hendrik van Roonhuyse in 1670 started to cut from inside outward because of all the pipes nearby. This operation was popular with fairground practitioners. All kinds of retentive splints were invented, leading Sayre to write in 1876: "Nearly all the complicated machinery which you may have seen in the shops for correcting wry-neck is of no use whatever."

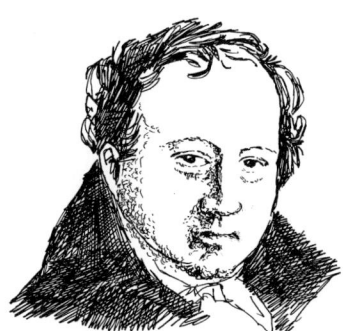

◆ Johann Christian Gottfried Jorg

Tuberculosis of the Cervical Spine

Old books are full of pictures of suspension of the head—like the one at the beginning of this chapter—because tuberculosis of the cervical spine was common. Today we see children with other kinds of instability walking around holding their head with their hands.

The Le Vacher Brothers: François-Guillaume (1732–1816) and Thomas (1738–1790)

François-Guillaume devised the jury mast seen at the beginning of this chapter and the Minerva cast. Thomas wrote a book about scoliosis and invented an extension chair with vertical traction and lateral pressure straps.

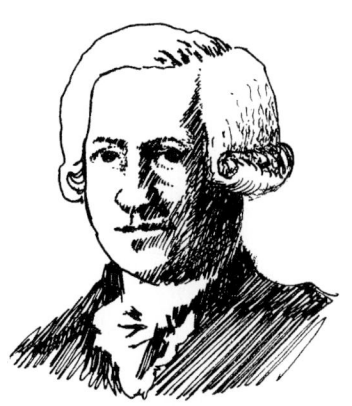

◆ François-Guillaume Le Vacher

Klippel-Feil Syndrome

A CASE OF ABSENCE OF CERVICAL VERTEBRAE WITH THE THORACIC CAGE ARISING TO THE BASE OF THE CRANIUM (THORACOCERVICAL CAGE)

MAURICE KLIPPEL AND ANDRÉ FEIL, 1912

"Anatomists have been interested in the study of variations for a very long time; but while formerly no special importance was attached to them other than caprices of nature, since Étienne Geoffroy St-Hilaire, a rational explanation has been sought for such occurrences. They are presented as variations of the human type which is not yet fixed, varying between what formerly existed and what we are to become, but evolving constantly toward a being more simple and more perfect.

"The syndrome which we report is an extremely rare example, perhaps unique, of a variant of the thoracic vertebrae, with congenital absence of the neck and the cervical vertebrae, ribs rising to the base of the skull to the degree that permits us to refer to a cervical thorax.

Observation

"Joseph, age 46, a tailor by profession, came to the Hospital Tenon on December 13, 1911, for pleurisy with pulmonary congestions and nephritis. On the first physical examination his appearance was striking. He appeared to have no neck; the head seemed to rest on the trunk. His appearance was quite unusual; there was absence of a neck, the head resting on his trunk astonished us. Nothing in his history or heredity had the least connection with this anomaly. The patient did not know whether the condition had been present at birth, he only knew that at about 7 years of age he had gone to a doctor who suggested an operation. At that time he presented apparently, besides the absence of a neck, a marked deviation of his head to the left, enough so that his ear touched the shoulder. This inclination lasted to the age of 12, slowly disappearing.

"His hair line went far down, occupying a triangular surface reaching to the third dorsal spinous process."

[He died of nephritis and the autopsy description follows.]

"**Vertebral Column.** There is a dorsolumbar scoliosis, concave laterally to the left.

"The first spinous process, the nearest to the cranium, is a bit larger, but especially larger than those below. It appears as if two spinous processes were soldered to each other. This process is separated from the occiput by a depression which increases with the head in hyperflexion and diminishes with the head placed in extension.

"There is a total absence of cervical vertebrae. There is no atlas, no axis, and that pivot which forms the odontoid process *of the axis is partly replaced by the interval which separates the occiput and the first spinous process.*

"This explains the limitation of movement of the head forward and backward, giving the impression of an articulation formed of two elements with the ample movement of a flexible vertebral column. The movement of the head is limited. Arms and legs are slightly atrophied but retain their normal movements . . . .

*"**Roentgenography.** The X-ray image is entirely characteristic. It confirms the complete absence of the cervical column. All the cervico-dorsal vertebrae carry ribs. The insertions of the first two ribs are so high that it is difficult to clearly see them attached to the vertebral column, they are partly hidden by the inferior maxilla in front, and by the base of the occiput behind.*

"The radioscopic examination, like the clinical examination, reveals a thoracic cage reaching to the base of the skull, occupied entirely by the two lungs whose superior lobes appear to mold themselves at the summit of the cage.

"Our patient is not only a curious example of an exceptional formation, but also serves as a deformity requiring clinical classification."

Maurice Klippel (1858–1942) was attending neurologist at Hôpital Tenon in Paris, and **André Feil** (b 1884) was his "intern" (today, probably resident) at the time this famous report was published. A rewriting of it appeared later that year in the *Bulletin of the Anatomic Society of Paris* (87:185, 1912).

In the latter third of the 19th and turn of the 20th century, comparative morphology was one of the most active disciplines in the scientific world of Europe, and the French were the leading exponents. Names such as Cuvier, Button, Geoffroy St-Hilaire, and Lamarck dominated the field and they sought to explain congenital malformations as links to an animal past. In this context, Klippel and Feil's report transcended the importance of a merely unique case. In the study of human congenital deformities, even as late as the 1930s, every attempt was made to relate them to some atavistic or ontologic precedent. In the present case the authors stress the fact that it bore no such relationship and suggest other possible causes for congenital deformity. Human genetics had not yet become a mature science.

References

Chapter references are located in Chapter 26.

◆ Chapter Nine

Infection

Infection was a frequent killer before antibiotics. One third of children died of infection, and the social impact was that parents did not dare to love them so much as they do today. Deaths of parents left many orphans and stepchildren. All kinds of infections spread as epidemics.

Today's major causes of death—heart disease, cancer, and trauma—were rarities. Staphylococci killed quickly and tuberculosis—the White Death—slowly. Bone and joint infections were seldom cured. Today, in the Third World this situation still persists, and patients with infections may fill a quarter of orthopaedic beds.

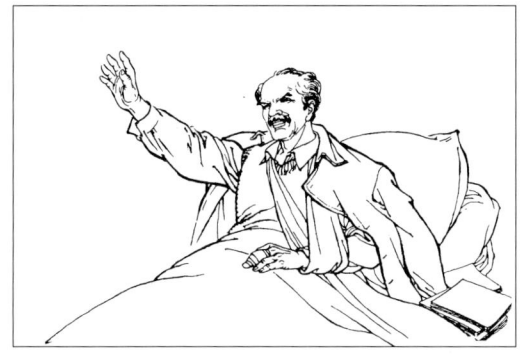

Norman Bethune, a Canadian surgeon, on his deathbed. Septicemia followed cutting his finger while operating on an infected patient. He was a surgeon with Mao in China in 1939.

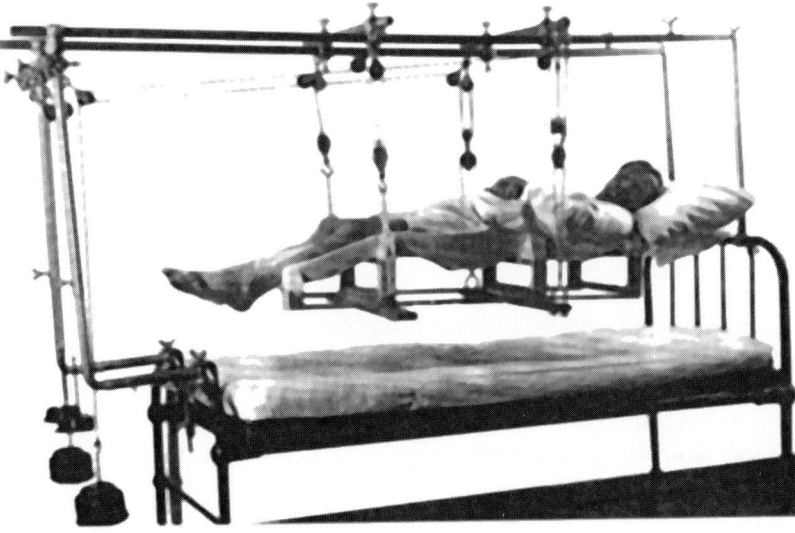

I remember building plaster beds for patients with spinal infections. The book, called "Nangle's Jangles," was indispensable and was the high-water mark of inventiveness. From Nangle EJ: Instruments and Apparatus in Orthopaedic Surgery. Oxford: Blackwell, 1951, Fig 791, p 90. Reproduced with permission.

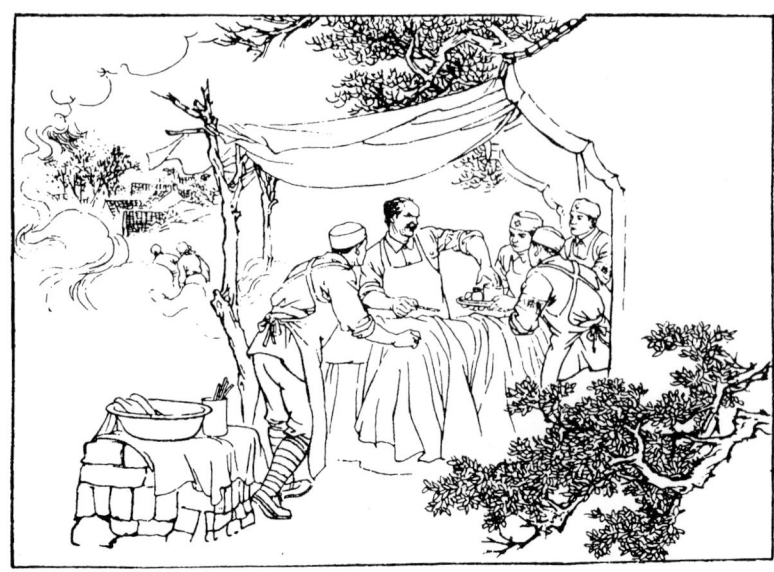

Norman Bethune (1890–1939). A Canadian hero, the subject of a chapter in Chairman Mao's *Little Red Book*. He trained as a surgeon in Montreal and went to China as an Army surgeon during the revolution. He was a firebrand and endured hardship. He was operating fast as the bombardment grew closer, cut his finger, dipped it in iodine, and worked on. Soon he died—because these were the days before antibiotics. Though human immunodeficiency virus (HIV) worries us today, the risk is less.

Until the 1950s, tuberculosis sanatoria were huge and were filled with spine and joint cases that employed many orthopaedic surgeons. The old image of an orthopaedic hospital was a hospital in the country where stay was measured in years and the patients were pushed outside all day, come rain or shine. The reduction in the length of stay that we have achieved with antibiotics for tuberculosis and osteomyelitis makes the reductions achieved by managed care today look minor.

Antibiotics have saved lives and have reduced disease. Chronic infection used to debilitate patients for months.

Surgeons who cut their fingers when draining abscesses were at risk of septicemia, leading to a severe illness or death. Paget thought he was going to die; Bethune did.

Tuberculosis

Tuberculosis (TB)—"The Captain of the Men of Death"—was long a problem that was made worse during the Industrial Revolution by the move to the cities and the overcrowding. A hacking cough filled a house or workplace with bugs enough to kill everyone around. Tuberculosis was the cause of 20 to 30% of deaths, and most patients with TB died. The treatment of bone and joint TB formed a large part of orthopaedic practice. With improved living standards and segregation of infected cases in sanatoria, the incidence began to fall, before streptomycin came on the market. In the 1950s, however, there were still many huge sanatoria, and

TB invalided a small proportion of medical students every year. Every orthopaedic ward had a patient with tuberculosis.

Effective treatment has eradicated TB from the First World, but it has always remained in the Third World and is becoming more common again because of human immunodeficiency virus.

TIMELINE OF TUBERCULOSIS
Paraplegia

300 BC	Hippocrates
1610	Dalechamps—early description
1610	Severinus—*De Recondite Abscessum Natura,* Naples, 1610
1744	Platner describes gibbus.
1779	Percival Pott provides such a clear description of paraplegia that it is called Pott's paraplegia. The alliteration ensures that every medical student will remember the name.
1779	Charles Hall
1779	Jean Pierre David writes in the same year as Pott, publishing a book in Paris.
1871	Michaud—Paris thesis
1880	Charcot—classic description

Pathology of Cord

1893	C. W. Burr—Patients died of paraplegia, providing this and the following writers the opportunity to study the histologic changes.
1897	V. P. Gibney
1898	W. G. Spiller
1898	S. Rosenheim
1923	E. Sorrel and Sorrel Dejerine classification
1935	Seddon and Butler classification

Medical Aspects

Hippocrates calls it phthisis, meaning the wasting disease, much the same as AIDS is called the slim disease in Africa today.

131	Galen says tuberculosis is contagious and that it is dangerous to live with consumptives.
1650	Royal Touch by a King is said to cure TB, known as scrofula.
1846	Klencke shows that cows can transmit TB—the incidence of human infection from drinking infected milk was reduced by pasteurization.
1850s	Death rate is 500 per 100,000.
1861	Pasteur—germ theory of disease
1865	J. A. Villemin: TB is a specific infection that is transmissible
1876	Dettweiller starts public sanatoria—they limit spread and provide better living conditions.
1882	Robert Koch discovers *Mycobacterium tuberculosis* while working as a country doctor.
1907	Jacob Riis starts to sell Christmas seals to finance TB care and research.
1910	Mantoux test

Box continued on following page

◆ **Jean-Pierre David (1737–1784)**
Professor of Anatomy and Surgery at Rouen and a proponent of rest for inflamed joints. He described tuberculous spine about the same time as Pott did, 1779. His dissertation was on rest and movement of joints.

1921	Immunization with BCG vaccine reduces the incidence of the disease.
1944	Streptomycin: Selman Waksman. In 1935 Waksman had been given the task of finding out what happened to tubercle bacilli in the soil. He found that saprophytic organisms led to their gradual disappearance but did not realize the significance of this. Even when a colleague brought him a culture of avian TB, which was killed by a contaminating mold, he did not wake up. Only when the concept of antibiotics was discovered did he start looking for an antituberculous organism in the soil. On August 20, 1943, he cultured a *Streptomyces* from a chicken's throat and found a substance that had antituberculous activity in vitro. In November 1944, the first patient was treated at the Mayo Clinic. In 1947, streptomycin became available to the general public. In 1952, Waksman was awarded the Nobel Prize.
1946	Lehmann—*p*-aminosalicylic acid (PAS)
1952	Isoniazid had been synthesized in 1912 but was tested only in 1952; it was found to have antituberculous activity by three drug companies simultaneously
1963	Death rate is 5 per 100,000: most sanatoria closed.

Surgical Aspects of Bone and Joint Tuberculosis

1000 BC	Mummy with tuberculosis
c 300–400 BC	Hippocrates gives a description of tuberculous spine
1676	Wiseman writes on tuberculous joints.
1705	Petit book on bone disease
1744	Platner on tuberculous gibbus—surgery for tumor
1779	Jean Paul David of Paris writes description of spine tuberculosis.
1779	Percival Pott advocates creating a draining sinus to decompress the abscess.
1813	Baynton—rest for tuberculous spine

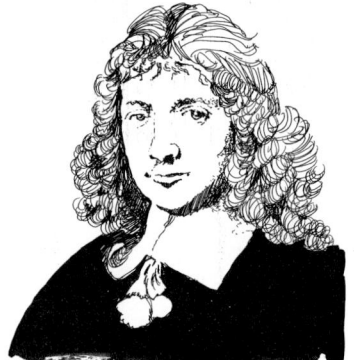

◆ **Richard Wiseman (1622–1676)**
Surgeon with the Royalists in the Civil War in Britain. He looked after gunshot wounds. He had an interest in tuberculosis and in his chirurgical treatise of 1676, entitled Several Chirurgical Treatises, he writes about tumor albus and warns against incising these swollen joints.

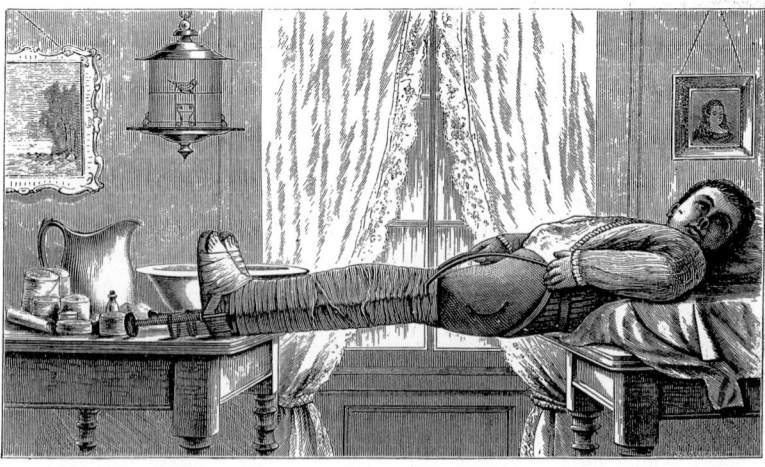

Redressing the wound after excision of the hip. Obviously home care was in vogue then too. From Sayre L: Lectures on orthopedic surgery. New York City, 1879.

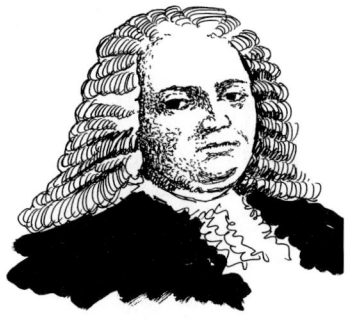

◆ **Jean-Louis Petit (1674–1750)**
French surgeon who used gravity to steady fractures—his inclined plane. In 1723 he wrote a book on bone disease, which included tuberculous spine.

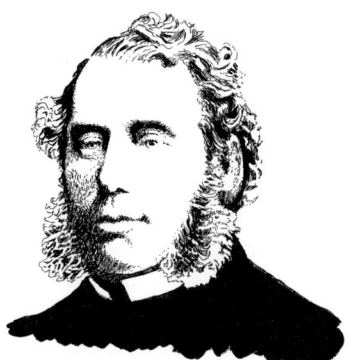

◆ **John Hilton (1807–1876)**
Surgeon at Guy's Hospital, who gave lectures entitled "Rest and Pain" in 1862, which became a book influencing us still today. He advocated rest and immobilization for painful joints. This may have encouraged infection to localize and discouraged systemic spread in the days before antibiotics, but now that we can kill bacteria early, movement is the best way to minimize local damage.

Treatment of Tuberculous Limbs

The original idea was to reduce deformity and immobilize the limb. There were fights between those who used traction, immobilizing splints, arthrodesis, and joint excision. This was one of the earlier examples of the difficulty of coming up with a consensus or a research answer in orthopaedics. There were many confounding variables, and there was a long delay between starting the treatment and knowing the result.

1806	Park and P. F. Moreau write about joint excision.
1829	Syme advocates joint excision and pseudarthrosis.
1845	Bonnet—*le grand appareil*—a complete wire exoskeleton
1845	A. Bonnet injects cadaver joints with fluid to discover what position the limb takes up and where the site of rupture lies (book, Paris)
1859	Bremer rest cure
1863	Hilton—*Rest and Pain*
1875	Thomas knee splint; although the older readers will remember using this for fractures of the femur, it was designed for tuberculosis of the knee.
1901	N. Senn (1844-1909) publishes one of the first big books on tuberculosis of bone and joint, in Philadelphia.
1932	Key—compression arthrodesis of knee
1940	Girdlestone hip excision in a book on tuberculosis of the bone

Treatment of Tuberculous Spine

Casts and Splints

Clearly splints and casts were often unsuccessful because they did not get to the cause of the problem. Variable results led to many acrimonious disputes between the protagonists of one method over another—e.g., Calot, Taylor, Sayre, Goldthwait, Bradford, Thomas, Whitman.

Drainage

Initially very few surgeons drained tuberculous abscesses because of the risk of introducing secondary infection. At first only a

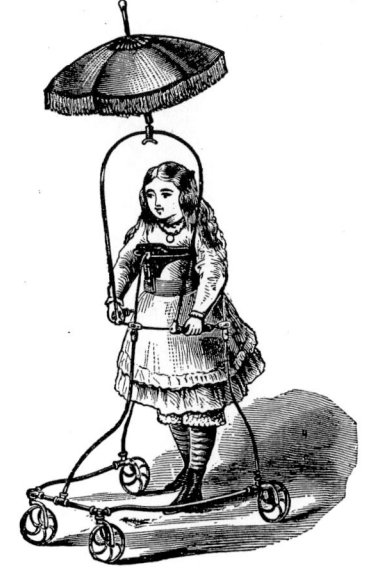

Ambulant treatment for spinal tuberculosis. From Sayre L: Lectures on Orthopaedic Surgery. New York: 1879.

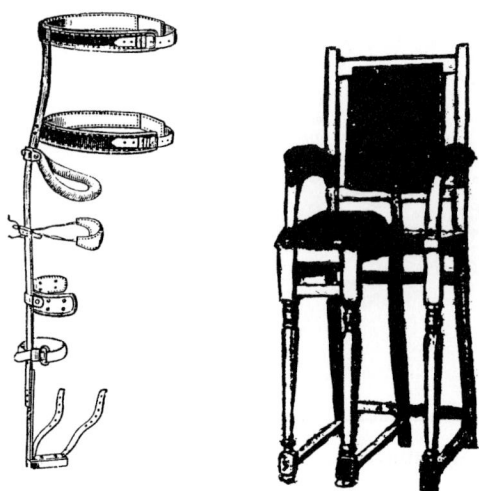

Special chair for the splint to immobilize a tuberculous hip. The patient sits on the sound side and rests the brace on the floor. From Sayre L: A Treatise on Orthopaedic Surgery, 1919.

few brave souls tried, but after antibiotics became available, drainage was on. Drainage removed the pus quicker than the body could absorb it.

Among the originators were Menard, Ito, Risko, Capener, and Hodgson.

Fig. 3
Schematic drawing to show the direct method of bone transplantation.

Anterior spinal fusion, 1933. From Ito H, Tsuchiya J, Asami G: New radical operation for Pott's Disease. J Bone Jt Surg Am 16:499-515, 1934. Reproduced with permission.

Fusion

A few surgeons fused the spine from behind in an attempt to reduce the risk of deformity and to provide immobility to achieve some healing. Later, anterior drainage and strut grafting were preferred—compression grafting is much sounder than tension grafting.

1891 Hadra advocates wiring a tuberculous spine from behind.
1893 A. Chipault uses fusion in Paris.
1902 Fritz Lange uses rods to fuse the spine.
1912 Hibbs does posterior fusion.
1914 Menard book on tuberculous surgery
1934 Hirumo Ito starts anterior debridement and strut grafting.
1938 Albee posterior strut grafts
1953 Johnson, Hillman, Southwick, etc., anterior surgery
1956 Hodgson and Stock advocate anterior spinal surgery.

Treatment of Paraplegia

1779 Pott drainage
1881 Macewen laminectomy
1891 Lane laminectomy
1894 Meynard costotransversectomy for cord compression
1954 Capener costotransversectomy
1956 Hodgson and Stock anterior decompression

Social Aspects

Many artists and writers had tuberculosis. Is there a link? Creative people with tuberculosis are thought to have been extra-productive because of a fevered imagination and the feeling that death lay ahead. If they didn't do it now they wouldn't have a second chance. There is the picture of Mimi in "La Bohème"; in orthopaedics there was Buckminster Brown; in poetry, Keats.

Volkmann on Hunchback

Richard von Volkmann (1830-1889) wrote fairy stories for his children during the Franco-Prussian War of 1870-1871, which eventually were printed and sold nearly a million copies in 31 editions and 5 translations. He used a pen name, "Richard Leander," which is Greek for Volkmann.

Here is one chilling example.

"Once upon a time there was a woman who had a child, a small pale girl who was unlike other children. When the woman took her for a walk, the people in the street stopped and whispered. When the little girl asked, 'Why do they look at me so strangely?' the mother answered, 'Because you wear such a very pretty new dress.'

"After a time the mother died, and the child had no one to take her walking. She became very pale and did not grow. A year later her father remarried, and the little girl fearfully asked if she might accompany her stepmother shopping. The stepmother cruelly replied, 'What would people say if they saw me walking with you. You're a hunchback and must stay at home!'

"The little girl often wondered about her hunch and what might be inside of it. Since she was never permitted to go out of doors again, she gradually grew paler and weaker and finally died. When an angel came to take her to heaven, she could not believe that hunchbacks go to heaven. The angel smiled and showed her that there were two magnificent white angel wings hidden in her hunch."

SPINAL TUBERCULOSIS
HIPPOCRATES, 3RD CENTURY BC

"The vertebrae of the spine, when contracted into a lump behind from disease, for the most part cannot be remedied; more especially when the gibbosity is above the attachment of the diaphragm to the spine.

"When the gibbosity occurs in youth before the body is fully grown, spinal growth stops, but the arms and legs are fully developed. And in those cases where the gibbosity is above the diaphragm, the ribs do not usually expand properly in width, but forwards, and the chest becomes short, pointed and not broad. They become affected by difficulty of breathing and hoarseness as the cavities which inspire and expire the breath do not attain their proper capacity. They generally have hard and

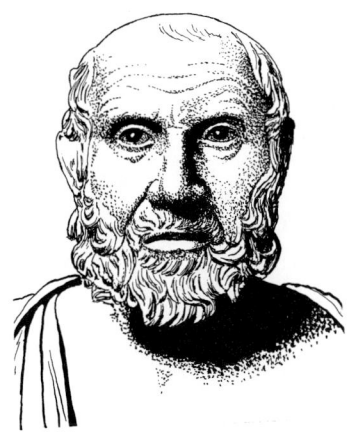

◆ **Hippocrates**

Hippocrates, about whom little is known and whose name is given to a wonderful collection of books written in the 3rd and 4th centuries BC. They are the first medical books of note and the most important works for the next two millennia. Most of today's aids to treatment have come in over the last 100 years: for example, anesthesia, X-rays, asepsis, antibiotics, blood transfusion; these developed over a period that is about one-twentieth of that during which Hippocrates' works remained standard teaching. Yet his works were not printed until the Renaissance and were not translated into English until the last century.

The legend is that he was born in Cos, an island in the eastern Aegean Sea off the Turkish coast, about 460 BC and later travelled widely, though living mainly in Cos, where, under a plane tree, he taught his students until his death about 355 BC. Portraits of him exist on coins.

Hippocrates was a very critical observer of disease; he wrote one book on fractures and another on articulations, which repay reading. They are systematic works containing so much of value that it is difficult to itemize.

unconcocted tubercles in the lungs, for the gibbosity and swelling in the neck are mostly produced by such Tubercles. When the gibbosity is below the diaphragm in some of these cases, nephritic diseases and affections of the bladder supervene, chronic abscesses that are difficult to cure occur in the loins and groins, and neither of these removes the gibbosity. In these cases the hips are more emaciated than when the gibbosity is seated higher up; the hair of the pubes and chin is of slower growth and less developed, and they are less capable of generation than those with the gibbosity higher up."

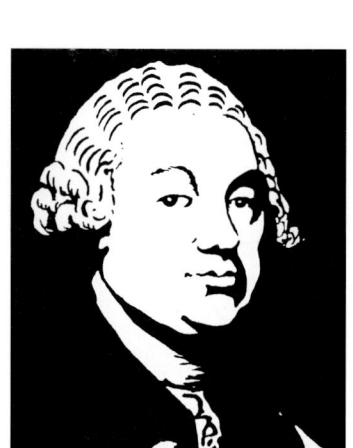

◆ **Percivall Pott (1714–1788)**
Pott's father came from a London family who were so prolific that it was a standing joke among their friends that although they were greengrocers by trade, they were the best Pott makers in London. Percivall Pott was a Cockney born in Threadneedle Street and was apprenticed to a surgeon at St. Bartholomew's Hospital. He obtained the Grand Diploma of the Barber Surgeon's Company in 1736, and was appointed to the staff of St. Bartholomew's 8 years later. He soon established himself as a teacher and a humane surgeon. His writing career started when he was recuperating from an open fracture of the tibia.

He wrote a classic monograph on head injuries and another on fractures and dislocations, drawing attention to the importance of relaxing the muscles that maintained deformity by correct positioning.

His account of tuberculous paraplegia was first published in 1779. He recognized the tuberculous nature of the disease but thought the paraplegia was due not to cord compression but to a distemper of the area. He advised drainage to stop the disease from progressing and allow bony healing to take place. He was a discursive writer, and this account is a curtailed version.

Pott on Paraplegia, 1779

REMARKS ON THAT KIND OF PALSY OF THE LOWER LIMBS, WHICH IS FREQUENTLY FOUND TO ACCOMPANY A CURVATURE OF THE SPINE AND IS SUPPOSED TO BE CAUSED BY IT, TOGETHER WITH ITS METHOD OF CURE

"The disease of which I am to speak is a disease of the spine, producing an alteration in its natural figure, and not infrequently attended with a partial, or a total loss of the power of using, or even moving, the lower limbs.

"From this last circumstance (the loss of the use of the limbs), it has in general been called a palsy, and treated as a paralytic affection; to which it is in almost every respect perfectly unlike.

"The occasion of the mistake is palpable; the patient is deprived of the use of his legs, and has a deformed incurvation of the spine; the incurvation is supposed to be caused by a dislocation of the vertebrae—the displaced bones are thought to make an **unnatural** *pressure on the spinal marrow; and a pressure on that being very likely to produce a paralysis of some kind, the loss of the use of the legs is in this case determined to be such. The truth is, that there is no dislocation, no unnatural pressure made on the spinal marrow; nor are the limbs by any means paralytic, as will appear to whoever will examine the two complaints with any degree of attention.*

"In the true paralysis, from whatever cause, the muscles of the affected limb are soft, flabby, unresisting, and incapable of being put into even a tonic state.

"In the present case, the muscles are indeed extenuated, and lessened in size; but they are rigid, and always at least in a tonic state, by which the knees and ancles acquire a stiffness not very easy to overcome. By means of this stiffness, mixed with a kind of spasm, the legs of the patient are either constantly kept stretched out straight, in which case considerable force is required to bend the knees, or they are by the action of the stronger

muscles drawn across each other in such manner as to require as much to separate them: when the leg is in a straight position, the extensor muscles act so powerfully as to require a considerable degree of force to bend the joints of the knees; and when they have been bent, the legs are immediately and strongly drawn up, with the heels towards the buttocks: by the rigidity of the ancle-joints, joined to the spasmodic action of the gastrocnemii muscles, the patient's toes are pointed downward in such manner as to render it impossible for him to put his foot flat to the ground, which makes one of the decisive characteristics of the distemper.

"The majority of those who labour under this disease are infants or young children: adults are by no means exempt from it; but I have never seen it at an age beyond forty.

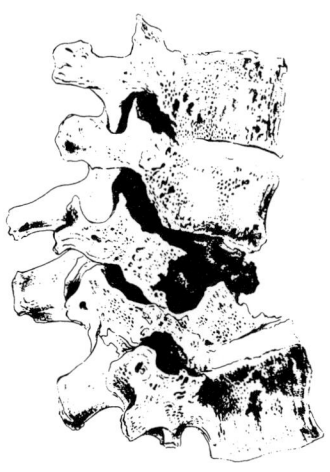

Pott's picture of a tuberculous spine, 1779.

"If the incurvation be of the neck, and to a considerable degree, by affecting several vertebrae, the child finds it inconvenient and painful to support its own head, and is always desirous of laying it on a table or pillow, or any thing to take off the weight. If the affection be of the dorsal vertebrae, the general marks of a distempered habit, such as loss of appetite, hard dry cough, laborious respiration, quick pulse, and disposition to hectic, appear pretty early, and in such a manner as to demand attention; and as in this state of the case there is always, from the connexion between the ribs, sternum, and spine, a great degree of crookedness of the trunk, these complaints are by every body set to the account of the deformity merely. In an adult, the attack and the progress of the disease are much the same, but there are some few circumstances which may be learned from a patient of such age, which either do not make an impression on a child, or do not happen to it.

"An adult, in a case where no violence hath been committed, or received, will tell you, that its first intimation was a sense of weakness in his back-bone, accompanied with what he will call a heavy dull kind of pain, attended with such a lassitude as rendered a small degree of exercise fatiguing; that this was soon followed by an unusual sense of coldness in the thighs, not accountable for from the weather, and a palpable diminution of their sensibility; that, in a little time more, his limbs were frequently convulsed by involuntary twitchings, particularly troublesome in the night; that soon after this, he not only became incapable of walking, but that his power either of retaining or discharging his urine and faeces was considerably impaired, and his penis incapable of erection.

"The primary and sole cause of all the mischief, is a distempered state of the parts composing or in immediate connection with the spine, tending to, and most frequently ending in, a caries of the body, or bodies, of one or more of the vertebrae: from this proceed all the ills, whether general or local, apparent or concealed; this causes the ill health of the patient, and, in time, the curvature. The helpless state of the limbs is only one consequence of several proceeding from the same cause: but though this effect is a very frequent one, and always affects the limbs in nearly the same manner, yet the disease not having its *origin in them, no application made to them only can ever be of any possible use.*

"The same failure of success attends the use of the different pieces of machinery, and for reasons which are equally obvious.

"They are founded upon the supposition of an actual dislocation, which never is the case, and therefore they always have been, and ever must be, unsuccessful.

"To understand this in the clearest and most convincing manner, we need only reflect on the nature of the disease, its seat, and the state in which the parts concerned must necessarily be.

"The bones are already carious, or tending to become so; the parts connected with them are diseased, and not infrequently ulcerated; there is no displacement of the vertebrae with regard to each other; and the spine bends forward only because the rotten bone, or bones intervening between the sound ones, give way, being unable in such state to bear the weight of the parts above.

"That is the case of carious spine, without curvature. It most frequently happens, that internal abscesses and collections of matter are formed, which matter makes its way outward, and appears in the hip, groin, or thigh; or being detained within the body, destroys the patient; the real and immediate cause of whose death is seldom known or even rightly guessed at, unless the dead body be examined.

"That what are commonly called lumbal and psoas abscesses, are not infrequently induced in this manner, and therefore when we use these terms, we should be understood to mean only a description of the course which such matter has pursued in its way outwards, or the place where it makes its appearance externally.

"That whosoever will consider the real state of the parts when a caries has taken place and the parts surrounding it are in a state of ulceration, must see why none of the attempts by swings, screws, etc., can possibly do any good but on the contrary, if they act so as to produce any effect at all, it must be a bad one.

"That the discharge, by means of issues produces a cessation of the erosion of the bones; that this is followed by an incarnation of the bones, by means of which the bodies of the vertebrae coalesce and unite with each other forming a kind of anchylosis."

Other Granulomatous Infections

When I was a student, there were still patients with tabes and syphilis of bone to be seen. This was as lethal in its day as AIDS is today. Columbus is said to have taken smallpox to the New World and brought back syphilis. Smallpox killed so many in the New World that the Spanish conquistadors (who were immune to smallpox) could colonize without much fighting. Syphilis became such a problem in the Old World that this was one reason why Puritanism took a strong hold.

Pyogenic Infection

TIMELINE OF PYOGENIC INFECTION

c 400 BC	Hippocrates recognized that pieces of bone lost their blood supply and were expelled as sequestra. Fistulas were probed in the 15th, 16th, and 17th centuries. Illustrations of bones with involucrum were made by Cheselden and Hunter in the 18th century.
1831	Nathan Smith on osteomyelitis—a good clinical description
1832	Brodie's abscess—subacute osteomyelitis
1844	The word osteomyelitis is invented by Nélaton
1874	Tom Smith—septic arthritis
1876	The birth of bacteriology: Robert Koch, a general practitioner in Wollstein in East Prussia, shows that he can culture an organism from a diseased animal and then inject the culture and produce the disease afresh in another animal.
1878	J. Rosenbach describes the experimental production of osteomyelitis.
1881	Robert Koch invents poured plates for culturing bacteria.
1883	Becker cultures organisms from osteomyelitis.
1893	Carl Garré classifies different forms of osteomyelitis.
1896	Lexer shows that experimental bone abscesses begin in metaphyses after intravenous injection of bacteria.
1921	Teruo Hobo in Japan finds that organisms are trapped in the vessels of the metaphysis.
1922	Starr advocates drainage of acute osteomyelitis. Irrigation protocols
1930	Winnett Orr writes a book on osteomyelitis and advocates drainage and immobilization.
1934	A. O. Wilensky book on osteomyelitis
1935	Sulfonamides provide the first systemic bacteriostatic drug. Hildegard Demargsk was dying of infection. Her father had been testing various compounds and gave her a sulfa compound as a last-ditch measure and saved her life.
1936	Report on mortality
1940	Penicillin is isolated and starts to be used for acute osteomyelitis.
1947	Chloramphenicol

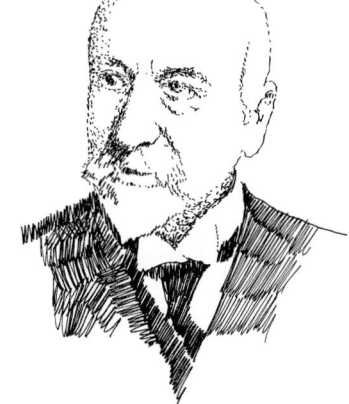

◆ **Carl Garré (1857–1928)**

Swiss-born, he became Professor in Bonn. He described 10 varieties of osteomyelitis: acute, chronic, multiple, a sclerosing nonsuppurative form that became known for him, and so on.

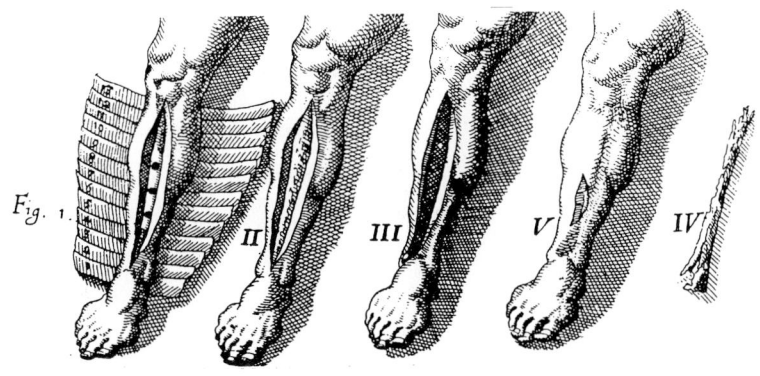

Sequestrectomy of the tibia. From Johannes Scultetus, 1593.

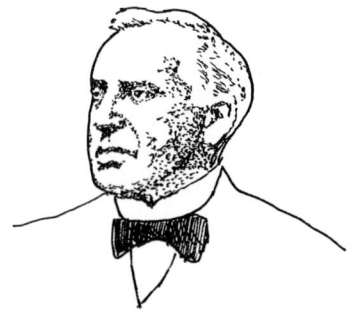

◆ **Auguste Nélaton (1807–1873)**
A Parisian surgeon, known for his line joining the anterior iliac spine to the ischial tuberosity: if the greater trochanter lies above the line, the hip is dislocated, varus, or fractured. He tended Garibaldi when Garibaldi was shot in the ankle, and he is said to have coined the word osteomyelitis.

Calvin Coolidge: American President (1923–1929)

In his autobiography, Coolidge blamed himself for his son's death in 1924. "If I had not been President, he would not have raised a blister on his toe, which resulted in blood poisoning, playing tennis on the South Grounds." His 16 year old son, Calvin Jr, was playing tennis with sneakers but without socks. The blister became infected and within a few days the boy died at Walter Reed Hospital. This story illustrates the change in outcome produced by antibiotics that we take for granted now.

President Coolidge was never the same again and came to be regarded as one of the least successful presidents. He wrote of his son, "When he went, the power and the glory of the Presidency went with him."

Likewise, acute hematogenous osteomyelitis was often fatal. When patients survived, they usually had a lifelong discharging sinus. The early descriptions focus on the chronic form with descriptions of large sequestra and massive involucra around them, of a kind not seen today.

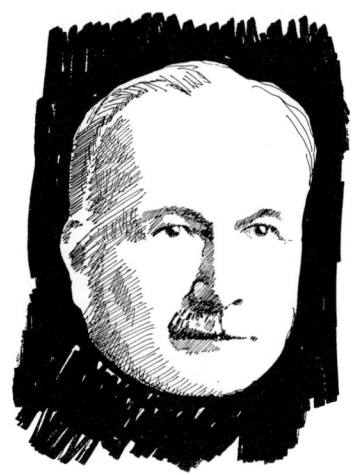

◆ **Clarence Starr (1867–1920)**
He was Chief of Surgery at the Hospital for Sick Children, Toronto, and led the Canadian Orthopaedic Services in World War I. He pointed out that radiographic changes are of no value in the early stages of acute osteomyelitis when drainage offers the best chance of success.

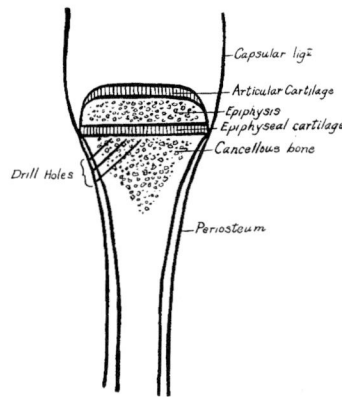

Clarence Starr was one of the first to advocate early operation for acute hematogenous osteomyelitis. If no subperiosteal abscess was present, he advised drilling the metaphysis. From Arch Surg 1922, 4, 597, Fig. 18.

Osteomyelitis

Acute hematogenous osteomyelitis is becoming quite uncommon as children are now treated early for the infections that would, in the past, have produced septicemia with seeding to the bone. Osteomyelitis either killed or produced the lifelong draining sinuses of chronic osteomyelitis. Most of the early descriptions are about the management of sinuses and sequestra in the survivors. Sinuses were probed, sequestra extracted, and abscesses laid open.

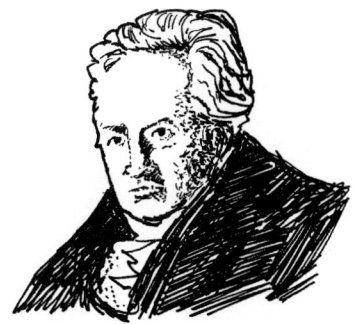

NATHAN SMITH, 1831

"Almost from the first commencement of the pain, there occurs severe symptomatic fever. The local affection generally terminates in suppuration, frequently as soon as the fourth or fifth day. The matter is at first deposited between the external periosteum and the bone. When the shafts of the long bones are the seat of the disease, there is formed a corresponding collection between the internal surface of the bone and the membrane surrounding the medullary substance. This fact, which I deem of great importance, as being essential to the correct treatment of the disease, I have ascertained in repeated instances, by the operation which I have performed for its relief, namely, trepanning the bone. Very soon after the attack, the whole limb swells, but there is no marked tumefaction immediately in the part affected, till after the matter makes its escape from the periosteum. Whenever this occurs, the extreme pain and symptomatic fever in some degree subside."

◆ **Nathan Smith (1762–1829)**

He grew up in Vermont, was apprenticed to the local doctor, and started a practice before going to the newly opened Harvard Medical School. He traveled widely and played a part in establishing several medical schools.

Brodie's Abscess, 1832

AN ACCOUNT OF SOME CASES OF CHRONIC ABSCESSES OF THE TIBIA
B. C. BRODIE

"I am not aware that any cases exactly similar to those which I am about to relate have been recorded by authors: and as they appear to me to throw some light on the history and treatment of a rare but very serious disease, I am led to believe that they are not unworthy of being communicated to the Medical and Chirurgical Society."

◆ CASE 1

"Mr. P., about twenty-four years of age, consulted me in October, 1824, under the following circumstances.

"There was a considerable enlargement of the lower extremity of the right tibia, extending to the distance of two or three inches from the ankle-joint. The integuments at this part were tense, and they adhered closely to the surface of the bone.

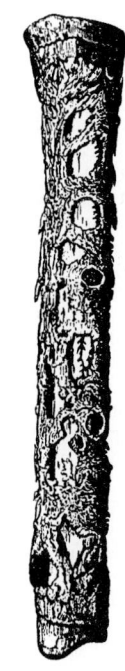

James Syme amputated the leg (illustrated) of a girl with osteomyelitis, 1835. This was the involucrum with the sequestrum imprisoned within. Only in the Third World can cases like this be found today. From Syme J: Observations in Clinical Surgery, 2nd Edition. Edinburgh, 1862.

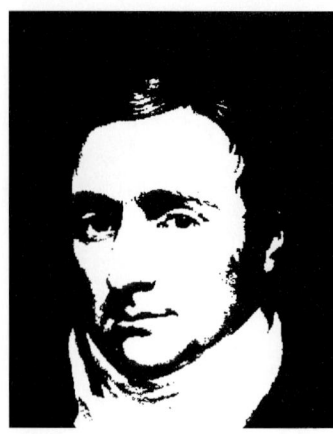

◆ **Sir Benjamin Brodie (1783–1862)**

A parson's son, Brodie was born at Winterslow, Wiltshire. After studying at Abernethy's School of Anatomy and the Great Windmill School he went to St. George's Hospital as a pupil of Everard Home (who is mainly remembered as the man who plagiarized John Hunter and later burned Hunter's manuscripts to avoid being rumbled). He qualified in 1805 and became Assistant Surgeon at St. George's at the age of 24. This involved a great deal of clinical work, as his chief's appearances were infrequent; further, at this period, outpatient departments were hardly a feature of hospital life.

He became one of the best-known surgeons of his day and attended many prominent people, including George IV. In 1818 his work on diseases of the joints appeared—though it does not seem original or fresh today, it was one of the early monographs and correlated pathologic and clinical aspects in a systematic manner with the object of distinguishing among different types of joint disease. In 1843 he introduced the Fellowship examination of the Royal College of Surgeons in an attempt to improve the education and standing of surgeons. In 1858 he was President of the Royal Society and in the same year first President of the General Medical Committee.

"The patient complained of a constant pain referred to the enlarged bone, and neighbouring parts. The pain was always sufficiently distressing; but he was also liable to more severe paroxysms in which his sufferings were described as most excruciating. These paroxysms recurred at irregular intervals, confining him to his room for many successive days, and being attended with a considerable degree of constitutional disturbance. Mr. P. described the disease as having existed more than twelve years, and as having rendered his life miserable during the whole of that period.

"In the course of this time he had been under the care of various surgeons, and various modes of treatment had been resorted to without any permanent advantage. The remedies which I prescribed for him were equally inefficacious. Finding himself without any prospect of being relieved by other means, he made up his mind to lose the limb by amputation; and Mr. Travers having seen him with me in consultation, and having concurred in the opinion, that this was the best course which could be pursued, the operation was performed accordingly.

"On examining the amputated limb, it was found that a quantity of new bone had been deposited on the surface of the lower extremity of the tibia. This deposition of new bone was manifestly the result of inflammation of the periosteum at some former period. It was not less than one-third of an inch in thickness, and when the tibia was divided longitudinally with a saw, the line at which the new and old bone were united with each other, was distinctly to be seen.

"The whole of the lower extremity of the tibia was harder and more compact than under ordinary circumstances, in consequence, as it appeared, of some deposit of bone in the cancellous structure, and in its centre, about one-third of an inch above the ankle, there was a cavity the size of an ordinary walnut, filled with a dark-coloured pus. The bone immediately surrounding this cavity was distinguished from that in the neighbourhood by its being of a whiter colour, and of a still harder texture, and the inner surface of the cavity presented an appearance of high vascularity. The ankle-joint was free from disease.

"It is evident that if the exact nature of the disease had been understood, and the bone had been perforated with a trephine, so as to allow the pus collected in its interior to escape, a cure would probably have been effected, without the loss of the limb, and with little or no danger to the patient's life. Such, at least, was the opinion which the circumstances of the case led me to form at the time; and I bore them in my mind, in the expectation that at some future period I might have the opportunity of acting on the knowledge which they afforded me for the benefit of another patient."

After the operation the patient suffered a reactionary hemorrhage and became delirious, dying on the fifth day. Brodie goes on to describe two further cases: he trephined both and both healed.

Here is Brodie's operation note of one of these.

"A crucial incision was made through the skin, the angles of which were raised so as to expose a part of the bone above the inner ankle, to which the pain was especially referred. A small trephine was then applied, and a circular portion of bone was removed extending into the cancellous structure. Other portions of bone were removed with a narrow chisel. At last about a dram of pus suddenly escaped and rose into the opening made by the trephine and chisel. On further examination a cavity was discovered from which the pus had flowed, capable of admitting the extremity of the finger. The inner surface of this cavity was exquisitely tender; the patient experiencing the most excruciating pain on the gentlest introduction of the probe into it.

"From the time of the operation, the peculiar pain from which the patient had previously suffered, was entirely relieved: and it was not long before he was quite restored to health, and able to walk and pursue his occupations without interruption. I have seen him lately, nearly two years from the time of the operation having been performed, and he continues perfectly well."

ON THE ACUTE ARTHRITIS OF INFANTS
TOM SMITH, 1874

"There have come under my observation during the last few years several cases of acute articular disease in infants, which differ so much in their progress and result from any of the recognised joint affections of childhood, that they seem to me to need what they have not hitherto received, namely, a special description.

"The disease to which I propose to direct attention, and which I shall call the acute arthritis of infants, probably owes its distinctive features more to the time of life at which it occurs than to any essential difference between it and other recognised joint-affections.

"It occurs, so far as my experience extends, within the first year of life, and is characterised by the suddenness of its onset and the rapidity of its progress and termination, whether the latter be of a fatal or a favourable kind. It is very dangerous to life, and intensely destructive to the articular ends of the bones, which, of course, at this period of life are largely cartilaginous. Lastly, I would mention as a feature of the disease, that it rarely produces anchylosis, but leaves a child with a limb shortened, by loss of part of the articular end of some bone, and with a weakened, flail-like joint.

"I have kept notes of many cases of the disease, twenty-one of which are here reported—they will serve to illustrate its principal characteristics.

"The fatal cases here reported, with one or two exceptions, are deficient in one important feature, namely, in the absence of

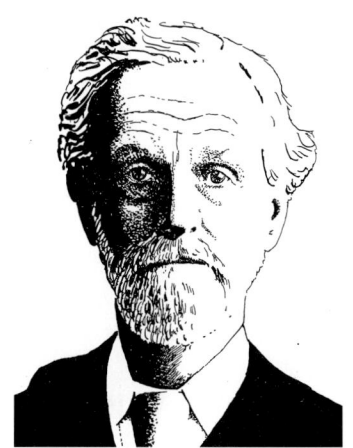

◆ **Sir Thomas Smith (1833–1909)**

Born in Kent and trained at St. Bartholomew's Hospital, Thomas Smith was later a surgeon there and at Great Ormond Street. He was a good and kindly man, who had no wish to write textbooks. He once said, "It is the men who don't get the cases who write the books about them."

His description of septic arthritis of infancy was written while he was an outpatient assistant at St. Bart's. He also described xanthomatosis of bone (Hand-Schüller-Christian disease) in 1865, long before this triumvirate noticed it.

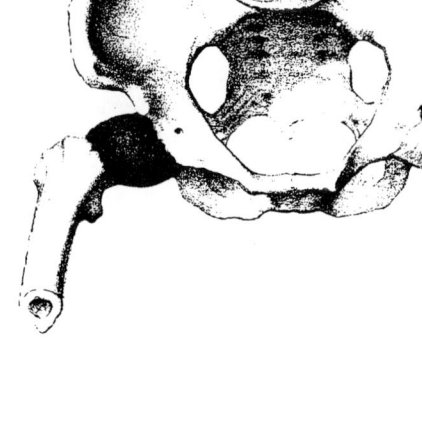

Amedee Bonnet injected joints in 1840. Injecting the hip causes flexion. He showed that effusions accounted for the position taken by infected joints.

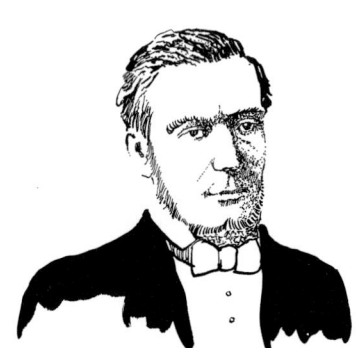

◆ Amedee Bonnet (1809–1858)

Chief surgeon at Lyons, France, who wrote two books on joint disease, 1845 and 1860. He injected cadaver joints with fluid to show how that dictated joint position. He rested inflamed joints and produced huge splints. He was followed at Lyons by Ollier.

any examination of the viscera. This arises from the fact that most of the infants were out-patients, and that consent to examine the local disease was only obtained on the express condition that the body should not be opened.

"In cases I have to relate, the disease first attacked either the shoulder, hip or knee, and often more than one joint was subsequently affected in the same infant.

"The disease was ushered in with restricted movement, and usually flexion of the joint affected, followed by pain, swelling, and rapid suppuration within the joint; the redness of the skin was often but little marked until the abscess was on the point of bursting. After the abscess had opened or had been punctured, if recovery took place, the discharge generally ceased to flow much sooner than is usual in ordinary cases of suppuration within the cavity of a joint. When death occurred, it resulted from exhaustion from local suppuration, or, as one may believe in certain cases, from this, together with a general condition of pyaemia, with secondary affection of internal organs.

"On post-mortem examination, I have found in all instances a considerable and rapid loss of substance in the articular end of one of the long bones entering into the joint affected. In some cases this absorption or ulceration has proceeded from the joint surface towards the deeper parts. In others, the destruction of tissue had commenced in abscess within the articular end of the bone, which, after excavating and destroying more or less of the interior of the bone, had burst into the joint by a small opening near the margin of the articular cartilage. In Case III, the existence of subarticular abscess was first discovered accidentally in making a section of the bone. I cannot doubt that, in times gone by, when I was unaware of this peculiar pathological condition, I have overlooked many instances of subarticular abscess from

Title page of Bonnet's book, 1845.

neglecting to make a section of the bone in cases of suppuration within joint cavities.

"It seems that in many cases, the formation of a subarticular abscess in the bone must have been the first step in the joint affection, since, while the articular end of the bone was extensively excavated, the aperture through which the abscess had burst into the joint was a mere pin-hole, and though the joint contained pus, the articular cartilage was apparently healthy.

"The following case will serve to illustrate the ordinary course of the disease in a well-marked case."

◆ CASE 2—Arthritis of the Knee in an Infant Four Weeks Old—Extensive Destruction of the Condyloid End of the Femur

"I saw Joseph Palmer at the Children's Hospital on March 21, 1866. He was four weeks old, and was the first child of apparently healthy parents. At his birth instruments were used, but no traction by the legs was employed. Four days after birth the left knee was noticed to be permanently flexed, and soon afterward the joint became swollen. When I first saw the child he was very ill, and the knee-joint was distended with pus; the abscess was opened, and a large quantity of matter escaped, and in a few days the child died.

"I have given the name subarticular abscess to abscess cavities formed beneath the articular cartilage, either in the cartilaginous or osseous structure of the end of the bone.

"On post-mortem examination the knee-joint was found full of pus, the cartilage over the tibia was healthy in appearance, as was also that covering the patella and external condyle of the femur. There was a large ragged hole in the cartilage of the internal condyle, large enough to admit one's finger; this led into a deep excavated cavity in the bone and ossifying cartilage; this cavity occupied a large part of the articular end of the femur, of which little remained but the shell."

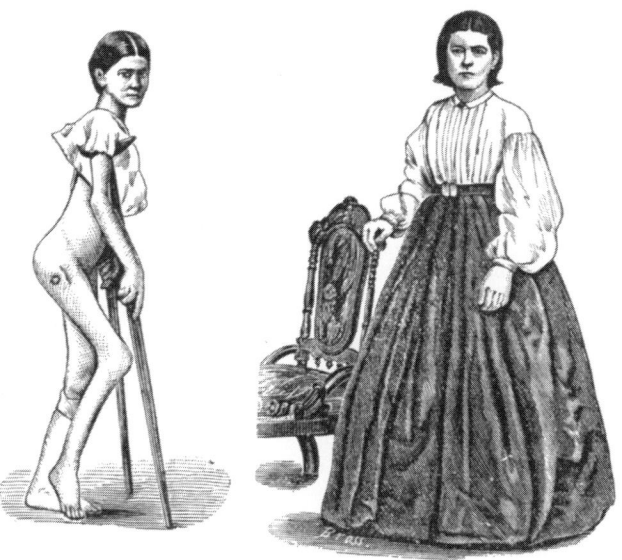

Matilda Hillory, age 14 years, from Iowa. She spent a year in bed with a tuberculous hip and discharging sinuses. On 3 July 1862, Sayre excised the hip, and she was able to go home 20 November 1862 with good hip movement and a 1-inch raise. She had gained 20 pounds in weight. Four years later she wrote that she "could run and dance as well as any girl in Iowa." From Sayre, 1879.

OTHER INFECTIONS

Syphilis

In the past this often caused large holes in bones (due to gumma) and neuropathic joints, particularly the knee, which were treated by fusion, often unsuccessfully.

1530	Frascatoro—poem on syphilis
1905	*Treponema* identified by Schaudinn
1945	Penicillin eradicates the problem.

Leprosy

Leprosy is due to an infection that damages the peripheral nerves, leading to paralysis, contractures, and loss of sensation. Ulcers followed, and loss of digits. It has been a worldwide problem.

Leprosy is mentioned in Bible: Leviticus, Chapters 13 and 14, Miracles in Luke 5:1.

1200+	In the Middle Ages, lepers were outcasts. A funeral service was read over them after diagnosis and they became the original "living dead."
1500+	Many leprosy hospitals provided lepers with a home and excluded them from society.
1873	The organism of leprosy is discovered in Norway by Armauer Hansen, hence the euphemism, Hansen's disease.
1921	Carville Leprosarium opened in the United States to centralize cases—closed in 1995.
1960s	Operations done to improve hand function and footware provided to reduce neurogenic ulcer problem. Sulfones are cheap and safe and are eradicating leprosy from all but the poorest countries.
1990s	There is still a training institute in Ethiopia to teach case finding, for treatment, and to provide orthopaedic care.

References

Chapter references are located in Chapter 26.

◆ Chapter Ten

Neuromuscular Disease

Much of the early success for orthopaedics came from tenotomy—as big a success in the last century as hip replacement is in this century. This success went some of the way toward levering orthopaedics free from general surgery. Today, neuromuscular disease has lost much of its importance because of the conquest of polio. Traumatic paraplegia is perhaps the major challenge, although surgical treatment plays only a small part.

Do not forget that muscle is the tissue that was the catalyst of our way of life. Galvani, an anatomist in Bologna, used muscle to show the existence of electricity in 1791. Without this we would still be living life simply. It is hard to imagine a world, or even medicine, without electricity.

Famous Patients

Richard III was born feet first with a hemiplegia. Shakespeare has him speak thus,

> *Deformed, unfinished, sent before my time*
> *Into this breathing world, scarce half made up,*
> *And that so lamely and unfashionable*
> *That dogs bark at me as I halt by them*

Tamberlane, or **Timur the Lame** (1336-1405), was named because his left side was disabled. This Turkoman Mongol conqueror created an empire that extended from India to the Mediterranean.

Franklin Delano Roosevelt (1882-1945) came from a distinguished family and studied at Harvard, becoming a lawyer and senator before being nominated as Democratic candidate for the vice presidency in 1920. The Republicans won, and he returned to business. In August, 1921, he went on a family holiday to Campobello Island in New Brunswick. One day he helped fight a forest fire, jogged home, and went for a swim. (The day before, he had visited a boys' camp.) The next day he had a fever and leg pain that progressed to paralysis. Eighty-three year old Professor Keen said it was a blood clot on the spine and sent in a bill for $600. Robert Lovett of Boston was summoned, who diagnosed polio. In secrecy Roosevelt was moved by private railway coach to New York. It was a year before he was up and about. His illness, said

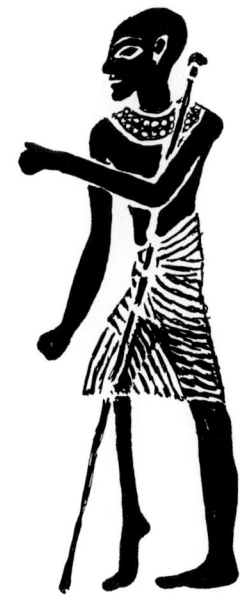

Is this polio? A stele from Egypt dated about 2000 BC and now in Copenhagen.

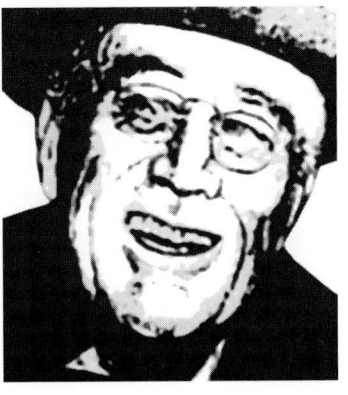

◆ F. D. R.

his wife, was "a blessing in disguise; for it gave him strength and courage he had not had before."

He developed contractures and had wedging casts. Later he used long leg braces to stand, and he needed help getting up from a chair. He could take only a few steps by pelvic hitching, using trunk muscles. He ran as a Democratic candidate for governor of New York in 1928 and told the press not to take pictures of him in a wheelchair or being lifted out of a car. Throughout his life this request was respected (or photographers had the film exposed by the Secret Service agents), and the public had no idea that he was so weak. "It is just as much a State duty to provide medical help as the providing of education," he said in one speech. He was president from 1933 until 1945. He expended much effort to conceal his disability on the one hand and to promote care for the handicapped on the other.

The Elephant Man. The story of Joseph Merrick is well known because of a movie called "The Elephant Man." He was born in 1860, and gradually his skin became thick, with folds. The original diagnosis of neurofibromatosis has been replaced by a diagnosis of the Proteus syndrome. He spent time in a freak show and was then befriended by a surgeon and lived his last years in The London Hospital. His story is well told in a short book; his autobiography ends with this poem:

> *Tis true my form is something odd,*
> *But blaming me is blaming God,*
> *Could I create myself anew*
> *I would not fail in pleasing you.*
> *If I could reach from Pole to Pole*
> *Or grasp the Ocean with a span*
> *I would be measured by the soul:*
> *The Mind's the measure of the Man.*

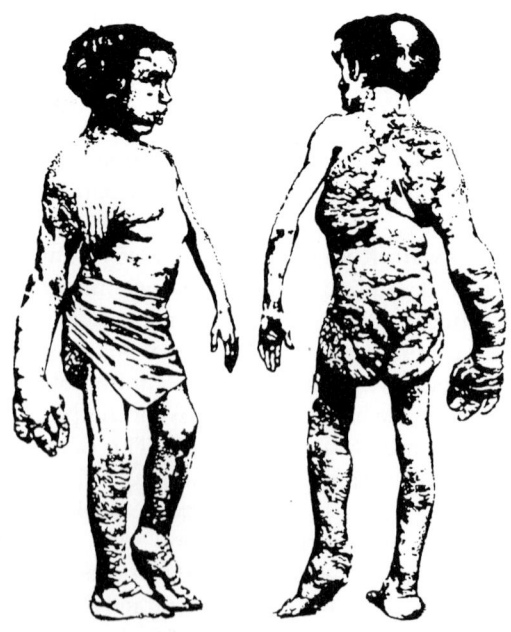

Joseph Merrick as a child.

TIMELINE OF NEUROMUSCULAR DISEASE

- 170 Galen experiments on cutting the spinal cord of pigs—complete section and hemisection.
- 1546 Estienne describes syrinx in book published in Paris.
- 1671 Willis—hysteria
- 1791 Galvani discovers electricity through muscle twitch.
- 1824 Ollivier d'Angiers coined the term syringomyelia.
- 1855 Duchenne uses electricity to diagnose and treat patients.
- 1855 Muscular dystrophy: Duchenne describes various kinds. Earlier descriptions by Conte in Naples and Meryon in the United Kingdom
- 1860 Brown-Séquard describes the clinical features of hemisection of the cord in English.
- 1861 Little—cerebral palsy
- 1862 W. Gull—syringomyelia
- 1863 Friedreich ataxia—picture of feet by Bouchard and Brissaud
- 1867 Duchenne—*Physiology of Movements;* founded kinesiology
- 1872 Mitchell—erythromelalgia
- 1875 Simon—syrinx
- 1879 Gowers' sign of muscular dystrophy
- 1886 Charcot-Marie-Tooth disease—now known as hereditary motor sensory neuritis
- 1886 Strümpell—hereditary spastic paraplegia
- 1891 Spinal muscular atrophy
- 1900 Amyotonia
- 1916 Guillain-Barré paralysis
- 1972 Brock and Sutcliffe—alpha-fetoprotein to screen for spina bifida
- 1991 Medical Research Council Report: Folate prevents spina bifida.

Poliomyelitis

Polio is the only disease that produces epidemics of sudden paralysis followed by muscle wasting in young people. One may think it has existed since the beginning of time. However, the disease was described recognizably only about 200 years ago, and

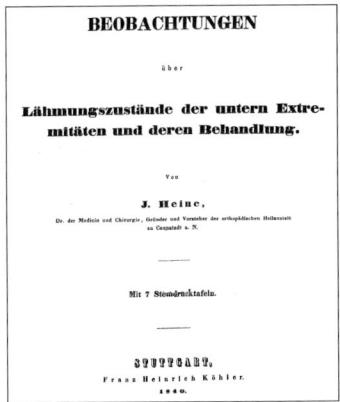

Title page of Heine's book, 1840.

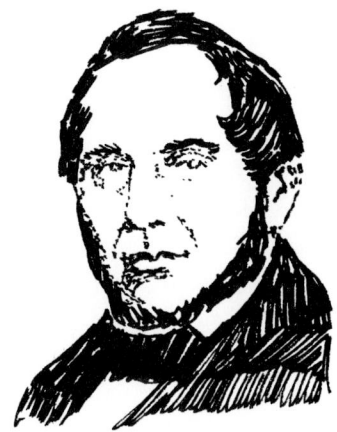

◆ Jacob Heine (1800–1879)

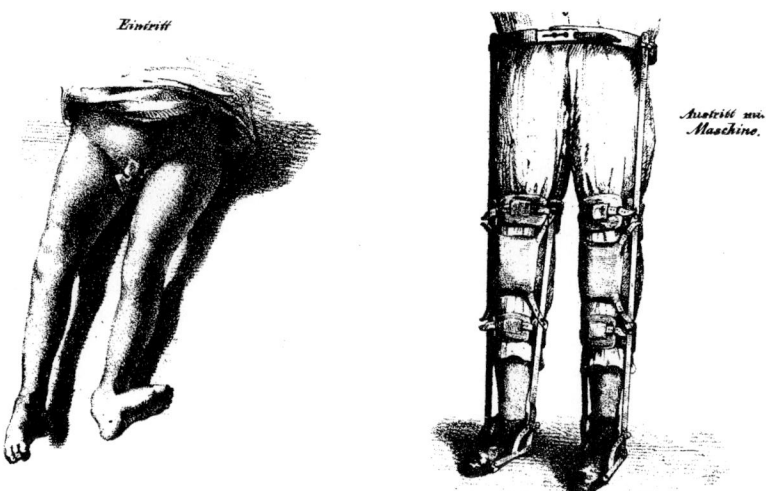

Jacob Heine wrote a book on polio and showed these braces—not so different from today's designs. The date was 1840.

only later were epidemics described. Polio may have come on the scene like HIV has in our generation. Now it is on the way out. A blip in human history.

Polio was everywhere until the 1950s and taught most orthopaedic surgeons everything they needed to know about neuro-orthopaedics. It was the University of Elective Orthopaedics. All the principles were worked out on polio. Since then the tide has been going out and one has to travel to the Third World to see new cases. In the 1960s I did a polio clinic before breakfast most mornings.

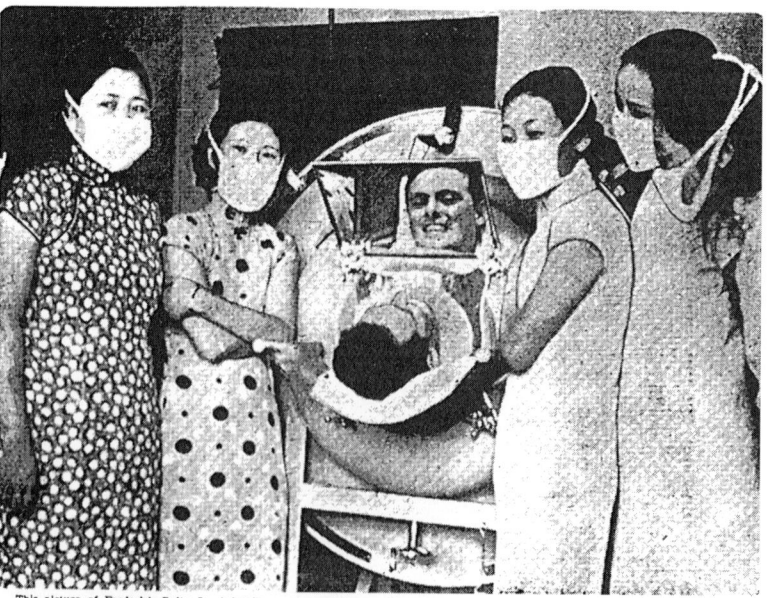

Polio often made front page news when epidemics swept through. As appeared in the Toronto Globe and Mail, 4 August 1937.

TIMELINE OF POLIOMYELITIS

5000 BC   Adult with a wasted calf and equinus pictured in an Egyptian tomb and generally assumed to be polio

400 BC   Not mentioned by Hippocrates!

1772   Walter Scott, later to become a famous Scottish writer, has a fever followed by paralysis at the age of 18 months. He is left with an atrophied leg and foot deformity for life. This may be the first documented case.

1789   Michael Underwood (1738-1810?) of London writes a pediatric text in 1784 that goes through 25 editions. In the second edition of 1789 he describes the clinical picture for the first time.

1813   Monteggia believes that his description is the first.

1828   J. Abercrombie reasons that it is a lesion of the anterior horn cell.

1840   Jacob Heine, member of a family with several generations of orthopaedic surgeons—they founded one of the first orthopaedic institutes at Cannstatt near Stuttgart, Germany—writes a 78-page monograph on polio. His treatment with exercises, simple operations, and braces remains unchanged in principle until polio is eradicated more than 100 years later. Leg irons remain unchanged until they are replaced by plastic braces in the early 1970s.

1867   C. F. Taylor, New York physician, publishes a 119-page book: *Infantile Paralysis and Its Attendant Deformities.*

1870   Charcot demonstrates the lesion in the anterior horn cells of the spinal cord.

1875   Adolphe Kussmaul names it: polio = gray, myelos = spinal cord, -itis = inflammation of.

1881   Epidemics of polio begin to be noticed—particularly in Scandinavia: Bull, 1868, in Norway; Bergenholtz, 1881, in Sweden; Medin, 1887, in Sweden.

1893-4   Epidemics in Boston and Vermont

1895   During the next 60 years many operations are invented for polio and are found to be useful for other problems. Polio surgery provides the training for orthopaedic surgeons and stimulates the organization of a nationwide charitable orthopaedic service.

1905   Huge Scandanavian epidemic of 1000 cases

1908   Landsteiner and Popper in Vienna show that an extract of the cord from a fatal case will cause the disease when injected into monkeys. They later prove it is a virus. This is the same Landsteiner who had discovered blood groups in 1901.

1910   Simon Flexner and P. A. Lewis produce experimental polio and find antibodies that neutralize the virus. They believe that immunization is just around the corner. In fact it is 40 years away.

   Multiple epidemics, and several false trails are explored.

1921   FDR has polio.

1927   Georgia Warm Springs Foundation starts as a philanthropic organization. Later it became a research foundation and was replaced by The National Foundation for Infantile Paralysis in 1938. President Roosevelt took office in 1933 and was its inspiration. The Foundation pioneered news re-

Box continued on following page

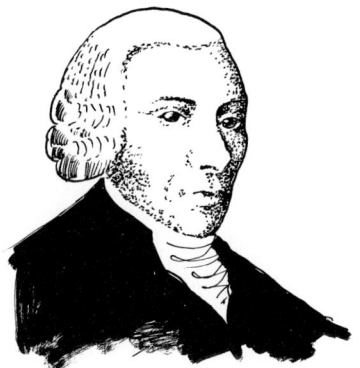

◆ Michael Underwood

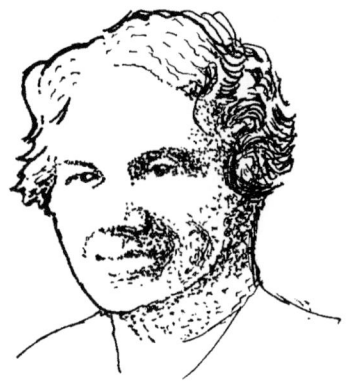

◆ Sister Kenny (1890–1952)

An Australian nurse in the Outback. Alone, and knowing little about paralysis, she massaged and moved the painful limbs of her patients with acute polio. This was the opposite of conventional wisdom—splinting the limbs to prevent contractures. Like Florence Nightingale, she pressed on and became a world-famous crusader for what is now called alternative medicine. She emerged on the American scene in 1942 and founded the Elizabeth Kenny Institute in Minneapolis.

◆ Albert Sabin

He was born in Poland in 1906 and came to the United States aged 15 years. He studied medicine at New York University and became a bacteriologist fascinated by polio and the epidemics that swept through New York. He worked at the Rockefeller Institute and then at the University of Cinncinati. During World War II he was in the Medical Corps working on immunization of troops against other viral diseases. Studies were done on citizens of the occupied countries in the postwar years. He favored living attenuated viruses for immunization. He later develops and runs trials on live polio vaccine, but it did not take off until 1957 when WHO called a meeting of its polio committee and international trials started. Many of these trials would not receive ethical approval today. Does this make important advances less likely?

	leases about medical breakthroughs to capture public attention and promote donations.
1929	Phillip Drinker at Harvard develops the iron lung and initiates an era of assisted ventilation, which we see in intensive care units today.
1940	Sister Kenny (1890-1952) comes to the United States from Australia. She is a nurse on a crusade to start moving paralyzed limbs early—contrary to the views of the orthopaedic establishment. Much controversy results. Survived by the Kenny Institute in Minneapolis.
1940s	Max Theiler attenuates polio virus.
1951	National Foundation forms a Committee on Immunization to use information from several attempts to make a vaccine.
1952	Tissue culture of polio virus in large amounts in Toronto provides the raw materials for a vaccine.
1953	Jonas Salk publishes a pilot trial of a vaccine prepared from formalinized dead poliovirus. It required injection.
1954	Field trial of the vaccine is a success. The formal trial is completed without incident; however, some children not in the trial develop polio soon after injection, giving the public reason for second thoughts.
	The incidence of paralytic polio in the United States drops from 14 per 100,000 in 1954 to 0.5 per 100,000 in 1961.
1962	Sabin had developed an oral live vaccine—attenuated through cell passage—about the same time as the Salk dead vaccine, but there was fear that it might become virulent. In 1962 a license was issued for general use, and it becomes the preferred vaccine.
1970	Polio largely disappears except in the Third World where poverty and the difficulties of getting refrigerated vaccine to remote areas prove too much.
2000	Rotary International plans to eradicate polio from the world by this date by paying for vaccination programs.

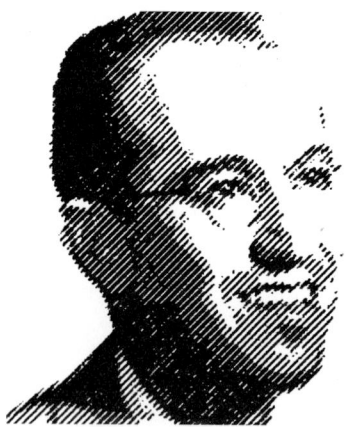

◆ Jonas Salk

In 1914 he was born in New York City and graduated in Medicine from New York University in 1939. He becomes a bacteriologist and takes part in large Army trials of a formalin-inactivated influenza vaccine before working on poliomyelitis virus typing. He moves to the University of Pittsburgh. He carried out the first trials on children convalescing from polio—something that would be banned today.

Michael Underwood, 1789

"... *It seems to arise from debility, and usually attacks children previously reduced by fever; seldom those under one, or more than four or five years old ... the first thing observed is a debility of the lower extremities, which gradually become more infirm, and after a few weeks are unable to support the body.*

... Nothing seems to do any good but irons to the legs ... enabling the patient to walk."

This seems like a description that might include rickets or tuberculosis or many other problems. It has one feature unlike polio. Polio usually causes sudden paralysis.

Monteggia, 1813

" ... In this connection should be mentioned a certain kind of paralysis limited to one or other of the lower extremities which I have observed several times in practice but have not yet found in the literature. It occurs in children who are nursing, or not much later; it begins with 2 or 3 days of fever, after which one of the extremities is found quite paralysed, immobile, flabby, hanging down, and no movement is made when the sole of the foot is tickled. The fever ceases very soon, but the member remains immobile and regains with time only an imperfect degree of strength."

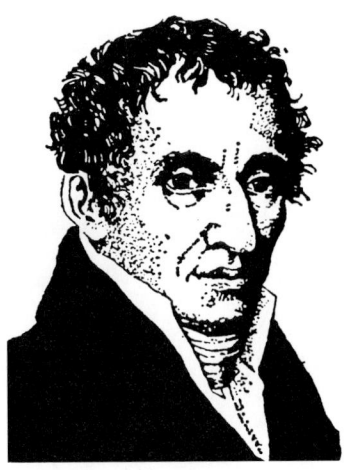

◆ Monteggia

Orthotics

They started as splints and then became braces and only in 1953 became orthotics—from *ortho,* straight in Greek.

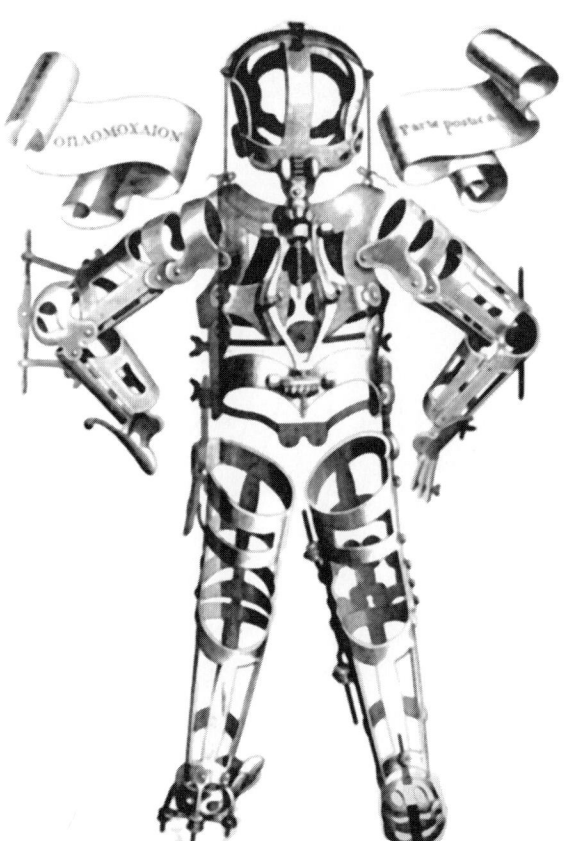

Makers of suits of armor were the forerunners of orthotists. This example was designed by Hieronymus Fabricius, 16th century.

TIMELINE FOR ORTHOTICS

1517 Hans von Gersdorff produces turnbuckle splints to correct deformities at joints.
1564 Ambroise Paré, an army surgeon, had the makers of armor shape sheet metal to brace the spine and foot.
1592 Hieronymus Fabricius publishes the *Hoplomochlion*, a composite of every kind of brace that can be built.
1650s Schott brothers set up scoliosis hospital.
1780 Venel starts a hospital in Switzerland for bracing the foot and spine.
1816 Heine in Germany builds a hospital for bracing.
1863 James Knight, founder of what is now called the Hospital for Special Surgery in New York. Formerly it was the Hospital for the Ruptured and Crippled. Operations were prohibited in favor of orthotics.
1870s Hugh Owen Thomas uses modular braces and fits them to each patient in a few minutes.
1940s Bunnell's hand splints
1948 American Board for Certification of Orthotists and Prosthetists
1964 Degree course in orthotics at New York University
1970 American Academy of Orthotists and Prosthetists

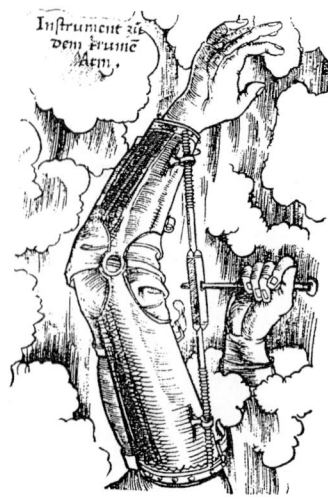

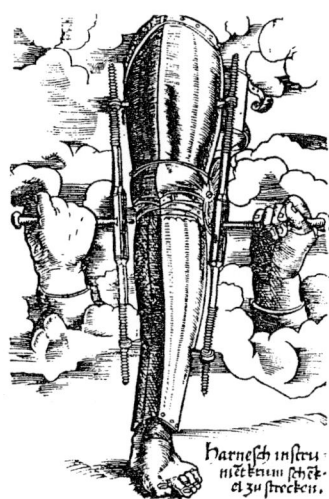

Turnbuckle correction of contractures is not new. Hans von Gersdorff, 1517.

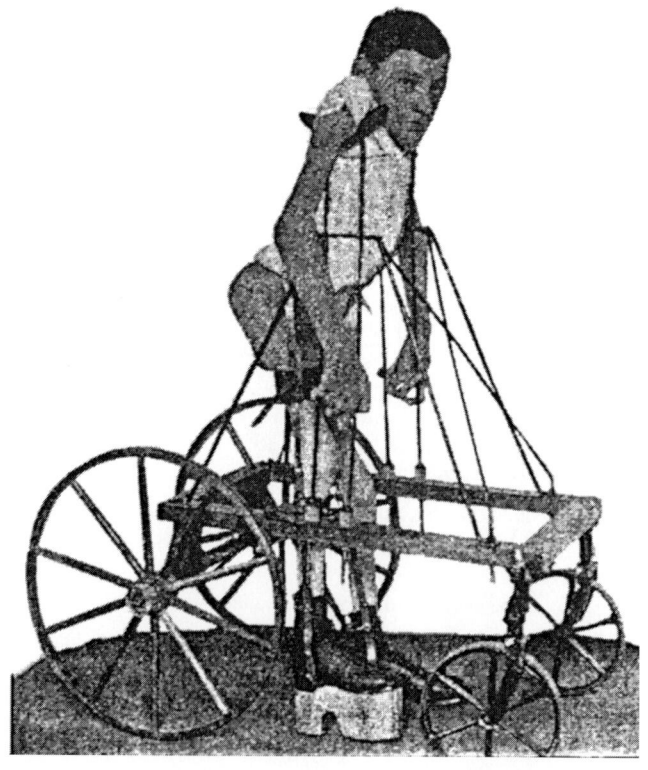

Willard's wheeled crutch. This sick-looking boy has a short leg, a flexed hip, and ulnar claw hands, suggesting tuberculosis of hip and spine. From Sayre L: Lectures on Orthopaedic Surgery. New York: 1879.

Cerebral Palsy

William John Little (1810–1894)

Little's life was largely shaped by the fact that he had polio as a child, resulting in a left talipes equinovarus deformity. He went to school in France, and after working for an apothecary for a while, studied at The London Hospital.

Two years after qualifying he went to the Continent, ostensibly to study. He had tried all sorts of mechanical contraptions to correct his deformity without success, and heard that Stromeyer was pioneering tenotomy for the condition in Hanover. Everyone told him it was dreadful and valueless, but after watching Stromeyer at work for some time, he decided that it was the treatment for him. He had an Achilles tenotomy, and his deformity was much improved. He helped in Stromeyer's clinic for a while and then started to tenotomize in Germany. He wrote a thesis for an M.D. degree on this, and returned to England to introduce the operation there. He persuaded his friends to subscribe to a hospital for him. This became the Royal Orthopaedic Hospital, which was amalgamated to form the Royal National Orthopaedic Hospital in London.

He had wanted to become a surgeon but was deterred when he missed a post at The London Hospital that he had coveted. Instead he decided to become a physician and after a period as Assistant Physician was elected to the staff of The London Hospital at the age of 35.

He wrote on all aspects of clubfoot. He advocated tenotomy of any tendon producing deformity, whereas Stromeyer had divided only the Achilles tendon; Stromeyer called him the "Apostle of Tenotomy." He also wrote on other deformities, such as knockknee and scoliosis; described the spastic state arising from birth damage of the brain, known as Little's disease or spastic paraplegia; and pioneered the use of intravenous saline and alcohol for dehydration.

At the age of 53 his private practice kept him too busy to go to The London Hospital, and he retired from there but kept his practice going for another 20 years.

It is interesting that his paper on cerebral palsy was read before the Obstetrical Society.

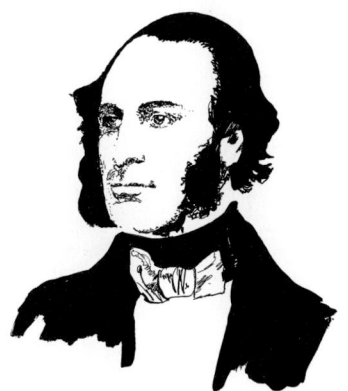

◆ William John Little

Little's Disease, 1862

ON THE INFLUENCE OF ABNORMAL PARTURITION, DIFFICULT LABOURS, PREMATURE BIRTH, AND ASPHYXIA NEONATORUM, ON THE MENTAL AND PHYSICAL CONDITION OF THE CHILD, ESPECIALLY IN RELATION TO DEFORMITIES

W. J. LITTLE, SENIOR PHYSICIAN TO THE LONDON HOSPITAL; FOUNDER OF THE ROYAL ORTHOPAEDIC HOSPITAL; VISITING PHYSICIAN TO THE ASYLUM FOR IDIOTS, EARLSWOOD

"Pathology has gradually taught that the foetus in utero is subject to similar diseases to those which afflict the economy at later periods of existence. This is especially true if we turn to the study of the special class of abnormal conditions, which are termed deformities.

"There is, however, an epoch of existence, viz., the period of birth, during which, at first sight, we might consider that the foetal organism is subjected to conditions so different to those of its earlier and of its prospective later existence, that any untoward influences applied at this important juncture would affect the economy in a manner different to the influences at work during the periods ordinarily characterised as those of before birth and after birth.

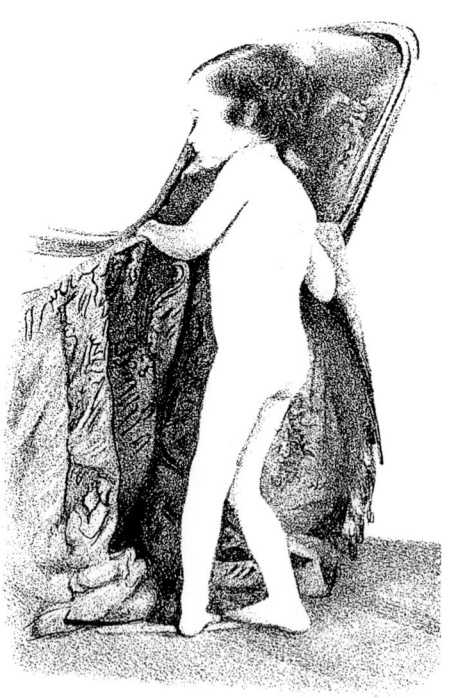
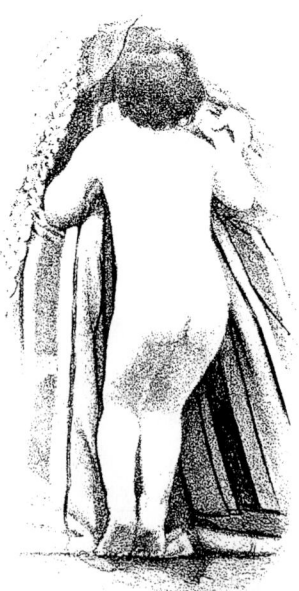

Spastic diplegia depicted by Little, 1862.

Cases of cerebral palsy with all these deformities are just the same today as when Bernard Brodhurst published this in 1871. *"Figure is taken from a cast which I placed in St. George's Hospital Museum in which are represented almost every possible deformity to which spastic rigidity can give rise."* The deformity is *"dependent alone on the structural shortening of the affected muscles."* From Brodhurst B: The Deformities of the Human Body. A System of Orthopaedic Surgery. London: 1871.

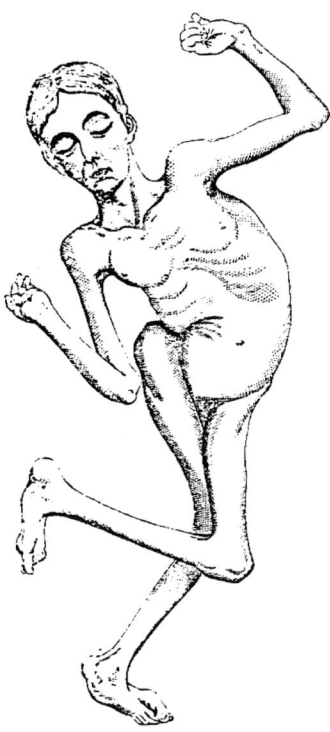

"The object of this communication is to show that the act of birth does occasionally imprint upon the nervous and muscular systems of the nascent infantile organism very serious and peculiar evils. When we investigate the evils in question, and their causative influences, we find that the same laws of pathology apply to diseases incidental to the act of birth as to those which originate before and after birth. We are, in fact, afforded another illustration that there exists no such thing as exceptional or special pathology.

"Nearly twenty years ago, in a course of lectures published in the Lancet, and more fully in a Treatise on Deformities, published in 1853, I showed that premature birth, difficult labours, mechanical injuries during parturition to head and neck, where life had been saved, convulsions following the act of birth, were apt to be succeeded by a determinate affection of the limbs of the child, which I designated spastic rigidity of the limbs of newborn children, spastic rigidity from asphyxia neonatorum, and assimilated it to the trismus nascentium and the universal spastic rigidity sometimes produced at later periods of existence.

"It is obvious that the great majority of apparently stillborn infants, whose lives are saved by the attendant accoucheur, recover unharmed from that condition. I have, however, witnessed so many cases of deformity, mental and physical, traceable to causes operative at birth, that I consider the subject worthy the notice of the Obstetrical Society. In orthopaedic practice alone, during about twenty years, I have met with probably two hundred cases of spastic rigidity from this cause. I omit reckoning the subjects of idiot and other asylums, in which probably such cases abound, but of which I have been able to attain no history. I revert to the subject at the present [that has been] been recognised as a genuine paralysis in the first instance, of which the rigidity of the muscles has been the sequel. Before the age of three or four months, though sometimes in slight cases not until ordinary time for walking arrives, the nurse perceives that the infant never thoroughly straightens the knees, that these cannot be properly depressed or separated, that she is unable to wash and dress the infant with the ordinary facility, that the hands are not properly used. The upper extremities recover before the lower limbs. Sometimes the trunk is habitually stiffened, so that the infant is turned over in the lap "all of a piece," as the nurse expresses it. Occasionally the head is habitually retracted. Where the symptom of convulsions or "inward convulsions" exists, the rigidity is attributed to the convulsions. In many cases convulsions have been absent. As the child approaches the period at

which the first attempts at standing and progression should be made, it is observed to make no use of the limbs, or he is incapable of standing except on the toes, or the feet are disposed to cross each other. Even children slightly affected rarely "go alone" before three or four years of age, many are unable to raise themselves from the ground at that age, and others do not walk, even indifferently, at puberty. On examination, the surgeon finds that the soles of the feet are not properly applied to the ground, that the knees always incline inwardly, and continue bent. When locomotion is accomplished, the movements are characterised by inability to stand still and balance the body in erect attitude. In the best recoveries from general spastic rigidity, even in the adult, the gait is shuffling, stiff; each knee, by forcible spastic rubbing against its fellow, obstructs progression.

"The external form of cranium occasionally exhibits departure from the normal or average type, such as general smallness of skull, depression of frontal or occipital region only, sometimes one lateral half of skull, sometimes of one half of occiput, or forehead only. In slight cases the head has been well developed.

"In cases even with great inertia as to exercise of volition in any part of the body, common sensibility appears little, if at all, deficient. The child often, indeed, manifests uncommon sensitiveness to external impressions, even when approaching adolescence he is alarmed at trifling noises. The sleep after the first weeks of life is light, easily disturbed. Often there is extreme sensibility to touch, the whole condition reminding the observer of tetanus. In a few cases a distinct resemblance to severe chorea is perceptible."

Sigmund Freud, 1897

Surprisingly, he wrote a 350-page book on cerebral palsy. He described hemiplegia beginning in infancy and genetic forms of diplegia. In these 350 pages there are only a few sentences on treatment. A true neurologist, he wrote "*Therapy of infantile cerebral palsy is a poor and hopeless subject in comparison to the great clinical interest it has aroused.... The treatment of the motor disturbance lies completely in the hands of orthopaedic specialists who have reported success by severing tendons and by supporting apparatus.*"

Christie Brown, 1954

This young boy with athetosis had his autobiography made into a movie, "My Left Foot."

"*I used to lie on my back all the time in the kitchen or out in the garden, a little bundle of crooked muscles and twisted nerves, surrounded by a family that loved me and hoped for me and that made me part of their own warmth and humanity. I was lonely, imprisoned in a world of my own, unable to communicate with others, cut off.*

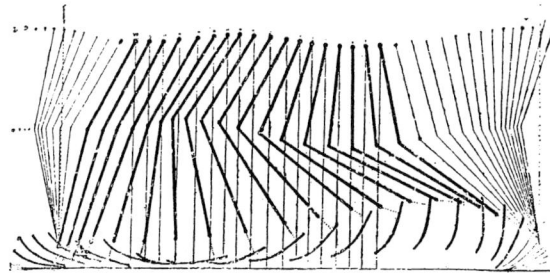

Marey calls this a geometric chronophotograph. Today Gait Laboratories produce similar records. From Marey EJ: Movement (trans by E Pritchard). London: 1895.

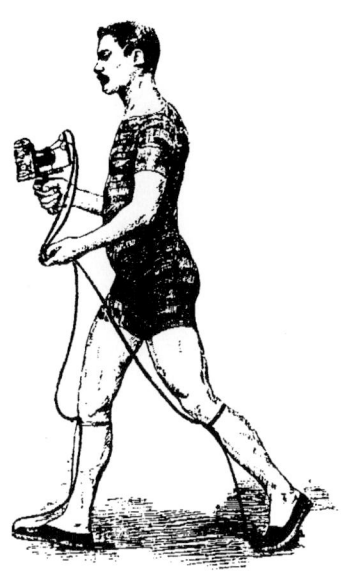

"Then suddenly it happened. I reached out and took the stick of chalk out of my sister's hand—with my left foot."

He learned to write and to paint with his foot and this opened up his world. Later he wrote a novel that was highly acclaimed, *Down All the Days.*

Étienne-Jules Marey (1830–1904) was an early student of making objective records. Here he records gait: *"Pedestrian furnished with special shoes and carrying a chronographic apparatus."* From Marey EJ: Movement (translated by E. Pritchard). London, 1895.

Motion Analysis

The objective recording of walking is playing a part in the surgical treatment of cerebral disorders. Video and computers put this within everyone's grasp. Muybridge was the first to take rapid-sequence photographs in California in the 1880s. Marey in France used graphing methods, and the German Army used these methods to improve marching and the design of knapsacks. Interest turned to making models with muscles to observe the amount of lengthening and shortening of each muscle on moving through a certain angle.

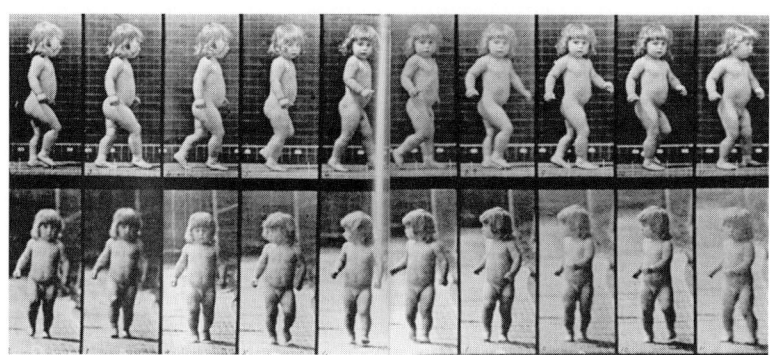

Eadweard Muybridge—an eccentric genius who was originally called Edward Muggeridge—invented a set of 24 cameras in 1877 that fired sequentially to freeze motion. He was bankrolled by a railway tycoon, Leland Stanford in California, to study racehorses. He later produced pictures of human movement and laid the foundations of cinematography and movement analysis, which provided many artists with ideas for paintings. From Animal Locomotion, 1887.

Neurofibromatosis
Robert William Smith (1807–1873)

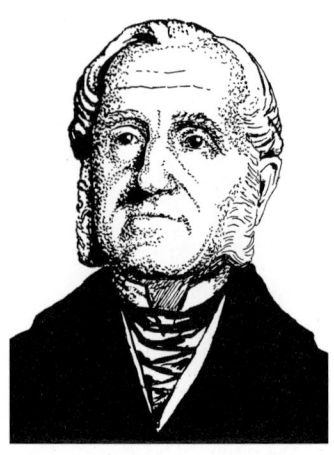

◆ Robert William Smith

Robert Smith was born in Dublin and studied and worked there, at a time when Irish medicine was very active: Stokes, Corrigan, Colles, Graves, and Adams set the pace. Smith was a surgical pathologist at heart—a great collector of specimens of bone pathology, especially fractures.

He founded the Pathological Society at Dublin, and when Colles died in 1843, Smith, at Colles' request, performed the autopsy, a report of which was published.

He had a small surgical practice and in 1847 wrote a very thoughtful book on fractures. In this he mentions the supination injury of the wrist, which is named after him, and a description of Madelung's deformity before Madelung described it. In 1849 he published a work on neuromata, which is said to be the largest book published in Ireland up to that time. When it is opened it is larger than an ordinary dining-room table. Smith wrote on neurofibromatosis very fully before von Recklinghausen described it in 1882, and for this reason his account is included.

He became Professor of Surgery at Trinity College, Dublin, and gave up his practice to teach.

A TREATISE ON THE PATHOLOGY, DIAGNOSIS, AND TREATMENT OF NEUROMA
ROBERT WILLIAM SMITH, 1849

"Although numerous instances of solitary neuroma have been placed on record, the annals of pathology contain as yet but few examples in which neuromatous tumours have been developed in almost countless numbers throughout the greater part of the nervous system: not only connected with the deep seated trunks, but visible in almost every superficial nerve of the body; not limited to the extremities, but likewise involving the nerves of the great cavities; not confined to the cerebrospinal, but also implicating the grand sympathetic system; not the seat of pain, but on the contrary, the source of no apparent injury to the patient; unaccompanied by any lesion of innervation, even when such nerves as the vagus and phrenic are involved from one extremity to the other.

"John McCann, 35 years of age, was admitted into the Richmond Hospital, under the care of Dr. Hutton, in 1840, having a large tumour on the right side of the neck, of a globular form, and equal to a moderate-sized coconut in magnitude; it extended from within the mastoid process to within a short distance of the sterno-clavicular articulation. It presented a uniform surface, and admitted of being moved freely in a transverse direction, but could neither be pushed upwards nor drawn downwards; the external jugular vein grooved its surface, the integuments did not adhere to it nor (although it obviously extended deep into the neck) did it appear to have contracted a close adhesion to

any important part. It was solid throughout and had existed for upwards of fifteen years, but it had never been painful nor was it now the source of much inconvenience to the patient.

"A second tumour, about as large as a walnut, existed underneath the left side of the tongue. (Treatment was decided against.)

"In 1843 he was again taken into hospital, having on the day previous ... been found ... lying upon the side of the road complaining of a pain in the left hip. A large solid tumour was discovered upon the back of the thigh, which the man stated had been growing for nearly two years. It exceeded in magnitude the size of the head of the patient. Its general surface was smooth. Several large veins ramified beneath the integuments, which were not adherent to the tumour. The patient suffered no acute pain. His general health had undergone a material alteration since the period of his first admission into hospital; he was now pale and greatly emaciated ....

"Upon the day succeeding that upon which the patient died I made a careful examination of the body.... The largest (tumour) was situated upon the posterior part of the right thigh, immediately beneath the lower margin of the gluteus maximus muscle; it was of an oblong form and considerably larger than a lemon. There was one upon the outer side of the right arm, near its centre, of the size of a pigeon's egg and another upon the front of the right forearm, immediately above the carpus, nearly as large as a hen's egg; they all admitted being moved in a lateral direction. The intercostal spaces upon each side, as well as the abdominal parietes and the right inguinal region, presented numerous tumours about the size of large peas.

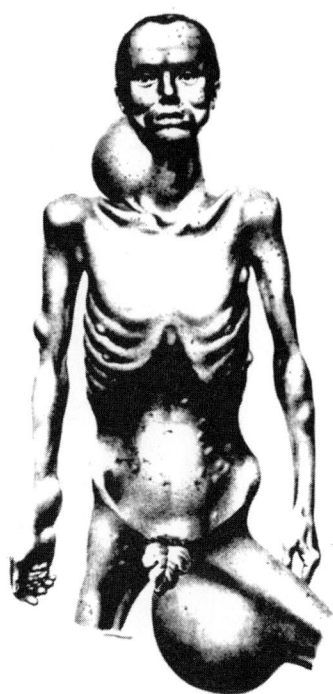

Neurofibromatosis. Robert Smith, 1849.

He then goes on to describe the detailed autopsy findings; he found 150 tumors on the right lumbar plexus and its branches, and similar numbers on the sciatic and brachial plexuses. One tumor on the sciatic nerve measured 11 by 10 inches.

"In this remarkable case the total number of tumours exceeded 800; they presented a striking uniformity, both in their external characters and the internal structure; their form was oval or oblong; their colour, a yellowish white; they were solid, and each surrounded by a capsule, which was continuous with the neurilemma; their surface was smooth; their long axis corresponded with the direction of the nerve on which they exist, and they were only movable from side to side. Their section exhibited an exceedingly dense, close texture, of a whitish colour, and a somewhat glistening aspect, presenting a uniform degree of solidarity, and remarkable for a total absence of vascularity. Examined by the aid of a microscope, they were found to be composed essentially of a fibro-cellular structure, the fibrous tissue predominating in by far the greatest number, the areolar predominating in a few; the fibres arranged in bands or loops, amongst which permanent oval or elongated nuclei became apparent on the addition of acetic acid. In no one instance was there any trace discovered of nerve tubes, nor any indication of malignant disease."

Spina Bifida

MYELOMENINGOCELE
G. B. MORGAGNI, PADUA, ITALY, 1761

"The life of the little patient is usually cut short by convulsions and other consequences of injury to the nerves. And these evils happen more speedily if the nerves are pricked in opening the tumor or if they are exposed to air. A boy was brought to me having a tumor on the lumbar vertebrae which was soft and in many places translucent. At birth it was small but within ten months it had grown to the size of a fist. The boy was strong and was well formed even in his lower limbs although they were weak. I cautioned the parents not to have the tumor opened. The surgeon, however, being ignorant of its nature, promised to cure the disease. He was permitted to thrust a knife into the middle of the tumour from whence it burst a considerable quantity of limpid fluid and toward the last some bloody fluid escaped. He afterward introduced a stent into the orifice. The child did not cease to cry, the body trembled, the face became pale and wrinkled, and death followed on the third day."

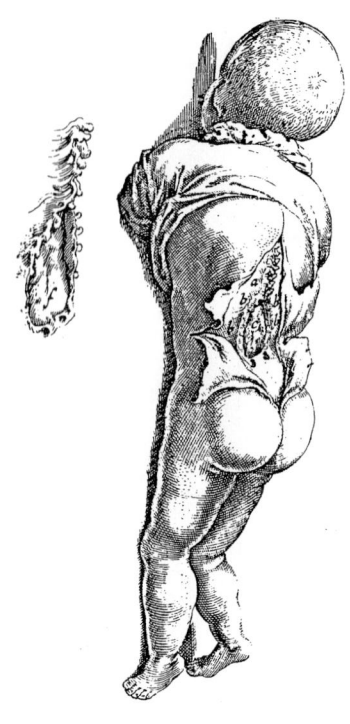

Nicholaas Tulp's engraving of myelomeningocele *circa* 1630. Tulp (1593–1674) was the Amsterdam doctor and anatomist who appears in Rembrandt's painting, "The Anatomy Lesson." His book contains an illustration of the autopsy findings of spina bifida.

The prevention of spina bifida has been a longtime goal. First came identification of affected fetuses by amniocentesis and ultrasound in the 1970s, and then in the 1990s came the means of reducing the chance of a fetus developing abnormally by giving the mother folate.

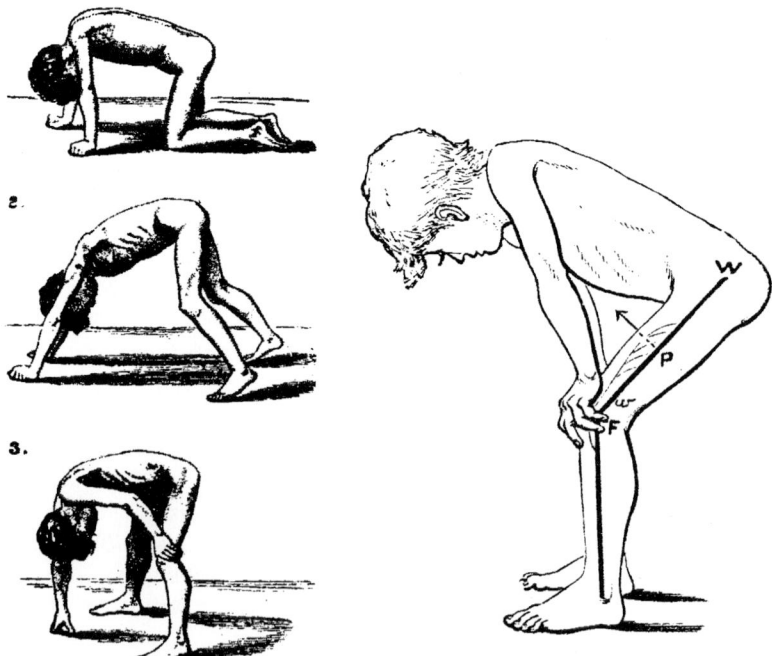

William Gowers' drawings of his sign of muscular dystrophy and his biomechanical explanation, 1888.

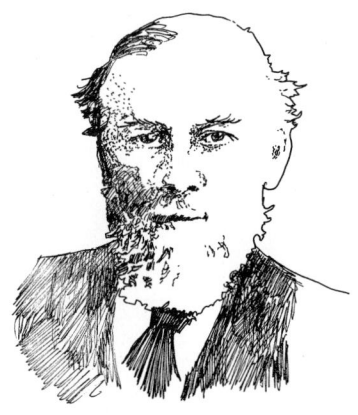

◆ **Sir William Gowers (1845–1915)**

He invented the device for measuring hemoglobin and counting red cells before he became the most famous neurologist of his generation. He wrote a bible of neurology in 1886 and is remembered for the first description of several diseases, as well as Gowers' sign.

Muscular Dystrophy

Duchenne on Dystrophy, 1858

"Pseudo-hypertrophic paralysis is a disease of infancy or youth, which I believe to be not very uncommon, but which nevertheless has not been yet described. This affection, serious from its very commencement, deceives the friends for a long time, and deludes them by giving the limbs an appearance of great muscularity.

"The prognosis is grave. I have always seen it progress steadily towards generalisation and terminate by complete loss of movement and death during adolescence."

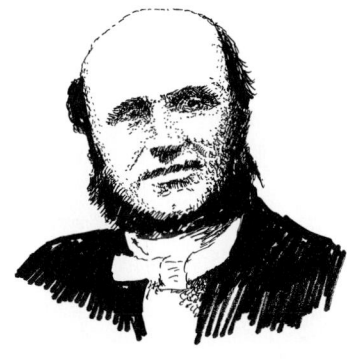

◆ **Guillaume Benjamin Armand Duchenne (also known as Duchenne du Boulogne) (1806–1875)**

He was a shy, strange, inarticulate man who used simple faradic stimulation of muscle to open new worlds. This was a new tool discovered by Faraday in 1831. He used it to discover the exact action of each muscle and the role of the muscles in producing facial expression, for diagnosis, and for treatment.

Duchenne was born in Boulogne where his family were ship's captains. He studied medicine in Paris when Laennec and Dupuytren were developing clinical science. He went back to Boulogne to practice. When his wife died in childbirth, much of him died with her. He neglected his practice and eventually left, penniless, for Paris. In the neurologic wards, he examined and recorded the findings of patients and followed them to autopsy. This was a time before examination had been systematized. Interns laughed at him, but Charcot called him The Master. His writings have kept his name alive—he described the commonest form of muscular dystrophy and various other conditions.

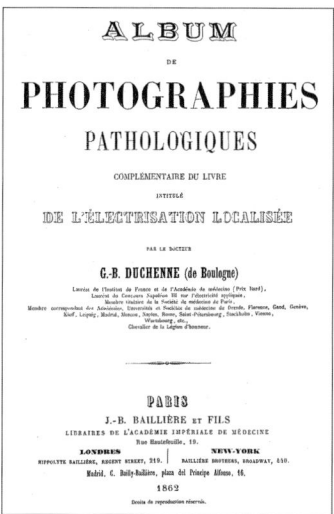

Title page of Duchenne's book, 1862.

238 Chapter 10 ◆ Neuromuscular Disease

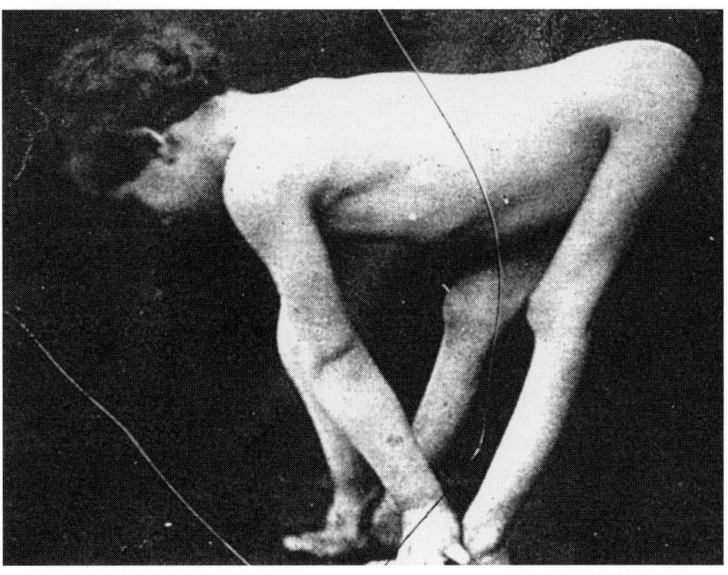

Duchenne's photograph of a boy who moved quickly, holding his feet with his hands owing to weakness, (?) spinal muscular atrophy. 1862.

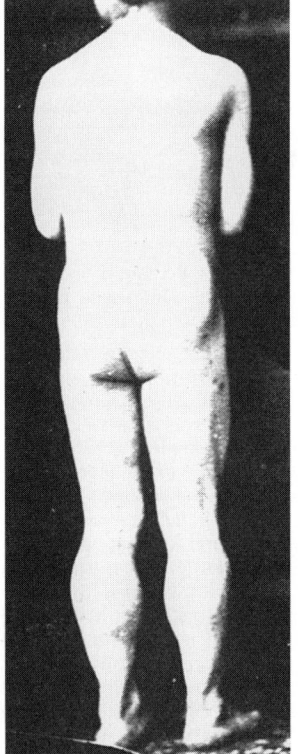

Duchenne's photograph of his form of muscular dystrophy. 1862.

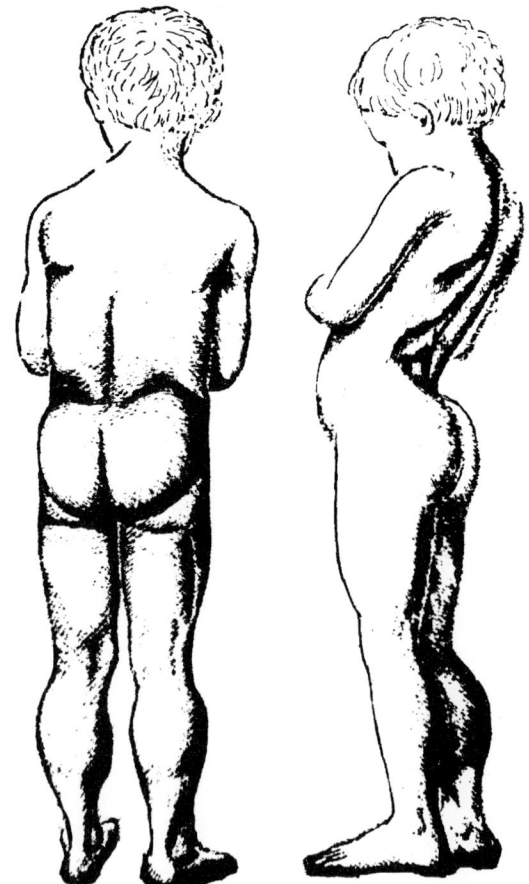

Drawings by Duchenne illustrating the features of pseudohypertrophic muscular dystrophy—the calves are large and there is a marked lumbar lordosis. 1858.

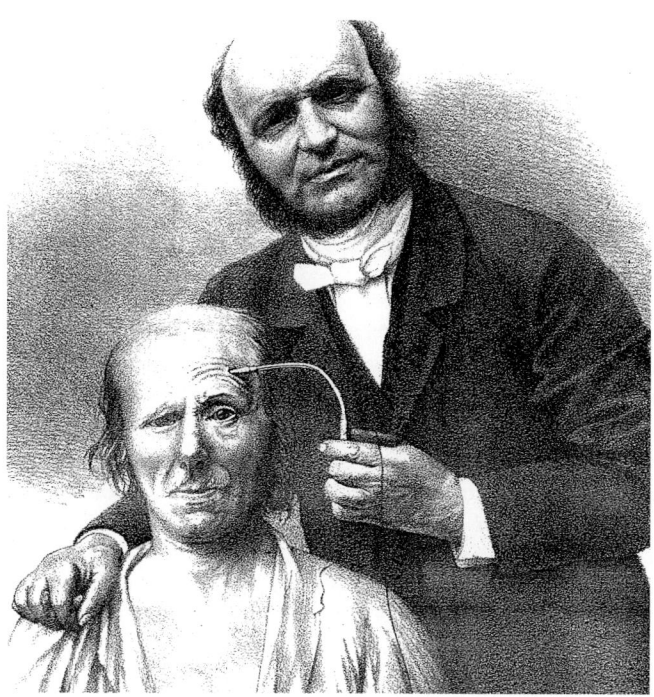

Duchenne pioneered clinical electrodiagnosis, and this picture is taken from the English translation of some of his work published in 1883. He studied the muscular basis of facial expression and limb movements. From Poor GV: Translation of Selections of Collected Works of Duchenne. London: 1883.

Arthrogryposis

Henry Mayhew was a Victorian journalist whose columns were collected into a book, *London Labour and London Poor*, which described the miserable lives led by the street people of the 1840s and 1850s. After Karl Marx read it, he started writing *The Communist Manifesto*. The engraving here looks to me like a person with arthrogryposis, and the following is an abridgement of his 4-page story.

The Crippled Street-Seller of Nutmeg-Graters, 1850

"I will now give an example of one of the classes DRIVEN to the streets by utter inability to labour. I have already spoken of the sterling independence of some of these men possessing the strongest claims to our sympathy and charity, and yet preferring to sell rather than beg.

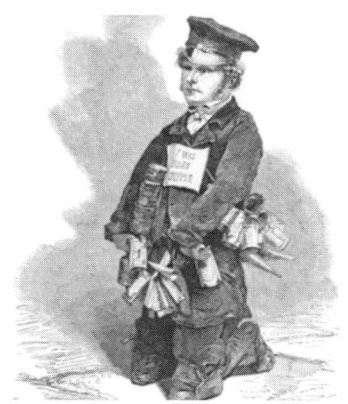

Arthrogryposis in the 19th century. The label reads: I was born cripple. From Mayhew, 1850.

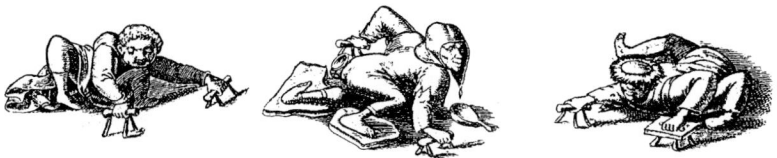

Hieronymous Bosch, a 15th century painter, drew these people with paralyzed legs dragging themselves around.

"His struggles to earn his own living (notwithstanding his physical inability even to put victuals to his mouth after he has earned them) are without a parallel. The poor creature's legs and arms are completely withered: indeed he is scarcely more than a head and a trunk. His thigh is hardly thicker than a child's wrist. His hands are bent inwards from contraction of the sinews, the fingers being curled up and almost as thin as the claws of a bird's foot. He is unable even to stand, and cannot move from place to place but on his knees, which are shod with leather caps, like the heels of a clog, strapped around the joint. His countenance is rather handsome than otherwise; his intelligence indicated by an ample forehead is amply bourne out by the testimony as to his sagacity in his business.

" 'I sell nutmeg-graters and funnels,' said the cripple to me, 'at 1 penny and 1½ pennies a piece. I buy them at 7 pence a dozen. Some days I sell only three though I am out from 10 till 6. The most I ever took was 3 shillings and 6 pence. Some weeks I barely clear my expenses—and they are between 7 and 8 shillings a week: for not being able to dress and undress myself, I'm obligated to pay someone to do it for me. When I don't make that much, I go without. I pay every night for my lodging as I go in, if I can: but if not my landlady lets it run a night or two.

" 'It's the Almighty's will that I am so, and so I must abide with it.

" 'I strive hard—and crawl about till my limbs ache enough to drive me mad—to get an honest livelihood.' "

His mother was a cook in a nobleman's house, and she paid 30 pounds a year to a lady to look after him as a child. His mother died and soon afterwards his foster mother. He had run a bed-repairing business, but he did not get paid and had to start selling in the streets. When he was sick, he was taken to the workhouse. It is a long, sad story.

References

Chapter references are located in Chapter 26.

◆ Chapter Eleven

Arthritis

In ancient times all joint pain was attributed to either infection or gout. "Gout" was the name given to every kind of nonsuppurative joint problem. In the 17th century, Ballonius introduced the term rheumatism—a word derived from the Greek *rheuma,* something that flows like a river; in olden times it was believed that bad humors flowed into the joints—perhaps not far from the truth. Hippocrates knew about rheumatic fever, which *"licks the joints and bites the heart"* in Bouillaud's 1840 quip.

Gradually several diseases were defined and separated—gonococcal arthritis by Pierre-Martin de la Martinière in 1664, chemical gout in 1797, rheumatoid arthritis in 1857, neuropathic joints in 1868, Clutton's syphilitic joints in 1886, and ankylosing spondylitis in 1898. Because there was no treatment for any of them, little was gained at first by separating them. They were managed with spa treatment, massage, bath chairs, crutches, and all kinds of useless and harmful medications. In the first half of the 20th century, patients were thought to be victims of focal sepsis by some leading surgeons; many were subject to removal of teeth, umbilicus, colon, and tonsils quite unnecessarily. I remember working as a general surgical resident and meeting a number of patients lacking an umbilicus for this reason.

Gout was the first disease to be successfully treated, with colchicine, in the 1770s. Rheumatoid arthritis was first treated with gold and steroids in the 1950s, and osteoarthritis waited until joint replacement was developed in the 1960s.

Although arthritis is such a big part of orthopaedics today, old orthopaedic textbooks had little to say about osteoarthritis. Whitman devoted only one page of 650 in 1901.

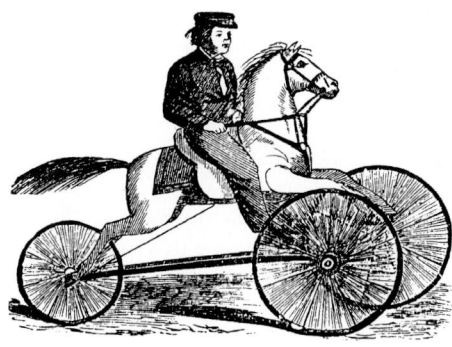

The locomotive cantering horse for mobilizing stiff hip and knee joints was used by James Knight in 1884. From his book *Orthopaedia.*

Famous Patients

Did **Emperor Constantine** (980-1055) have rheumatoid arthritis? At the age of 63 he developed a polyarthritis affecting feet, hands, shoulders, and knee His friend Michael Psellus wrote, *"I myself saw his fingers, once so beautifully formed, completely altered from their natural shape, warped and twisted with hollows here and projections there, so that they were incapable of grasping anything at all. His feet were bent and his knees, crooked like the point of a man's elbow, were swollen making it impossible for him to walk steadily or to stand upright for any length of time. Mostly he lay on his bed..."*

Christopher Columbus had attacks of swollen painful joints, as well as fevers and eye problems.

Mary, Queen of Scots. She was afflicted with rheumatoid arthritis in 1566. When she was beheaded, she needed two people to help her walk. Because of her well-known disability, she was known as Marie Malade (malade is French for sick). Some say marmalade derives its name from her. Others say this is rubbish and the word is derived from the Greek for quince.

Peter Paul Rubens. If you look at the later paintings of this 18th century painter, you will notice that the hands often resemble those of someone with rheumatoid arthritis, with the posture and the swellings. He is known to have suffered from some kind of arthritis—every joint problem was attributed to gout then—and the hands in his paintings may have been autobiographical.

Pierre Auguste Renoir. The impressionist painter had to have brushes taped to his fingers in old age because of his rheumatoid arthritis. I think his painting suffered.

Raoul Dufy. The French artist used to paint jolly paintings. He developed rheumatoid arthritis and the paintings became simpler and lacked detail. Then, when cortisone first came on the market, he was offered treatment in the United States. Portraits at this time show him with cherubic cheeks. But he started to paint black pictures and died in 1953.

TIMELINES
Gout

3rd century BC	Hippocrates describes gout clearly—"the most violent, tenacious and painful of joint affections."
100	Rufus of Ephesus: treatise on gout.
circa 600	Alexander of Thralles uses colchicine with benefit, but then this knowledge is lost.
1531	Paracelsus: book on diseases of "Tartar." Gout due to a chemical deposition in the joint.
1684	Leeuwenhoek sees under the microscope that tophi contain urate crystals.
1689	Sydenham writes the classic on gout.
1763	Storck reintroduces colchicine in Vienna.
1797	Woolaston: urates in gouty deposits.

1819 Brodie: classic treatise on joint disease.
1854 Alfred Garrod devises a test for urates in blood and postulates that acute gout is due to precipitation of urate in the joint.
1913 Folin and Denis test for urate in blood.

Rheumatoid Arthritis

123 *Caraka Samhita,* an Indian book, describes incurable polyarthritis.
1642 Guillaume de Baillou of Paris distinguishes between gout and rheumatic fever in his book on rheumatism, becoming the Father of Rheumatism. Others, such as Cullen (1785) and Pitcairn (1788) provide descriptions of rheumatic fever.
1676 Thomas Sydenham's account of rheumatoid arthritis.
1770 Heberden: rheumatoid arthritis.
1800 A.J. Landre-Beauvais' account of rheumatoid arthritis in a thesis.
1818 Benjamin Brodie's classic treatise, *On the Pathology and Surgery of Diseases of the Joints.*
1828 Jean Cruveilhier: atlas of anatomy has clear pictures of rheumatoid arthritis and gout affecting the hands.
1857 Robert Adams in Dublin distinguishes chronic rheumatoid arthritis from osteoarthritis.
1859 Sir Alfred Garrod invents the name rheumatoid arthritis. His classic work is published: *The Nature and Treatment of Gout and Rheumatic Gout.* The second edition calls it Rheumatoid Arthritis.
1876 Maclagan uses acetylsalicylic acid for rheumatoid arthritis.
1884 Strümpell describes ankylosing spondylitis, as do Bechterew (1897) and Marie (1898).
1890 Archibald Garrod (son of Alfred): book on rheumatoid arthritis.
1891 Bouchard: infection theory.
1896 Still describes juvenile arthritis.
1896 Ballantyne: treatise on the pathology of rheumatoid arthritis.
1901 William Hunter's focal sepsis theory leads to removal of all kinds of organs.
1904 Sir William Gowers coins the word fibrositis—perhaps the worst thing he did.
1916 Hans Reiter describes an officer in the German Army with diarrhea, conjunctivitis, urethritis, and arthritis and on the basis of this single case gives his name to a syndrome. Brodie had mentioned it in 1818.
1928 International League Against Rheumatism formed.
1934 American Rheumatism Association founded and starts to publish the Primer.
1935 Jacques Forestier tries gold treatment. It was fashionable for TB, and so it seemed reasonable to give it a try in rheumatoid arthritis.
1940 Waaler finds rheumatoid factor.
1942 Concept of collagen disease: Klemperer.
1948 LE cell test: Hargreaves.

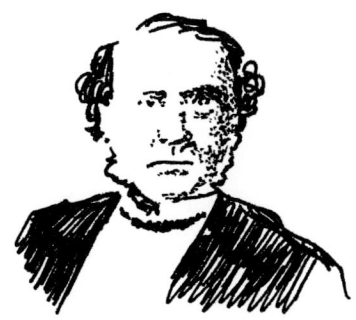

◆ **Alfred Baring Garrod (1819–1907)**

London physician who devoted his life to the study of gout and was one of the first metabolic physicians. In 1859 he devised a chemical test pathognomonic for gout.

◆ **Sir Archibald E. Garrod (1857–1936)**

The son of Sir Alfred, he started modern rheumatology, separating osteoarthritis from rheumatoid arthritis.

Box continued on following page

> 1948 Hench and Kendall use cortisone with benefit.
> 1975 Lyme disease. Two mothers in the town of Old Lyme, Connecticut, complained to the public health department about a cluster of cases of juvenile rheumatoid arthritis. The incidence was supposed to be 1 in 100,000, but this community of 12,000 had 39 children and 12 adults with the disease. Eventually a veterinary pathologist in Montana identified the spirochete—*Borrelia burgdorferi*—carried by a deer tick.

Gout

Derived from the latin *gutta,* drop. The ancients, who believed that the four humors were the cause of all disease, believed that a drop of phlegm distilled by the brain could arrive in the joint and make it swell.

Famous Patients

King Phillip 2 of Spain (1527–1598) was a religious and political despot. His father died of gout, and he suffered from attacks of gout and then from chronic arthritis. He regarded gout as God's punishment for not exterminating the heretics. He therefore pressed on with the Inquisition and sought to replicate the pain of gout on transgressors.

William Pitt, Earl of Chatham was prime minister of Britain during the troubles with the Americans in the 18th century. He had gout that put him out of action during crucial periods—the imposition of the Stamp Tax and the Tea Tax. If these taxes had not been imposed, there would not have been the Boston Tea Party in 1773, and perhaps things would have turned out differently.

He had wanted to take colchicum, but it had given his doctor, Dr. Sydenham, diarrhea, and so Pitt was advised against it. When Franklin and Chatham met, they discussed gout.

Benjamin Franklin introduced colchicum to the United States and wrote a "Dialogue with Gout":

"Midnight, October 22, 1780

Franklin: Eh! Oh! Eh! What have I done to merit such cruel sufferings?

Gout: Many things; you have ate and drank too freely, and you too much indulged those legs of yours in their indolence.

Franklin: Who is that who accuses me?

Gout: It is I, even I, the Gout.

Franklin: What, my enemy in person?

Gout: No, not your enemy.

Franklin: I repeat it; my enemy; for you would not only torment my body to death, but ruin my good name; you reproach me as a glutton and a tippler; now all the world that knows me, will allow that I am neither one nor the other."

Gout continues to chide him for 8 more pages, leading Franklin to promise to live better.

Comments on Gout

S. Smith

"I thought it a bargain of nature that men should have the gout and ladies produce the children." 1800

Hippocrates

"Eunuchs do not take the gout nor become bald.

"A woman does not take the gout, unless her menses are stopped.

"A young man does not take the gout until he indulges in coition."

Original Papers

GOUT
THOMAS SYDENHAM, 1683

"Either men will think that the nature of gout is wholly mysterious and incomprehensible, or that a man like myself who has suffered from it for thirty-four years, must be of a slow and sluggish disposition not to have discovered something respecting the nature and treatment of a disease so peculiarly his own. Be this as it may, I will give a bona fide account of what I know. The difficulties and refinements relating to the disease itself, and the method of its cure, I will leave for Time, the guide to truth, to clear up and explain.

"Concerning this disease, in its most regular and typical state, I will first discourse; afterwards I will note its more irregular and uncertain phenomena. These occur when the unseasonable use of preposterous medicines has thrown it down from its original status. Also when the weakness and langour of the patient prevent it from rising to its proper and genuine symptoms. As often as gout is regular, it comes on thus. Towards the end of January or the beginning of February, suddenly and without any premonitory feelings, the disease breaks out. Its only forerunner is indigestion and crudity of the stomach, of which the patient labours some weeks before. His body feels swollen, heavy and windy—symptoms which increase until the fit breaks out. This is preceded a few days by torpor and a feeling of flatus along the legs and thighs. Besides this, there is a spasmodic affection, whilst the day before the fit the appetite is unnaturally hearty. The victim goes to bed and sleeps in good health. About two o'clock in the morning he is awakened by a severe pain in the great toe; more rarely in the heel, ankle or instep. This pain is like that of a dislocation, and yet the parts feel as if cold water were poured over them. Then follow chills and shivers and a little fever. The pain, which was at first moderate, becomes more intense. With its intensity the chills and shivers increase. After a time this comes to its height, accommodating itself to the bones and ligaments of the tarsus and metatarsus. Now it is a violent

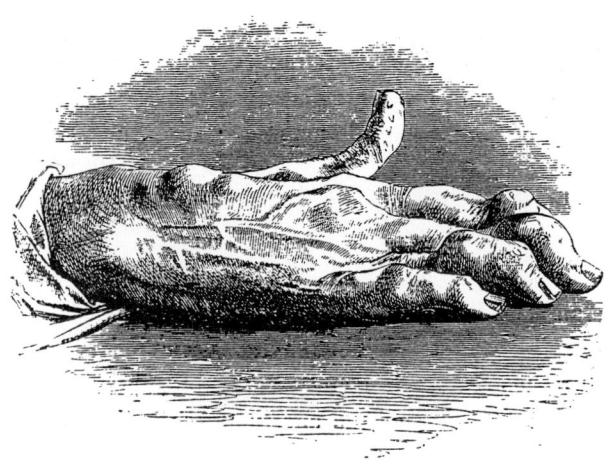

A hand affected by gout. *"There can be no doubt that the essential component of gouty deposits is urate of soda, which always assumes a crystalline form."* From Garrod AB: The nature and treatment of gout and rheumatic gout. London: 1859. Reprint of Garrod AB: A Treatise on Gout. *In* Clin Orthop Related Res 1970, 71, 3-13.

stretching and tearing of the ligaments—now it is a gnawing pain and now a pressure and tightening. So exquisite and lively meanwhile is the feeling of the part affected, that it cannot bear the weight of the bedclothes nor the jar of a person walking in the room. The night is passed in torture, sleeplessness, turning of the part affected, and perpetual change of posture, the tossing about of the body being as incessant as the pain of the tortured joint, and being worse as the fit comes on. Hence the vain effort, by change of posture, both in the body and limb affected, to obtain an abatement of the pain. This comes only towards the morning of the next day, such time being necessary for the moderate digestion of the peccant matter. The patient has a sudden and slight respite, which he falsely attributes to the last change of position. A gentle perspiration is succeeded by sleep. He wakes freer from pain, and finds the part recently swollen. Up to this time, the only visible swelling had been that of the veins of the affected joint. Next day (perhaps for the next two or three days), if the generation of the gouty matter had been abundant, the part affected is painful, getting worse towards evening and better towards morning. A few days after, the other foot swells, and suffers the same pains. The pain in the second foot attacked regulates the pain in the first one attacked. The more it is violent in the one, the more perfect is the abatement of suffering, and the return of strength in the other. Nevertheless, it brings on the same affliction here as it had brought on in the other foot, and that the same in duration and intensity. Sometimes, during the first days of the disease, the peccant matter is so exuberant, that one foot is insufficient for its discharge. It then attacks both, and that with equal violence. Generally, however, it takes the feet in succession. After it has attacked each foot, the fits become irregular, both as to the time of their accession and duration. One thing, however, is constant—the pain increases at night and remits in the morning. Now a series of lesser fits like these constitute a true attack of gout—long or short, according to the age of the patient.

"Gout produces calculus in the kidney. The patient has frequently to entertain the painful speculation as to whether gout or stone be the worst disease.

"It makes life worse than death, and finally brings in death as a relief."

Sydenham (1624-1689) has a quality in common with Hippocrates: his writings cover a wide field, with the accent on personal observation rather than quasiscientific theorizing, and, as with Hippocrates, little is known of his life.

He was born at Winford Eagle and studied at Oxford, but his studies were interrupted by the Civil Wars, during which he served in the Parliamentarian Army with the rank of Captain. On his return to Oxford he was made a Bachelor of Medicine by the Parliamentarian Chancellor of the University himself, by some very irregular procedure; he had studied medicine only for a few months altogether. He continued his studies at Montpellier and then set up in practice in London.

He was a friend of the chemist Robert Boyle and John Locke. He wrote on the exanthems of childhood and the use of quinine in malaria. He suffered from gout for many years, and his description of the disease is among his best work. *"Gout kills more rich men than poor, more wise than simple."*

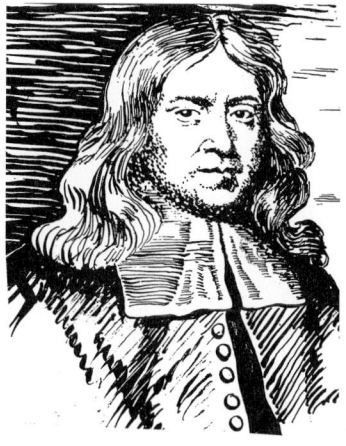

◆ Thomas Sydenham

Ankylosing Spondylitis

At the end of the 17th century, Bernard Connor, an Irishman who became physician to the King of Poland and died of malaria at the age of 32 in London, came across *"an extraordinary human skeleton, whose vertebrae of the back, the ribs, and several bones down to the os sacrum, were all firmly united into one solid bone, without jointing or cartilage."*

He concluded that this person must have been incapable of motion, unable to bend or stretch, and that his respiration was limited. The dramatic picture of fully developed ankylosing spondylitis was the subject of several case histories. Delpech in 1828 gives a good account, and Paget noticed it in 1877, but it was not until the late 19th century that much interest was aroused.

Adolf Strümpell, in 1884, wrote: *"As a remarkable, and, it would seem, definite disease, we might now draw attention to a form of illness in which there supervenes, progressively and without pain, a complete ankylosis of the entire spine and both hip joints, in such a manner that the head, the trunk and the thighs become fused and completely rigid, while the other joints retain their normal mobility. It goes without saying that, as a result of this fusion, very definite alterations of posture and gait make their appearance. We ourselves have seen two identical cases of this singular condition."*

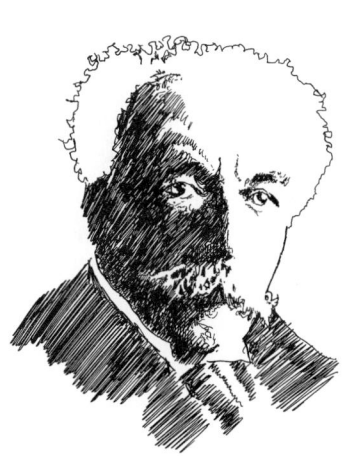

◆ Adolf Strümpell (1853-1925)

Pierre Marie in 1898 gives a textbook description of the disorder. Eight years later he filled in the details in a paper with Leri. The disease was first called ankylosing spondylitis by C. W. Buckley in 1935.

SPONDYLOSIS RHIZOMYELIQUE
PIERRE MARIE, 1898

"A particular characteristic of this disease is the occurrence of complete fusion of the spine together with a more or less pronounced ankylosis of the joints at the bases of the limbs, while the small joints remain unaffected.

"We are going to examine each of the phases of this definition separately:

"The Fusion of the Spine is complete, at least in the lower half; slightly higher, and especially in the cervical region, the spinal column may retain a certain mobility for some time. The rigidity thus produced is such that the spine would fracture rather than allow the slightest movement in it.

"The position in which this fusion of the spine occurs is worth nothing; in rhizomelic spondylosis the kyphosis is above all due to a definite and rather acute bend at the cervical section of the spine, and also a little of the upper dorsal spine, while the lumbar and lower and middle dorsal sections of the spine often continue almost in a straight line. What considerably exaggerates the kyphotic appearance of these patients is the ankylosis of the hip joint in flexion, so that the trunk seems to be thrown further forward than it is in fact.

"The fusion of the spine with the sacrum is complete . . . it seems that at this . . . level even a bony proliferation may be formed; in particular one may encounter osteophytic promi-

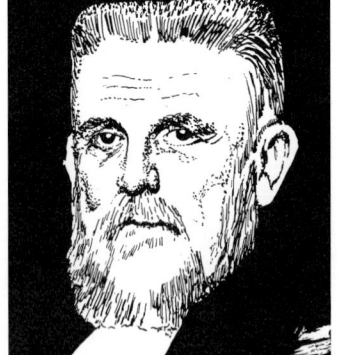

♦ Pierre Marie

♦ Pierre Marie (1853–1940)

A great teacher. His square-cut hair, square-cut beard, and striking personality indicated his severe, dignified, and authoritarian manner in public, but at home, where he collected painting and sculpture, this thawed. He had no longing for honors or titles, being happy enough to devote his life to neurology and arouse the same enthusiasm in others.

Marie was born in Paris near Place de la Concorde when this area had fields nearby. At his father's insistence he read law and was called to the bar, but then followed his own desire to study medicine. He became an intern under Charcot and continued to work for him for many years. In his doctoral thesis he first described the tremor of thyrotoxicosis. He had a succession of distinguished appointments: Physician at the Bicêtre, a mental hospital, Professor of Pathological Anatomy, and Professor of Clinical Neurology at the Salpêtrière, following Charcot and Dejerine.

Many of his original ideas were presented at his lectures and in consequence these talks were well attended. He kept up the Charcot tradition of attracting large numbers of postgraduate students.

His middle age was his most productive period, but his old age was a succession of personal tragedies. His wife died, his daughter died of appendicitis, and finally his son, who was studying botulism at the Institut Pasteur, contracted the disease and died.

What were Marie's contributions? Within three years of qualification he had described peroneal muscular atrophy. (Tooth described it in the United Kingdom in the same year.) He made the first observation of acromegaly in 1886 and observed the pituitary tumor.

Marie described hypertrophic pulmonary osteoarthropathy in 1890. In 1898 he published the first account of craniocleidal dysostosis and wrote the accompanying account of ankylosing spondylitis. His only other contribution of interest to orthopaedic surgeons was his continued belief that poliomyelitis was infectious.

nences at the level of the sacroiliac joint. Furthermore, the hyperostoses do not appear to be limited to the lower posterior section of the spine, for one finds, by feeling within the mouth, that bony protuberances on the anterior surfaces of the vertebral bodies are palpable through the posterior pharyngeal wall. It is most likely that the difficulty, which some of these patients experience when swallowing, is due to the irregularity at this level."

"***Ankylosis of the Joints of the Limbs.*** The joint which is most affected, and the only one which is really the site of complete ankylosis, is the hip joint. In this joint there may be complete loss of movement, with the joint fixed in some flexion and adduction.

"The Scapulo-Humeral Joint is much less frequently affected than the hip joint and does not suffer comparable ankylosis. Nevertheless movements were considerably reduced in two of our patients. Neither of them can lift their arms above the horizontal; when they are told to put a hand on their head—if they can manage it—it is due to the kyphosis which pushes their head forward and to the swinging movement of the scapula. When these two patients carried out passive movements gross crepitus could be observed at the site of the acromio-coracoid arch.

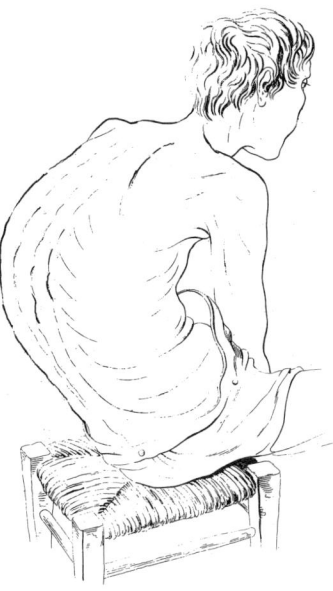

Delpech: ankylosing spondylitis, 1828.

"The Knee is another joint in which symptoms may require study. At first sight movements appear to be completely normal and patients do not mention their knees; nevertheless if they are asked to bend their knees as much as possible, it can be seen that movement is limited to a greater or lesser extent; in no case is it sufficient for the heel to touch the buttock.

"The other joints appear undamaged.

"The appearance of the patient is profoundly altered by a singular and very marked flattening of the pelvis and thorax. It is difficult to say whether the flattening of the pelvis is due only to atrophy of the buttocks or whether the bones themselves participate; this latter hypothesis is not unlikely. The thorax is, like the pelvis, flattened in the antero-posterior diameter; here, too, muscular wasting of the back muscles may play a certain part, though the skeleton shares in the deformity. This is very clear when one looks at the patient from the side.

"In addition to this deformity there is extraordinary respiratory immobility of the chest; the ribs (except occasionally for the lowest ones) do not move during respiration, which is almost entirely abdominal.

"Obviously such gross disease of many of the principal joints will lead to functional disabilities. In order to stand, the patients are forced to resort to a trick—they keep their knees in some flexion. Indeed, without this expedient, the trunk, leaning noticeably forwards as a result of the fixed, flexed hips, would bowl the patient over and make him incapable of keeping his balance. The flexion of the knee joint remedies this and compensates for the hip flexion. The occurrence of flexion at the two principal joints of the lower limbs has the result that these patients, on standing, resemble a letter Z. When they have to remain in this position for some time they are forced to make use of a stick, or else to lean forward with the hands resting on the front of the thighs.

"In bed they cannot lie as they would like, for if they lay flat on their back in bed the fixed flexed spine would tend to lift up the pelvis and lower limbs. The only position in which one patient can get to sleep is on his side; another has constructed above his bed an iron bracket to which a sling is attached—this passes under his occiput, holding his head and shoulders well above the level of the bed, on which his lower limbs are resting.

"As for walking: this too has a peculiar appearance because the hip joints are not functional. Progress forwards depends on movements at the knee and ankle joints. The patients look like wooden dolls, in which the leg movements occur about one transverse axis through the two knees. Though it is possible for them to walk unaided, they prefer to use two sticks or crutches because it is both difficult and painful.

"It would be foolish to lay down any rules concerning the aetiology and natural history of the disease as we have seen only a small number of cases. However some points may be made at this stage.

"All the cases I have been able to review have been men—is this simply a coincidence?

"It is a disease which begins in early adult life, though it can begin in adolescence."

OSTEOTOMY OF THE SPINE FOR CORRECTION OF FLEXION DEFORMITY IN RHEUMATOID ARTHRITIS
M.N. SMITH-PETERSEN, CARROLL B. LARSON, and OTTO E. AUFRANC, 1945

"Osteotomy of the Spine is a slightly misleading title for this paper, but it is an intriguing one, effective in stimulating interest and curiosity. The operative procedure is confined to the laminae and articular facets and does not involve the vertebral bodies."

*"**Summary of Recent Progress in Surgery of Rheumatoid Arthritis.** In 1941 the authors were granted the assignment of Operative Procedures for the Prevention and Correction of Deformities in Rheumatoid Arthritis, at the Massachusetts General Hospital.*

*"**Analysis of Development of Flexion Deformity and Its Surgical Correction.** Recumbency in the position of minimum pain commonly results in a flexion deformity of the spine sufficiently marked to interfere with the function of the lower extremities in standing and walking, and to make the sitting position one of strain and discomfort. Manipulation, followed by support, will improve many of these patients; it will not be of benefit after bony ankylosis of the articular facets and calcification of the longitudinal ligaments have occurred. Patients with ankylosis of both hips not infrequently present this latter extreme condition of the spine. After arthroplasties, the flexion deformity of the spine interferes to such an extent with function of the lower extremities that the problem of correction becomes most im-*

portant. Analyzing the obstacles to correction, we came to the conclusion that the ankylosed facets, surrounded by overgrowth of bone, offered more resistance than any of the other spinal structures. Any surgical procedure for correction of the flexion deformity must, therefore, be aimed at the facets, articular processes, and adjacent laminae; osteotomy of these structures, with excision of sufficient bone, should allow corrective leverage to be transmitted to the intervertebral discs and longitudinal ligaments, overcoming whatever resistance these may present.

"Preceding the first operation, a diagram was made and the operative steps were outlined. It is rare that a surgeon is able to carry out a preconceived plan of operation, but in this case that was true; furthermore, the operation is even now essentially the same. Only six cases have been done; further experience may, and probably will, bring about improvement in the operative technique.

"The lumbar region is more favorable than the thoracic, since the latter commonly presents ankylosed costovertebral joints rendering correction difficult, if not impossible. Thoracic osteotomy has been done in only one case; it resulted in subjective improvement, but there was no objective evidence of it.

"Selection of the lumbar level or levels at which the osteotomy is to be performed depends on the roentgenographic findings; the less marked the ossification, the better the chance of correction.

"1. The operative procedure must not be belittled; there are many points in the technique that we have found difficult.
"2. Osteotomy of the spine, performed in a small series of six cases, has yielded satisfactory results."

Rheumatoid Arthritis

Guillaume de Baillou (1538–1616) was the first to use the word rheumatism in the modern sense in 1642. *"The joints are wracked with pain. Those who suffer two or three times from rheumatism can scarcely hope to escape chronic arthritis."*

Jean-Baptiste Bouillaud (1796–1881) in 1836 published a book, *New Research on Articular Rheumatism.*

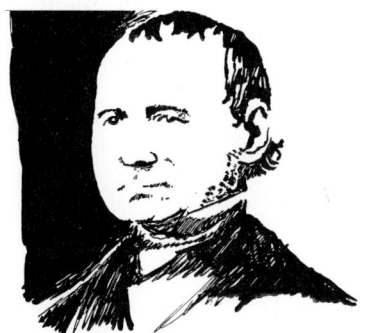

♦ Jean Baptiste Bouillaud

♦ Guillaume de Baillou

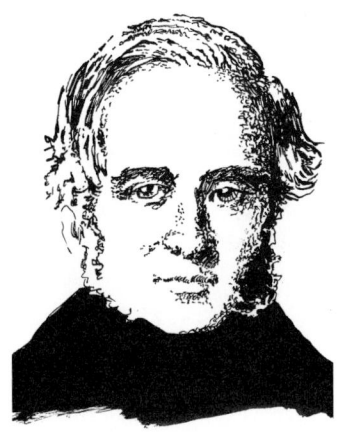

◆ Robert Adams (1791–1875)

ON CHRONIC RHEUMATIC ARTHRITIS
ROBERT ADAMS, 1857

"Those of the lower order who are thus afflicted with this as a general constitutional disease soon become incapable of earning their bread, and most of such in this country are consequently at last found inmates of our Poor-houses. In these asylums they usually spend much of their time during the winter months in their beds, and even here complain much of the cold. From want of exercise, the circulation of blood through their limbs becomes languid; the joints become rigid as well as painful; the surrounding muscles, through disuse, fan into a state of atrophy. The bones and the cartilages also degenerate, and in some cases, from constant immobility of the joints for years, we have found the articular surfaces to have in points coalesced with each other, and in these points of contact a species of red vascular union of the surfaces to have taken place (see case of M'Garry). When all the joints of the lower extremities are the seat of the disease, the patient frequently becomes altogether bedridden, and the knee-joints and those of the feet become distorted, and even dislocated. The former joints are habitually kept semiflexed, the leg becomes rotated out-wards, and under these circumstances we have known partial luxations of the patella occur. The patient usually becomes much stooped in his figure, the spinal column being flexed forward. The neck often becomes rigid, and this state of things, too, is sometimes found associated with a rigid condition of all the joints, great and small, of the upper extremities. Now, the patient, although he has laid before him food convenient for him, soon becomes really incapable of feeding himself, and thus in a certain sense becomes wholly dependent on others. I have observed many unhappy victims of this disease, the inmates of Poor-houses, who, had they been placed in more favourable circumstances as to fuel and clothing, might have lived for years with this malady, carried off unexpectedly during the winter months by sudden attacks of other diseases, such as dysentery or diarrhoea, produced by cold. Some have died of acute inflammations of some of the viscera; others of chronic phthisis.

"Those who are placed in better circumstances, who can provide themselves with the comforts and conveniences of life, who can clothe themselves warmly, and who, although unable to walk, can be daily furnished with the means of taking, exercise in the open air—these, so far as my observation goes, seem to live as long as any of those of the same period of life who are free from the disease."

Title page of Adams' book.

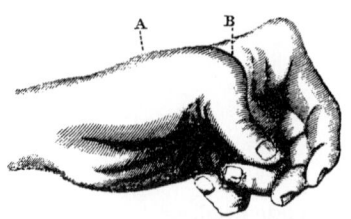

A hand affected by rheumatoid arthritis, from Robert Adams' *Treatise*, 1857.

Still's Disease

Today juvenile arthritis is subdivided into several forms—polyarticular, pauciarticular, and this condition.

ON A FORM OF CHRONIC JOINT DISEASE IN CHILDREN

GEORGE F. STILL, Medical Registrar and Pathologist to the Hospital for Sick Children, London, 1897

"The occasional occurrence in children of a disease closely resembling the rheumatoid arthritis of adults has been recognised for several years. The identity of the disease seen in children with that in adults has never, so far as I am aware, been called in question.

"The purpose of the present paper is to show that although the disease known as rheumatoid arthritis in adults does undoubtedly occur in children, the disease which has most commonly been called rheumatoid arthritis in children differs both in its clinical aspect and in its morbid anatomy from the rheumatoid arthritis of adults.

"The cases hitherto grouped together as rheumatoid arthritis in children include, therefore, more than one disease; and it will be shown that there are at least three distinct joint affections which have thus been included under the one head, Rheumatoid arthritis.

"The paper is based on a study of 22 cases, almost all of which have been in the Hospital for Sick Children, Great Ormond Street. Nineteen of these I have had under personal observation.

"The disease may be defined as a chronic progressive enlargement of joints, associated with general enlargement of glands and enlargement of spleen.

"The onset is almost always before the second dentition; ten out of twelve cases began before the age of six years, and of these, eight began within the first three years of life; the earliest was at fifteen months. Girls are more commonly affected than boys.

"The onset is usually insidious; the child, if old enough, complains of stiffness in one or more joints, which slowly become enlarged, and subsequently other joints become affected; but occasionally the onset is acute, with pyrexia and, it may be, with rigors.

"I wish to lay some stress on the character of the enlargement of the joints. It feels and looks more like general thickening of the tissues round the joint than a bony enlargement, and is correspondingly smooth and fusiform, with none of the bony irregularity of the rheumatoid arthritis of adults.

"The absence of osteophytic growth and of anything like bony lipping, even after years have elapsed since the outset, is striking.

"There is, I believe, never any bony grating, although creaking, probably either of tendon or of cartilage, is frequently present. There is no redness or tenderness of the joints, except in very acute cases. The absence of pain is generally striking, but it

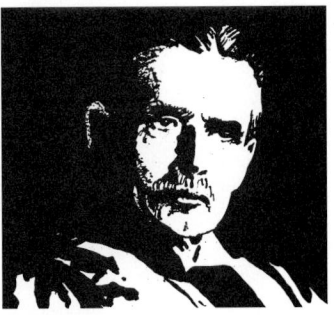

◆ **Sir George Still (1868–1941)**

Still was born at Holloway, the son of a surveyor of Customs, and after taking a first in Classics at Cambridge, he trained at Guy's Hospital. He went to work at the Hospital for Sick Children and remained there all his life—one of Britain's first full time pediatricians.

He quickly became successful because of two good pieces of work written while he was young: he described the disease known after him, and he recognized an organism of meningitis. He became the children's physician of his age. Outwardly he was industrious, distant, and impersonal in his dealings with adults; with children he was relaxed and placating. In addition to writing a standard textbook, he wrote a scholarly *Anthology of Paediatrics,* in which he reviewed the history of child care.

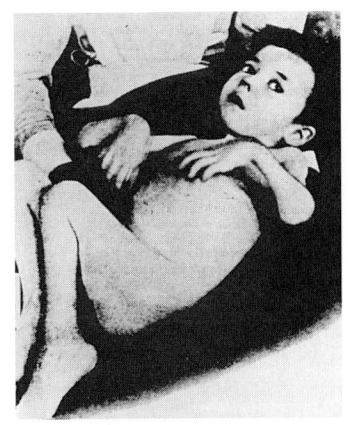

Still's disease from his article.

may be present in slight degree, especially on movement. Limitation of movement, chiefly of extension, is almost always present; the child may be completely bedridden owing to more or less rigid flexion of joints.

"Those most common so far as I have seen are, flexion of the wrist with slight deviation of the hand to the ulnar side, and slight flexion of the proximal, combined sometimes with slight flexion of the distal, interphalangeal joint.

"The joints earliest affected were usually the knees, wrists and those of the cervical spine; the subsequent order of affection being ankles, elbows and fingers. The sternoclavicular joint was affected in two out of twelve cases; the temporo-maxillary in three. The affection is symmetrical. There is no tendency to suppuration nor to bony ankylosis. The muscles which move the diseased joints show early and marked wasting, which contrasts often strongly with the good nutrition of the rest of the body.

"Perhaps the most distinctive feature in these cases is the affection of the lymphatic glands. The enlargement is general, but affects primarily and chiefly those related to the joints affected. The glands are separate, rather hard than soft, not tender, and show no tendency to break down. They may become so large as to be visible, but more often do not become larger than a hazel-nut. The enlargement seems to bear a definite relation to the progress of the disease in the joints. Slight affection of the glands is found very soon after the first symptoms of the joint affection, and as the latter increases the glands become larger. If the joint affection subsides, the glands become smaller, increasing again in size if the joints become worse.

"It will thus be seen that the enlargement is general; and I may add that it is constant; it was found in all the twelve cases mentioned.

"Enlargement of the spleen is also a striking feature of these cases. It is, of course, not always easy to be certain of splenic enlargement, but it was definite and considerable in nine out of twelve cases, the edge of the spleen being felt one to two fingers' breadth below the costal margin. The enlargement of the spleen seems to be roughly proportionate to that of the glands, and like that of the glands has been observed to increase as the joint condition became worse.

"A remarkable feature in these cases is the general arrest of development that occurs when the disease begins before the second dentition. A child of twelve and a half years would easily have been mistaken for six or seven years, while another of four years looked more like two and a half or three years.

"The arrest is, however, of bodily rather than of mental development, and hence although backward in some respects from the enforced absence from school, the child often appears by comparison with its size to be rather precocious than backward.

"The course of these cases is slow. Improvement may occur for a time under treatment or spontaneously, but the disease soon progresses again until a condition of general joint disease is reached which seems to be permanently stationary.

"The morbid anatomy of this disease is gathered from three postmortems. The joints show marked thickening of the capsule and of the connective tissue just outside this. There is also thickening and vascularisation of the synovial membrane, and fibrous adhesions are sometimes present.

"The cartilage may be perfectly normal, as in two cases that had lasted nearly one and a half years; but in a case that had lasted three years it showed pitting of its surface as if from pressure, with little processes of the thickened synovial membrane fitting accurately into the pits, which were situated chiefly at the margin of the cartilage; otherwise, however, the cartilage was healthy—there was no fibrillation, no osteophytic change, no exposure or eburnation of bone.

"In each case the pericardium was universally adherent; there were also pleural adhesions.

"This disease has hitherto been called rheumatoid arthritis, but it differs from the disease in adults, clinically in the absence of bony change, even when the disease is advanced, and in the enlargement of glands and spleen, and pathologically in the absence, even in an advanced case, of the cartilage changes which are found quite early in that disease, and also in the absence of osteophytic change."

Hemophilic Arthritis

This odd name—meaning blood loving—was first used in 1828 for a disease known from the early days of circumcision. Royalty made it famous. Queen Victoria was a carrier; her daughter married Tsar Nicholas of Russia and their son Alexis, born in 1904, was affected. Movies and books have told his story. He had repeated, painful joint bleeds. When Nicholas should have been attending to social injustice in Russia, he was under the shadow of Alexis, his

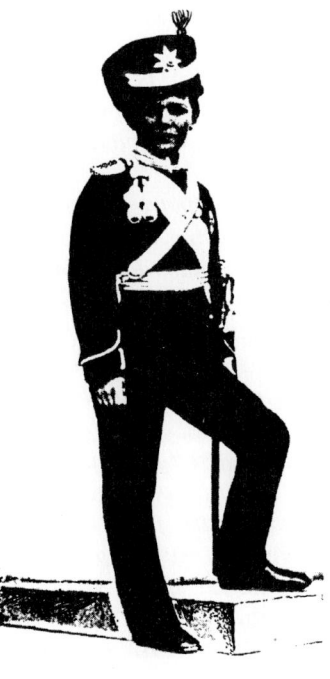

Tsarevich Alexis, aged 10. The photographer has cleverly disguised his severe hip and knee flexion contractures due to hemophilic arthropathy.

wife, and the awful Rasputin. Hemophilia impaired mediation and was one of the causes of the Russian Revolution. There was no treatment. The mechanism of blood clotting was unknown. The understanding of the clotting defect has been accumulating in the past 50 years. All kinds of compounds were tried at first, and factor VIII dates from the 1950s.

Neuropathic Joints

JEAN-MARTIN CHARCOT
1868

"I desire, at present, to insist upon an affection, whose existence I have pointed out, and which I am accustomed to designate, in order to prejudge nothing, by the name of arthropathy of ataxic patients.

"To my mind, and I hope to make you share my way of looking at it, we have here one of the manifold forms of spinal arthropathy. What is spinal arthropathy, some amongst you may ask? I have proposed to designate by this name a whole group of articular affections, which appear to depend directly on certain lesions of the spinal cord. The irritative lesions of the spinal cord, especially those which occupy the grey substance, react sometimes, you are aware, on the periphery, and determine various nutritive disorders, either in the skin or in the deeper parts, such as the muscles. The bones and articulations do not appear to escape this law.

"Ataxic arthropathy is evolved with clinical characteristics, altogether its own, as you will soon see, which cause it to constitute a really distinct disorder.

"I would also add that there is no question here of an extremely rare and exceptional phenomenon. I can show you five examples of these arthropathies in about fifty ataxic patients, whom I know in this refuge. Five cases in fifty, is already a respectable number. Taking my own experience, I have observed this complication of ataxia, perhaps thirty times, in private practice and in hospital.

"A woman aged 49 was admitted to the Salpêtrière on May 1, 1867. She had begun to suffer from symptoms of locomotor ataxy ten years previously, and she had been bedridden for the past four years. She noticed on awakening in the morning of June 9, 1860, that her left shoulder was swollen, the swelling getting progressively less until it reached the wrist. She was not feverish, there was no pain, and she was quite unable to account for the swelling.

"Three days later the swelling had disappeared from the arm and the forearm, but the shoulder still remained larger than normal, and there was marked creaking when the joint moved.

"On June 18, in addition to the general swelling of the shoulder, there was a rounded swelling about the size of an orange situated in front of the joint. It fluctuated, and appeared to be a distended subdeltoid bursa. The creaking in the joint was

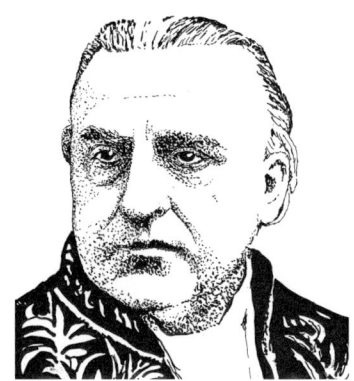

◆ Jean-Martin Charcot (1825–1893).

Charcot was the son of a Parisian coachbuilder of limited means. Legend has it that Father sent his three sons to school for a year. The son who did best could have higher education, the middle son would be trained for the army, and the son who came bottom would follow his father's footsteps as a coachbuilder.

Jean-Martin came top and graduated in medicine. While working as an intern at the Salpêtrière, he wrote a thesis in which he distinguished between gout and rheumatoid arthritis for the first time. He spent the rest of his life at the Salpêtrière, becoming, in 1882, the first professor of nervous diseases in the world. He was world famous in his own day largely because of the splendid demonstrations and lectures that he devised. He was one of the first to break away from the tradition of bedside teaching. He gave a lecture in a hall, well lighted and equipped with a magic lantern, and brought the patients to illustrate points in his lecture, which he demonstrated in a most theatrical manner; he started the fashion, which is so well kept up by neurologists today, of imitating any neurologic disturbance, from a minor nerve palsy to grand mal epilepsy.

He wrote a great deal; in his lectures and papers can be found first descriptions of intermittent claudication, disseminated sclerosis, amyotrophic lateral sclerosis, intermittent hepatic fever, neuropathic joint disease, and oddities such as herpes zoster due to compression of the posterior root ganglion.

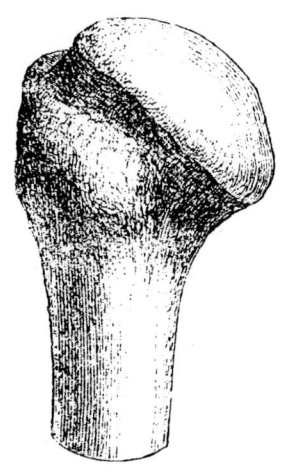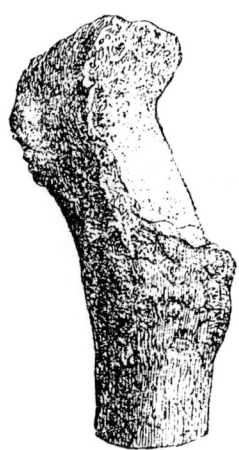

Charcot shoulder joint, 1868.

still more marked. Matters remained in this state until August 2, when the patient was seized with diarrhoea, choleraic in character, of which she died on August 15. The swollen shoulder became much smaller a few days before death.

"A post-mortem examination made on August 16 showed that the capsule of the joint was much thickened, and contained some bony plates in its substance. The synovial membrane was also thickened, and was slightly reddened on its inner surface. The cavity of the joint contained a little transparent yellow fluid, and there were intraarticular loose bodies. The head of the humerus had undergone the remarkable changes [shown in the accompanying figure]. *Although the arthropathy had only lasted nine weeks, a large part of the head of the bone had disappeared as if it had been rubbed away by friction. There was no trace of the articular cartilage, and the globular head was replaced by a flat or slightly concave surface, worn away and roughened in some parts, smooth and eburnated in others. A few small rounded osteophytes surrounded this surface, but they were quite unlike the bony edges which surround and enlarge the joint surfaces in osteoarthritis.*

"The glenoid cavity showed similar changes. The surface was worn away like the head of the humerus, but to a lesser extent. Every trace of articular cartilage had disappeared, and there was no lipping of the bone. The clavicle and acromion were normal in appearance. The posterior columns of the spinal cord showed in a high degree the lesions of grey degeneration with atrophy, more especially in the dorsal and lumbar regions. The cervical cord was affected in the same way, but to a less extent. The posterior nerveroots were clearly atrophied and of a greyish colour. There were slight traces of a posterior spinal meningitis.

"I shall confine myself, gentlemen, to this summary exposition, which suffices, indeed, to make you familiar with the principal aspects of the arthropathy. . . .

"A. To sum up: without appreciable external cause, without blow or fall, apart from any traumatic accident whatever, the

local affection appears. At this moment the incoordination is not yet marked, the patients do not fling about their legs, in a disorderly manner. I must insist on this detail, because it answers an objection made by Herr Volkmann, which has been repeated by other surgeons, who refuse to see, in the arthropathy of ataxic patients, anything else than a traumatic arthritis caused by the mode of locomotion peculiar to these patients. . . .

"F. With respect to the question of frequency, the order of preference begins with the knee, then comes the shoulder, next the elbow, the hips, and the wrists. But the small articulations are not always spared."

Osteoarthritis

Unlike rheumatoid arthritis, osteoarthritis is to be seen in prehistoric skeletons. Osteoarthritis and rheumatoid arthritis were words used interchangeably for many years, and diagnosis did not matter much before there was any treatment. In 1831 Robert Adams started to use the term morbus coxae senilis—not a name that would go down well today—to describe hip osteoarthritis. About the same time, Charcot used arthritis deformans to include both rheumatoid arthritis and osteoarthritis. The word osteoarthritis was first used by Spender in 1889, but he couldn't separate osteoarthritis from rheumatoid arthritis! Not until 1907 did Sir Archibald Garrod get them sorted out.

Colles did an autopsy of a Dr. Percivall who had bilateral osteoarthritis. *"There was flattening of the heads of the bones, the ivory deposit replacing the absorbed cartilage, a similar deposit on the acetabulum: total absence of the ligamentum teres."*

If you look at the proportion of the population who survived into the osteoarthritis age group, you will see why this condition has become important only recently. In the year 1693 the proportion of people who died before 40 years of age was 65%. In 1838 it was 46%, rising in 1900 to 38%, in 1928 to 24%, and now to less than 5%.

Spas

The name spa comes from a town in Belgium, but the Babylonians had spas in 2000 BC just as we have Jacuzzis today. They were good for aching muscles and joints, as well as being good for the skin and for sex. They were fashionable as well. Immersion in water has always been a religious rite. Foul-tasting spa water was drunk to cure all kinds of disease. With so many benefits, spas were very popular. In the United States, catalogues of spas were published; in France, they are a social security benefit still. In Britain, the first hospital specializing in arthritis was the Royal Mineral Water Hospital at Bath, founded in 1742 at the site of the Roman Spa.

Today hydrotherapy still has a role, because water supports the weight of the body and reduces the load on joints so that active movement is easier. Perhaps therapy on the moon will be the next fashion.

Spa Life in Saratoga, 1827

"The pleasure parties and balls every evening in this village engross the attention of the old and young, sick and well, and this village place I fear will prepare more souls for destruction than these efficacious waters will ever heal infirm bodies."

Reference

Chapter references are located in Chapter 26.

◆ Chapter Twelve

Tumors

In ancient times our forebears knew only of malignant tumors. Sarcoma is an ancient term. Pictures of huge, slowly growing tumors adorn old books. Old case reports of ulcerating osteosarcomas describe the kind of patient seen now only in the Third World. Small benign tumors were largely unknown until X-rays revealed them at the turn of the 20th century.

The modern treatment of tumors starts with making an exact diagnosis of the type and extent of the tumor. This did not happen overnight. More than 100 years passed between the beginning of histologic diagnosis and the recognition of many common tumors.

One of the major advances was the development of a tumor registry so that surgeons could agree on a common vocabulary and begin to do statistical studies. Before Ernest A. Codman achieved this in the 1920s, there had been more ego than fact.

Until recently, malignant tumors killed every patient. This led to nihilism about everything—even biopsy. Chemotherapy has enabled patients' lives to be saved, and now all the ingenuity that went into the treatment of benign tumors is now applied to malignant tumors. This includes such forms of salvage surgery as resection and grafting or prosthetic replacement.

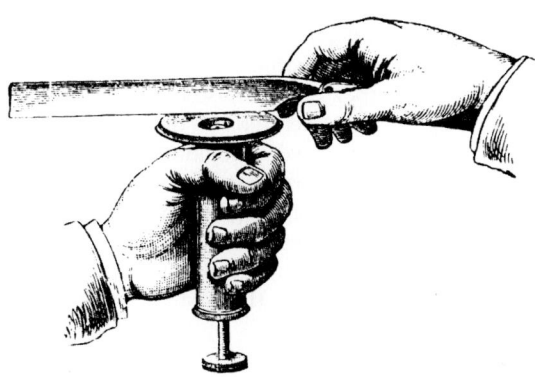

A hand microtome in 1892. The difficulty of cutting and staining sections, especially bone, did not help progress.

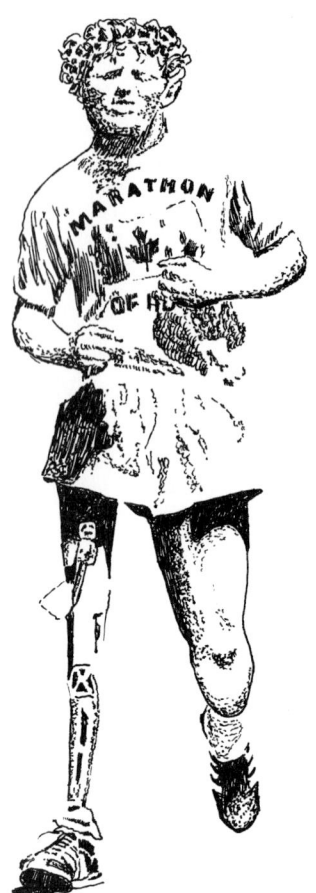

◆ Terry Fox

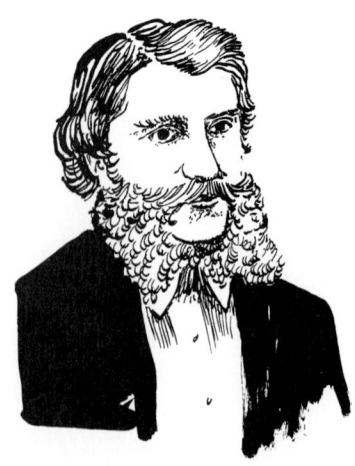

◆ Herman Lebert

Famous Persons

Terry Fox (1958–1981)

Terry was a Canadian teenage athlete studying kinesiology when he was found to have an osteosarcoma in his leg in 1977. He had an above-knee amputation and then decided to run across Canada to raise money for cancer research—The Marathon of Hope, he called it. At first he had little support but, as the run progressed, he became a Canadian folk hero. His run was chronicled on television every night. He started in Newfoundland on April 12, 1980, and his disease caught up with him in Thunder Bay in September after his unique hop and jump had covered 5373 kilometers, averaging 40 kilometers a day. He raised $1.7 million, and this was matched with $27 million from his fans. He soon died, but the Terry Fox Run is now an annual event and a major fundraiser for cancer research.

TIMELINE OF TUMORS

Before 1900

1802 In London, The Society for Investigating the Nature and Cure of Cancer is founded. They circulated questions to drum up interest.

1802 Alexis Boyer divides bone tumors into two species: solid osteosarcoma and blood-containing cystic lesions—spina ventosa.

1804 John Abernethy defines sarcoma as a kind of tumor with a firm and fleshy feel. These solid tumors were distinguished from hollow, hemorrhagic tumors (mostly giant cell tumors, perhaps aneurysmal bone cysts and unicameral bone cysts as well), which had been called spina ventosa or bag of wind. In 1830 in his collected works he wrote, "An Attempt to Form a Classification of Tumors According to Their Anatomical Structure."

1818 Astley Cooper and Benjamin Travers classify bone tumors in a book.

1829 J. C. Récamier distinguishes between primary and secondary bone tumors, coining the word metastasis.

1829–1842 Jean Cruveilhier, a student of Dupuytren, publishes two volumes on pathologic anatomy.

1830 Lister Senior—father of Lord Lister, the inventor of aseptic surgery—invents the achromatic microscope lens for the microscope. This improves resolution enormously and paves the way for histologic diagnosis.

1838 Johannes Müller starts histologic study of tumors.

1845 Herman Lebert advances histologic technology. Until this time sections were cut by hand, and fixation, embedding, and stains were unknown. He used microscopic appearance to classify tumors.

1847 Founding of the journal that came to be known as Virchow's Archives—allowing information sharing.

1845 Paget lectures on pathology.

1847 Dupuytren: studies of osteosarcoma
1854 Louis Marie Michon: synovial tumors
1860 Auguste Nélaton: monograph on giant cell tumor
1863-1867 Rudolf Virchow writes a three-volume book on tumors and writes much on sarcomas.
1869 The medical school at Harvard starts laboratory learning with microscopes, chemistry, and physiology. The basic sciences become a part of education. No longer is it enough to walk the wards.
1876 Morris resects a giant cell tumor from the wrist.
1879 Sam W. Gross published a classic review of 165 sarcomas of long bones—70 were giant cell tumors. This was the first focused review, about 80 pages long.
1892 Bloodgood begins studies on giant cell tumor. This tumor had provided surgeons with a chance to show ingenuity. After curettage, a variety of methods were used to kill the remaining tumor cells—iodoform, cyanide, phenol, and liquid nitrogen. Salvage surgery needed more ingenuity than amputation.

After 1900

1909 Codman's triangle described—a diagnostic sign of osteosarcoma
1920 Broders' grading system; he describes the degree of malignancy.
1920 Codman starts a bone tumor registry to produce uniform nomenclature and define pathologic features.
1921 Because of the poor success of surgical treatment of malignant tumors, William B. Cooley used bacterial toxins and published a book. He started this after observing that an attack of erysipelas had caused an inoperable recurrent sarcoma to disappear.
1921 Ewing's tumor described.
1921 Bloodgood publishes on giant cell tumor.
1931 Codman describes chondroblastoma.
1931 Geschickter and Copeland: book on tumors.
1932 First paper to distinguish giant cell tumor from osteosarcoma—Kirklin
1935 Jaffe describes osteoid osteoma.
1940 Jaffe: eosinophilic granuloma
1941 Jaffe and Lichtenstein: nonossifying fibroma
1941 Jaffe, Lichtenstein, and Sutro: pigmented villonodular synovitis
1952 Lichtenstein: book on tumors
1952 Jaffe describes aneurysmal bone cyst.
1953 Arthur Purdy Stout writes a fascicle on soft tissue tumors for the Armed Forces Institute of Pathology.
1955 Ottolenghi: needle biopsy for the spine
1957 Dahlin at the Mayo Clinic writes a monograph on more than 2000 tumors.
1958 Jaffe publishes a book on bone tumors.
1958 George T. Pack and Irving M. Ariel publish *Tumours of Soft Tissues*. They codified tumors difficult to categorize and emphasized en bloc resection of the compartment.
1980 Enneking: surgical staging
1981 Scaglietti: injection of bone cysts.

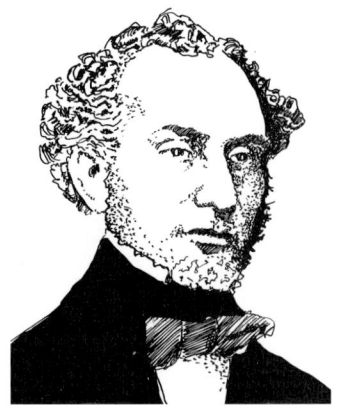

◆ **Sam W. Gross (1837–1889)**

Son of famous Sam D. Gross who was featured in Thomas Eakins' painting "The Gross Clinic." He graduated from Jefferson in Philadelphia, and joined the Union Army in the Civil War. He followed father as professor of surgery at Jefferson. He died of infection; his widow married Sir William Osler.

◆ **Henry J. Jaffe (1896–1979)**

He became pathologist to the Hospital for Joint Diseases, New York, in 1928 and added to our repertoire of diseases. He wrote textbooks and provided a reference service to patients around the world. He described osteoclastoma in 1932, osteoid osteoma in 1935, eosinophilic granuloma in 1940, pigmented villonodular synovitis in 1941, chondroblastoma in 1942, nonossifying fibroma in 1942, chondroid myxofibroma in 1948, and aneurysmal bone cyst in 1952—many with Lichtenstein. (Not to be confused with Norman Jaffe—no relation.)

◆ **Louis Lichtenstein (1906–1977)**

He was pathologist for 12 years at The Hospital for Joint Diseases. He wrote two textbooks and unified histiocytosis X.

A Brief History of Pathology

The ancient Egyptians had a wonderful opportunity to become experts on gross pathology. For 50 centuries bodies were embalmed—the viscera were removed from millions of corpses. It was a potential autopsy for everyone—the key to correlating the clinical state with pathology, but nothing was learned, nothing was written. Think how much we have learned in just one century and multiply the opportunity they had by 50. Remarkable people though they were in many ways, they certainly had an aversion to medical knowledge. A parallel can be found in the thousand-year tradition of bloodletting in Europe. Nothing was learned about the chemistry of the blood or about hypertension until the time the practice came to an end around the end of the 19th century.

The Greeks burned their dead and early Christians considered an autopsy to be sacrilegious, so that no progress was made by them either. All kinds of stray observations were made. But pathology became a recognizable subject only when Faculties of Medicine became enlightened after the French Revolution, and when Lin-

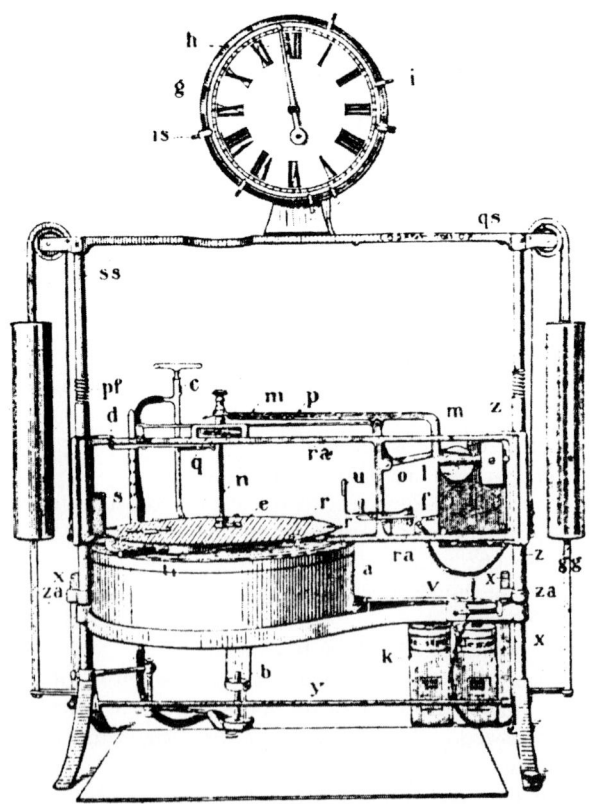

Arendt's automatic tissue processor, 1909.

naeus showed the way to classify biologic material. Many patients died of their diseases in these days, so that it was a golden time to compare the clinical and pathologic appearances.

Although Leeuwenhoek started to look down a microscope and identify cells in 1677 and Johannes Müller wrote a book on the finer structure of tumors in 1838, histologic technique was not advanced enough to be useful. Not until 1858, in Würzburg, Germany, was the cellular theory written by Virchow, which changed pathology forever. The compound microscope was invented by Lister's father in 1830. Tissue sections were cut with freezing microtomes after Benedikt Stilling left a piece of spinal cord by a window in the winter of 1842 and found it easier to section. Bone was decalcified with acid from 1848 onward. Fixation with formaldehyde goes back to Blum in 1893. Paraffin embedding started in 1881. All kinds of colors for staining the tissues were tried in the 1870s and 1880s.

Suddenly, looking down a microscope helped make a diagnosis. Until this time it had been a basic science tool that advanced knowledge but could not be applied to help individual patients. Pathology moved into routine clinical practice.

The phrase "Come in for a biopsy" was first heard around 1870.

The most benefit to orthopaedics has been in the field of tumors, and many benign and malignant forms have been differentiated.

The electron microscope, invented by Canadian James Hillier in 1937, showed a submicroscopic world, and now molecular pathology is the hot interest because of monoclonal antibodies and other techniques.

Broders' Classification, 1920

This is included because it illustrates how a concept that has proved useful for years can start with a simple intuitive, untested idea. Broders was working in the department of surgical pathology at the Mayo Clinic on epitheliomas of the lip.

"In studying these epitheliomas it occurred to me that they should be graded according to differentiation and mitosis, special stress being laid on the former. The grading was made on the basis of 1 to 4, and absolutely independent of the clinical history. If an epithelioma shows a marked tendency to differentiate, that is, if about three quarters of its structure is differentiated epithelium and one fourth undifferentiated, it is graded 1; if the differentiated and undifferentiated area are about equal, it is graded 2; if the undifferentiated epithelium forms about three fourths and the differentiated area about one fourth, it is graded 3; if there is no tendency of the cells to differentiate, it is graded 4. Of course the number of mitotic figures and the number of cells with single, large, deeply staining nucleoli play an important part in the grading."

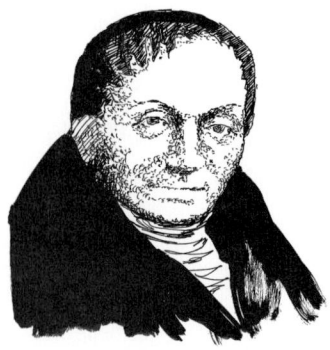

◆ Alexis Boyer (1757–1833)

Title page of Boyer's book.

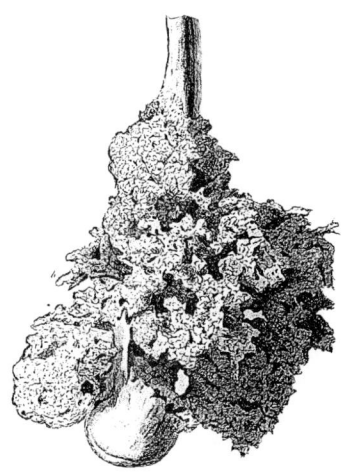

An osteosarcoma. From Boyer, 1804.

Osteosarcoma

Alexis Boyer
1804

Boyer's lectures on bone disease had a chapter on osteosarcoma and distinguished between osteosarcoma and giant cell tumor.

"The first variety, which merits particularly the name of osteosarcoma, which signifies, in itself, the conversion of an osseous substance into flesh: it may be doubted, however, if the name of flesh be properly applied to this substance, which resembles rather a scirrhus of soft parts than flesh, and which presents no mark of organization. The soft parts which surround a bone participate in the disease, which is always announced by very acute pains, and which originates sometimes from an internal disease, and particularly from the cancerous virus; at other times, from an external cause, as a violent contusion; in many cases it can be traced to no cause.

"The second species, named spina ventosa, or poedarthrocace, consists in a swelling of the head or body of a long bone, in such a manner as that its cancelli become very much enlarged. The medullary membrane which lines these cancelli becomes thick, and granulations sprout from it, which destroy by their growth the substance of the bone, so that there only remains an external shell filled with small holes.

The osteosarcoma, of whatever species, is in general a dangerous disease, and often requires amputation of the part."

Codman's Triangle
1909

"The reactive triangles at the bases of osteogenic sarcomas are normal new bone with which nature endeavours to check the progress of the disease. In the macerated specimen, it is seen that this triangle, since it is present at the periphery from all angles, really forms a trumpet-shaped affair which holds the old shaft as a candlestick holds a candle. This collar of bone is constantly being absorbed and renewed at a lower level."

Enneking Staging
1980

In 1959 the American Joint Committee for Cancer Staging and End Result Reporting started work but failed to produce a satisfactory system for musculoskeletal tumors. The system produced by Enneking, based on a huge collection of carefully studied cases, became the accepted method.

"A surgical staging system for musculo-skeletal sarcomas is most logically accomplished by assessment of the surgical grade (G), the local extent (T) and the presence or absence of regional

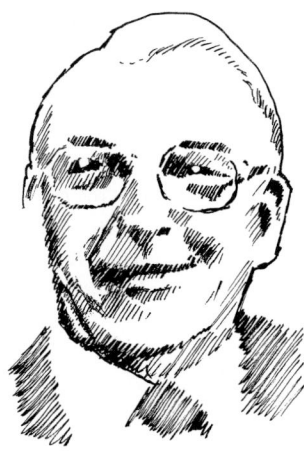

◆ **William Enneking**
Until recently he was the professor at Gainesville, Florida. After training with Hacker, he became a surgeon-pathologist. He built a unit that studied every tumor and used the information for research, a museum, books, instructional courses, and a video disc. Many contemporary tumor surgeons have studied with him.

or distant metastases (M). Neoplasms are divided into two grades: low (G1) and high (G2). The anatomic extent or setting (T) indicates how the surgical procedure is likely to be accomplished or even whether the desired margin can be achieved at all. Therefore the two stages are subdivided by whether the lesion is intracompartmental (A) or extracompartmental (B)."

He defined what was meant by different margins removed during operation and showed that the system correlated well with outcome.

Codman's Register
1920

"In August 1920, the following letter was sent as a circular to every member of the American College of Surgeons:

"Dear Doctor: Have you any living cases of bone sarcoma? Include in this question, recent cases which are now under treatment and also any cases which you may consider as having recovered.

"I have a patient with a sarcoma of the ilium, who is having treatment with radium, and I am most anxious to get in touch with other surgeons who have similar cases, whether of the ilium or of other bones, or whether their treatment is by surgery, by Coley toxins, by radium, or by other agencies.

(He asks for clinical information only because, at this time, biopsy was thought to provoke metastases.)

"We feel that these cases are too rare for each individual clinic to work alone, and that the plan outlined will bring before surgeons in general, in the most rapid possible manner, the facts as they develop.
"E. A. Codman, M.D."

His patient died and proved to have a metastatic lesion in the ilium, but in the meantime he had 454 replies of which only four were cases surviving more than 5 years.

"So it occurred to us to continue this clinical research as a permanent Registry of Bone Sarcomata." And he persuaded the College to fund and promote it. He noted that many surgeons were treating just a few cases and the outcome was unknown. Each case was like an unscientific experiment involving amputation or radium burns. *"The public would be horrified if a laboratory was planning such an aimless and cruel series of experiments by hundreds of different experimenters who were not even intending to record their experiments so that their errors might not be repeated."*

Ewing's Sarcoma

James Ewing (1866–1943)

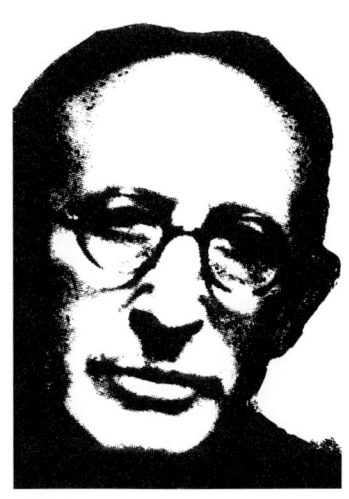

◆ James Ewing

He was born in Pittsburgh on Christmas Day. When he was 14 years old he had osteomyelitis of the femur and spent 2 years in bed. He had a tutor and entered a competition to make the largest number of words from the word Constantinople. He won the prize, a microscope, which shaped the rest of his life. He had a limp and draining sinus all his life. He studied medicine in New York.

His wife died of eclampsia, and Ewing raised his child, never remarrying.

While working in a pathology laboratory at Bellevue, he interested a philanthropist, James Douglas, in tumors, which led to the founding of the Memorial Hospital for the Study of Cancer and Allied Diseases. He was pathologist to the hospital and gained a huge experience that led to his book, *Neoplastic Diseases,* published in 1919.

In 1920 he described the tumor that bears his name. A story circulates in our hospital that our pathologist sent him a slide for confirmation of what he took to be a Ewing sarcoma. Ewing sent it back with a note, "This is not a Ewing sarcoma and I enclose a slide of a typical example." To our pathologist, they looked the same. After some days of thought he soaked the label off the slide he had been sent, put his own label on, and mailed it back to Ewing. It came back with the same note and another slide.

Ewing appeared on the cover of Time magazine January 12, 1931.

DIFFUSE ENDOTHELIOMA OF BONE
EWING'S SARCOMA, 1921

"For some years I have been encountering in material curetted from bone tumors a structure which differed markedly from that of osteogenic sarcoma, was not identical with any known form of myeloma, and which had to be designated by the vague term 'round cell sarcoma' of unknown origin and nature. I had no opportunity of following the course or learning the outcome of these cases, as most of them were treated by amputation of the limb.

"Recently a case came under observation at the Memorial Hospital which revealed that this tumor is highly susceptible to radium, a fact that convinced me that the disease was entirely different from osteogenic sarcoma, which resists treatment by the physical agents.

"The story of this case is briefly as follows:

"A fourteen-year-old girl had been treated by an outside physician in 1918 for nasal discharge and occasional bleeding. Some ocular symptoms led to the suggestion of congenital lues, and a Wassermann reaction being weakly positive, salvarsan was administered. In November, 1918, while pulling on a rope, a spontaneous fracture of the ulna recurred and continued with pain and disability until a well-marked tumor occupied the upper part of the arm. This tumor was noted to fluctuate in size. The veins of the skin were dilated, and the appearance led to the diagnosis of osteogenic sarcoma. Eight injections of Coley's toxins were administered at Mount Sinai Hospital, without notable effect.

"On April twelfth at the Memorial Hospital a radium pack of 12,760 millicurie hours was applied to the arm and followed by two other packs at intervals of two weeks. The tumor began to recede at once and at the end of five weeks no external swelling remained.

"On admission the radiograph showed a peculiar diffuse fading of the upper half of the shaft of the radius, and a faint line from the old fracture. The outline of the slightly swollen shaft was smooth; there was no bone formation, no point of perforation, or area of erosion of the shaft, all of which features told against osteogenic sarcoma. The prompt recession under radium was also quite unlike our experience with osteogenic sarcoma. With the recession of the tumor the shaft was well restored and normal function regained. The patient left the hospital with instructions to return weekly for observation, which was continued for several months.

"The patient then came under the care of her original physician who noted persistence of the nasal and ocular symptoms and regarding the tumor of the radius as luetic, he instituted vigorous treatment by salvarsan. The injections, however, were followed by severe toxic symptoms, vomiting, bloody urine, collapse, and progressive anemia. Later injections of cacodylate of sodium were administered for the anemia. The patient failed steadily and the tumor of the arm began to reappear. There was now an irregular fever up to 103 °F. The urine failed to show Bence Jones protein.

"In October 1920, the patient returned to the Memorial Hospital with a definite recurrence of the tumor, and owing to the conflict of opinion, a portion of tissue was removed for diagnosis. It proved to be a round cell growth of the abovementioned type. Other tumors had now appeared plainly in the skull. There was exophthalmos. The eye grounds showed choked disc and nerve atrophy. The radiograph of the lungs was negative. Anemia and cachexia progressed rapidly and death occurred on December 23, 1920. The total duration was about thirty months.

"During the past four months I have seen six other cases of this disease. They occurred in subjects from fourteen to nineteen years of age. The bones affected were tibia, ulna, ischium, parietal, and scapula. The tumors grew rather slowly, requiring some months to attract attention, but they were accompanied by attacks of pain and disability.

"The radiographs gave characteristic features on which a diagnosis may be based with considerable certainty. A large portion or the whole of the shaft is involved, but the ends are generally spared, contrary to the rule with osteogenic sarcoma. The shaft is slightly widened, but the main alteration is a gradual diffuse fading of the bone structure. Bone production has been entirely absent. Some of the bones appeared honeycombed. Perforation of the shaft and sharp limitation of the process are wanting. The central excavation with widened bony capsule, as seen in benign giant cell tumors, is missing. The radiograph is therefore rather specific.

"Under radium treatment the tumor recedes and the shaft gradually becomes well defined with little deformity and no eccentric bone formation.

"In seven cases the tissue was examined microscopically, and in all the structure was nearly identical. The growth was composed of broad sheets of small polyhedral cells with pale cytoplasm, small hyperchromatic nuclei, well-defined cell borders, and complete absence of intercellular material. Hydropic degeneration often affects large islands of cells, in which only nuclei and cell borders are visible. Necrosis occurred after radium applications. There is very little desmoplastic quality, but the tumor cells readily infiltrate muscle and pass along the fasciae. In none were pulmonary or other forms of metastases observed. In the case cited the tumors of the skull were regarded as primary and of long standing. In some sections the cells were of increased size, while in others they were smaller and more compact, and approached the morphology of plasma cells. However, no definite areas of plasma cells have been seen in any case.

"The probable endothelial nature of the tumor was suggested by the form of the cells, and especially by the appearance in broad sheets of polyhedral cells without intervening stroma. This origin, however, did not seem to be fully supported until I encountered sections in one case in which the cells were found to line a complex series of fine channels enclosing intact blood. Here the endothelial character of the cells was quite pronounced, but they were much smaller than those occurring in angioendothelioma, with which this tumor is doubtless closely related. In other portions of the same growth the cells appeared in diffuse sheets without capillary lumina, as seen in other tumors of the series.

"The exact point of origin of the growth is not clear, but the early rarefaction of the bone indicates that the disease begins in the blood vessels of the bone tissue. Yet an involvement, simultaneous or early, of the vessels of the bone marrow cannot be excluded. In the discussions of multiple endothelioma in the literature some authors thought they could trace the origin to the vessels, blood or lymph, of the periosteum. Many multiple endotheliomas, as in Marckwald's case, have appeared well within the bone marrow.

"The designation of the tumor as endothelioma rather than as myeloma seems advisable, since myeloma is properly reserved for tumors derived from the specific cells of bone marrow.

"The main point of the present communication lies in the demonstration that there is a rather common tumor occurring in young subjects, commonly identified with osteogenic sarcoma, and usually called round cell sarcoma, which is really of endothelial origin, and which is marked by such peculiar gross anatomical, clinical, and therapeutic features as to constitute a specific neoplastic disease of bone."

Giant Cell Tumor

Joseph Bloodgood
1912

Bloodgood noticed that there was something different about patients with giant cell tumor. When he wrote to them in a follow-up study, *"Practically all of these patients answered the letters. Most of the other cases of bone sarcoma had died of the disease. . . . I have been able to study pretty carefully 52 cases. . ."*

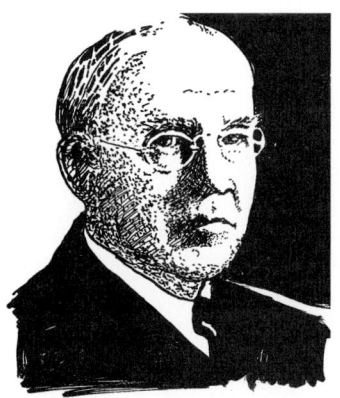

◆ **Joseph Bloodgood (1867–1935)**
Surgeon at Johns Hopkins and Director of surgical pathology.

"*In conclusion we may emphasize the following points:*

"*1. Up to the present time we have no proof that the pure giant-cell sarcoma ever metastasizes. It is a question, therefore, whether it should be called a sarcoma.*
"*2. Conservative treatment is justifiable. Curetting should, in some localizations of the tumor, be the operation of choice. But in those localizations where resection in continuity does not interfere with function, resection becomes the operation of choice; for example, upper end of fibula, lower end of ulna.*
"*3. It is justifiable to attempt curetting to preserve function, even when conditions suggest a great probability of recurrence. There is no position where curetting is not justifiable as a first attempt. It has succeeded when the entire lower end of the femur was involved.*
"*4. Among 26 cases subjected to curetting there were five recurrences: one has remained well after a second curetting; three after resection; and one after an amputation. I am confident that the number of successful cases of curetting will depend chiefly on the number of attempts.*
"*5. Twenty-two cases were subjected to primary resection: one recurred and was cured by amputation.*
"*6. As I found only five cases in the literature of giant cell sarcoma subjected to primary amputation, and there*

are nine in my own list, one can feel pretty certain that many of these cases are not reported, except in statistical studies from large clinics.

"7. After curetting or resection, the wound should be disinfected with pure carbolic acid followed by alcohol or chloride of zinc solution. The operation should always be done, if possible, under an Esmarch.

"This procedure is not indicated because of the malignancy of the giant-cell tumor, but because in curetting we leave cells and disseminate cells, while in resection we may inadvertently cut into the tumor. There is apparently no danger in recurrences, except that they subject the patient to a second operation and perhaps more mutilation.

"8. It is not necessary to perform the bone transplantation at the primary operation unless a single bone like the humerus or femur is divided in its continuity. In simple cases there is no reason why the transplantation should not be performed at the same time, but in some cases the resection may be tedious and bloody, and the patient may not be in good condition. In such cases it will be safer to transplant at a second operation.

"9. I think I am the first to recommend and to practise direct transplantation into the bone cavity after curetting. I am sure that this procedure will grow in value and importance as we attempt curetting more frequently.

"10. My experience teaches me that it is simpler, when possible, to get the bone for filling the defect by splitting the bone which has been resected. This can be accomplished through a single wound. When this cannot be done on account of the large defect, one can remove the upper third of the fibula without injury to the function of the limb, or chisel large pieces from the tibia without destroying the continuity of the bone.

"11. In every case in which the X-ray shows a medullary shadow the urine should be examined for Bence Jones bodies; the latter indicate the presence of a multiple myeloma, or metastatic carcinoma.

"12. I should caution against the surgeon making a positive diagnosis of either a bone cyst or a giant-cell sarcoma. The more X-rays I see, the less confidence I have in my ability to make a differential diagnosis, except in the later stages.

"13. The positive diagnosis must be made at the exploratory incision. The bone cyst as a rule can be recognized by its blood-stained contents; the giant-cell sarcoma by its red, vascular tissue, which looks like granulation tissue. But the giant-cell tumor often has white areas of ostitis fibrosa and the ostitis fibrosa often red giant-cell areas. The two are often mixed. One tissue, however, predominates. The less experienced surgeon should always aid himself with a frozen section."

Chondroblastoma, 1931

Codman was the first to describe this tumor. His first case had been published as a sarcoma, then as a giant cell tumor, and it was even reported as a benign tumor. Several eminent pathologists flip-flopped. Such was the state of diagnosis. He looked after none of these nine patients himself—they were all from the registry he started. Their similarity was evidence for the recognition of a new species of bone tumor. It was a fruit of his tumor registry.

Treatment of Tumors

At first malignant tumors were treated by amputation or local resection; the results were dismal.

In the 1920s there was a move away from surgery to such an extent that some surgeons avoided even biopsy. Radiation followed by amputation for the survivors had a vogue. Coley's toxin was a primitive attempt at chemotherapy.

Chemotherapy for various cancers started with nitrogen mustard, which had been developed for chemical warfare, but nothing was effective against osteogenic sarcoma. Methotrexate was discovered in 1948 but was ineffective in conventional dosage. Then in 1972 methotrexate with citrovorum rescue was reported by Djerassi for lung tumor patients with success. Norman Jaffe started to use the combination at the Children's Hospital, Boston, in 1971, beginning with children with pulmonary metastases. The good results prompted a trial on patients without visible metastases. The results were published in 1974, and the graph tells the tale. The goal changed from lifesaving to limbsaving.

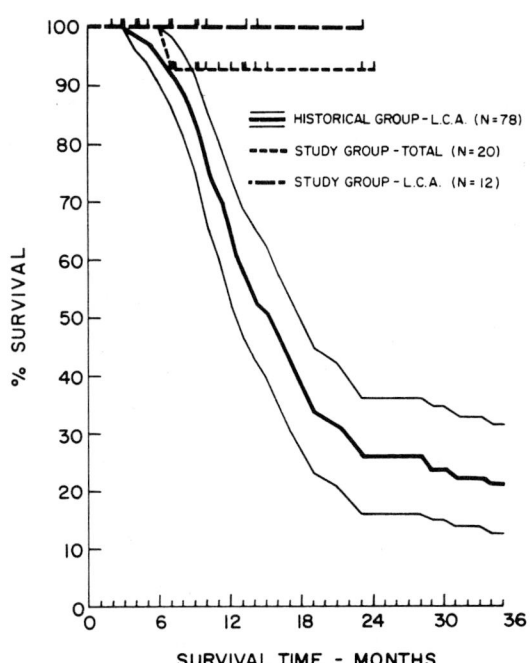

Survival with and without chemotherapy. The beginning of a new era. From Jaffe N, Frei E, Traggis D, Bishop Y: N Engl J Med 1974, 291, 994-997, Fig. 3. Reproduced with permission.

Amputation for Tumor

Obviously, extensive amputations were done mostly for wounds, with a few for infection, and the examples given here were done for tumors. This is not a history of amputations.

Forequarter Amputation

    1838   Philadelphia: George McClellan
    1893   Paul Berger

Hindquarter Amputation

    1895   Charles Girard
    1916   J. H. Pringle
    1940   Gordon Gordon-Taylor

Radiation and Amputation of Survivors

    1940   Albert Ferguson
    1955   Stanford Cade

TIMELINE OF SALVAGE SURGERY

1828 Valentine Mott: clavicle for osteosarcoma—patient died
1876 H. Morris: distal forearm resection for giant cell tumor
1889 Volkmann curetts bone tumors.
1894 Clutton excises giant cell tumor of radius.
1895 J. Mikulicz: excision of the distal femur and fusion of the remaining femur to the tibia
1907 Erich Lexer: transfer of whole joints
1912 Joseph Bloodgood: reconstruction with what remains after excision
1922 F. Saurbruch: "Turn-up-plasty" of tibia after excision of the femur
1928 B. E. Linberg: excision of the scapula
1930 Borggreve: femoral rotationplasty
1936 Albee: bone grafts
1940 Phemister: bone grafts
1943 Moore and Bohlmann: hip prosthesis for giant cell tumor
1950 Cornelius Pieter Van Nes: rotationplasty
1960s Jackson Burrows: massive resections and prosthetic replacement for aggressive tumors
1966 Parrish: bone grafting
1970s Massive allografts: Volkov, Nilsonne, Koskinen, Ottolenghi, Mankin
1974 Marcove: cryosurgery
1977 Enneking: resection arthrodesis of the knee
1977 Taylor: replacement with vascularized fibula
1982 Kotz: rotationplasty for distal femur

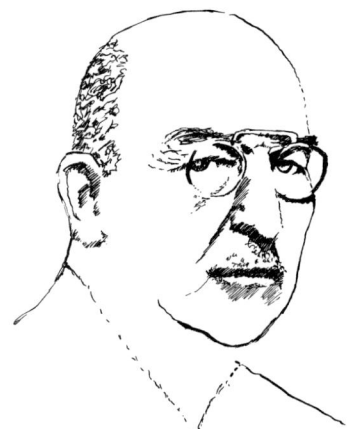

◆ **Erich Lexer (1867–1937)**
He studied in Würzburg and worked in Berlin and Munich. He had many original ideas. He did whole joint transfers.

SALVAGE SURGERY FOR OSTEOSARCOMA

DALLAS PHEMISTER, 1925

"In carefully selected cases, resection of bone sarcoma and repair of the defect with a bone graft is a justifiable procedure

which may save an extremity and carries only slightly more risk to life than does an amputation. . . . A limited percentage of extremities could be saved that are now being sacrificed by amputation."

Conclusions

The methods of operating have really not changed much in 100 years. Limb-saving surgery—developed for benign tumors—is now used for malignant tumors. The big change has been in the repertoire of tumors that have been identified and in the use of chemotherapy. This supports the general contention that the advances that have made a difference have come from outside orthopaedics.

References

Chapter references are located in Chapter 26.

◆ Chapter Thirteen

General Bone Diseases

Bones are like the walls of a house; everything takes shape from the skeleton. Galen

Not so long ago there were more young children with rickets than without. Every child with crooked limbs was thought to have rickets. Until the 1920s, rickets made up a large part of children's orthopaedics. Only after it became known how to prevent rickets in the 1920s were other dysplasias discovered. Then, Sir Thomas Fairbank put together a collection of funny looking radiographs under the title *An Atlas of General Affections of the Skeleton* in 1951; some order was made of chaos. These individually rare, but collectively common, bone dysplasias changed from being curiosities to being a diagnostic and therapeutic challenge. Radiologists led the field in separating them. Advances in biochemistry in the 1960s carried knowledge forward but reached a blank wall until DNA sequencing started the race to identify the gene.

At the other end of life, osteoporosis is a big concern. This was overlooked in the past because people seldom lived long enough to develop it.

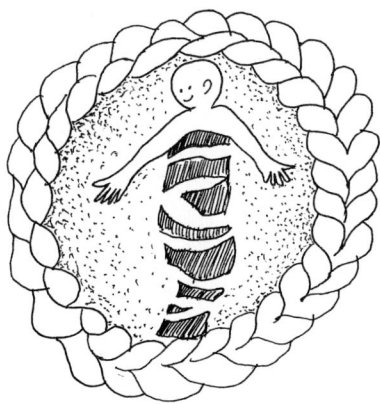

The swaddled child is a common symbol of idyllic childhood. The original piece of art was produced by Luca della Robbia for Brunelleschi's Hospital for Infants in Florence in 1445. Children were swaddled for two reasons—first, to prevent limb deformities due to rickets and second, to stop them from crawling, which was viewed as animal behavior. Only later was swaddling incriminated as a risk factor for hip dislocation. This symbol is going out of favor.

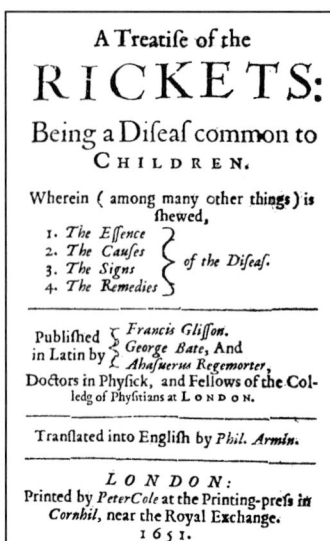

Title page of book of Glisson and associates, 1651.

Levacher's book on rickets, 1772. This is the younger brother of the Levacher who is mentioned in Chapter Six on the cervical spine.

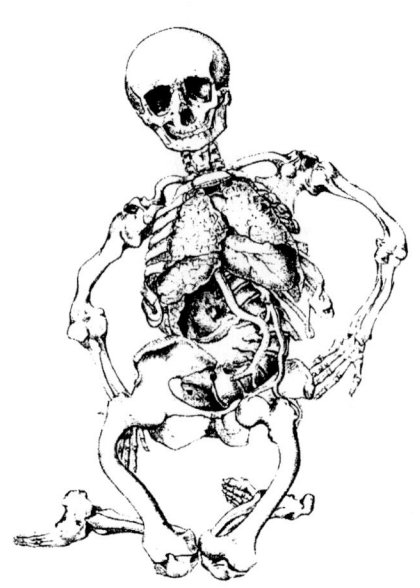

Rickets. Bouvier: 1858

Rickets

During the Industrial Revolution, rickets affected the majority of children. Frequent deformities resulted from the smog that filtered sunlight and a diet with so much bread that calcium and vitamins were inaccessible. Many osteotomies were done. Only in the 1920s did rickets begin to disappear as a result of dietary supplements. Starvation in times of war causes a resurgence. At these times, crooked legs in children spell rickets—hence there should be no surprise that small children with crooked legs are still viewed so seriously by elderly relatives.

Rickets affected more than half the children born before 1920. The deformities in weight-bearing bones were dramatic. From Kirmisson E: Acquired deformities of the locomotor system in infants and adolescents. Paris: 1902.

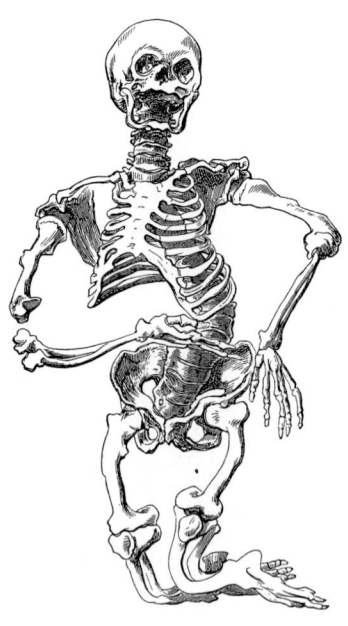

A rachitic skeleton: Humphry

TIME LINE OF RICKETS

- 300 BC — Lu Pu Wei describes crooked legs and hunchback.
- 200 BC — Soranus of Ephesus
- 180 AD — Galen describes rickets.
- 1230 — Bartholomeus Anglicus: *"The limbs of the child may easily and soon bend and take diverse shapes. And therefore children's members and limbs are bound with bandages that they be not crooked or evil shaped."* This was the origin of binding infants, which created the symbol of some old Italian children's hospitals. It also stopped infants from crawling, which was thought to be a throwback to our animal past.
- 1634 — The word rickets was first used in London, Bill of Mortality.
- 1645 — Daniel Whistler; book on rickets provides a clinical description but does not attract the attention of Glisson.
- 1650 — Francis Glisson wrote a book on rickets, calling it rachitis, which is Greek for spine. Rickets is an old word related to the phrase, "He ricked his ankle," meaning to twist or bend and injure it.
- 1669 — John Mayow (1643-1679)—a Brit who wrote a monograph on rickets
- 1696 — The window tax in Britain. Government started taxing properties on the number of windows. The citizenry responded by bricking up windows. Dark, airless houses are thought to have contributed to increased rickets and tuberculosis.
- 1742 — Nicholas Andry writes about rickets but does not add anything useful.
- 1800s — Delpech and Bouvier draw skeletons of rachitic patients.
- 1824 — Schutte: empirical discovery that cod liver oil protects against rickets
- 1883 — Thomas Barlow distinguishes between acute scurvy and acute rickets for the first time. Both produced children with limb pain, inability to walk, and deformity. When X-ray was discovered 12 years later, the distinction became easy.
- 1894 — Bethnal Green study shows a high incidence of tuberculosis, rickets, and scurvy in schoolchildren.
- 1899 — Theodor Escherich in Vienna: 97% of infants aged 9-15 months have rickets.
- 1900 — J.L. Morse finds that 80% of all infants under 2 years have rickets in Boston.
- 1904 — Askanazy: parathyroid tumors cause osteitis fibrosa
- 1908 — L. Findlay produces rickets in puppies raised in the dark.
- 1909 — Schmorl finds at autopsy that 89% of children aged 2 months to 4 years have signs of active or healed rickets.
- 1917 — Alfred Hess and L.J. Unger describe prevention with cod liver oil or by ultraviolet radiation.
- 1921 — Hess notes that 75% of children in New York have rickets.
- 1921 — Sir Edward Mellanby experiments on puppies and produces nutritional rickets.
- 1922 — Vitamin D was identified in fat by McCollum at Johns Hopkins.
- 1925 — Collip identifies parathormone.
- 1949 — McCune: vitamin D-resistant rickets

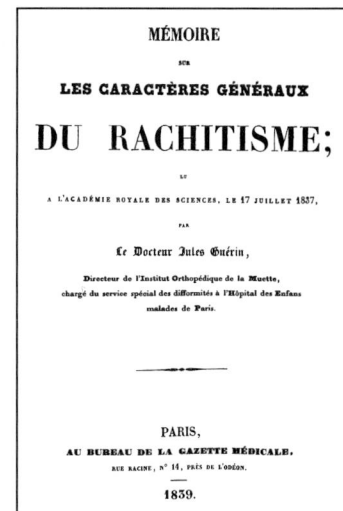

Title page of Guérin's book on rickets, 1839

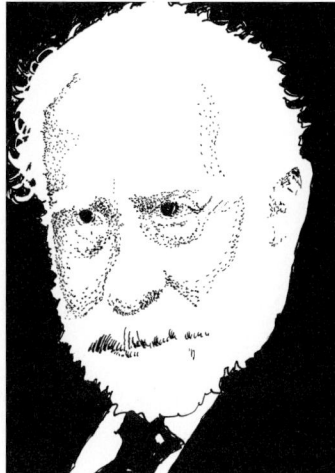

◆ Thomas Barlow (1845–1945)

Born at Lancaster. He studied at University College Hospital, London, England and joined the Staff of Charing Cross and The Hospital for Sick Children, Great Ormond Street, London. Physician to Queen Victoria during her last illness. Lived to be 100. At UCHI was given the Thomas Barlow prize for Medical History—fostering a lifelong interest.

◆ **Daniel Whistler (1619–1684)**

He studied at Merton College, Oxford, and took his medical degree in Holland at Leyden. His thesis was on rickets. He became a president of the Royal College of Physicians in London, a founder of the Royal Society, and a friend of Pepys. Something bad happened and he died in debt and was buried secretly for fear his creditors would seize his body.

Daniel Whistler qualified at Leyden in 1645 with a thesis entitled, *The Disease of English Children Called in the Vernacular—Rickets.* These are some of the features he describes.

"1. Distension of the abdomen
2. The epiphyses at the joints are massive and large out of proportion to the age
3. Knotty swellings also grow out on the sides of the chest where the cartilaginous parts join the bony
4. The whole bony system is in truth flexible, like wax that is rather liquid, so that the flabby and toneless legs scarcely sustain the weight of the superimposed body, so that the tibiae yield to the weight and become bent; for the same reason the thighs above are curved and the back, through the bending of the spine, projects hump-fashion in the lumbar region."

Francis Glisson wrote in 1650 that if rickets begins in the first year, the children walk late: "*They speak before they walk, which amongst us English men, is vulgarly held to be a bad omen.*" His account is too long and rambling to print here.

Surgical Treatment of Rickets Deformity

Closed osteoclasis was never very popular because the bone did not break as intended. Fierce machines—osteoclasts—were invented, perhaps by the same folk who invented cranioclasts for obstetricians. They would break the bone without opening the skin, avoiding the risks of infection.

Open osteotomy arrived with anesthesia but carried a death rate due to infection. Only after Lister did it become popular. Then some surgeons did a vertical femoral intercondylar osteotomy, before a transverse metaphyseal osteotomy became the accepted technique. In 1875 Volkmann describes two osteotomies using the aseptic system of Lister, and by 1880 Macewen had enough experience to write a book about osteotomy.

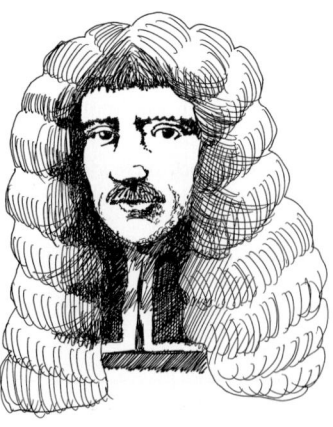

◆ **Francis Glisson (1597–1677)**

Born in Dorset, educated at Oxford and Cambridge, he became professor of physic at Cambridge, founder and member of the Royal Society. An anatomist, he described Glisson's capsule, which is in liver. Described rickets from autopsy findings.

Vitamin C Deficiency

Scurvy was a brake on exploration. Sea voyages that lasted longer than a person's stores of vitamin C—about 3 weeks—killed many sailors until lime juice was used to protect against scurvy. Only after lime juice was introduced did intercontinental passenger traffic become safer.

> **TIMELINE OF SCURVY**
> 1753 James Lind: *A Treatise on Scurvy* (book)
> 1898 Report of the American Pediatric Society on scurvy
> 1928 Ascorbic acid synthesized by Albert Szent-Gyorgi
> 1933 Leonard G. Parsons uses ascorbic acid with success for a child at Birmingham Children's Hospital.

Jacques de Vitry was born near Paris; he became a priest and went to the Orient during the Crusades. He died in 1244. He wrote about scurvy in his history of the Crusades.

"A large number of the men in our army were attacked also by a certain pestilence, against which the doctors could not find any remedy in their art. A sudden pain seized the feet and the legs: immediately afterwards the gums and teeth were attacked by a sort of gangrene, and the patient could eat no more. Then the bones of the legs became horribly black, and so, after having suffered continued pain, a large number of Christians went to rest on the bosom of the Lord." (The skin changes were purpura.)

King Louis of France became a Saint because of his pursuit of the Crusades. His army fell to scurvy. **Jean, Sire de Joinville** in the 13 century, wrote:

"We were attacked with the army sickness, which was such that our legs shrivelled up and became covered with black spots ... The gums became putrid with sores and no man recovered of that sickness. It was a sure sign of death when the nose began to bleed ... The proud flesh in our men's mouths grew to such excess that the barber-surgeons were obliged to cut it off, to give them a chance of chewing their food or swallowing anything. It was piteous to hear through the camp the shrieks of the people who were being operated for proud flesh, for they shrieked like women in childbirth."

Scurvy in the New World

Jacques Cartier, a Breton explorer, discovered what became the St. Lawrence River and Montreal in 1536. During this voyage his crew developed scurvy, and a cure was found. This is Hakylut's description.

♦ **James Lind (1716–1794)**
He was born in Edinburgh and at age 15 was apprenticed to a surgeon. He joined the Navy as surgeon 8 years later. He saw two severe outbreaks of scurvy; in one there were 80 cases out of 350 sailors. At the naval hospital in the south of England he had up to 100 cases of scurvy under his care at a time. He wrote about the appalling conditions at sea and how they may be improved: *An essay on the most effectual means for preserving the health of Seamen in the Royal Navy, 1757*. He saw many tropical diseases and in 1768 wrote a book on diseases incidental to Europeans in hot climates.

♦ **Julius Moller (1819–1887)**
From Konigsberg in East Prussia. He described acute rickets in 1859, which was in fact scurvy.

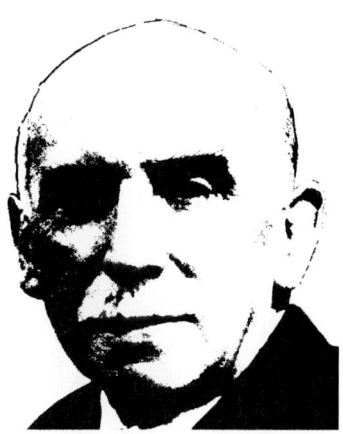

♦ **Leonard Gregory Parsons (1879–   )**

(He describes the hemorrhagic rash and swollen gums.)

"This sickness spread itself in our three ships. Of about 110 persons, there were not more than 10 whole, so that one could not help another.... There were already 8 dead and more than 50 sick and as we thought, past all hope of recovery."

(The Captain did an autopsy of one man ... Then the Captain went ashore and saw a person who recovered after having been very sick with scurvy.)

"He had taken the juice and sap of a certain tree ... ameda or sassafras tree."

(The rest of the crew recovered after taking this remedy.)

"If all the physicians of Montpelier and Lovaine had been there with all the drugs of Alexandria, they would not have done so much in a year as that tree did in six days."

Until Vitamin C was added to diets, long voyages were hazardous.

Paget's Disease of Bone

On a Form of Chronic Inflammation of Bones (Osteitis deformans)

James Paget
1877

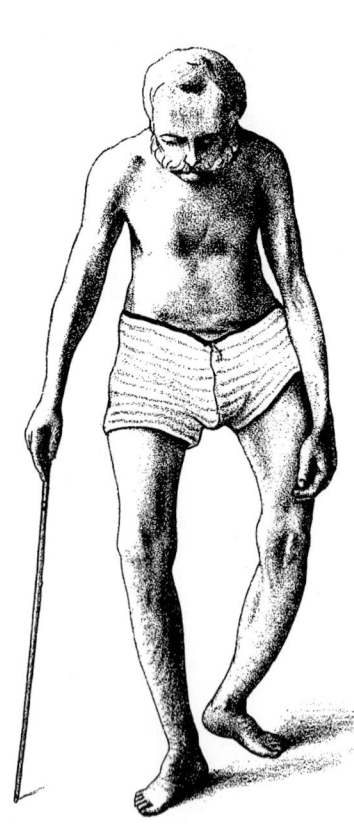

Paget's patient, 1877

"I hope it will be agreeable to the Society if I make known some of the results of a study of a rare disease of bones. The patient on whom I was able to study it was a gentleman of good family, whose parents and grandparents lived to old age with apparently sound health, and among whose relatives no disease was known to have prevailed. Especially, gout and rheumatism, I was told, were not known among them; but one of his sisters died with chronic cancer of the breast.

"Till 1854, when he was forty-six years old, the patient had no sign of disease, either general or local. He was a tall, thin, wellformed man, father of healthy children, very active in both mind and body. He lived very temperately, could digest, as he said, anything, and slept always soundly.

"At forty-six, from no assigned cause, unless it were that he lived in a rather cold and damp place in the North of England, he began to be subject to aching pains in his thighs and legs. They were felt chiefly after active exercise, but were never severe; yet the limbs became less agile or, as he called them "less serviceable", and after about a year he noticed that this left shin was misshapen. His general health, however, was quite unaffected.

"I first saw this gentleman in 1856, when these things had been observed for about two years. Except that he was very grey and looked rather old for his age, he might have been considered as in perfect health. He walked with strength and power, but somewhat stiffly. His left tibia, especially in its lower half, was broad, and felt nodular and uneven, as if not only itself but its periosteum and the integuments over it were thickened. In a

◆ **Sir James Paget (1814–1899)**

Paget bears many similarities to Dupuytren—he had a clinicopathologic approach and recognized several conditions for the first time. His descriptions are so full and accurate that they have not been bettered. He was born in Yarmouth, the son of a brewer and shipowner of varying fortunes. After he had been apprenticed to the local surgeon for four years, he went to St. Bartholomew's Hospital. As a student he discovered that the little calcific deposits in the muscles of cadavers were due to a parasite, later identified as *Trichina spiralis*. His father's money ran out and he could not afford a surgical dressership. He does not seem to have occupied any surgical post until he was elected a consultant in 1847. He was curator of the museum and a demonstrator in morbid anatomy, supplementing his meager income as part-time subeditor of the *London Medical Gazette*. As a result of these difficulties he was not a brilliant operator but rather a sound clinician and a good orator.

"The popularity of Sir James Paget is unbounded. When it is known that he is to address a meeting, the hall in which he is announced to appear is crowded with an earnest, intelligent audience, which realises that it has come to be instructed and pleased, and that its expectations will not be disappointed. His manner of speaking is entirely free from that drawl and hesitation which are so common to many of his countrymen. So great is his reputation for versatility and for the rapid acquisition of knowledge, that it has been said of him, 'Give him six weeks and he will lecture on Oriental languages'."Samuel D. Gross (1805-1884).

In 1851 he was elected to the Royal Society and became president of the Royal College of Surgeons in 1875. He nearly died in 1871 as a result of an infected cut he suffered while carrying out a postmortem—this led to his resignation from Bart's. He was one of the many surgeons who nearly died of infections in the days before antibiotics. The risks were greater for them than AIDS is for us.

Good literary style is seldom found between medical covers: the accompanying excerpt from Paget's first paper on osteitis deformans is an outstanding example of style. He unfolds the narrative as a story.

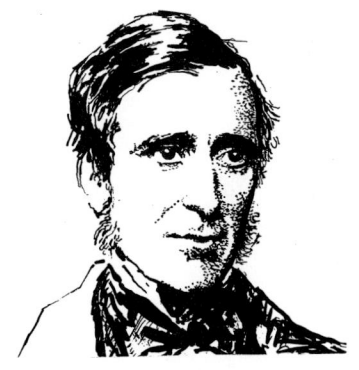

◆ Sir James Paget (1814–1899)

much less degree similar changes could be felt in the lower half of the left femur. This limb was occasionally but never severely painful, and there was no tenderness of pressure. Every function appeared well discharged, except that the urine showed rather frequent deposits of lithates. Regarding the case as one of chronic periostitis, I advised iodide of potassium and Liquor Potassae; but they did no good.

"Three years later I saw the patient with Mr. Stanley. He was in the same good general health, but the left tibia had become larger, and had a well-marked anterior curve, as if lengthened while its ends were held in place by their attachments to the unchanged fibula. The left femur also was now distinctly enlarged, and felt tuberous at the junction of its upper and middle thirds, and was arched forwards and outwards, so that he could not bring the left knee into contact with the right. There was also some appearance of widening of the left side of the pelvis, the nates on this side being flattened and lowered, and the great trochanter projecting nearly half an inch further from the middle line. The left limb was about a quarter of an inch shorter than the right. The patient believed that the right side of his skull was enlarged, for his hats had become too tight but the change was not clearly visible.

"Notwithstanding these progressive changes, the patient suffered very little; he had lived actively, walking, riding, and engaging in all the usual pursuits of a country gentleman, and, except

that his limb was clumsy he might have been indifferent to it. He had taken various medicines, but none had done any good, and iodine, in whatever form, had always done harm. In the next seventeen years of his life I rarely saw him, but the story of his disease, of which I often heard, may be briefly told and with few dates, for its progress was nearly uniform and very slow. The left femur and tibia became larger, heavier, and somewhat more curved. Very slowly those of the right limb followed the same course, till they gained very nearly the same size and shape. The limbs thus became nearly symmetrical in their deformity, the curving of the left being only a little more outward than that of the right. At the same time, or later, the knees became gradually bent, and, as if by rigidity of their fibrous tissues, lost much of their natural range and movement.

"The skull became gradually larger, so that nearly every year, for many years, his hat, and the helmet that he wore as a member of a Yeomanry Corps, needed to be enlarged. In 1844 he wore a shako measuring twenty-two and a half inches inside; in 1876 his hat measured twenty-seven and a quarter inches inside. In its enlargement, however, the head retained its natural shape and, to the last, looked intellectual, though with some exaggeration.

"The changes of shape and size in both the limbs and the head were arrested, or increased only imperceptibly, in the last three or four years of life.

"The spine very slowly became curved and almost rigid. The whole of the cervical vertebrae and the upper dorsal formed a strong posterior, not angular, curve; and an anterior curve, of similar shape, was formed by the lower dorsal and lumbar vertebrae. The length of the spine thus seemed lessened, and from a height of six feet one inch he sank to about five feet nine inches. At the same the chest became contracted, narrow, flattened laterally, deep from before backwards, and the movements of the ribs and of the spine were lessened. There was no complete rigidity, as if by union of bones, but all the movements were very restrained, as if by shortening and rigidity of the fibrous connections of the vertebrae and ribs.

"The shape and habitual posture of the patient were thus made strange and peculiar. His head was advanced and lowered, so that the neck was very short, and the chin, when he held his head at ease, was more than an inch lower than the top of the sternum.

"The short narrow chest suddenly widened into a much shorter and broader abdomen, and the pelvis was wide and low. The arms appeared unnaturally long, and, though the shoulders were very high, the hands hung low down by the thighs and in front of them.

"Altogether, the attitude in standing looked simian, strangely in contrast with the large head and handsome features.

"All changes of shape and attitude are well shown in sketches from photographs taken six months before death. Only the lowering of the necks of the femora is not shown. In measurement after death the axes of the shaft and neck of the right femur

formed an angle of only 100 degrees instead of 120 degrees or 125 degrees, and this change of shape added to the appearance of increased width of the pelvis.

"But with all these changes in shape and mobility of the head, spine, and lower limbs, the upper limbs remained perfect, and there was no disturbance of the general health.

"In 1870, when the disease had existed sixteen years, the left knee joint was, for a time, actively inflamed and its cavity was distended with fluid. But the inflammation soon subsided, only leaving the joint stiffer and more bent.

"About this time some signs of insufficiency of the mitral valve were observed, but the patient now lived so quietly, and moved with so little speed, that this defect gave him no considerable distress.

"In December, 1872, sight was partially destroyed by retinal haemorrhage, first in one eye, then in the other, and at nearly the same time he began to be somewhat deaf. In the summer of 1874 he had frequent cramps in the legs, and neuralgic pains, which were described as 'jumping over all the upper part of the body except the head', but change of air seemed to cure them.

"In January, 1876, he began to complain of pain in his left forearm and elbow which, at first, was thought to be neuralgic. But it grew worse, and swelling appeared about the upper third of the radius and increased rapidly, so that, when I saw him in the middle of February, it seemed certain that a firm medullary or osteoid cancerous growth was forming round the radius.

"An attitude somewhat similar is given by a rare form of what I suppose to be general chronic rheumatoid arthritis of the spine involving its articulations with the ribs. The spine droops and is stiff, the chest is narrow, the ribs scarcely move, the abdomen is low and broad, but there is no deformity of head or limbs.

"Still, the general health was good. Auscultation could detect mitral disease, but the appetite and the digestion were unimpaired, the urine was healthy, the mind as clear, patient, and calm as ever. As letters about him at this time said his general health has been excellent; he is free from pain except in the left arm; he sleeps well, enjoys himself, and does not know what a headache is.

"After this time, however, together with rapid increase of the growth upon the radius, there were gradual failure of strength and emaciation, and on the 24th March, after two days of distress with pleural effusion on the right side, he died."

At autopsy Paget found a malignant tumor of the radius that had metastasized to the lungs and skull.

"The periosteum was not visibly changed, not thicker or more than usually adherent. The outer surface of the walls of the bones was irregularly and finely nodular, as with external deposits or outgrowths of bone, deeply grooved with channels for the large periosteal blood-vessels, finely but visibly perforated in every part for transmission of the enlarged small vessels. Everything

seemed to indicate a greatly increased quantity of blood in the vessels of the bone.

"The medullary structures appeared to the naked eye as little changed as the periosteum. The compact substance of the bones was, in every part, increased in thickness.

"The thickening of the walls of the shafts of the bones appeared due chiefly to outward expansion and some superficial outgrowth. In some places there were faint appearances of separation of parts of the outer layers of the walls, and of these becoming thick and porous, while the corresponding parts of the inner layers were less changed; but in the greater part of the walls the whole construction of the bone was altered into a hard, porous or finely reticulate substance, like very fine coral. In some places, especially in the walls of the femur, there were small, ill-defined patches of pale, dense, and hard bone looking as solid as brick.

"In the compact covering of the articular ends of the long bones, and in those of the neck and great trochanter of the femur, and in the patellae the increase of thickness was due to encroachment on the cancellous texture, as if by filling of its spaces with compact porous, new-formed bone.

"Holding then the disease to be an inflammation of the bones, I would suggest that, for brief reference and for the present, it may be called after its most striking character, osteitis deformans. A better name may be given when more is known of it."

Osteoporosis

Today the commonest generalized bone disease is postmenopausal osteoporosis. This was not recognized for years because of short life expectancy and limited means for estimating bone mass.

The interest toward the end of the 19th century was in rickets and the distinction from hyperparathyroidism, which produced bent bones in young people. Osteomalacia was a problem in the days before contraception, when women had the calcium drain of yearly pregnancies. The words osteoporosis and osteomalacia were used interchangeably until metabolic studies began in the 1930s, when serum calcium and potassium began to be measured. They were normal in osteoporosis, and so the loss of height and the fractures of osteoporosis were thought to be due to aging.

Fuller Albright built up one of the first Metabolic Wards at Massachusetts General Hospital and wrote a classic book in 1948. He pointed out that female sex hormones were responsible for putting the shell on a bird's egg—the reason for the gender predilection of osteoporosis.

"Postmenopausal osteoporosis, although frequently overlooked in treatises on bone diseases, is the commonest of all forms of osteoporosis; indeed it is the commonest of all systemic osteopathies."

Surprisingly, this is one of the first mentions of the condition.

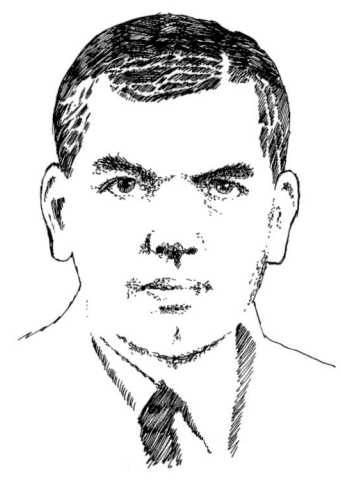

◆ **Fuller Albright (1900–1969)**
He was born in Brookline, Massachusetts, and studied at Harvard. After a residency in internal medicine at Johns Hopkins, he went on to develop a clinical endocrinology unit at Massachusetts General Hospital. He described Albright's syndrome—polyostotic fibrous dysplasia with skin pigmentation and precocious puberty in girls—in 1937. In 1942 came pseudohyperparathyroidism and in 1952, pseudo-pseudohyperparathyroidism. The poor man developed Parkinson's disease in his thirties; he had stereotactic surgery at age 56 and was never the same again.

Skeletal Dysplasias

Fairbank was one of the first to put together this miscellaneous group of conditions. Each condition is rare but together they are common. Although in the past experts frequently disagreed about the diagnosis, with the new molecular approach to disease, diagnosis is more exact, and these conditions have become a window on the control of the body as a chemical factory. Dysplasias have taken on a new interest.

1951	Sir Thomas Fairbank: *An Atlas of General Affections of the Skeleton*
1955	Victor McKusick introduces the term hereditable disorders of connective tissue and changes it to heritable when his book is published in 1956.
1964	Phillip Rubin: Dynamic classification of bone dysplasias. This tried to explain dysplasias using knowledge of bone formation and remodeling.
1966	McKusick: *Mendelian Inheritance in Man*

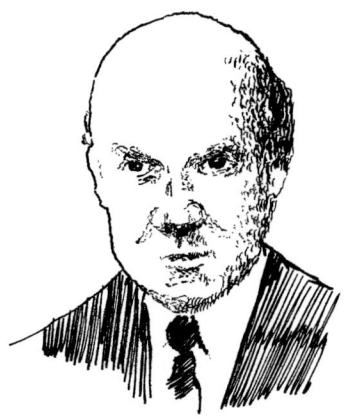

◆ **Sir Thomas Fairbank (1876–1961)**

A London orthopaedic surgeon who worked for Lane and then went to Great Ormond Street. World War I had him on the front line teaching mules to carry packs and teaching surgeons in wound care. It is not clear which was easier. He returned to King's College Hospital and became known for his expertise on dysplasias. He was interested in Erb's palsy and sectioned the subscapularis muscle for subluxations. He excelled at keeping records of interesting cases. His son is an orthopaedic surgeon.

Dyschondroplasia: Ollier's Disease
1899

"M. Ollier described under this name a new type of disease which he has been able to determine by means of clinical observation and radiography. It consists of the irregular formation and development of cartilaginous tissues which have a tendency to delayed ossification.

"This differentiates it from the chondroplasia of Parrot, in which there is atrophy or lack of development of the bone, and brings it closer to multiple osteogenic exostoses.

"The first case observed by M. Ollier in June, 1897, was a little girl of 6 who presented with an inturned forearm and femur, exostoses of the femur of a cartilaginous appearance, and deformities of the fingers, which were shorter, thicker and soft on pressure. Radiography showed a series of irregular spaces that were radiotranslucent and cartilaginous in the diaphyses of the phalanges.

◆ **Louis Ollier (1830–1900)**

Ollier was one of the great men of orthopaedics. He devoted his life to his work; in addition to writing several important clinical papers, he carried out research on normal and pathologic bone growth, considering it not only as a structure but also as a tissue. He was born at Vans in Ardeche and studied at Lyons and Montpellier. At the age of 30 he became senior surgeon at Lyons. In the 1870 war he was a battle surgeon, looking after the wounded of both sides. In 1894 he was decorated with the Order of Knight of the Legion of Honour by the French President. A few hours after the ceremony the President was assassinated and Ollier was called to him, but his injuries were too severe for Ollier to be able to save his life.

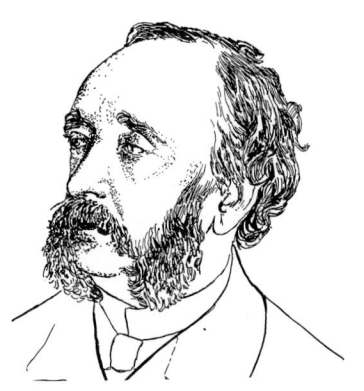

◆ **Louis Ollier (1830–1900)**

"A little later M. Ollier observed an analogous case in a young girl of 9. The femora were curved in; the upper end of the fibula, which was slightly atrophic, carried a mass resembling cartilage. Radiographs of the fingers presented the same abnormal appearance of cartilaginous spaces in the phalanges.

"Since then, M. Destot has seen and radiographed a third case. The disease appeared to have been present for a long time, developing without pain, with a tendency to delayed ossification, and the persistence of the initial deformities. This affection does not resemble osteomalacia, nor rickets, nor the chondromata which have no tendency to ossification. There is a need for further observation to define its place; but it appears to M. Ollier to be a completely new disease entity, which must be given a new name, that of Dyschondroplasia."

In the discussion that followed the presentation of his paper, Ollier put forward the view that the difference between dyschondroplasia and osteogenic exostoses was *"a difference of form and situation, but not of nature."* He hoped that it might eventually be possible to treat the cases by stimulating the cartilage to ossify.

Short Stature

Famous People

People with short stature have always excited unwelcome attention that makes it difficult to live a normal life. Velázquez painted the dwarfs of the Spanish Court, who were confidants because they could not hide. Others could only earn a living in the circus.

General Tom Thumb was one of the most famous. He was born in Bridgeport, Connecticut, in 1832 and was only 27" tall at the age of 13—becoming 40" and weighing 70 pounds as an

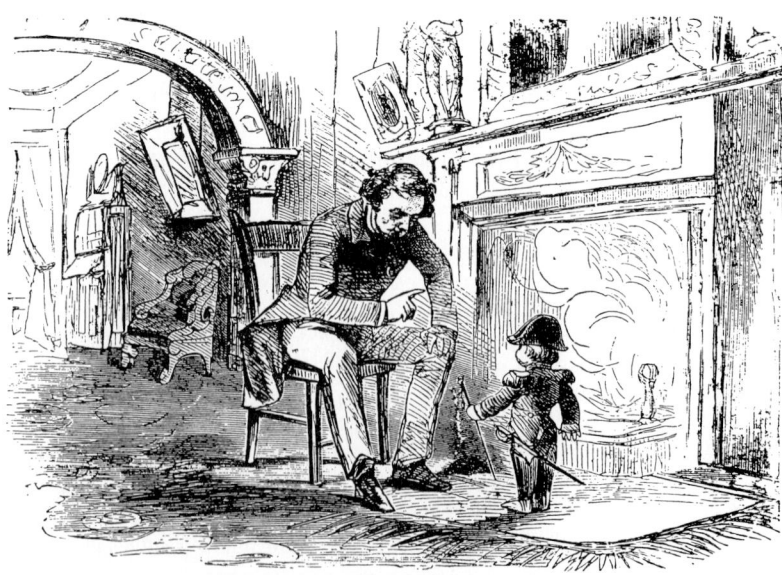

Tom Thumb learning his role as Napoleon, about 1850

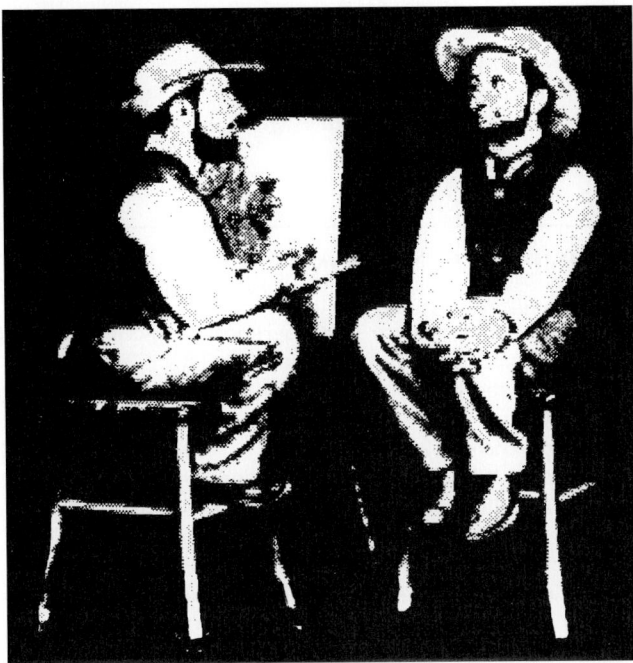

Toulouse-Lautrec had a skeleton dysplasia, causing repeated fractures in childhood and disproportionate stature. The diagnosis is still a matter of argument.

adult. He was a prisoner in his home until Barnum, the exploitive showman, heard of him and gave him a job. He made a fortune by the age of 20 and retired in luxury. He toured the world and met many famous people. He married in a famous wedding held in the biggest church in New York.

What was the strange disease of **Toulouse-Lautrec?** This wonderful painter had multiple fractures in childhood and was of disproportionate short stature. There is talk of checking the DNA of his surviving relatives to make a diagnosis because, like many people with a syndrome, he is not a perfect fit for anything—not even pyknodysostosis, the current favorite.

Syndromes

This comes from the Greek word meaning to run together, or concurrence. If you see one person with some apparently unconnected clinical features, you may be on the way to describing a syndrome. In the past this was called a case report, now it is called an "anecdote." Two people with the same features is "case after case," and three people is a "series." Because it is often difficult to find a single word to describe all the features, the use of someone's name is popular.

If a syndrome is to be remembered, it needs a memorable name. Some alliterate, like Sprengel's shoulder. Some need explaining to every new generation, like the VATER syndrome—"No, it is not anyone's name, the V stands for vertebral," and so on. Some

Title page of Saint-Hilaire's book on experimental teratology. Etienne Geoffroy Saint-Hilaire carried out experiments in development and moved the subject beyond the description of monsters in the 1820s. His son Isidore carried on his work and published the first volume of this three-volume work in 1836 before he was 27 years old.

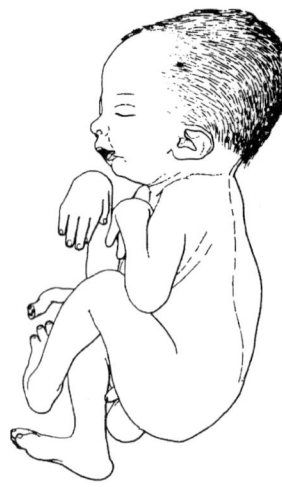

Arthrogryposis: Otto, 1841

have fuzzy edges—like Marfan's syndrome—and can be thrown in as a differential diagnosis quite frequently.

If you really want to give your name to something you can still go for a new syndrome—they are being described more frequently now than in the past.

TIME LINE OF SYNDROMES

- 1733 Jean-Louis Petit—radial club hand
- 1841 Adolph Wilhelm Otto—arthrogryposis, described as a "human wonder with incurved limbs"
- 1841 Poland—absent pectoral muscles, syndactyly, and short middle phalanges
- 1866 Down—trisomy 21
- 1881 Mafucci—hemangioma plus enchondroma
- 1882 Von Recklinghausen—neurofibromatosis. This disease had been described before.
- 1882 Gaucher's disease
- 1896 Marfan—genetic disorder of elastin. There is a lot of confusion about the early descriptions.
- 1899 Ollier—dyschondroplasia or multiple enchondroma
- 1900 Klippel-Trénaunay—hemangioma plus leg length inequality
- 1901 Ehlers-Danlos—collagen disorder producing joint laxity and stretchable skin, and much more
- 1906 Apert—syndactyly and craniostenosis
- 1912 Klippel-Feil—the man without a neck due to congenital cervical fusions
- 1938 Louis Lichenstein—polyostotic fibrous dysplasia
- 1950 Loren Larsen—multiple congenital dislocations with a characteristic facial appearance
- 1972 VATER, described by Linda Quan and David Smith—radial club hand and other lesions

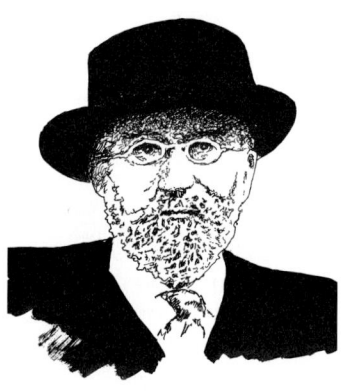

◆ Angelo Mafucci (1845–1903)

Marfan's Syndrome

A Parisian pediatrician, Antoine Bernard-Jean Marfan, described a 5-year-old girl with long, stiff fingers in 1896. She does not fit today's description of this syndrome. This particular child would be diagnosed as having congenital contractural arachnoidactyly. In 1902 Emile Charles Archard described a girl with long, flexible fingers that he called spider fingers, or arachnoidactyly. This would not be called Marfan's syndrome today. The real Marfan's syndrome was described by a Cincinnati ophthalmologist in 1876, Dr. E. Williams.

Neurofibromatosis

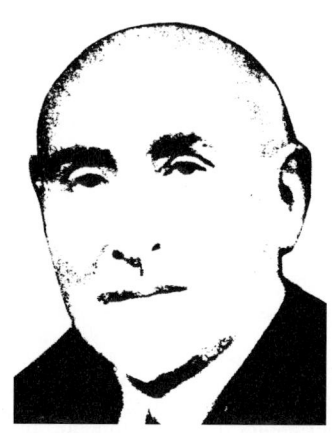

◆ Bernard Marfan (1858–1942)
Parisian pediatrician

This disease captured the imagination of the public with the sad story of "The Elephant Man," who died in 1890. A movie and a book have described his life. He probably suffered from Proteus syndrome.

One of the first descriptions of neurofibromatosis was by Tilesius in 1793 and was published in a book in Leipzig (*Historia Pathologica*). I like the 1849 description by Robert Smith from Dublin (see Chapter 10).

Ehlers-Danlos Syndrome

Job van Meekren, who appears elsewhere in this book, noted the stretchable skin of George Albes in 1657 in Leiden.

This was described in Russia by a dermatologist, A.N. Chernogubov, in 1881. Edvard Ehlers, a Dane, noted the stretchable skin in 1901, and Henri Danlos, a Frenchman, noted the fragility of the skin in 1908. The different types of this syndrome are now a laboratory for studying collagen genetics.

Congenital Malformations

"Lycurgus made a law for the guidance of the Greeks, in which it was decreed that all children born with deformity or defect should be destroyed. Its object was to preserve and improve the form and physical capacity of the Spartan children, so that he could rely on them, when they reached man's estate, as protectors of his government." James Knight: The Improvement of the Health of the Children and Adults by Natural Means. New York, 1875

Malformations were regarded in medieval times as the sins of the fathers being visited on the children. Studies were limited to descriptions of monsters. Etienne Sainte-Hilaire was the first experimentalist, doing various things to incubating chicken eggs. He changed the interest from cataloguing anomalies to discovering mechanisms. His son published a three-volume account in 1836, coining the word teratology.

References

Chapter references are located in Chapter 26.

◆ Chapter Fourteen

Amputations and Prostheses

It is no small presumption to dismember the image of God.
John Woodall: The Surgeon's Mate, 1617

Pull on a lizard's tail and it falls off without losing a drop of blood—no need for a surgeon. Then it grows back—no need for a prosthetist. Evolution took a backward turn when we lost these abilities.

Amputation was more commonly performed in olden days than today. Many open fractures and battle wounds that would be repaired today were treated by amputation amidst scenes of gore, and screaming and the stink of pus.

In medieval times, gangrene due to poor food storage—ergotism—produced another reason for amputation that no longer exists. Tumors and infections of bones and joints were treated by amputation. So amputations were common and frequently fatal.

Famous Amputees

The Above-elbow Amputation of Lord Nelson

In 1779, Admiral Horatio Nelson wanted to seize the treasure ships in the harbor of Teneriffe in the Canary Islands. The trip had not gone well, and he launched a commando-style raid in rowing boats. The Spanish were waiting and opened fire as the British

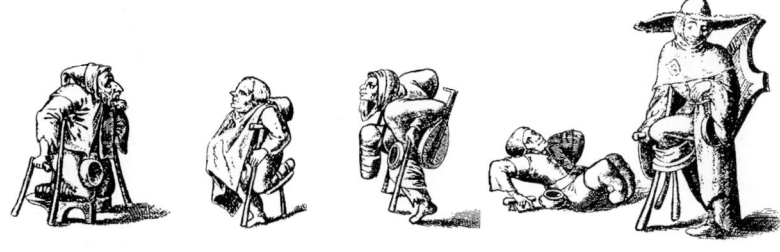

After amputation, kneeling prostheses were used. They are still used in third world countries today because construction is simple. Hieronymous Bosch, about 1500.

landed. Nelson stood on the beach and reached for his sword. A grape shot struck him in the right arm. He cried out, "I am shot through the arm. I am a dead man." His stepson put a bandage round the arm and got him back on the ship. "Tell the surgeon to make haste and get his instruments. I know that I must lose my right arm and the sooner it is off the better."

The 28-year-old surgeon wrote in the log, which still exists, "Admiral Nelson, 25 July 1797. Compound fracture of the right arm by a musket ball passing thro' a little above the elbow: an artery divided; the arm was immediately amputated." He ligated the artery. The arm was thrown in the sea.

"Discharged on board the Sea Horse 20th August. The sore reduced to the size of a shilling, in perfect good health one of the ligatures not come away."

The fee for the surgeon was 36 pounds and for the assistant, 24 guineas.

Nelson went back to active duty. Statues of him are to be found in many former British ports, and all depict him as an amputee—perhaps the most sculpted amputee ever.

Whitejacket, 1850

Herman Melville in the novel *Whitejacket* (published in 1850) describes a poor result from a high thigh amputation. Melville had shipped as a sailor on a U.S. frigate in 1843, and this is a fragment of the tale.

A sailor had suffered a gunshot fracture of the thigh and, after a few days, amputation was carried out on the deck. A board was balanced between 2 gun carriages for the operating table, and there was quite an audience.

"They say he can drop a leg in one minute and ten seconds from the time the knife touches it," whispered one of them to another. *'We shall see,' was the reply, and he checked his watch. The patient was brought up and the surgeon removed his wig, glass eye, false teeth and coat. He addressed the patient.*

"I would advise perfect repose of your every limb, my man. The precision of an operation is often impaired by the inconsiderate restlessness of the patient. It is better to live with three limbs than to die with four." (The surgeon begins a lecture to the audience and talks about red hot knives and boiling oil until the patient faints. The patient faints again when the risk of death is discussed. The amputation is carried out while the patient's mates pin him down. Then he is carried to the sick bay while the surgeon continues a bragging lecture which is terminated only by the news that the patient has died.)

TIMELINE OF AMPUTATIONS
Until 1000 AD

Neolithic times: amputation carried out for injury, disease, to appease the gods, for punishment, and for beautification

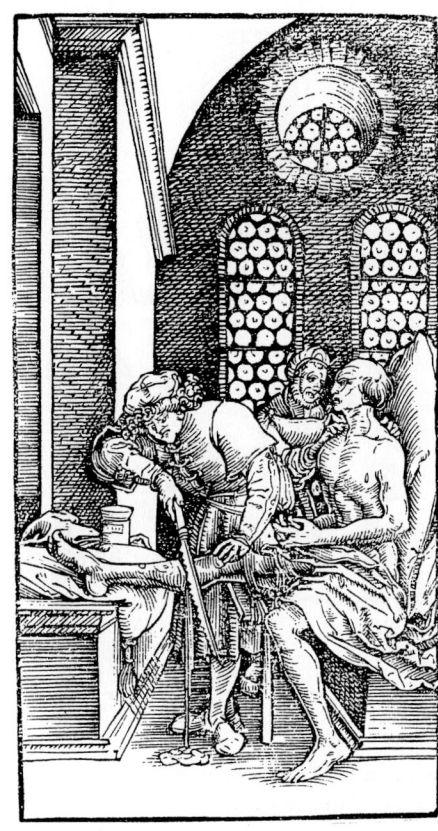

Cicero underwent amputation in the 1st century BC.

484 BC Herodotus, the Greek historian, writes about Hegistratus who was imprisoned, presumably manacled by his ankle. He escaped by cutting off his foot and made his way to a town 30 miles away where he fitted on a wooden foot, which worked well until he was imprisoned again.

400 BC Hippocrates: *"When gangrene supervenes on a fracture, the soft parts separate quickly. But the bones separate slowly. Remove the dead tissues."*

30 AD Celsus: *"Between the sound and the diseased part, the flesh is to be cut through with a scalpel down to the bone, but this must not be done actually over a joint, and it is better that some of the sound part be cut away than that any of the diseased part should be left behind. When the bone is reached the sound flesh is drawn back from the bone and undercut from around it, so that in that part also some bone is bared; the bone is then to be cut through with a small saw as near as possible to the sound flesh which still adheres to it; next the face of the bone which the saw has roughened, is smoothed down, and the skin drawn over it; this must be sufficiently loosened in an operation of this sort to cover the bone all over as completely as possible. The part where the skin has not been brought over is to be covered with lint; and over that a sponge soaked in vinegar is to be bandaged on."* Clearly

Box continued on following page

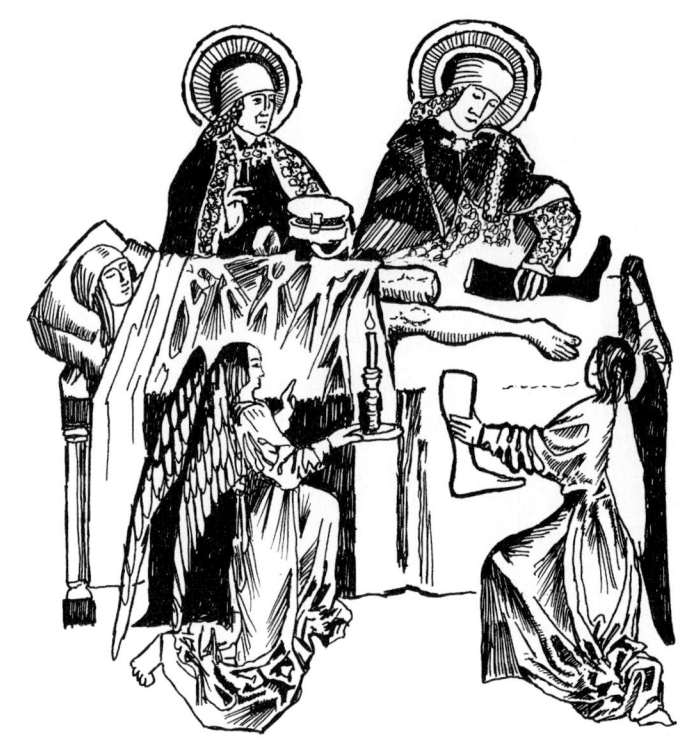

The story of Saints Cosmos and Damien. In about 300 AD they replaced the gangrenous leg of a white man with the leg of a dead black Moor. They are patron saints of medicine—Arab by birth, physicians by occupation, and martyred by Diocletian.

he used flaps to achieve closure without the bone being a problem. In the Dark Ages this was forgotten until 1700 or later.

- 100   Technique is well advanced. Archigenes and Heliodorus use tight bandages to control bleeding and ligate vessels.
- 300   The Dark Ages sees methods fall back. Leonides of Alexandria uses red hot irons to stop bleeding, and this continues for centuries.
- 850   Poor grain storage leads to ergotism, which causes vasoconstriction. Limbs became gangrenous, resulting in many amputations.

Amputations from 1100 Until 1800

- 1170   Roger and, in 1230, Roland both introduce the idea of laudable pus, provoking pus to encourage healing.
- 1346   Cannon shot introduced at the Battle of Crecy
- 1364   Half-pound gunshot introduced at Perugia. Battlefield injuries were more mutilating then, and battlefield surgery was the result.
- 1517   Gersdorff publishes the first illustration of an amputation.

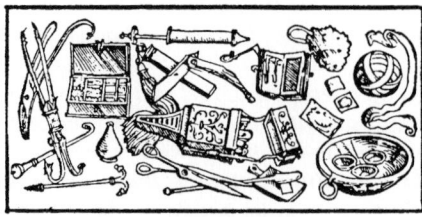

The surgeon's instrument table, Gersdoff, 1517

Chapter 14 ♦ Amputations and Prostheses

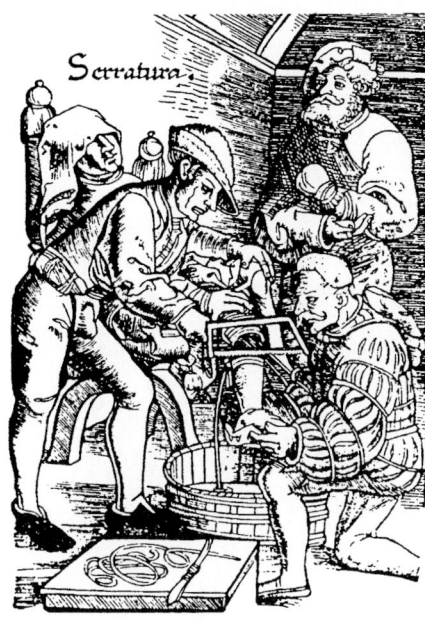

Amputation scene, Gersdorff, 1517

1536 Ambroise Paré becomes a battle surgeon and performs the first elbow disarticulation.
1552 Paré reintroduces ligatures. He stops the use of boiling oil to sterilize the wound because the pain and damage are increased. He invents spring-loaded artery forceps.
1588 William Clowes describes above-knee amputation.
1593 Fabry: monograph on gangrene. First amputation through the thigh. Uses tourniquet.
1596 Peter Lowe, Scotland: first English language description of ligatures
1616 Harvey's discovery of the circulation provides a rationale for tourniquet: 1674, Morel's Spanish windlass; 1718, Petit's tourniquet

Box continued on following page

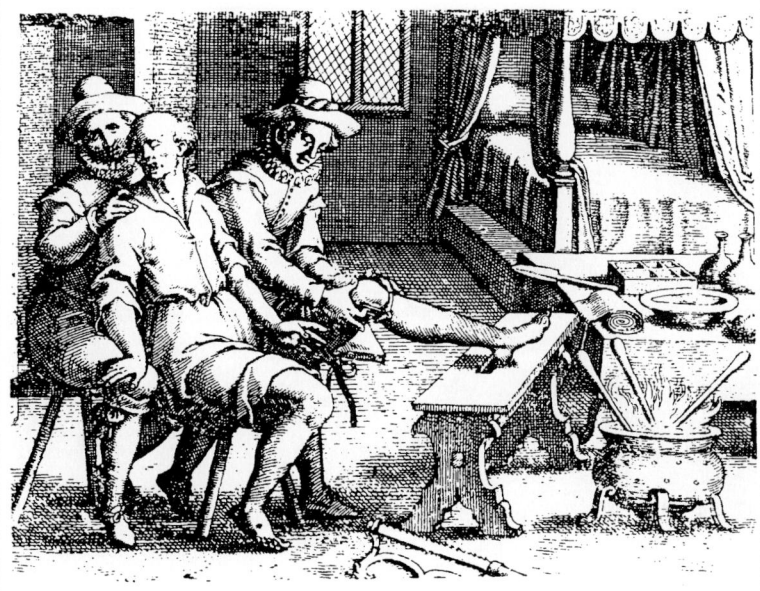

Amputation scene, Fabricius Hildanus, 1646. The cautery irons are heating up. The line of amputation is above the line of demarcation. From J Bone Jt Surg Br 1949, B, 474.

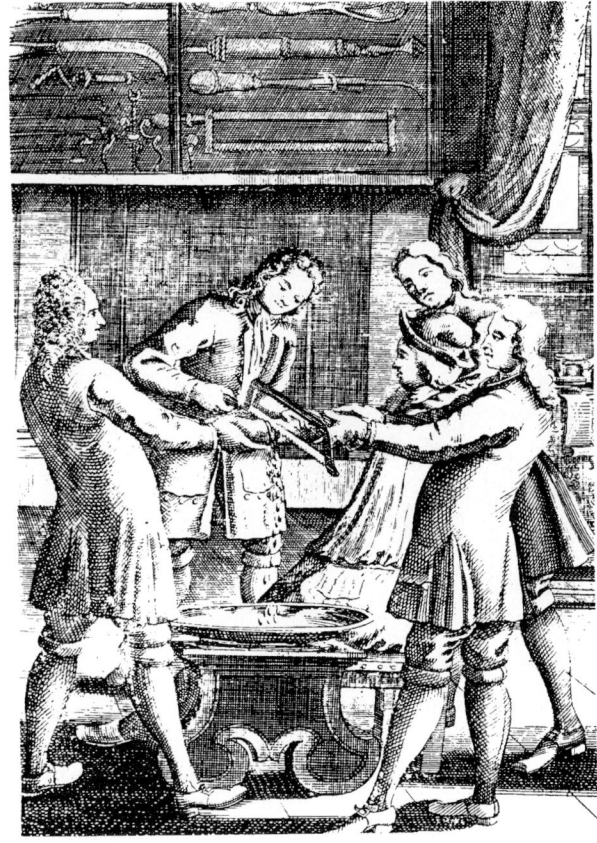

Amputation scene, Lorenz Heister, 1724. The distal forearm and hand are being removed. There are so many surprising things about these pictures. Why were they engraved? They are not instructive, nor are they pretty. Why is the patient sitting? Did this make fainting more likely—as a kind of preanesthetic oblivion? The blood bowl is common to most pictures. J Bone Jt Surg Br, 1949.

1672	Richard Wiseman encourages use of cautery.
1696	Verdun of Amsterdam uses flap method.
1739	Rovaton: flaps
1765	Vermale: flaps
1779	Alanson of Liverpool and Hey of Leeds, 1803: triple incision. Cut the skin and fascia with the first cut and retract proximally. Cut the bone with a saw. Close soft tissue over the bone.
1792	Fourcroy-Chopart amputation

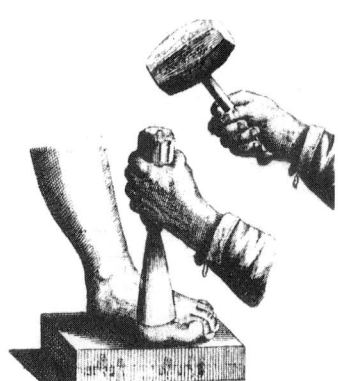

Scultetus, 1672.

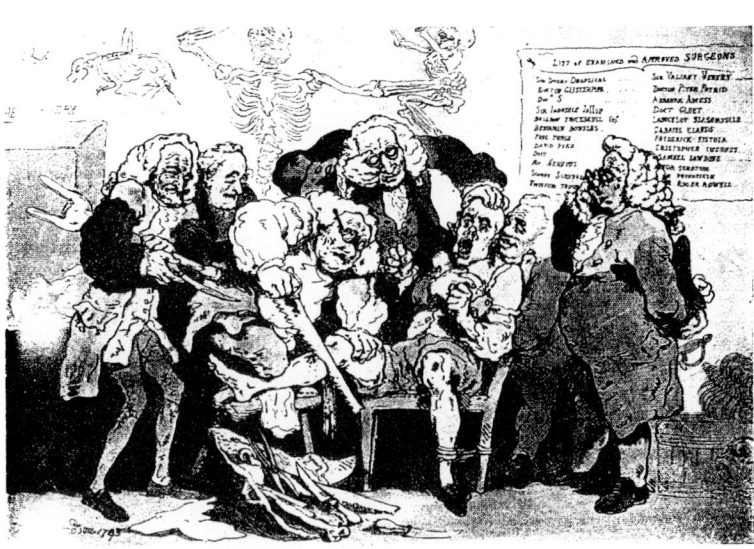

Amputation scene, 1793. This is Thomas Rowlandson's satire.

Amputations from 1800 Until 1900

1803   Larrey, Napoleon's surgeon, gains a lot of experience because he amputated for all open fractures, all joint injuries and joint fractures, and large wounds involving nerves and arteries. Wounds were left open and closed with tape later.

1808   Ralph Cuming carries out a forequarter amputation at the Naval Hospital, Antigua.

1815   J. Lisfranc de St. Martin publishes a book in Paris on partial amputation through the foot.

1825   Nathan Smith in America develops through-knee amputation.

1830   Velpeau writes about through-knee amputation.

1837   Liston popularizes flaps. Malgaigne advocates racquet incision.

1842   Dupuytren had 62% mortality from thigh amputations.

1844   James Syme describes disarticulation through the ankle.

1846   Anesthesia reduces suffering and reduces the need for speed. In the past Charles Bell had said that "the knife should be handled more like a sabre than a surgeon's scalpel."

1854   Pirogoff worked in the Crimean War. Some idea of the speed of these surgeons can be gleaned from his description of how he avoided secondary hemorrhage. *"In the Crimea War we had to perform hundreds of amputations. I covered the wounds of the first 20 to 30 amputees with wet sponges and left them in place while performing a subsequent 20 to 30 operations. In the meantime, patients in the first group were given warm tea or wine. If there was no hemorrhage, I bandaged the wound. About an hour elapsed between the amputation and the application of the bandage."*

Box continued on following page

Title page of Lisfranc's book, 1815.

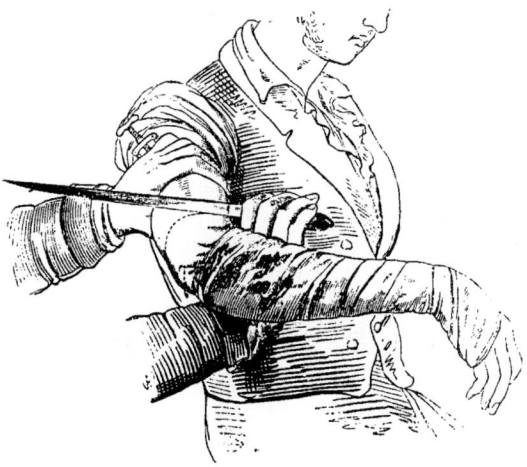

Amputation scene, William Fergusson, 1852. The tour de maître. This grip on the knife allowed a quick encircling incision without pause. Another 40 years would pass before surgeons and patients took off their best clothes. As late as 1852, pictures of amputation of limbs of fully dressed patients by fully dressed surgeons still appear in books. From Fergusson W: A System of Practical Surgery, 3rd ed. London: 1852.

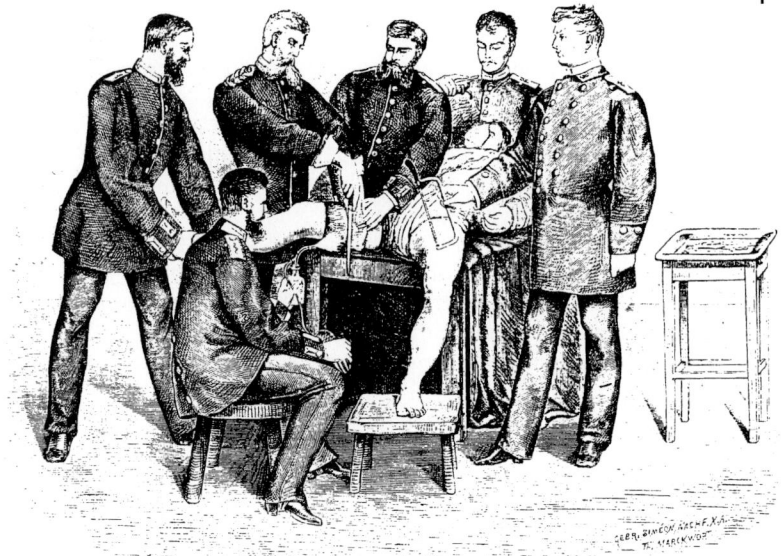

Amputation after the invention of anesthesia, Esmarch, 1884. The seated doctor is using Lister's spray. A tourniquet prevents bleeding—gone is the blood bowl. Still the staff is dressed for parade.

1857 Gritti: supracondylar amputation fusing the patella to the end of the femur after removing the articular surface. The result was an end-bearing stump but not easily fitted with a prosthesis.
1867 Lister's paper on asepsis. The U.S. Army adopts the principles in 1877. The American Surgical Association follows in 1883.
1870 Stokes modifies Gritti's amputation in the United Kingdom.
1873 Esmarch: rubber bandage, makes amputation safer. Thomas Spencer Wells invents artery forceps while at the Crimean War to make control of hemorrhage easier.
1883 Neuber: sterile gowns and caps
1894 Jaboulay: hindquarter amputation
1895 Girard: hindquarter amputation
1897 Mikulicz: face masks

Amputations from 1900

1900 Cineplasty. This idea came about because the Abyssinians amputated the hands of Italian prisoners of war in 1897–1898. Vanghetti realized that the muscles were working and could be harnessed to a prosthesis. Ceci of Pisa did the first operation. Others made tunnels to hold rods.
1917 Krukenberg's amputation turned the radius and ulna into chopsticks, which looks ugly but provides good grasp and pinch.
1930 Borggreve carries out femoral rotationplasty for overcoming leg length discrepany due to resection.
1950 Van Nes of Leiden, Holland, reports it for proximal focal femoral deficiency.
1959 Weiss: myoplasty is "*the fixation of the sectioned muscle groups at a proper tension to the bone stump.*" This provided a stump with good cover, sensation, and strength. It was used by Diderich in Germany and later by Weiss in Poland.
1961 Thalidomide causes phocomelia.

TIMELINE OF PROSTHESES

- 300 BC   artificial leg found in Italy
- 200 BC   Marcus Sergius, a Roman general, is fitted with an iron hand.
- 1509   Gottfried von Berlichingen, a German Knight, loses his right hand in Bavaria. An armorer makes a hand with movable fingers. When someone is offended because he offers his left hand to be shaken, he says, *"My right hand, though not useless in war, is insensible to the pressure of love. It has rendered more service in the fight than it ever did in the original flesh."*
- 1564   Paré describes arm and leg prostheses in his book. No active movement was possible. Breughel illustrates knee pads worn by below-knee amputees to enable them to get about.

Box continued on following page

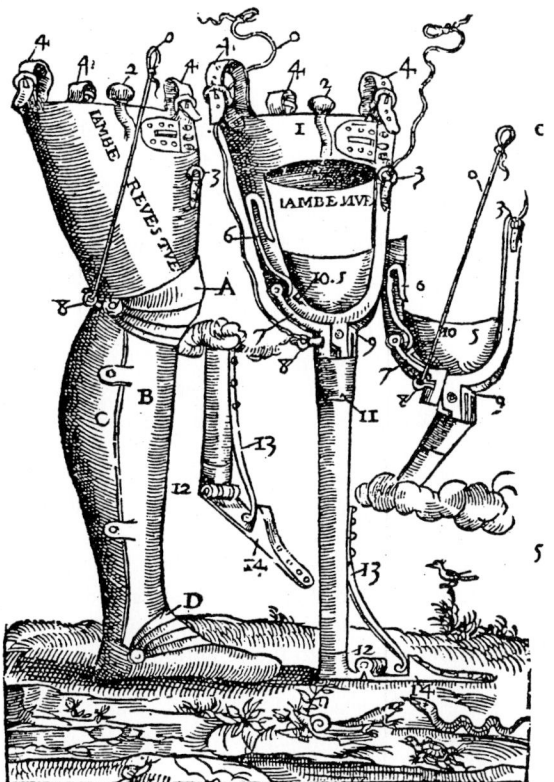

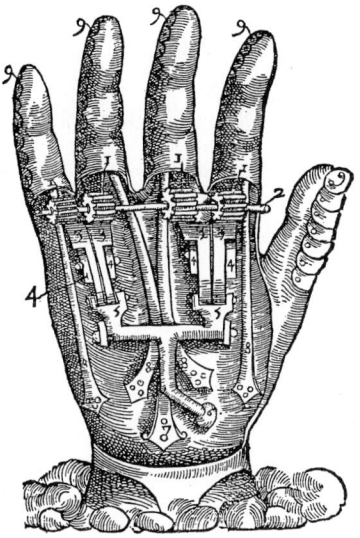

Paré: articulated hand. The fingers could be passively flexed to hold a sword. 1579.

Paré: articulated prosthesis with a spring ankle and a knee joint which can be locked. For a knight in armor it could be considered to have a cosmetic cover. 1579.

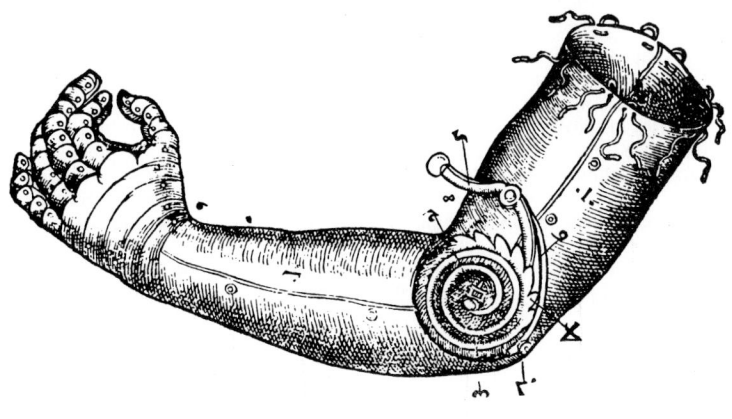

Paré designed several prostheses.

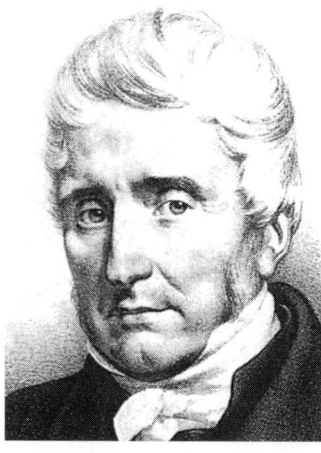

◆ Jacques Lisfranc

◆ **Jacques Lisfranc (1790–1847)**

He was a surgeon in Paris. It is not clear whether he did anything more than write a short monograph on his amputation in 1815.

1658	The Prince of Homburg had his leg blown off at the Siege of Copenhagen. He completed the amputation himself. He wore a prosthesis for 50 years. The ankle had a spring to provide power. It was called "the silver leg."
1696	Verdun of Holland developed a below-knee prosthesis. Before this the knee was flexed.
1800	The Anglesea limb. The Marquis of Anglesea lost his leg at Waterloo. James Pott made him a limb with a knee joint and an ankle joint that were linked with cords so that they moved together.
1818	Peter Baliff, a Berlin dentist, introduces a shoulder harness to provide power to move the fingers.
1831	Goyrand: ischial weight bearing for an above-knee amputee
1844	Van Peeterssen, a Dutch sculptor, uses a shoulder harness to power the elbow in an above-elbow amputation.
1863	Dubois Parmalee introduces and patents the suction socket, but it is forgotten.
1864	The American limb is patented. Selpho and then Palmer add bumpers to the ankle joint.
1867	Comte de Beaufort of France writes a booklet on prostheses. He uses cords for powering fingers and a rocker bottom foot to improve gait.
1886	Clasen: heavy-duty hand
1904	Carnes: sophisticated hand and wrist with wrist movement and pronation and supination
1912	Dorrance devised a split hook for his own use.
1940s	Committee on Prosthetic Devices formed in the United States, which funded university and industry research and moved the subject into the scientific age.

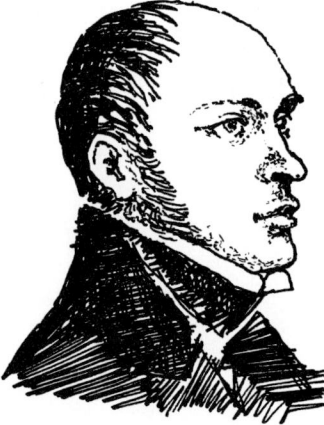

◆ Nikolai Pirogoff

◆ **Nikolai Pirogoff (1810–1881)**

A child prodigy, he was born in Moscow; he became professor of surgery at the Academy of Military Medicine at St. Petersburg. This Russian surgical genius is known for his amputation at the ankle but little else because his work has not been translated into English. In 1843 he wrote an anatomy text and later a three-volume text on surgery. In 1854 he described an amputation in which he took off the distal tibia and fibula and fused it to a sliver of os calcis—anchoring the heel pad.

Between 1852 and 1859 he published an *Atlas of Cross-Sectional Anatomy,* based on sawed frozen sections. He produced the views we see today on MRI and CT scans. He invented plaster bandages about the same time as Mathijsen. In 1856 he was forced to resign as Professor on the trumped-up charge that he was insane because he tried to improve conditions in the military hospital. He wrote *Principles of General Military Field Surgery* in 1864, based on the Crimean War, in which his side opposed that of Florence Nightingale. He introduced nurses on the battlefield at the same time. He gave up surgery for a job in education and wrote a long autobiography available in English translation.

He called war "a traumatic epidemic."

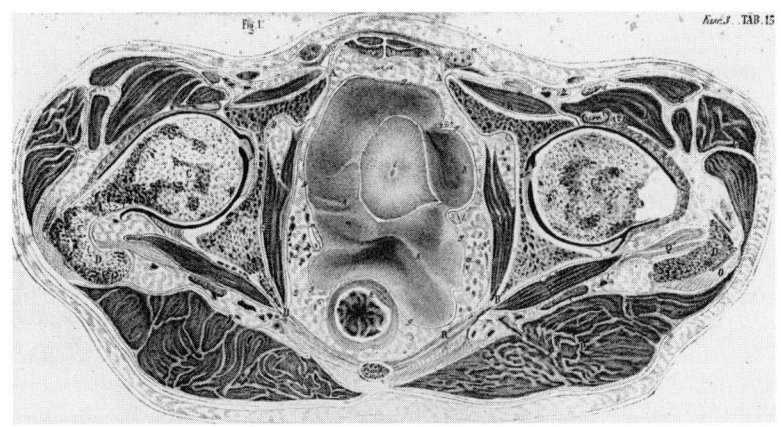

Pirogov gave his name to an ankle-level amputation. Here is a plate from his atlas of cross-sectional anatomy, published in 1852. These are the hips. His study was done on frozen corpses during a Russian winter. Only the advent of computed tomography has enabled us to see the body like this.

1946 Suction socket developed by a group for the U.S. Academy of Sciences. Major research and development centers were established in America and were very productive. One product was the patellar tendon-bearing prosthesis.
1960 Myoelectric controls for upper limb prostheses developed by Russians
1966 Marian Weiss in Poland reports success with instant fit of prostheses.

Thalidomide

This drug was introduced in Germany in 1956 especially for the nausea of pregnancy. It came to Britain in 1958 but was kept out of the United States by Dr. Frances Kelsy of the Food and Drug Administration.

Thalidomide is such a powerful teratogen that it has been estimated that every mother who took it between the 35th and 50th day produced an abnormal child. There was an epidemic of children born without arms and legs. Dr. W. Lenz observed that the incidence of phocomelia at the Children's Hospital in Hamburg went from zero in the 10 years before 1959 to 154 cases in the year 1961. He suspected thalidomide and told his friends. He read a paper to pediatricians in 1961, and within 7 days the drug was withdrawn. More than 8000 affected children were born. Special prostheses were designed, and research was advanced. A class action against the manufacturers provided some compensation.

Syme's Amputation at the Ankle, 1842

"Caries is frequently seated in the articular surfaces of the joint between the astragalus and os calcis, where it may seem to be of limited extent, and occasion no formidable symptoms, but

nevertheless exhibits its characteristic obstinacy, and resists all means of remedy except amputation. A succession of such cases painfully impressing me with the imperfection of surgery which afforded no milder means of remedy than removal of the leg, suggested the idea of operating, at the ankle, so as to preserve the thick integuments of the heel, and lessen the extent of mutilation.

"J.W., aged 16, recommended to my care by Mr. Aitchinson of Dunbar, and admitted into the hospital on the 5th of September, 1842, afforded me an opportunity of trying this plan. He was suffering from disease of the foot, which, in consequence of a sprain sustained twelve months before, had suppurated and ulcerated, so as to admit a probe into the joint between the os calcis and astragalus. I performed the operation without any difficulty, and as the ankle joint remained sound, did not remove the articulating surface, further than by taking away the malleolar projections of the tibia and fibula. The patient went home on the 2nd of December, and did well afterwards, as appears from the following extract of a letter which Dr. Aitchinson sent me four years subsequently to the operation: 'He tells me he suffers no inconvenience from the stump, or the slightest tenderness. He has become a country tailor, and often has ten or fifteen miles a day to go to his work'."

Syme describes the details of the operation and points out that the flap will slough if the vessels are scored crosswise. He continues to describe its advantages and some case histories.

"The advantages of this operation are, in the first place, its facility and simplicity, requiring no tourniquet, and being completed, so far as the disarticulation is concerned, without any hurry, in less than a minute; secondly, its not implicating any large blood-vessels or nerves so as to expose the patient to the risk of suffering from hemorrhage or nervous pains; thirdly, its protection against the chance of exfoliation by the spongy nature of the bone divided; and fourthly, its affording a stump so perfect as to give the requisite support without any extraneous assistance. No other stump of the lower extremity can bear pressure on its face sufficiently for supporting the body but the one in question, or at least be so used without inconvenience; and there was a man lately at the hospital, who, after having both of his feet amputated, could not only stand, but walk and run without aid of any kind whatever."

Marian Weiss
1966

As far back as the Napoleonic Wars distinguished surgeons and even military leaders tried to persuade amputated soldiers to attach temporary prostheses to their stumps, so that they could escape the enemy. During World War I, the French surgeon Martin introduced the 'Operating Table Prosthesis' in field conditions. In recent years Berlemont proved that an early outfitting of amputees with prostheses stepped up the healing process.

◆ **Marian Weiss**
Marian Weiss was a Polish orthopaedic surgeon who developed a large rehabilitation hospital in Constantine. Somehow he survived Nazi occupation and Communism. He pioneered immediate-fit prostheses and was very active in treating spinal cord injury.

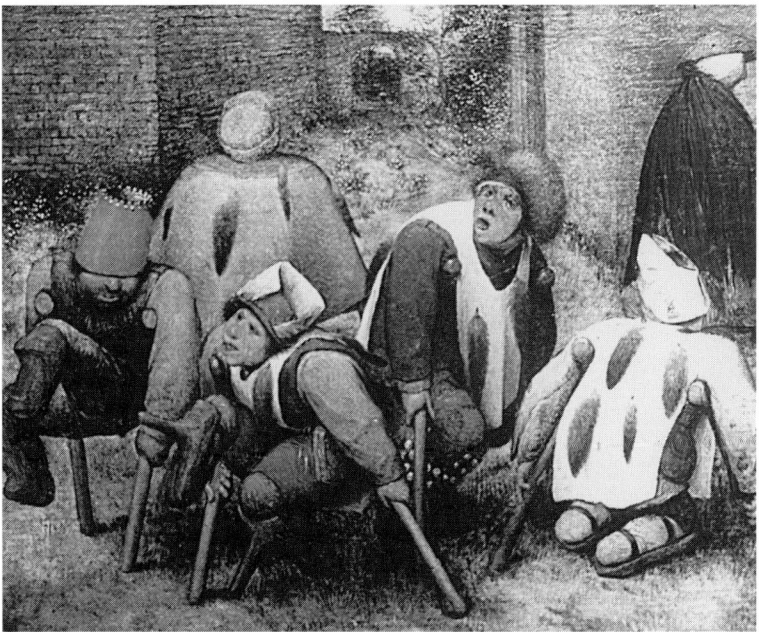

The artist Pieter Brueghel depicted amputees with their primitive prostheses. It is believed that ergotism was the cause of loss of many limbs. The crutches had no cross-bar and must have been hard to use. *circa* 1550.

In 1963 we performed the first operations which confirmed the correctness of our concept...myoplastic surgery, immediate fitting, ambulation.

About the same time Burgess in Seattle was exploring the same ground.

Crutches

The Pyramids have pictures of crutches. Until recently people on crutches were a common sight because of problems getting leg fractures to heal well and because of arthritis and tuberculosis. Now most people use them only on a short-term basis. Walking frames, or "walkers," for the elderly are a recent invention.

Old-time crutches were a pole with a T-piece at the top to fit under the armpit. Artists such as Bosch and Breughel included them in drawings and paintings. There was nothing but the pole for the hand to grasp so they must have been tiring to use. About 1800 the saw made it possible to split the pole and insert a transverse hand piece. Canadian forearm crutches came much later.

References

Chapter references are located in Chapter 26.

◆ Chapter Fifteen

Orthopaedic Treatment

As for those "surgeons" who cannot read and write I would advise them to peruse the 6th commandment, "Thou shalt not kill."
John Jones, first American fracture textbook, 1776

The object of treatment is the restoration of complete function with least risk and inconvenience to the patient and with least anxiety to the surgeon.   Robert Jones, 1913

The aim of an operation is to speed up slow treatment by mechanical orthopaedics.   Georg Stromeyer, about 1840

In the beginning, orthopaedic treatment meant nonoperative treatment—corrective shoes, corrective braces, black boxes, and bizarre exercises of all kinds. Today we chuckle when practitioners of alternative medicine extol our cast-off methods. We have moved on to operative treatment.

We all envy neurosurgeons and cardiac surgeons who have neurologists and cardiologists to look after the nonoperative aspects of disease. Physiatrists have not filled this role for us. We have only ourselves to blame. Our forefathers fought internists who believed that surgeons should be technicians working under their direction; our forefathers knew that the selection of patients for operation was more important than technical performance of the operation.

A large part of our job is patient education. In the past a surgeon might say, "I'll fix it. You will be all right . . . don't worry. I will put you down on the operation waiting list." That would be the end of discussion. Today, patients want information as much as treatment. Giving information takes a lot of time—almost as much time as it takes to do many operations. We are as much in the information business as the operating business.

The first book on orthopaedics was written more than 250 years ago by Andry for parents, not for doctors. It was a self-help book. As public education improved the need for information increased, and we now have a legal obligation to discuss risks and options and benefits of management. Now we have handouts and videos, and even video evidence that these discussions have taken place.

Title page of book by Park and Moreau, 1806.

Operating Room Methods

Esmarch's Tourniquet

On the Artificial Emptying of Blood-Vessels in Operations, 1873

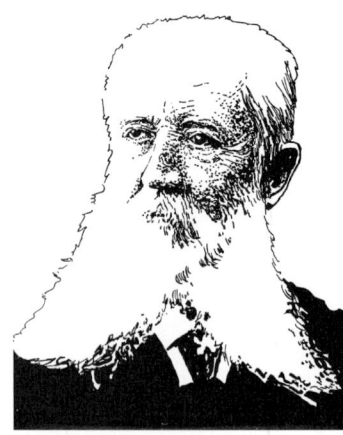

◆ Johann Friedrich August von Esmarch (1823–1908)

A military surgeon who was concerned with blood loss and first aid. He was born at Tonning, Schleswig-Holstein, at a time when the province was struggling for freedom from Denmark. The son of a doctor, he studied at Göttingen and Kiel, becoming an assistant to Langenbeck.

During the insurrection against Denmark in 1848–1850 he began surgery; he also organized the resistance movement. In 1857 he became professor of surgery at Kiel, succeeding Stromeyer, the tenotomist, and marrying his daughter. He was engaged in military surgery again between 1866 and 1871 in the wars with Austria and France; in 1871 he became Surgeon General of the army. Soon after, in 1873, he married again—this time a princess of Schleswig-Holstein. In the same year he published his description of the bandage that bears his name. He used this to produce a clear, bloodless field for surgery and to diminish the blood loss during amputations in particular. His contributions to medicine were mainly derived from his battlefield experiences.

In 1869 and 1883 he published handbooks on first aid and founded the Samaritan's Schools, based on the St. John's Ambulance Brigade, to teach first aid throughout Germany. "When I look back on my career as a surgeon I can say with truth that many and many are the times I have deplored that so very few people know how to render the first aid to those who have suddenly met with some injury. This specially applies to the field of battle; of the thousands who have flocked thither in their desire to help, so few have understood how to render aid." His program of education has improved the situation.

"Gentlemen—You all witnessed yesterday a difficult and tedious operation, in which the patient lost a very large quantity of blood, in spite of all the care that was taken to prevent it.

"What, more than all, rendered the operation difficult, was the profuse haemorrhage.

"You will remember that, with almost every incision, although I took care to make them as slight as possible, one or more arteries spurted, or veins poured out their dark blood over the field of the operation. You saw how I sought to check the hemorrhage as much as possible by taking up the bleeding vessels, after each incision, with bulldog forceps, and left these hanging in the wound while I went on with the operation. More than once there were hanging in the wound all the twenty-four pairs of forceps which I always have at hand in great operations, and I was compelled first to tie the vessels already divided before I could cut deeper. When the operation was at last finished, I had applied altogether more than fifty ligatures, of which, however, fifteen were applied on the tumour itself, so that only thirty-five remained in the wound.

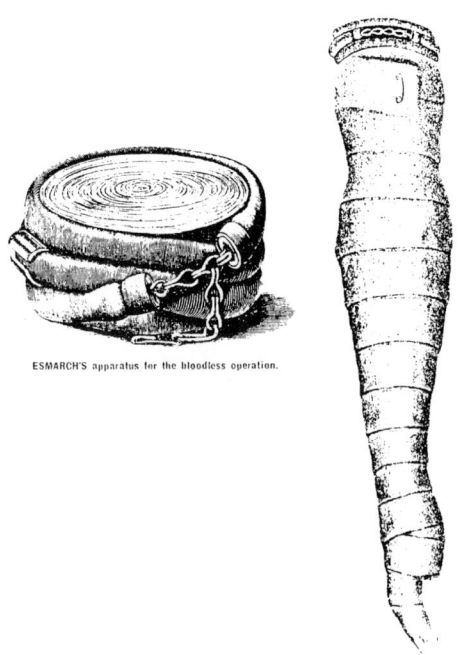

ESMARCH'S apparatus for the bloodless operation.

Esmarch's tourniquet and bandage, 1884.

"I cannot make any guess as to the exact quantity of blood lost, since it was constantly removed with sponges; but we could judge that the patient had very little blood left in her body by the wax-like paleness of the skin, the small, weak pulse, and the laboured respiration.

"Most of you will, no doubt, have said to yourselves that you would not desire to commence your career as operators with such an extirpation. And, in fact, it is just the 'demoniac' blood, as Dieffenbach called it, which not infrequently deters the young practitioner from performing an important operation, especially when he cannot command sufficient and reliable assistance. And yet he only becomes a good operator who has learnt calmly to enter into the struggle with haemorrhage.

"I need not explain to you here how important the question of haemorrhage is in almost every operation. In many cases the limit we put to our operative undertakings is determined by the extent of the haemorrhage to be expected. We do not venture to undertake many operations against which no other contra-indication exists, because the operation would last so long that we can foresee that the patient would bleed to death before it was completed, or because we consider him already too weak to survive the unavoidable loss of blood.

"I shall perform an operation today in which the loss of blood would be still greater than in that of yesterday, if I did not adopt a procedure before commencing it which enables us to prevent the haemorrhage entirely. In the patient about to be placed upon the operating table, there is almost total necrosis of both tibiae, resulting from an acute osteomyelitis, which followed a severe cold more than twenty years ago. You see that on the anterior surface of both legs numerous fistulae openings exist, which discharge a large quantity of pus, and, through which the probe comes everywhere upon roughened, moveable bone. . . . I think it best to convert the bony cavity into a broad trough, by taking away the whole anterior wall, so that no adjacent cavities may remain to retard the healing process. Those amongst you who have already seen similar operations will remember what profuse haemorrhage accompanied them, and how greatly the performance of them was rendered difficult and protracted by the loss of blood. Our patient is still tolerably well nourished, and not exactly to be called anaemic but I do not believe that I should have ventured formerly to undertake both operations at one sitting, because I should have feared that the loss of blood would have placed the life of the patient in great danger. With the aid of the process which I am about to show you, I do not hesitate to undertake both the operations simultaneously, and to spare the patient thereby a second operation, and a second long confinement to bed. My assistant, Dr. Petersen, will operate upon the right leg at the same time and in the same manner as I do on the left.

"While the patient is being put under the influence of chloroform, the leg is first wrapped in waterproof varnished silk-paper, to prevent the bandages from being soiled by the discharge from the fistulous openings; both legs are then firmly bandaged from the points of the toes to above the knee with these elastic bandages, which are made of woven India rubber, the uniform compression from which drives the blood out of the vessels of the limb. Immediately above the knee, where the bandage ends, we now apply this India rubber tubing, well drawn out, four or five times round the thigh, and connect one end with the other by means of a hook and brass chain attached to them respectively. The India rubber tubing so thoroughly compresses all the soft parts, including the arteries, that not a drop of blood can enter the part so treated. This has the special advantage over the tourniquet, that we can apply it at any part of the limb, and need not be concerned about the position of the main artery. Even in the most muscular and stoutest individuals we are able thoroughly to control the supply of blood by this simple process.

"We now remove the bandages first applied, together with the varnished silk-paper, and you see that both legs below the tubing resemble completely those of a corpse and with their pale colour contrast almost uncomfortably with the rosy colour of the rest of the surface of the body. You will observe, also, that we operate precisely as on the dead subject.

"We both now divide the soft parts along the whole anterior surface of the tibia down to the bone; a few drops of blood ooze from the bone and are wiped away with a sponge. From that time no more blood is seen. The periosteum, divided in the long direction, is now pushed back so far on both sides that the whole anterior surface of the thickened, uneven bone, with its numerous fistulous openings, is freely exposed. . . .

"We now, first, slowly remove the compressing India rubber tubing. You see how the pale skin of the foot becomes red, first in spots, then uniformly everywhere, and soon even presents a darker red colour than the other parts of the body. Observe the dressing of the wound under the transparent paper; you nowhere see blood oozing through the gauze bandage. The patient has, therefore, not lost more than a teaspoonful of blood. And now, observe the still quietly sleeping patient; he has, even now, the same red cheeks as before the operation; his pulse is full and strong, and the recovery in his case will, no doubt, be much quicker and more certain than if we had removed the bone in the usual manner."

◆ Arnold K. Henry (1886–1962)
An Irishman who trained in surgery in Dublin and then served in the Serbian Army until the country was overrun. He joined the French Army for the latter part of World War I. He spent a few years back in Dublin before becoming the professor of surgery in Cairo in 1925, where he wrote the first version of his book. He subsequently worked at the Hammersmith Hospital before going back to Dublin as Professor of Anatomy. He developed surgical approaches to the long bones and is also remembered for the master knot of Henry seen during clubfoot surgery.

Surgical Exposures

Long ago, a circumferential incision for an amputation and an x over an abscess were all that a surgeon needed to know. In the future, endoscopy portals may be the extent of knowledge, but, at present, there are a thousand different approaches to reach deep inside without doing damage. Kocher, in Switzerland, worked out new approaches every day before breakfast, and Henry, in Cairo, wrote *Extensile Exposure*.

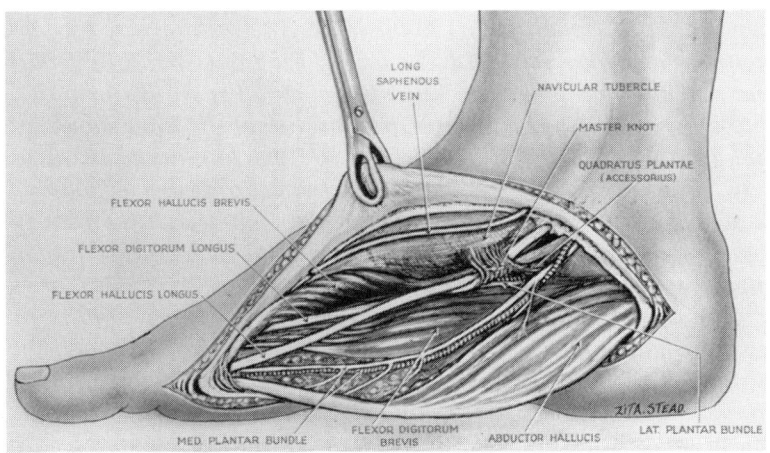

Master knot of Henry from *Extensile Exposure*, 1945.

Operations on Bone

CORRECTIVE OSTEOTOMY
JOHN RHEA BARTON, 1837

"The object of my treatment was to remove deformity, and to restore to usefulness a limb which had unfortunately been suffered to become anchylosed in a mal-position. The following will, I trust, satisfactorily explain the operation and the after treatment of the case, as well as the principles by which I was guided in the management of it.

"S.D., M.D., formerly of Charleston, S.C., but now a resident of Alabama, when a youth of about nine years of age unluckily had his knee joint involved in inflammation and suppuration so extensively as to occasion the destruction of the synovial membranes, the ligaments, cartilages, and in short, every struc-

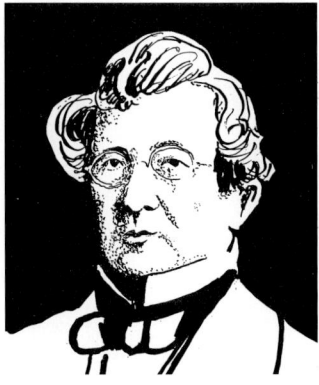

◆ **John Rhea Barton (1794–1871)**

It is unusual for a surgeon to develop two entirely new principles of treatment and to realize the significance of the innovations himself. Barton introduced both arthroplasty and corrective osteotomy for limb deformities. His ideas have been elaborated and applied to a wide range of situations.

He was born in Lancaster, Pennsylvania, the son of a judge (who designed the United State seal) and studied at the Pennsylvania Hospital in Philadelphia. He later worked for the Father of American Surgery, Dr. Physick, who was one of Hunter's pupils, before being elected to the surgical staff himself at the age of 29. He is said to have possessed great manual dexterity, and was ambidextrous, with the result that once he had positioned himself for an operation he was not always shunting about.

In 1854 he wired a fractured patella but lost the patient to sepsis. His name is attached to a fracture he described—carpal subluxation with a marginal fracture of the articular surface of the radius.

There is a marble bust of him at the College in Philadelphia, and the University of Pennsylvania to this day has a Barton Professor of Surgery, endowed by his widow.

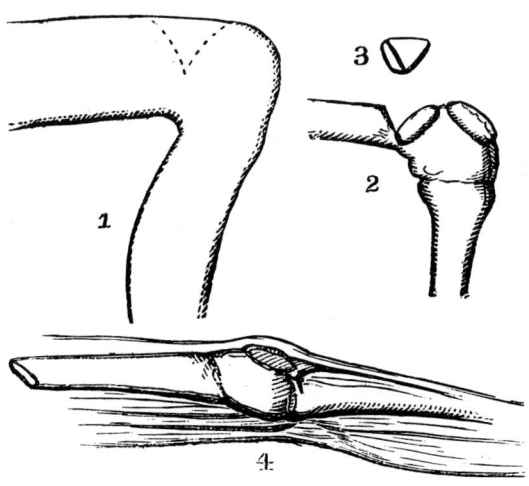

Corrective wedge osteotomy of Barton, 1837.

ture peculiarly appertaining to the joint. After a protracted suffering he finally recovered with the loss of the joint; the tibia, femur and patella having become united to each other in the form of a true anchylosis. The loss of the articulation of the knee, however, though a misfortune, did not constitute the sadness of his case. It was caused by the mal-position of the limb; the leg having been flexed upon the thigh to a degree somewhat less than a right angle. Hence the only alternatives of which he could avail himself to aid him in walking were, either to use crutches, or to employ a very high block-sole boot, and to lower his stature by flexing the sound limb, in order that both feet might reach the ground. The latter expedient he adopted. The long continued pressure and weight of the body sustained by this defective limb, acting under such great mechanical disadvantages, had at length caused some protection of the instep, and other irregularities, which it is unnecessary to particularise.

"This supposed irremediable condition of his limb, with all its ills, the young gentleman endured during the period of about sixteen years. In the meantime he graduated in medicine, and became a successful and highly respectable practitioner; but as his professional labours increased, he found the condition of his limb to be an obstacle not only to his further success, but also a source of unceasing annoyance and vexation. Whereupon, with a resoluteness not surprising to those who knew the strength of his mind, the firmness of his character, and the abundance of his manly courage, he repaired to Philadelphia in order that some relief might be obtained, if it were possible. When consulted by him I found him fully prepared to learn that no benefit was to be expected from any heretofore known practice, and that if he could be relieved it must be by some novel expedient and treatment.

"After a candid and full disclosure of my views of his case, and of the means by which I thought he might be benefited, his own judgment accorded with mine; and believing in the feasibility of the plans, he became urgent for the undertaking. It was accordingly commenced on the 27th day of May, 1835, and pursued as follows: Two incisions were made over the femur, just above the patella. The first commenced at a point opposite the upper and anterior margin of the external condyle of the femur, and, passing obliquely across the front of the thigh, terminated on the inner side. The second incision commenced also on the outer side, about two and a half inches above the first; and passing likewise obliquely across the thigh, terminated with the other in an acute angle. By these incisions were divided the integuments, the tendon of the extensor muscles of the leg, at its insertion into the upper part of the patella, and some of the contiguous fibres of the rectus and crureus muscles themselves, a greater part of the vastus internus, and a portion of the vastus externus muscles. A flap, composed therefore of this structure, was elevated from the femur close to the condyles. The soft parts were next detached from the outer side of the bone, from the base of the flap toward the ham, by passing a knife over the circumference of it, so as to admit of the use of a saw. The flap

then being turned aside, a triangular or wedge-like piece of the femur was easily removed by means of a small narrow bladed saw; such as was used in the operation at the hip. This wedge of bone did not include the entire diameter of the femur at the point of section; so that a few lines of the posterior portion of the shaft of the bone remained yet undivided. By slightly inclining the leg backward, these yielded, and the solution was complete. This mode of effecting the lesion of the bone was designedly adopted, and constituted what I conceived to be a very important measure in the operation. Important, because it rendered a popliteal artery free from the danger of being wounded by the action of the saw, and subsequently the interlocking of the fractured surfaces tended to retain the extremities of the divided bone in their positions until the harshness of their surfaces had been overcome either by the absorption of their angles, or by the deposition of new matter upon them—a change essential to the safety of the artery during the subsequent treatment of the case. Not a blood-vessel was opened which required either a ligature or compression. The operation, which lasted about five minutes, being thus ended, the reflected flap was restored to its place, the wound lightly dressed, and the patient was put to bed, lying on his back, with the limb supported upon a splint of an angle corresponding to that of the knee previous to the operation. This position was maintained until it was believed that the asperities of the bone had become blunted, and were not likely by their pressure to cause ulceration of the artery beneath them. This first splint was then removed, and another having the angle slightly obtuse was substituted. In a few days a third splint, with the angle more obtuse than that of the second, supplied its place. Others, varying in degrees of angularity, in like manner came in their turn to support the limb until it had attained a position almost straight. It was then unchangeably continued in that line until the contact surfaces of the bone had united and securely fixed the limb in this the desired direction.

"During the treatment of the case, especial care was bestowed in protecting the popliteal vessels against any injurious encroachment upon them. With that view, all antagonising pressure on the soft parts in the ham was carefully avoided. The limb was rested on two longbran bags, laid upon the splint, with their ends apart—a vacancy of four or five inches being left between them opposite the lesion of the bone. The interspace was lightly filled with carded cotton, so as to afford a safe support. Every symptom of pain or uneasiness in this part was promptly attended to. The occasional issue of a drop or two of blood from the corner of the sore, during the process of dressing the limb, caused me some solicitude in this case; whereas, ordinarily I should have considered it as a matter of no moment—it being so frequent an occurrence during the dressing of wounds, owing to the disturbance of the granulations, especially in compound fractures. The wounded soft parts finally healed and quieted his anxiety. The straightening of the limb having been very cautiously and by degrees effected, the first two months elapsed during the accom-

plishment of this object. Having then reduced it to the desired position, means were carefully observed to retain it so until the reunion of the bone had been fully completed; which occupied two months longer. The constitutional symptoms were such as usually occur in compound fractures—somewhat severe, but at no time alarming. Throughout the whole treatment it was not found necessary to bleed him, or to have recourse to any very active constitutional measures. He was occasionally indisposed from irregularity in the digestive functions, but was always speedily relieved by resorting to mild and appropriate remedies.

"At the end of about four months from the date of the operation my patient stood erect, with both feet in their natural position, and the heels resting alike upon the floor, although a slight angle had been designedly left at the knee, in order that there might not be any necessity for throwing the limb out from the body in the act of walking, which is always the case when the knee is quite straight. After this period, the use of shoes of the ordinary shape was resumed, and the limb was daily exercised with increasing strength and usefulness. On the 19th of October, the Doctor took his departure for the South, bearing with him the injunction to continue the support of a small splint and the aid of a crutch or cane, until he should acquire sufficient confidence in the strength of the limb to justify him in laying them aside.

"I was subsequently advised of his improvement—but was resolved not to give publicity to the case until the full and entire benefit of the operation could be ascertained. The wide distance which afterwards separated us prevented me from obtaining the necessary and direct information until within a recent period. I have the pleasure now not only to afford this intelligence, but to present it in the most satisfactory manner. Having written to the doctor for the information, and to learn from him in what manner it might be agreeable that I should refer to him as the subject of the case, the following clear, satisfactory, and well-written answer was promptly received. As the letter is full of interest in the case, I must be excused if I publish it almost entire, even though it contain some flattering sentiments for the one to whom it is addressed. That part only has been omitted which is in courtesy to my family.

"Charleston, November 6th, 1837

"My dear Sir,

". . . I have the satisfaction and pleasure of saying to you now, that the operation you performed on my leg has been completely successful, and has more than realised my most sanguine anticipations. The small abscess, which you dressed the day before we parted at Norfolk, continued open, and threw out, from time to time, small pieces of bone, until the August after, when the last piece was discharged; the orifice then closed, and I have suffered no material inconvenience from it since. From the January previous, however,

I was going about and attending to my professional business; and early in the summer, when our sickly season commenced, I was on horseback daily, riding from thirty to fifty miles a day; without more than the ordinary fatigue or inconvenience. I am at present well; the wound sound; and I feel no other inconvenience in riding or walking, than what arises from my knee joint being stiff, which was the case before you performed the operation. I walk without a stick or other aid, with the sole of the foot to the ground, and my friends tell me, with but a slight limp; and I have great pleasure in adding that the leg and foot have increased considerably in size, so as now to be nearly equal to the other. When I think of what I was, and what I am; and that to your firmness, judgment, and skill, I am indebted for the happy change, I want words to express adequately all that I feel. I will not attempt it, but believe me, my dear sir, I feel it not the less.

"I shall remain here for a week or two longer, and if you wish any further information on my case, do write me, and I will give it most cheerfully. After that period I cannot say where a letter would reach me. Adieu...and am, my dear sir, very sincerely, your friend,

"Seaman Deas"

In 1845 Gurdon Buck improved on this procedure. Barton's operation produced angular deformity just above the knee so that the line of the tibia was some inches in front of the femur. The artist who drew Barton's illustration has concealed this by extending the leg at the knee joint and not at the osteotomy.

Buck performed the osteotomy through the knee joint.

Closed Osteoclasis

Many designs were popular before sterile surgery became universal.

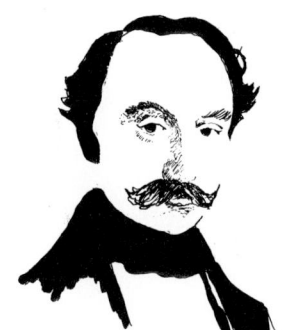

◆ **Francesco Rizzoli (1809–1880)**
Professor of surgery and obstetrics at Bologna. He willed his estate to found the Institut Rizzoli, which became home to Codivilla and Putti and a showplace of Italian orthopaedics. He used his osteoclast for leg equalization. He fractured the long leg and allowed it to shorten.

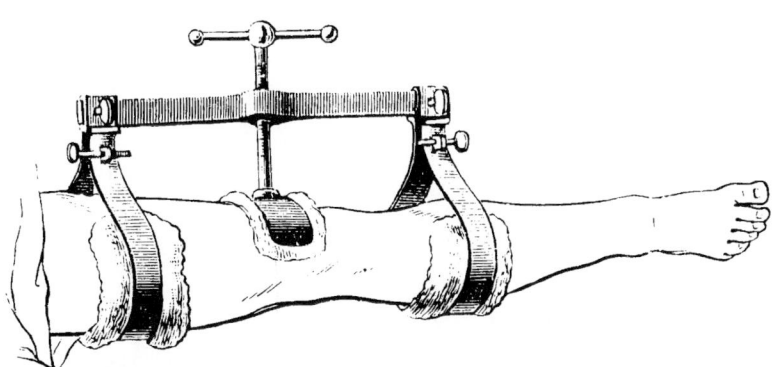

Rizzoli's osteoclast. Closed osteoclasis was safer than open osteotomy until aseptic surgery was universal. Many osteoclasts were designed. In the days before aseptic surgery and after anesthesia, this seemed like a good idea. From Young JK: Orthopaedic Surgery. Philadelphia, 1894.

Corrective Osteotomy

OPERATION FOR KNOCK-KNEES
MAYER, 1853

"To the Editor of The Lancet

"Sir,

"The following case of operation for knock-knees is reported by Dr. Mayer, of the Orthopaedic Hospital at Wurzburg, in the proceedings of the Medical Society of that place (lately published), and seems well worth recording in your pages.

"Your most obedient servant,

"F. A. B. Bonney

"Knightsbridge, April, 1853

"John II, a strong and healthy-looking boy of fifteen, son of a baker, and employed in his father's business, was found, on admission into the Orthopaedic Hospital at Würzburg, to have the right leg diverging about seven inches, and the left about eight, from the direction of the corresponding thigh.

"On the 14th of August, 1851, the lad having been put under the influence of chloroform, Dr. Mayer made an incision beginning three-quarters of an inch below the insertion of the ligamentum patellae, and curving downwards so as nearly to surround the front and inner (or mesial) side of the head of the tibia. He then turned the flap upwards, and divided the periosteum in the line of the first incision, and afterwards, with Heine's

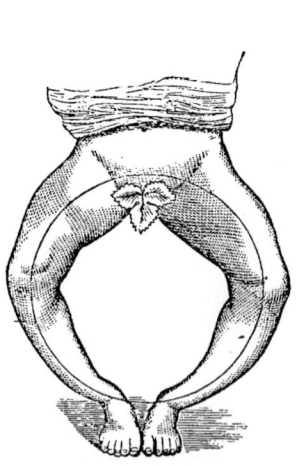 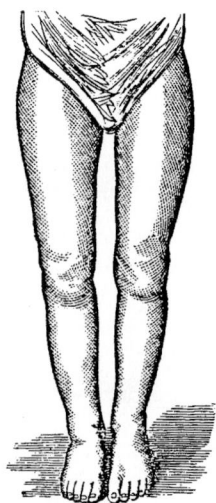

Osteotomy of Mayer for bow legs, 1853.

cutting-needle, separated the periosteum from the outer and posterior surface of the tibia, so as to prepare for the use of the saw. To protect the soft parts in that situation during the sawing, a strip of watch-spring, about half an inch wide was introduced between the denuded bone and the periosteum. Dr. Mayer, then, with a round saw, made two incisions converging towards the posterior part of the tibia, and meeting about a line and a half from the surface, without therefore quite cutting the bone in two. The wedge thus excised was about five lines thick at its base, and was easily removed by forceps. The wound was cleared of bone-dust by forcible injections of cold water, after which, through the flexibility of the remaining isthmus of the tibia and the mobility of the fibula, no difficulty was found in bringing the cut surfaces of bone into close apposition. The outer wound was brought together with the greatest accuracy by needles and ligatures (as for hare-lip), the haemorrhage being quite inconsiderable. The leg was then put into one of Boyer's hollow splints, used for fracture of the patella.

"Half an hour after the operation as, through the perfect apposition of the divided parts, no discharge of any kind was visible, the wound was covered with a thick layer of collodium, and upon this drying the ligature and needles were removed. The traumatic reaction was very slight, and on the fourth day the external wound (five inches long) had perfectly united. The leg was now left quiet in the splint for twenty-three days, when Dr. Mayer had the pleasure of finding that the incised surfaces of bone had united also. The next day the patient was allowed to walk in his room with crutches, and a few days afterwards in the garden without any artificial support whatever.

"On the 3rd of October the other leg was operated on in the same manner and with the same success. He left the hospital, free from deformity, and with a firm and natural gait, on the 19th of November."

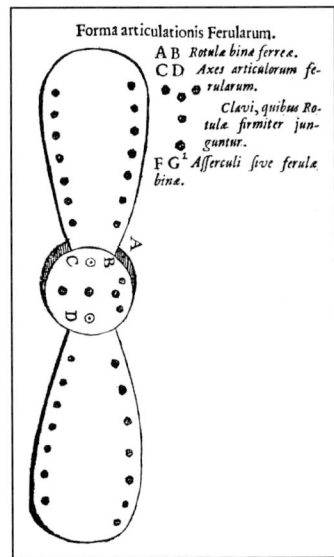

Glisson's splint for rachitic knee deformities, 1651. This was all that could be done before operations began.

Bone was initially cut with a chisel. Bernard Heine invented a clever little chain saw worked by hand in 1830. The idea was to protect soft tissues. Later, Macewen invented the osteotome we use today—sharpened both sides, it cuts straight.

Supracondylar Osteotomy, 1878

CLINICAL LECTURE ON ANTISEPTIC OSTEOTOMY DELIVERED AT THE ROYAL INFIRMARY, GLASGOW, BY

WILLIAM MACEWEN, M.D., SURGEON AND LECTURER ON CLINICAL SURGERY AT THE INFIRMARY

"Gentlemen, For some time past those of you who attend my wards have seen under treatment two patients on whom osteotomy was performed for the relief of knock-knee, and, as I intend performing a similar operation this morning, you will allow me to bring the subject of antiseptic osteotomy briefly under your notice.

♦ **Jean-Louis Mallet (1790–1847)**

It is said he was a protegé of Larrey, a military surgeon, during the heyday of battlefield amputations. He was left to deal with partial hand and foot amputations and tired of using a cannon ball to hammer an axe blade through the tissues. He introduced a chisel and a specially shaped hammer, which came to be known by his name.

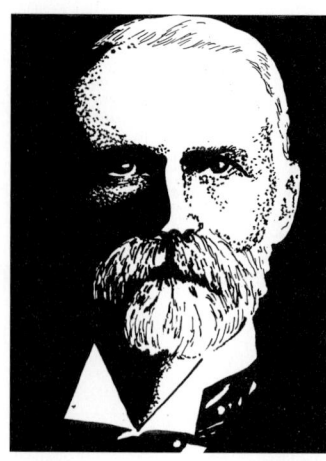

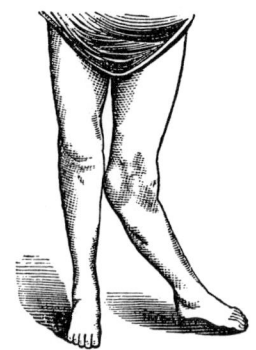
After first operation on right leg; the left leg in natural state.

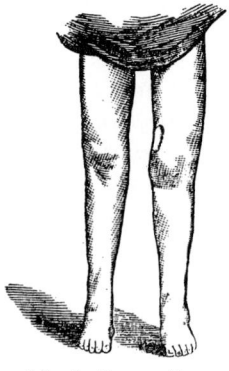
After both operations.

These woodcuts are taken from photographs.

Osteotomy by Macewen.

◆ **Sir William Macewen (1848–1924)**

The youngest of 12 children, he was born on the Isle of Bute and was graduated from Glasgow in the time of Lister and Syme. At the age of 28 he was elected to the surgical staff of the Royal Infirmary.

The new concept of antiseptic surgery was quickly assimilated by Macewen and enabled him to work up experimental operations so that they were safe, gave consistent results, and were no longer a desperate remedy but a widely applicable technique. For example, in 1877 he first performed subcutaneous osteotomy for genu valgum using an antiseptic technique; only seven years later he reported a series of 1800 osteotomies for this condition without any serious infection in a single case. There were, of course, a large number of cases of rickets in Glasgow at this time.

He found a chisel unsuitable for cutting bone transversely and devised a special instrument sharpened on both surfaces so that it did not deviate to one side, for which he coined the word "osteotome."

He was a pioneer of chest surgery and neurosurgery and introduced bone grafting and invented the endotracheal tube. Bone growth was his main research interest and he made many contributions; he made a special study of antler formation to further his knowledge of prodigious rates of bone growth.

"We may date the introduction of osteotomy, in its modern acceptation from the time when a firm faith in the value of antiseptics had gained possession of the minds of some surgeons who saw that they thus possessed a power enabling them with safety and surety to undertake operations which otherwise would be so dangerous to life that they were never contemplated."

Bone Grafting

For nearly three centuries osseous defects have been replaced by bone grafts. Perhaps the first person to do this was Dutch surgeon Jobi Meekren in 1682. He replaced a defect in the cranium of a soldier with a piece of dog's skull; the implant is said to have healed in perfectly. However, Jobi Meekren was required by the church authorities to remove the graft, under the ban of excommunication, as they refused to recognize such unchristian methods of treatment. This is recorded, not in the surgical literature, but in church records.

At the beginning of the 19th century, several surgeons transplanted bone with occasional success. A little later in the century Ollier performed a great volume of experimental work but was discouraged because his grafts were absorbed through being put in the soft tissues. Bone grafting, though it was clearly possible, did not become a practicality until the advent of antiseptic surgery. Macewen, who had studied under Lister and was fascinated by bone growth, produced some spectacular results, and a few surgeons copied him with varying success.

In about 1911 bone grafting became an accepted technique owing to the work of Fred Albee of New York (1876–1945). Albee used cortical bone grafts accurately carpentered to produce a cabinetmaker's joint. He moved away from the tools of a sculptor and introduced electrical saws. Looking back, it is surprising that bone grafting should have come into its own with cortical grafts

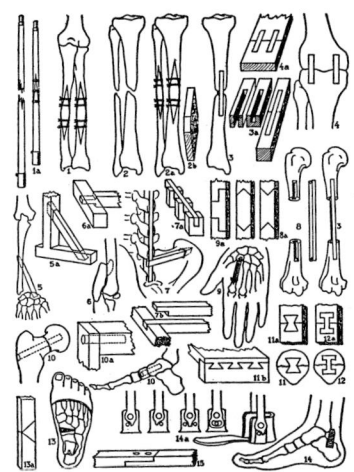

This drawing illustrates the precision joinery elements made possible by the electrically driven bone mill in bone surgery. The examples are self-evident analogies. Nos. 11 and 12 are keyed in members to hold in tension broken knee-caps which will not unite. No. 14 is a stop at the ankle joint itself, made of the patient's own bone, to prevent the foot from dropping, thus discarding metal brace, No. 14-a. No. 10 illustrates an un-united fracture of the hip with bone graft peg which has been shaped in the lathe component of the mill of an automatic size to the drill that made the hole for it.

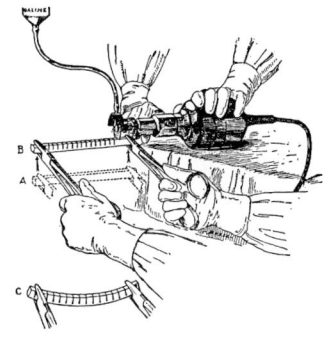

The power saw that allowed Albee to cut bone accurately.

Albee was the great bone grafter in the 1920s and 1930s. He was the most aggressive, egotistical surgeon of the day. From Albee FH: A Surgeon's Flight to Rebuild Men. An Autobiography. New York, 1943.

as these are looked upon today as not only more difficult to insert but also as less reliable than cancellous grafting.

Phemister in 1931 wrote the paper that coupled his name with cancellous grafting of ununited fractures. But in fact the paper is a very matter-of-fact comparison of different methods of treatment rather than an encouraging account. In 1933 Ghormley used iliac grafts for lumbosacral fusion but few surgeons followed him. The value of cancellous bone grafting was not widely appreciated until World War II when, perhaps, fixation was better and the graft was not required to provide both fixation and new bone. Rainsford Mowlem, a plastic surgeon, showed the clear supremacy of cancellous grafting for ununited fractures for the first time in 1944.

Macewen pointed out that deer can produce new bone to form a new pair of antlers in a few months, so our attempts to create bone seem clumsy by comparison. It seems likely that alternatives to bone grafting as a means of stimulating formation will be found. Bone marrow, bone morphogenic protein, and distraction osteogenesis are our current best hopes.

OBSERVATIONS CONCERNING TRANSPLANTATION OF BONE, ILLUSTRATED BY A CASE OF INTER-HUMAN OSSEOUS TRANSPLANTATION WHEREBY OVER TWO THIRDS OF THE SHAFT OF THE HUMERUS WAS RESTORED
BY WILLIAM MACEWEN, 1881

"William Connell, aged three years, was admitted into the Royal Infirmary, Glasgow, under my care, on July 17, 1878, in a much emaciated and exhausted condition arising from suppura-

tion in connection with necrosis of the right humerus. On August 7, 1878, the part of the necrosed bone exposed at the operation was divided by the bone forceps. The upper part of the shaft was then caught by lion forceps, rotated in order to loosen its periosteal attachments, and then pulled out. The lower portion was similarly dealt with."

The arm healed but was useless and the parents wanted amputation, but Macewen encouraged them to allow him to try to improve it.

"Transplantation of two wedges of bone on November 9, 1879 (one year and three months after the removal of the necrosed shaft): An incision was made down to the extremity of the upper fragment. This extremity was found to be cartilaginous for fully a quarter of an inch. This cartilaginous spike was removed leaving then a portion of bone which measured 1 3/4 inches from the tip of the acromion process. From this point a sulcus about 2 inches in length was made in a downward direction between the muscles. The former presence of bone was nowhere indicated, and the sole guide as to the correct position into which the transplant was to be placed was an anatomical one. After the sulcus was formed, the haemorrhage was fully arrested and an aseptic sponge was placed in the gap, which was then ready to receive the bone.

"Two wedges were then removed from the tibia of a patient six years of age, affected with anterior tibial curves. The last of these osseous wedges consisted of the anterior portion of the tibia, along with its periosteum, the wedges gradually tapering towards the posterior part of the tibia.

"They were removed, then cut into small fragments with the chisel, and immediately thereafter deposited into the sulcus in the boy's arm. They were kept under the spray while they were removed from the tibia until they were covered by the soft parts of the arm and its antiseptic dressing. . . . " [He repeated the graft on February 1 and July 9, 1880.]

"At the beginning of March, 1881, the bone was found firmly united, from the head to the condyles, and measured 6 inches, while the left humerus measured 6½ inches, that is to say half an inch longer than the transplanted one. The patient could lift his arm to his head and otherwise use it."

Macewen published a follow-up note in 1909.

"It is now thirty years since the humeral shaft was rebuilt and during the greater part of this period the man has depended on his physical exertions for the earning of his livelihood. He has worked as a joiner for many years and is now an engineer's pattern maker. His grafted arm has increased in length but not proportionate to the sound one. Measurements: The grafted humerus measures from the tip of the acromium to the tip of the *external condyle 10" but following the curve in the bone it is 11" long. The sound humerus from the same points measures 1¾" longer than the other."*

After this William Connell served in World War I.

Power Tools

Cortical bone is hard and needs to be worked like metal rather than wood. Chisels and osteotomes tend to split and break it unpredictably. The hand saws used for amputation needed more space than was permitted by the keyhole incisions of early surgeons scared of introducing infection. Heine in Germany produced a tiny chain saw worked like a hand drill. But anyone who has used a hand drill knows how difficult it is to be precise. Powered equipment is more accurate. An assistant using a dental drill with a foot treadle was the starting point. Then came fast-turning circular saws run by cables. This is what Albee used with such success. But other surgeons found them difficult to handle—I remember one fellow who touched the drapes with the spinning blade; the drapes were whisked off the patient and were spun like a huge flag over the open wound. Little wonder that oscillating blades were so welcomed.

Percutaneous fixation of fractures became popular only after air-powered drills and image intensifiers became available.

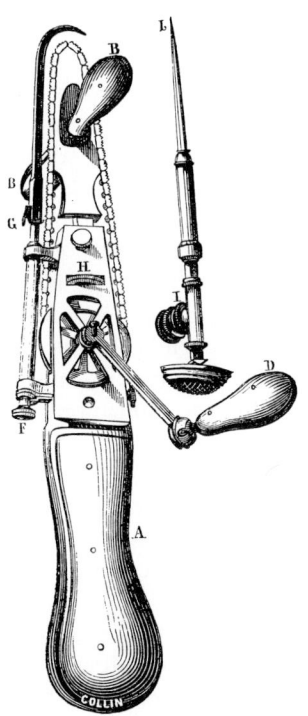

Heine's osteotome. It works like a small chain saw. From Ollier L: Traite des Resections. Paris, 1885.

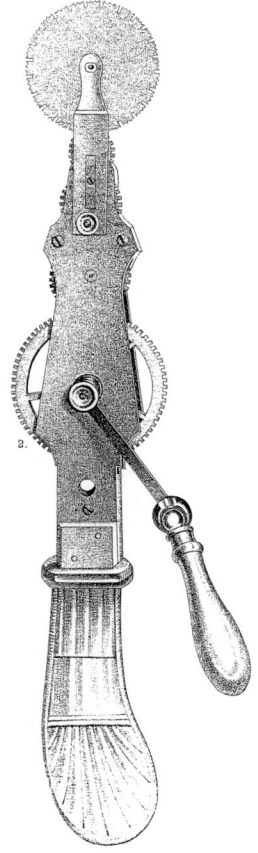

Mollett's saw, 19th century. When osteotomies were done, the kind of carpenter's saw used for amputations became unsuitable. From Medical and Surgical History of the War of Rebellion.

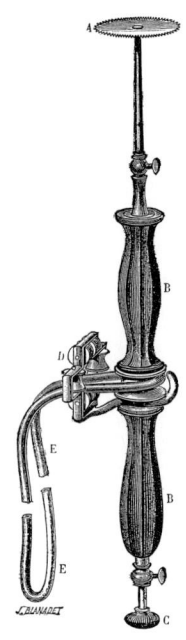

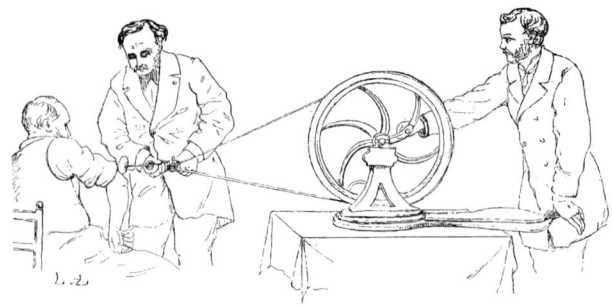

A circular saw with a rubber drive appears to be a challenge. Ollier, 1885.

Operations on Joints

Arthroplasty

Of all formal orthopaedic reconstructive procedures, the construction of new, movable joints was one of the first suggested. In Greek mythology, Pelops had a shoulder replaced by Klotho after Demeter had eaten it by mistake. The new shoulder was made of ivory. But excision arthroplasty generally preceded joint replacement.

In 1536, Ambroise Paré excised the elbow of a patient that had been destroyed by infection. In 1762, Filkin took out a knee joint damaged by tuberculosis in Norwich. In 1770, Charles White proposed excision of the head and neck of the femur, but did not carry it out except on cadavers. After this priorities are difficult to elucidate; one school developed arthroplasty for fixed joint deformities, and the other, larger school excised infected or severely damaged bone in the vicinity of the joints, and accepted the movement that occurred as a bonus. The instigators of each school lived on opposite sides of the Atlantic.

In 1822, Anthony White excised a hip joint at the Westminster Hospital, London, for sepsis, and for five years afterward the hip preserved good movement. John Rhea Barton performed an intertrochanteric osteotomy of the femur in Philadelphia in 1825 for a fixed flexed hip, and succeeded in producing a pseudarthrosis.

Similar operations were carried out in small numbers, and in 1831 Syme published a little book summarizing the indications for the procedure. Thirty years later, Hodge in America produced an excellent review but noted that the mortality from excision of the hip was about 50%, though this compared with a mortality rate of nearly 100% for amputation at the level of the hip. This encouraged Hugh Owen Thomas and others to advocate nonoperative treatment for infective hip conditions as far as possible.

After these early attempts at arthroplasty, stiffness seems to have been the main problem; further advances used devices to keep the raw bone ends apart. Carnochan used wood in 1840, Verneuil interposed muscle in 1861 and this remained popular,

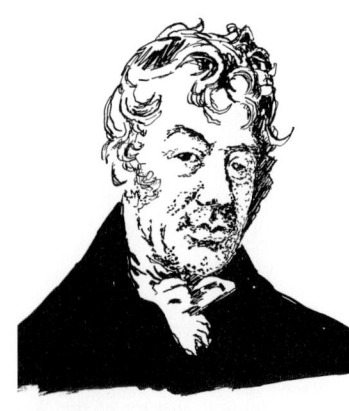

♦ Charles White (1728–1813)

but surgeons tried fascia, skin, oil, rubber, celluloid, ivory, and membranes whose origins would satisfy any witch doctor.

Themistocles Gluck experimented with bone cements to hold ivory prostheses. In 1890 he implanted a knee and a wrist. He presented these at one meeting and wanted to present them at an international meeting. He was not allowed to by his ex-chief, who said, "As the leader of German surgery I cannot allow you to discredit German science in front of a platform of international surgical specialists." A year later Gluck was pressured into reporting that his results in tuberculous joints were a failure, but 30 years later he reported success and he was honored.

J.E. Pean in Paris produced an artificial shoulder joint in 1893. It was made of rubber and platinum. He implanted it into a tuberculous shoulder and it lasted for 2 years. Pean removed it because of infection and ectopic ossification. The prosthesis can be seen at the Smithsonian Institution.

The Colonna capsular arthroplasty was described in 1932, based on principles laid down by Hey Groves. Subsequently, distraction proved sufficient to produce a pseudarthrosis after joint excision, and Robert Jones in 1921 and Girdlestone in 1945 became the principal advocates of this.

Excision arthroplasty, while satisfactory from many points of view, produced undesirable instability. Smith-Petersen of Boston realized that if the joint was to retain stability a proper congruous mechanical bearing was needed. This was the very situation in which the joint was most likely to fuse solid. He therefore introduced his cup to serve as an interposition membrane. At first he looked upon it as a mold—to mold the fibrocartilage as it developed over the raw bone ends—and planned to remove the mold when it had served its purpose. He spent a long time finding a suitable material from which to form a mold; he started with glass in 1923, then used viscalloid (an early form of plastic), Pyrex, and bakelite. Not until 1938 did he use vitallium. This became the arthroplasty of the 1940s.

In the 1950s the Judet brothers, Robert and Jean, dominated the scene with a new idea; replacement arthroplasty. The first one was carried out in 1946, and their experience appeared in book form in 1952. Their choice of material, acrylic, proved as unfortunate as Smith-Petersen's choice of his earlier materials, but it was forced on them because stainless steel and other metals were not available in France just after the war. The failures of the acrylic, and the difficulties with the nearly horizontal stem, paved the way for the development of the Austin Moore and Thompson prostheses with their stronger materials and better stem design. The relative softness of the head of the acrylic prosthesis had not revealed another potential difficulty of a replacement arthroplasty that has become apparent with metal prostheses—the acetabulum wears out in certain cases. Replacement of both the acetabulum and femoral head followed and is discussed in Chapter 2.

Silicone spacers for small joints began life in Alfred Swanson's laboratory in 1962 and were implanted in the first patient in 1966.

Parallel to the developments in the formation of false joints and new joints has been other attempts to revitalize joints by means of osteotomies. Kirmisson in 1894 suggested high femoral

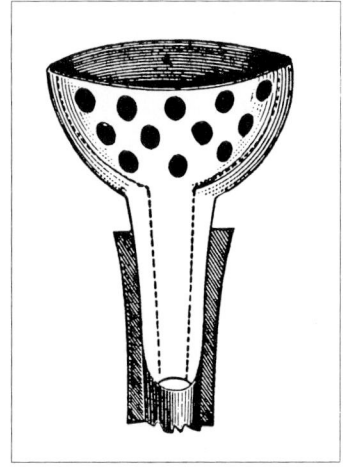

The ivory prosthesis designed by Gluck for the upper end of the tibia, to be used in arthroplasty of the knee. From Senn N: Tuberculosis of the Bones and Joints. Philadelphia: F. A. Davis, 1901.

osteotomy for long-standing irreducible dislocation of the hip. Lorenz in 1919 treated this condition by femoral section at the level of the acetabulum and displaced the distal fragment into the acetabulum to form a new joint. Shanz in 1922 described a lower osteotomy with angulation at the osteotomy site so that the upper fragment lay parallel to the pelvic wall, acting as a slight support.

This type of operation found a new use in 1935 when McMurray and Malkin independently published a small series of osteotomies for the deformities of osteoarthritis of the hip. The pain was relieved. This operation has been largely replaced by hip replacement.

EXCISION ARTHROPLASTY
ANTHONY WHITE, 1822

The first successful excision of the head of the femur was performed in Britain's Westminster Hospital by Anthony White in April, 1822.

"John West, when nine years old, slipped down stairs, and slightly hurt his left hip. After a few weeks, he was observed to limp in his gait, and complained of stiffness and pain in his groin, and subsequently he lost the power of locomotion, had the usual symptoms of disease in the hip-joint, and the head of the thighbone became displaced, and rested far back on the dorsum ilia. He suffered very acutely, and underwent the usual treatment of cupping, blistering, and every other method of local and constitutional treatment for many months, but without benefit, and after a time suppuration in the joint took place, which was evacuated from the front and upper part of the thigh. Temporary relief was thus obtained, but during two years a succession of similar abscesses formed around, and small portions of bone were frequently protruded through the sinuses which remained, and more especially, from those formed over the pubes. At the end of the third year, he was in the greatest possible state of emaciation, no longer suffering acute pain, but exhausted by the previous suffering, and by an overwhelming discharge from numerous apertures. The integuments over the displaced bone had become at various parts absorbed, and the bone at these points was readily found to be in a state of superficial caries. The knee had been long imbedded and immovably fixed on the inner side of the opposite thigh, and the right side on which he could alone lie, was cruelly galled with bedridden ulcerations. The formation of fresh abscesses had for some months ceased and further diseased processes were not apprehended. In the month of April, it was determined, in consultation with Travers, to remove the head of the bone; the circumstances of his health, with the exception of great emaciation, not forbidding it."

White made an incision, divided the bone 2 inches below the greater trochanter, and removed the upper end of the femur. The leg now became straight, and John West was nursed on his back with his leg in bandages.

The wound quickly healed; the various sinuses soon ceased to discharge; and the health of the patient speedily improved. Within 12 months he enjoyed the most useful compensation for the loss of the original joint, had perfect flexion and extension of the thigh, and every other motion except for turning the knee outward. The limb, of course, remained shorter, by as much as had been cut off from the top of the thigh bone.

He died of phthisis five years after the operation, and an opportunity was thus obtained to study the parts. The specimen, which was put in the museum of the Royal College of Surgeons, showed a fibrous ankylosis.

ON THE TREATMENT OF ANCHYLOSIS, BY THE FORMATION OF ARTIFICIAL JOINTS. A NEW OPERATION, DEVISED AND EXECUTED BY

J. RHEA BARTON, 1825

"I beg leave to call the attention of my professional brethren to the following paper, believing that it contains some new views, in relation to a deformity and lameness, hitherto, I think, excluded from the surgeon's list of curable complaints, and one of the opprobria of our art; I allude to a firm, bony anchylosis of the human joints.

"John Coyle, native of Philadelphia, twenty-one years of age, sailor on board the schr. Topaz, Captain Schyler, states, that on the 17th day of March, 1825, he fell from the hatchway into the ship's hold, upon the end of a barrel, a distance of about six or

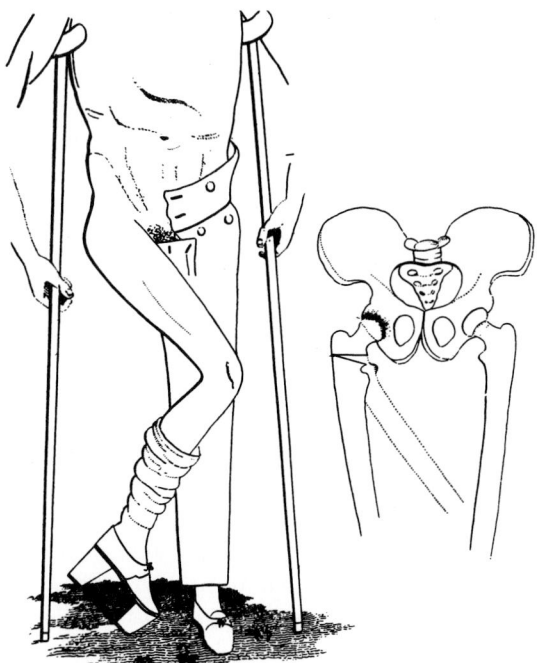

Hip arthroplasty. John Rhea Barton, 1825.

seven feet; that the force of the fall was sustained on the outside of his right hip; violent pain was the immediate consequence, and much tumefaction ensued; that after the injury, he arose with difficulty, and attempted to walk, thinks he made one or two steps, but was compelled to retire to his hammock, where he laid contracted for the space of about eighteen days; was then taken into Porto Cavello, and conveyed to the hospital. When lodged upon his bed, he placed himself on his side, with the injured limb uppermost, drawing the thigh to a right angle with the axis of the pelvis, and the knee resting on the sound side. In this posture he continued, without any material alteration, for the space of about five months, enduring all the suffering attendant upon a high degree of inflammation of one of the largest joints in the human body, and unalleviated by the support of splints, or a judicious antiphlogistic course of treatment. As might naturally be expected, a rigid and deformed limb was the result of such disease, combatted only by the administration of some simple liniment.

"*With regard to the real nature of the primary injury sustained, little can be said. The opinion on this point, of the medical attendant, under whose special care the patient was placed in the hospital, is not known. Dr. Murphy, surgeon general, who occasionally saw him, believed it to be a dislocation. On board of the Topaz, previous to his removal to the hospital, two physicians, belonging respectively to an English and French vessel of war, laying in port, inspected the limb, in company with the American Consul, Dr. Litchfield. Two of these gentlemen thought there was fracture; the French physician believed it to be some form of luxation. It is certain therefore, from the difference of sentiment, that there was much obscurity in the case.*

"*In October, 1825, Coyle returned to Philadelphia, having been sent home by our Consul.*

"*Early on his arrival, he exhibited himself to me. He was then supported by crutches, having the thigh drawn up nearly to a right angle with the axis of the pelvis, and the knee turned inward, and projecting over the sound thigh; so that the outside of the foot presented forward. There was considerable enlargement round the hip, which so much obscured the case, even at this date, as to prevent me from forming any positive opinion as to the real nature of the original injury. From the fixed and immovable condition of the limb, it was impossible to ascertain whether, in a straight position, there would be shortening, and, if any, to what extent. The general feature of the limb bore somewhat the resemblance of that resulting from a dislocation into the ischiatic notch; yet the position in which the great trochanter stood, in relation to the superior anterior spinous process, discouraged such a belief. All things considered, I was rather inclined to the opinion, that there had been neither fracture nor luxation; but that the violence of the fall had produced an extensive contusion of the round ligament and joint, and that disorganisation had followed the consequent inflammation. On this point, whatever might have been the nature of the accident, I thought I might feel assured, that now all articular movement* was gone, and that true anchylosis had taken place. Trusting, however, to the fallibility of my judgment, and wishing, for the patient's sake, that it might prove erroneous, I was induced to admit him into the Pennsylvania Hospital, with the view of employing extension on the limb for some weeks, in hopes that its malposition might thereby be corrected. A perseverance, however, in this treatment, only proved the unalterable state of the hip-joint, and confirmed my early formed opinion. He subsequently fell under the care of my estimable friends and colleagues, Drs. Hewson and Parrish, in their respective tours of surgical attendance in the hospital, where we several times considered his case in consultation, and were united in our final decision, that any further attempt to release the joint would be useless.

"Finding Coyle still in the hospital, a year after his admission, much reflection on his case led me to propose to my colleagues, the following operation, viz. to make an incision through the integuments, of six or seven inches in length, one half extending above, and the other below, the great trochanter; this to be met by a transverse section, of four or five inches in extent; the two forming a crucial incision, the four angles of which were to meet opposite to the most prominent point of the great trochanter; then to detach the fascia, and, by turning the blade of the scalpel sideways, to separate anteriorly all muscular structure from the bone, without unnecessarily dividing their fibres. Having done this, in like manner, behind and between the two trochanters, to divide the bone transversely through the great trochanter, and part of the neck of the bone, by means of a strong and narrow saw, made for the purpose; this being accomplished, to extend the limb, and dress the wound. After the irritation from the operation shall have passed away, to prevent, if possible, by gentle and daily movement of the limb, etc., the formation of bony union; and to establish an attachment by ligament only, as in cases of ununited fractures, or artificial joints, as they are called.

"In this proposition, four material points presented themselves for consideration, viz. the practicability of the operation; the degree of risk to life, consequent thereto; the probability of being able to arrest ossific re-union; and the reasonable prospect of benefiting the patient thereby.

"These views were fully explained to my colleagues, and were accompanied by the assurance, that my patient had been fairly apprised of his present condition, and of the nature and intentions of the operation proposed; that he had not merely acceded to it, but that, after placing his sufferings, the difficulties, risks to life, the chances of failure, and the dangers eventually of aggravated lameness, in the strongest and most exaggerated light, he had expressed his willingness to endure any pain, or duration of suffering, and to subject himself to all hazards, for the remotest prospect of relief.

"Accordingly, on the 22nd day of November, 1826, assisted by Drs. Hewson and Parrish, I proceeded to the operation publicly in the Pennsylvania Hospital.

"To a large medical class, and many respectable physicians, assembled, I again represented the nature of the case, and of the operation, and the views and course of reasoning which induced me to adopt it, stating likewise, that I wished it to be distinctly understood, that a submission to my contemplated plans had not been urged upon my patient by any false or delusory promises; but that an explanation of his existing condition, and of the means proposed to be attempted for his relief, were fully made to him, in language adapted to his right comprehension of the matter, as well as by my colleagues, as by myself; and that he had authorised me thus publicly to state, that he was prepared to assume all and the exclusive responsibility for the issue.

"With this exculpation, therefore, the operation, as already detailed, was put into effect. The integuments and fascia being divided and raised, the muscles in contact with the bone, around part of the great trochanter, were carefully detached, and a passage thereby made, just large enough to admit of the insinuation of my fore-fingers, before and behind the bone; the tips of which now met around the lower part of the cervix of the femur, a little above its root. The saw was readily applied, and, without any difficulty, a separation of the bone was effected. The thigh was now released, and I immediately turned out the knee, extended the leg, and placed the limbs side by side; by a comparison of which, in reference to length, the unsound member betrayed a shortening of about half an inch. This might have been caused partly by a distortion of the pelvis. Not one blood-vessel required to be secured. Union by the first intention was not attempted; the lips of the wound were only supported by adhesive plaster and slight dressings. The patient was put to bed, and Dr. Sault's splints were applied, to support the limb.

"The operation, though severe, was not of long duration, it being accomplished in the space of about seven minutes."

Postoperatively, the patient kept the leg still for nearly six weeks, and then began to move it in bed. By nine weeks the wound was soundly healed and he stood out of bed on crutches. A few days later he took a few steps and developed good control over the false joint.

Ten years later Barton gives a follow-up report about him.

"The patient, upon whom this operation was performed, enjoyed the use of his artificial joint for six years; during which period he pursued a business (trunk-making) with great industry, earning for himself a comfortable subsistence, and a small annual surplus.

"Pecuniary losses however, through the reverses of those in whose hands he had confided his means, sunk him into a state of despondency and desperation, followed by habits of intemperance. This, with its train of evils, abuse of health, etc., was, no doubt, the cause of the change which afterwards took place in the artificial joint. It gradually became more and more rigid, and finally, all motion ceased in the part. With this exception, the benefits of my operation were retained and fully appreciated *until the period of his death; for as the limb had been freed from deformity and restored to a useful position, he had no occasion even for a cane to aid in walking. During an attack of the Asiatic cholera, he expressed a desire that I should be sent for, in order that he might renew his bequest to me of the parts interested in the operation. He recovered from the cholera, but subsequently died of phthisis pulmonalis. The autopsy exhibited the parts as described in the published case, but with the artificial joint ancholysed; a change which had been effected within the two years previous to his death. With ordinary care, in all probability, this would not have taken place.*

"The final history of this case presents now the important fact, that benefit had resulted, which fully requited the individual for the pains he had endured, and were considered by him, even after the closure of the joint, yet all ample reward for the operation he had undergone."

In the original article he goes on to explore the possibilities of arthroplasty.

"Having now established the fact, that an artificial joint can be substituted for the loss of the natural articulation at the hip, it becomes a matter of importance to ascertain how far the same principles are applicable to the formation of new joints in other parts of the body, where natural motion has been lost. My reflections on the point, have not presented any forbidding circumstances but it is not in every joint, that the loss of motion would be sufficiently important to call for the aid of a painful operation. The most serious evil is sustained by the loss of the hip, knee, shoulder, elbow, great toe, and finger joints, and of the lower jaw, and these, I believe, may all come within the reach of amendment by operation, if the muscles which move these respective joints are in a sound and efficient state. If they have been lost, it would be palpably wrong to form a joint, since its unrestrained motion would be more troublesome than a rigid limb. A transverse section of the bones would be proper, if the operation were to be attempted at the shoulder, knee, fingers, or toes; but an angular division would be necessary at the elbow, in order to preserve some resemblance to the natural joint at this part.

"I hope I will not be understood as entertaining the belief, that this treatment will be applicable to, and judicious in, every case of anchylosis. I believe the operation would be justifiable only under the following circumstances, viz., where the patient's general health is good, and his constitution sufficiently strong; where the rigidity is not confined to the soft parts, but is actually occasioned by a consolidation of the joint; where all the muscles and tendons, that were essential to the ordinary movements of the former joint, are sound, and not incorporated by firm adhesions with the adjacent structure, where the disease, causing the deformity, has entirely subsided; where the operation can be performed through the original point of motion, or so near to it, that the use of most of the tendons and muscles will not be lost; and, finally, where the deformity, or inconvenience, is such, as

will induce the patient to endure the pain, and incur the risks of an operation."

ON THE DISEASES AND INJURIES OF THE JOINTS IN WHICH EXCISION MAY BE PERFORMED
JAMES SYME, 1831

"Owing to the improvements of modern surgery, more particularly in the treatment of aneurysms, fractures and necrosis, amputation of the extremities is now very seldom performed in civil practice except in cases of disease or injury of the joints.

"Though amputation is a measure very disagreeable both to the patient and to the surgeon, it has hitherto, with hardly any exception, been regarded as the only safe and efficient means of removing diseased joints which do not admit recovery. The idea of cutting out merely the morbid parts and leaving the sound portion of the limb, seems to have hardly ever occurred, or to have met with so many objections that it was almost instantly abandoned."

Arthrodesis

Perhaps the first person to carry out an arthrodesis for deformity was Henry Park in Liverpool in 1781. The son of an apothecary in Liverpool, he was apprenticed to Pott, to whom he dedicated the technique. Apart from describing arthrodesis, his other chief claim to fame is that he delivered Gladstone, a Victorian British Prime Minister.

AN ACCOUNT OF A NEW METHOD OF TREATING DISEASES OF THE JOINTS OF THE KNEE AND ELBOW IN A LETTER TO MR. PERCIVALL POTT
BY H. PARK OF LIVERPOOL, 1781

Joint infections all too often ended in amputations; he thought that there were other untried surgical methods that would produce a better result.

"The resource I mean is the total extirpation of the articulation, or the entire removal of the extremities of all the bones which form the joints, with the whole, or as much as possible, of the Capsular ligament; thereby obtaining a cure by means of Callus or by uniting the femur and tibia, when practised on the knee; and the Humerus, Radius and Ulna, when at the elbow, into one bone, without any movable articulation.

"The practicability of such an operation, with a probability of success, occurred to me some years ago; but as the undertaking appeared liable to many difficulties and objections, I wished to avoid being too precipitate in the attempt, and therefore frequently made it a subject of conversation with different Gentle-

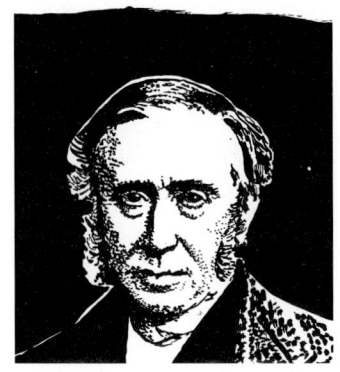

◆ **James Syme (1799–1870)**
Born in Princes Street, Edinburgh, the son of a lawyer. While a student at Edinburgh University, he found a way of dissolving rubber and discovered that when this was applied to material it became waterproof. Had he realized the commercial value of this, his name, and not that of Mackintosh, would have been attached to this product.

After qualifying, he opened a school of anatomy and later a very successful private clinic. For a short while he was professor of surgery at University College Hospital. He found it difficult to get on the staff of the hospital at Edinburgh; however, the professor of surgery eventually agreed to retire at the age of 81 on the condition that his successor paid him a pension. Syme acquiesced and obtained hospital beds. Later Lister became his assistant and married his daughter.

Syme is remembered for the introduction of conservative alternatives to major amputations. In 1831 he published a booklet on joint excision as an alternative to amputation for grossly diseased joints. Later, joint excision fell into disrepute because it tended to supplant all other methods of treatment for tuberculous joints, and the succeeding generation of surgeons decried it in favor of rest. He introduced his amputation in 1844 as an alternative to below-knee amputation, which was then the standard level.

men of the Profession. The principal difficulties that occurred, either from my own reflections, or the observations of my friends were as follows, viz.: the hazard of wounding the principal blood vessels; the great inflammation and large suppurations usually consequent on wounds of the articulations; the uncertainty of obtaining a firm callus; the loss of the insertions of the extensor muscles; the doubt respecting the utility of the limb, provided a cure could be obtained; the uncertainty of removing the whole disease when caries gave rise to operation; and, when undertaken on account of a scrophulous affection of the joints, the hazard of return of the same disease."

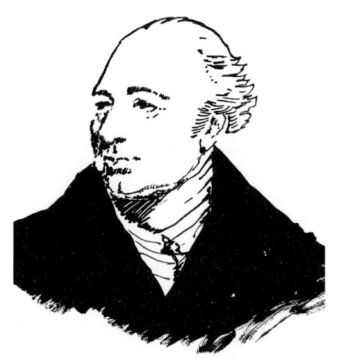

◆ Henry Park (1745–1831) Liverpool surgeon.

These difficulties he considered and finally discounted after rehearsing the procedure on cadavers. He decided to put the operation into practice.

"I had under my care in the Infirmary, Hector M'Caghen, a strong, robust, Scotch sailor, aged 33, who was admitted for a diseased knee of ten years standing. The joint, though pretty considerably enlarged, was by no means so much so as is frequently met with in scrophulous affections; yet the integuments were so tense as to appear incapable of further distension; the contraction of the Flexor Muscles was such as to draw back the leg, so as to form a right angle with the thigh, in which position it was immovably fixed; apparently some degree of union had begun to take place, but this could not yet be determined with certainty, as every attempt to communicate to the joint the smallest amount of motion, gave him the most excruciating pain."

Conservative treatment did not help, and the patient's pain led him to request amputation. Park suggested his operation, and carried it out on 2nd July, 1781. He made a cruciate incision, removed the patella, and sawed off 2 inches of femur and 1 inch of tibia, making transverse cuts. This was just enough to allow the sawn ends of the bones to be in close contact, held by the contracted hamstrings. He inserted a few skin sutures, applied a minimum of dressings, and placed the leg in a case of tin.

The wound discharged profusely for some time and did not heal for about three months. The patient started to go about on crutches, and by five months after the operation union was strong enough for him to lift the leg up straight, and in another month it felt solid. He subsequently had 3 inches shortening, and wore a raised shoe and a protective leather support. Hector M'Caghen returned to sea once more with a leg that felt strong. (In the same letter Park describes an arthrodesis of elbow.)

Syme gives a little more of the history of Hector M'Caghen. He continued as a sailor and was shipwrecked twice without his leg causing any trouble, finally drowning in the Mersey when a boat overturned.

MOREAU, 1782

P. F. Moreau's father wrote, but did not publish, the following idea:

[1782: The elbow joint.] *"The caries should affect the whole of the joint. I would not hesitate to cut it out. I would bring the cut ends of the bone together; and while the contraction of the muscles would retain them in contact, I would keep the limb fixed, as in cases of fracture. and wait patiently, till nature should unite the bones together by callus."* He did an excision of the shoulder joint in 1786 and reported it. But his Medical Society suppressed the report. In 1792 he excised a knee joint, and this was reported by his son.

Exactly 100 years later Albert of Vienna suggested arthrodesis as a means of treating flail limbs.

SOME CASES OF ARTIFICIALLY PRODUCED ANKYLOSES IN PARALYZED LIMBS
E. ALBERT, 1881

"I have tried the idea of making paralysed legs, especially those incapable of bearing weight due to poliomyelitis, more useable and more independent of appliances by artificial ankylosis in the following cases and found it successful:

"Josef F., aged 22; admitted 20 July 1881. Left leg, especially calf, grossly wasted. Muscles of hip joint functioning perfectly. Knee and foot completely flail; foot in slight equinus. This leg which was attacked by poliomyelitis in childhood is notably shorter.

"20 July. Resection of the knee joint through Volkmann's incision and division of the patella. Removal of the capsule. Enough cut off the femur to allow the level of section to pass through the fossa intercondyloideus; a thin disc cut off the tibia. Two bone sutures between femur and tibia, and one between the two halves of the patella. Sutures, drainage, Lister bandage, and splint fixation.

"The wound healed mostly per primam, but in a few places with some sepsis.

"2 September. Erysipelas was in the wound.

"11 September. Abscess opened below tuberosity. Erysipelas faded.

"15 October. Firm joint confirmed.

"2 November. Silver wires removed; joint solid and immoveable.

"After the patient had walked around for some time on crutches he was, at the end of November, given a support which was fixed to the unstable foot by means of a lace-up boot and two side irons. The irons pass above the knee so as to protect the rigid knee joint from accidental injury for some time. At discharge on 12th December the knee is completely ankylosed.

"Another knee fusion. Successful.

"Another knee fusion. Some movement remained.

"Therese W., aged 11. Struck down by poliomyelitis aged 1 year. Left leg almost 3 cm short, wasted. Calf much more wasted than the thigh. Hip and knee joint normally actively mobile. Foot in fixed equino-varus position. Pronounced hump on the dorsum of the foot. Toes capable of active flexion and the existing plantar

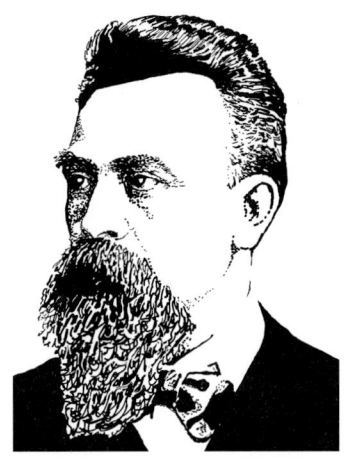

◆ **Eduard Albert (1841–1900)**

Born in Bohemia and studied in Vienna. He became professor of surgery at Innsbruck in 1873 and later transferred to Vienna. An excellent teacher and man of ideas, he described arthrodesis to improve the function of flail limbs, synovectomy, the transplantation of nerves, sciatic scoliosis, and Achilles bursitis.

flexion could be increased. The dorsal group of muscles paralysed. The foot completely unstable, walking difficult.

"29 December, 1881. Achilles tenotomy, then the ankle joint opened up through a dorsal incision which also divided the attenuated tendons of the toe extensors. The cartilage covering the talus and the articular surface of the fibula removed. The cartilage was extraordinarily easy to peel off, as is almost always the case with paralysed extremities. Wound sutured, Lister bandage, plaster cast.

"On the sixteenth day erysipelas spreading only over the calf and disappearing by the 23rd day. In order to relieve the equinus deformity of the foot and to ankylose it in the neutral position of the ankle joint the plaster cast had to be removed several times and replaced after further correction. When the last cast was applied it appeared that slight overcorrection had been produced so that a minor degree of pes calcaneus seemed to have developed. In order to achieve better control, the leg was fixed to a splint, of which the longer part was fixed to the calf and the shorter to the foot, fixing the two at right angles. After 6 weeks the patient could put her weight on the foot. She was discharged 9 weeks after operation; the talus and lower leg were firmly united; the foot was in a position of very slight pronation; in walking the leg moved in one piece, but the foot was no longer unstable and the patient was plantigrade. She was given a supporting appliance (a lace-up shoe with a side iron).

"The cases I report can only be regarded as encouraging; the expected results were achieved, in fact one might say that the results exceeded expectation since one might have doubted whether bone might be expected to fuse in a paralysed leg.

"But nor should these cases be considered more than encouraging; only further experience can show how one should plan the operative technique and how applicable this method is to other joints."

Joint Transplantation

There was a flurry of interest in joint transplantation at the beginning of the 20th century in Europe. Joint surfaces from cadavers were used, cartilage from old dislocations was removed and reapplied to the reconstructed joint, and toe joints were put somewhere more important.

JOINT TRANSPLANTATION AND ARTHROPLASTY

ERICH LEXER, 1907

"The first case of half joint transplantation operated upon by me in 1907 was a cystic sarcoma in the upper third of the tibia. The transplant, which was taken from a freshly amputated leg, took exceptionally well with very good motion and capacity for weight bearing. In spite of the fact that the joint surfaces did not articulate exactly, since the transplant had to be taken from

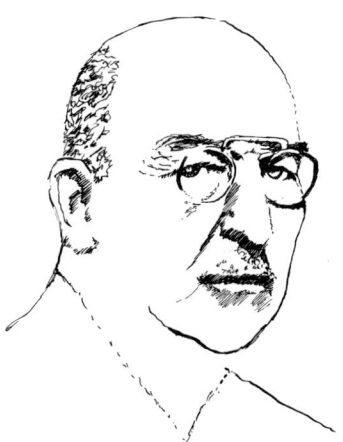

◆ **Erich Lexer (1867–1937)**
Leaving painting for the study of medicine, he became professor of surgery at several German universities. He was a researcher and especially interested in transplantation of all kinds of tissues. He wrote several textbooks, including a textbook of general surgery, which was translated into English and published in New York.

a leg which did not correspond as to right and left, only at the beginning was there noticed, on bearing weight, a slight looseness. In spite of the best clinical results an amputation had to be performed 1 year and 5 months later because of religious convictions of the patient's. The specimen showed complete union with the diaphysis. There were no adhesions in the joint. The crucial ligaments were united with the tibia. The joint cartilage was everywhere well maintained.

"*In my first case of knee joint transplantation which was operated upon in 1907, there is still after 16 years, painless and good weight-bearing and joint motion sufficient for going up and down stairs. The patient was caught in the Russian drive on East Prussia and had to march days at a time.*

"*A total of 300 cases of large joint have been operated upon of which 242 are very good or good, 34 are failures, and 24 are questionable.*"

Most of Lexer's writings, including a book on transplantion, are in German.

Operations on Tendons

If it were not for tenotomy, we would still be nomads and hunters. Why? Because the first step in domesticating wild animals was to cut their tendo Achillis so that they could not run away. Later, the tendons of enemy soldiers were cut to make them useless. The heelcord was cut so that they could not walk for a while, and the flexor of the thumb was cut so that they could not raise a sword. There are many stories of tenotomy in mythology.

The ancients are said to have repaired tendons and nerves, but as they did not distinguish between these structures until the Renaissance, information is a little uncertain.

Tenotomy was the operation that put orthopaedics on the map. Why? It could be done without anesthesia and asepsis. The risk of infection was small, and the gain could be large.

In the 17th century, tenotomy began to be practiced in Holland. Isaac Minnius performed a tenotomy for torticollis in 1685. A hundred years later Lorenz of Frankfurt treated a clubfoot by division of the tendo Achillis. Delpech of Montpellier repeated this on several occasions between 1816 and 1823 but gave it up because of complications, leaving it to Guérin and then Stromeyer to popularize it from 1831 onward. It was brought to England, as will be described, by Little, and was soon to be used for a range of fixed deformities—even for squint.

Myotomy came into vogue soon afterward but floundered after a period of trial on the posterior vertebral muscles in the treatment of scoliosis.

Tendon transfers filled the needs of the thousands of patients with infantile paralysis, but not until after the invention of aseptic surgery toward the end of the 19th century. Then the procedure took off and its success contributed to the movement to separate

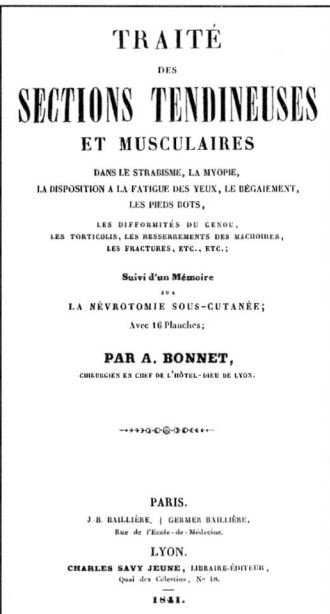

Title page from book of Bonnet, 1841.

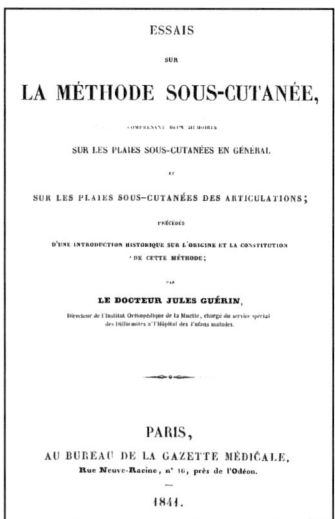

Title page from Guérin's book on tenotomy, 1841.

musculoskeletal surgery from generaly surgery. Many new operations were invented, which are now forgotton, along with polio.

Tenotomy

CLUBFOOT AND ITS TREATMENT BY TENOTOMY
WILLIAM JOHN LITTLE, 1839

"In most cases of talipes equinus, and in many of T. varus, which require an operation, the tendo Achillis only is required to be divided. In other cases of Talipes equinus I have sometimes found it necessary likewise to divide the tendons of the tibialis posticus and flexor longus pollicis muscles. In severe long-standing cases of Talipes varus the section of the tendons of the anterior tibial, posterior tibial, extensor proprius and flexor longus pollicis muscles is requisite, in addition to division of the tendo Achillis, in order to facilitate the restoration of the foot to its natural shape and position. The case of congenital Talipes valgus already mentioned will indicate the parts which it may be found necessary to divide in that form of disease.

"As I regard Stromeyer to be the originator of this important addition to our means of curing club-foot, with other contractions of the ankle, and similar deformities of various parts of the body, and having experienced in my own person the success of his method of treatment, corroborated by the numerous cases which I have cured by the same means, I shall here only briefly enumerate the principles recommended by Stromeyer to be followed.

"The tendons of the muscles which maintain the deformity should be divided with as little injury as possible to the skin and neighbouring parts.

"No attempt should be made to force the foot into its natural shape immediately after the operation; but the necessary extension for that purpose should be commenced as soon as the external punctures are completely healed; this occurs about the second or third day.

"The lymph which is effused between the ends of the divided tendon or tendons, with the muscles that are not divided, and the ligaments and fasciae which may impede the replacement of the foot, must be gradually extended until the foot assumes its natural shape, and the ankle can be bent to its fullest extent.

"The application of the apparatus by which extension is effected must be continued for a certain period after the cure, notwithstanding that the patient has been enabled to stand firmly, and has improved in walking, in order to obviate the tendency to contraction evinced by the intermediate substance or lymph effused between the ends of the divided tendon."

Little quotes the technique of tenotomy from Stromeyer:

"The operation must invariably be effected by puncture, with-

out external incision. A very small cutting instrument should be selected—a small, moderately curved, sharp-pointed bistoury is adapted for most occasions. The limb should be extended, in order to produce the necessary projection of the tendon, when the instrument should be passed behind it, the point perforating the opposite skin; division of the tense resisting tendon being effected rather by pressure of the edge than by its slow and cautious onward movement. The skin, being elastic, yields to the pressure of the knife, the two punctures not exceeding its width. I have frequently divided the tendo Achillis in this manner without producing a second puncture; but this is of little moment, as two minute punctures heal as quickly as a single one. The division of the tendon is known by an accompanying sound, which can scarcely be mistaken. The performance of the operation with the point of the instrument is less to be relied on, partly from its being too weak, and also because the operator can be less certain of not causing injury io other structures in the event of the patient not remaining quiet throughout the operation. . . . The attempt to commence extension directly after the operation, and the endeavour immediately to restore the limb to its natural position, which will very seldom succeed, and, as the case of Sartorius proves, can only be effected by great force, is neither necessary nor advisable. The commencement of extension before cicatrisation of the wound in the integuments is unadvisable even when possible, as it may produce inflammation and suppuration not confined to the vicinity of the wound; it is unnecessary, inasmuch as the tension of the divided muscle is not restored during the gradual mechanical extension applied subsequently to the healing of the wound, but occurs after the complete reunion of the tendon and after the necessary motions of the limb during exercise have acted as a stimulus to its contractility."

Tendon Transfer

Many cases of polio provided a fertile field for the development of tendon transfers—it was one of the commonest operations.

SIR ROBERT JONES (1857–1933)

Robert Jones is a name that keeps recurring in British orthopaedics because he built up a school of orthopaedics, because he built up a system of organization for the care of orthopaedic patients, and because he made many contributions over the whole field. Most of all he is remembered because he was liked, and popularity provides opportunities denied other men.

Robert's father, destined by the family to be a prosperous architect, gave up everything to write, and in consequence was poor and found it difficult to support his children. When Robert was 16, he went from his home in London to live with his uncle Hugh Owen Thomas in Liverpool, who sent him to medical school. He had been at Thomas' house before with his brother on a famous

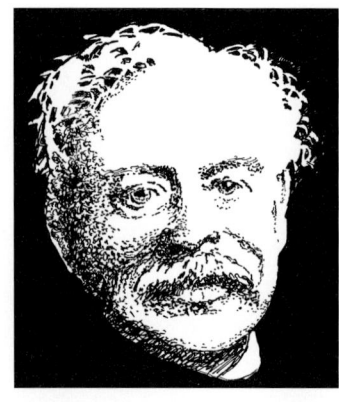

◆ Sir Robert Jones (1857–1933)

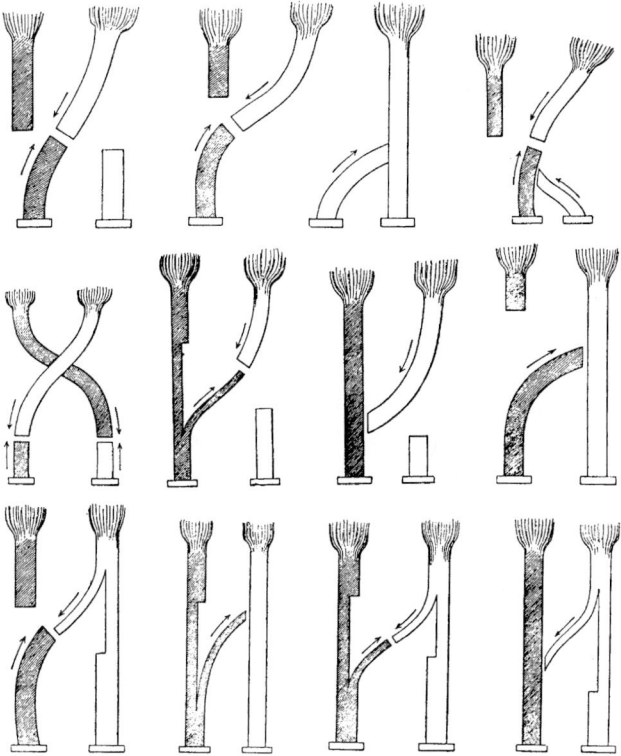

Tendon transplantation, 1906. From Young JK: Orthopaedic Surgery. Philadelphia, 1906.

occasion when he and his brothers had decided to become sailors. Robert's father had asked Thomas what he should do about this. Thomas, who had shares in some ships, put the boys on the ship with the most disagreeable captain. Robert's brother took along a gun to shoot birds, but at an early stage in the voyage put a shot through the mate's hat. If the result of that did not put them off the sea, a storm shortly afterward did so. They did not complete the voyage but landed prematurely, and Robert was pleased to look forward to a medical career.

He qualified in 1878, and worked part-time with Thomas, in general practice, until the latter's death in 1891. He was appointed General Surgeon to the Royal Southern Hospital, Liverpool, in 1899, but restricted himself to orthopaedics from 1905. In the early nineties he organized and administered the Casualty Service during the building of the Manchester Ship Canal.

In 1900 Agnes Hunt opened the Basechurch Home. It was a farmhouse and stables in which she looked after a few crippled children. When they needed surgery, she sent them to Liverpool. In 1903 her own stiff hip began to give her trouble, and she consulted Robert Jones. Soon afterward she interested him in these children, and from this small, informal beginning there grew the Robert Jones and Agnes Hunt Orthopaedic Hospital at Oswestry, serving most of the center of England and Wales.

When World War I broke out, Jones was aged 57—a man whose reputation was international. At first he cared for 500 orthopaedic casualties at Alder Hey, Liverpool, and published an excellent book on injuries to joints in 1916. He quickly ascended the military hierarchy and became Director General of Military Orthopaedics. He organized a scheme for disabled servicemen at Shepherd's Bush, London.

Soon after the war ended, he put the camaraderie which had been engendered to good use, forming the British Orthopaedic Association, and set out on the third stage of his career. He had shown the path for the overall care of crippled children at Basechurch, and for disabled servicemen at Shepherd's Bush; he now set himself the task of a national scheme for the detection, treatment, and training of cripples. He helped found the Central Council for the Care of Cripples and altered everyone's approach to the problem.

"If I were made dictator, I would have an accident centre in each large city, where cases could be properly treated, and for as long as necessary. I would have beds for adults in each orthopaedic hospital and small county hospital to act as casualty clearing stations."

His literary output was considerable, averaging about four papers a year on every aspect of orthopaedics, and it is difficult to select one particular extract for inclusion.

Robert Jones made orthopaedics a specialty.

A typical half-day operating list shows how things have changed since his day:

Royal Southern Hospital Liverpool
3rd September 1913
Mr Robert Jones 2 PM

1. Adhesions L shoulder joint
2. Old Colles fracture. Manipulation
3. Genu varum. Moulding
4. Old fracture radius and ulnar. Manipulation
5. Genu varum. Osteoclasis
6. Talipes equinovarus. Tenotomy & Wrenching
7. Infantile paralysis. EHL to MI. Peroneus longus to scaphoid
8. Pes calcaneo-cavus
9. Loose body outer side left knee joint
10. Pes calcaneo-cavus
11. Metatarsalgia
12. Spastic paraplegia
13. Removal nodule scapula
14. Genu varum. Wedge from tibia
15. Excision TB knee
16. Cong dislocation hip
17. Cong dislocation hips
18. TB tarsus
19. Malunion Potts
20. Elbow fracture
21. Cleft palate
22. Nephropexy

Robert Jones' Rules for Tendon Transfer

His rules appear in several forms and demonstrate the rapid changes in attitude that occurred in the first few years of the 20th century. The rules he enunciated in 1908 are given first, and then a later edition of them prepared for his textbook of orthopaedics by McMurray in 1921.

1908 Version

In tendon transplantation one must insist on:

1. *The over-correction of deformity as a preliminary measure.*
2. *The removal of skin flaps to secure uninterrupted continuity of the over-correction. Ellipses of skin were removed from the paralysed side of a joint and the incision closed to hold the over-corrected position.*
3. *The direct and not angular deflection of the tendon.*
4. *The free tunnelling in the one plane through soft tissues.*
5. *The firm suturing into periosteum or bony groove.*
6. *The careful choice, tension, and nursing of the transplanted tendon.*
7. *The maintenance of the hypercorrected position until voluntary power is assured to the tendon.*
8. *The deflection of body weight during walking from the reinforcing tendon.*

In addition to these, it may sometimes be well to shorten the paralysed tendons and prevent the overaction of their opponents by tenotomy.

All my hospital transplantations are treated as out-patients, and return to their homes on the day of operation, and no difficulties of any kind arise therefrom.

1921 Version

Certain rules for tendon transplantation:

First: *The joints upon which the transplanted tendons are called upon to act must be rendered as mobile as possible.*

Second: *The muscle and tendon for transplantation must be of sufficient strength to accomplish the action for which it is to be employed.*

Third: *The transplanted muscle and tendon must pursue a straight course between its origin and its insertion, and should not work obliquely or round an angle.*

Fourth: *The transplanted muscle must be attached under slight tension.*

TIMELINE OF TENDON TRANSFERS

1770 Missa transferred the extensor tendon of the index finger to the middle finger after injury

Box continued on following page

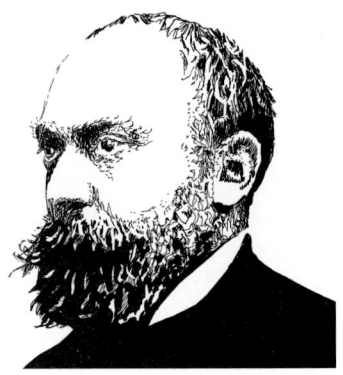

◆ **Carl Nicholadoni (1847–1902)**
Professor of Surgery at Innsbruck.

1873 Polaillon: after rupture of the extensors of the index, middle, and ring fingers, he attached the distal end to the extensors of the thumb and little fingers.
1874 Tillaux did something similar.
1875 Duplay and Tillaux: extensor carpi radialis to extensor pollicis longus
1881 Nicholadoni: transferred peroneal tendons into the tendo Achillis for paralytic equinus. The long-term result was poor.
1892 Milliken and Parrish of New York suture the extensor digitorum longus to the tibialis anterior without dividing it. The results were mediocre.
1892 Drobnik in Poland did some foot transfers and a transfer for radial nerve palsy. His results were better.
1894 Goldthwait: like the others he believes he is doing something new when he repeats Nicholadoni's operation. Francke and 2 years later Eulenberg use tendon transfers in cerebral palsy.
1902 Waterman reviews the history of transfers.

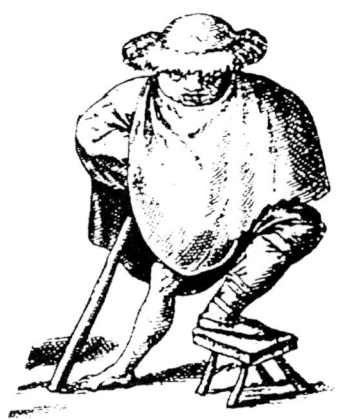

◆ **Hieronymus Bosch**

Limb Length Equalization

Polio resulted in many children with a short leg, and equalizing length by something better than a shoe lift was a challenge. In the 1920s, attempts were made to stimulate growth by increasing the blood supply to the growth plate by playing tricks on it, but the results were disappointing.

The idea of arresting growth had occurred to Ollier, but it was Phemister who first carried it out in Chicago in 1933.

Blount popularized equalization by staple epiphyseodesis in 1949. The timing of this operation was crucial, and, beginning in 1947, Green and Anderson produced graphs of the growth of the lower limbs to improve the accuracy of discrepancy prediction. Today these graphs could not be produced. No ethics review board

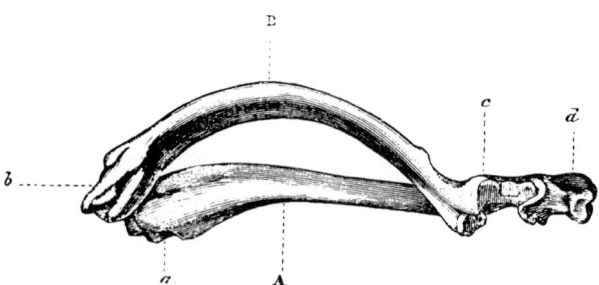

Experimental growth arrest of the ulna after excision of the distal growth plate. The radius becomes bowed. Ollier, 1885.

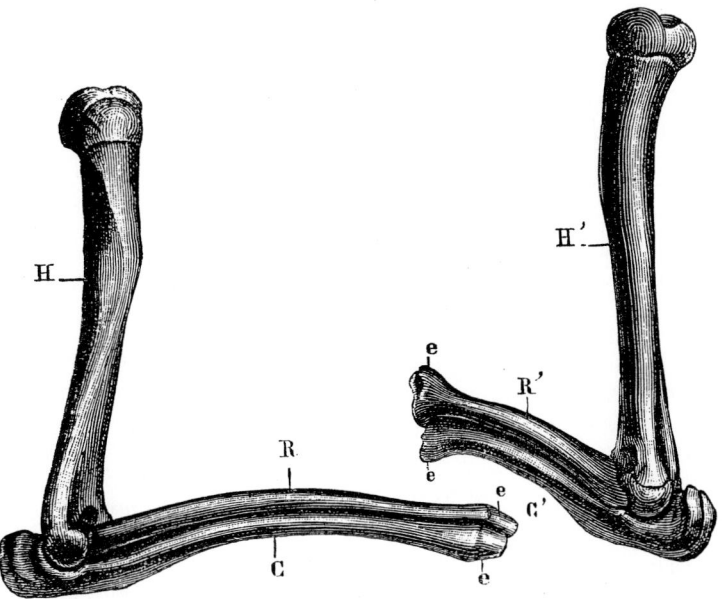

Experimental growth arrest of the distal radius and ulna by Ollier. He considered putting this to clinical use. From Treatise on Resections and Conservative Operations on the Osseous System, 1885.

would allow yearly radiographs of 100 normal children for this purpose.

Their graphs are still used. *"We do not attempt to reduce predictions of the result to a precise, mathematical formula. With the knowledge of the range of the possible effect and of the factors affecting the range, however, the timing of an arrest becomes a practical clinical decision for the individual child."*

The only way to make up big differences without loss of stature is by limb lengthening—by cutting the bone and distraction during healing.

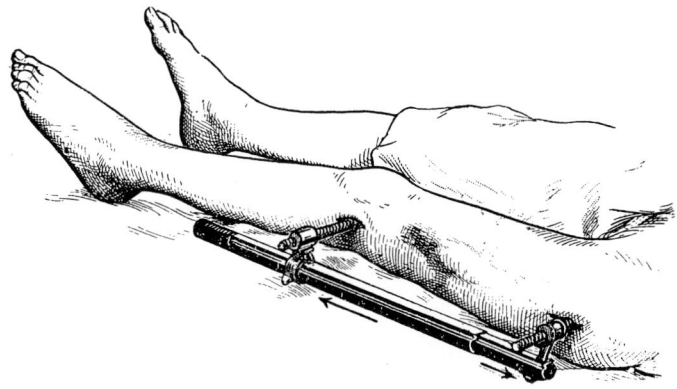

Femoral lengthening. Putti, 1920. From Jeanbrau E, et al: Chirurgie Reparatrice et Orthopaedique.

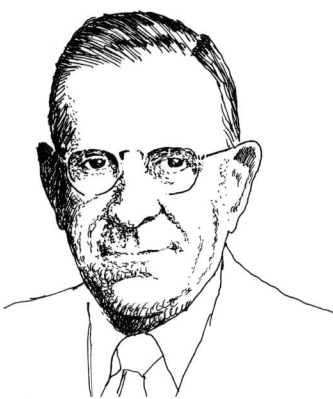

◆ **William T. Green (b 1901)**

He trained in general and orthopaedic surgery in Detroit and was chief at the Children's Hospital in Boston from 1946. He was President of the American Academy of Orthopaedic Surgeons in 1957. He had an enormous influence on the training of orthopaedic surgeons in children's surgery. He was tough on trainees and was famous for going round the ward in the middle of the night and putting a cross on casts that had to be changed before morning. It was rumored that there were more cast rooms than operating rooms. The prediction of lower extremity growth was his main claim to fame. He was active in cerebral palsy care and the transfer of the flexor carpi ulnaris to the back of the wrist is known after him.

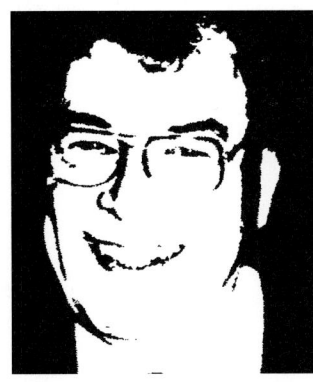

◆ **Heinz Wagner (contemporary)**

Professor at Altdorf. A great technical surgeon who invented osteotomies for the sequelae of developmental dislocation of the hip and stimulated interest in leg lengthening. His fixator was excellent, but the idea of delaying lengthening until callus formed had not dawned, so grafting and plating were usually required.

TIMELINE FOR LIMB EQUALIZATION

- **1840s** Bernhard Heine proposes bone shortening to equalize length.
- **1847** Francesco Rizzoli in Bologna shortens a femur to equalize length. Others consider this unwise.
- **1877** Ollier proposes epiphyseodesis.
- **1905** Codvilla of Bologna lengthens by oblique osteotomy, and an acute lengthening using a calcaneal pin and cast.
- **1908** Paul Magnusson shows that the soft tissues accommodate to lengthening in dogs. He lengthened a patient by up to 4 inches acutely, and one died of shock.
- **1911** Lambret of Lille, France: two transfixion pin leg distraction
- **1914** Arbuthnot Lane notes that staples across the growth plate halt growth.
- **1916** R. Tunstall Taylor: shortening osteotomy using a double-step cut
- **1921** Vittorio Putti in Bologna uses a monolateral fixator and gains 3 to 4 inches in the femur.
- **1927** Leroy Abbott frame for lengthening the tibia. He performed a tendo Achillis lengthening and divided the fibula and the periosteum.
- **1929** Bohlman uses foreign material implanted near the growth plate to stimulate growth.
- **1929** Jones and Lovett: Z osteotomy with distractor
- **1930** Harris uses sympathectomy to stimulate growth.
- **1932** Other frames published using K wires
- **1933** Phemister stops epiphyseal growth by operating on the growth plate.
- **1936** Compere writes about complications.
- **1939** Abbott and Saunders add massive releases.
- **1947** Green and Anderson: growth charts to predict the timing of epiphyseodesis
- **1948** Allan's apparatus using K wires on a frame. He did an oblique osteomy and fixed this with screws when he had gained length.
- **1949** Blount and Clarke: staple epiphyseodesis
- **1950** Janes at the Mayo clinic begins a long flirtation with producing arteriovenous fistulas to promote growth.
- **1951** Ilizarov: Circular frame for distraction osteogenesis. The principle of delay to allow callus formation before distraction and slow lengthening several times a day avoids the problem of nonunion. The method does not become known in the West for 30 years.
- **1952** Anderson apparatus: His frame was the standard for many years. He fixed the fibula to the distal tibia and carried out a drill osteotomy with preservation of the periosteum. Patients were bedfast.
- **1958** Soffield, Blair, and Millar have many complications.
- **1963** Wagner distractor: this was the first that allowed the patient to get out of bed. Most patients need plating and bone grafting.

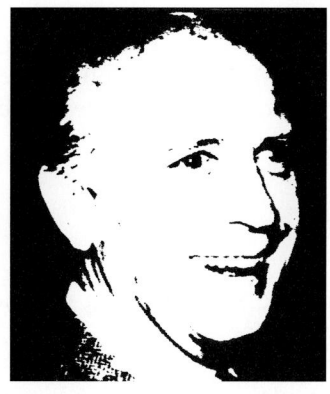

◆ **DeBastiani**
Until recently he was professor in Verona, where he developed callotasis and a very adaptable lengthener.

1965 Kuntschner: closed shortening over intramedullary nail.
1986 DeBastiani develops the Orthofix and promotes growth plate distraction as well as callotasis (callus distraction).

Gavriil A. Ilizarov

"The Principle of Tension-Stress that governs the response of tissues to elongation: living tissue, when subjected to slow steady traction, becomes metabolically activated in both the biosynthetic and proliferative pathways, a phenomenon dependent on vascularity and functional use."

Rehabilitation

The word means making patients self-sufficient after injury or disease. The word shares its origin with the gown worn by a monk—the monk's "habit." So rehabilitation means putting on the clothes of rank again and getting back to work. It is not an old idea.

In the past, the prospect of rehabilitating the battle-injured was so bleak that many were put out of their misery by a killing blow—the coup de grace. Then came an era of convalescent homes in which people rested while recovering from postoperative anemia and malnutrition. Told to "take it easy," many remained disabled permanently. Rehabilitation is demedicalizing patients so that they build up their muscles and build up their spirits.

An orthopaedic enthusiast was Sir Reginald Watson Jones, famous for the telling phrase:

The average man who lies in bed for weeks and months, asking for this, ordering that, commanding the other, becomes the king of a little universe which revolves around him. The germ of chronic invalidism is easily implanted.

Getting fit is a whole time job.

Real rehabilitation is getting into the mind of a man, finding out what his anxiety is, and his worry and fear, and removing them.

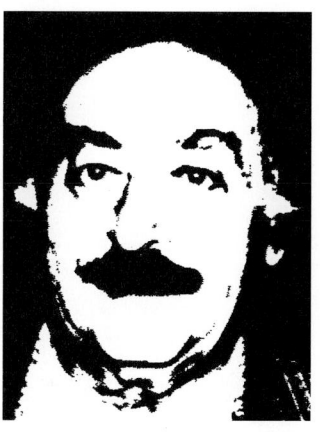

◆ **Gavriil Ilizarov**
Born in the Caucasian Mountains and did not attend school until he was 12. During World War II he was evacuated to Dolgovka, near Kurgan, and ran a hospital single-handed. Injured Russian soldiers came through the village, and this is when he started developing his apparatus. He patented it in 1952 and moved to Kurgan, which was rebuilt in 1984.

Watson Jones ran a rehabilitation service for the Royal Air Force based on cheerfulness and physical activity. Later, he worked hard to establish services for civilians; these began only when employers became responsible for the social consequences of the industrial diseases and injuries of their workers.

Compensation

Compensation for injury goes back to the beginning of time. But fortunately it has evolved beyond eye for an eye.

The Romans had a schedule to be paid for loss of a body part. King Canute paid in schillings: 100 for total paralysis due to a neck fracture, the same as for death. A thumb was 30, and fingers ranged between 18 and 9. In the Muslim world today the rates of compensation are laid down.

In the past, railway injuries attracted all the compensation interest that injuries due to car accidents do today.

References

Chapter references are located in Chapter 26.

◆
◆
◆ PART TWO

The Story of Fractures

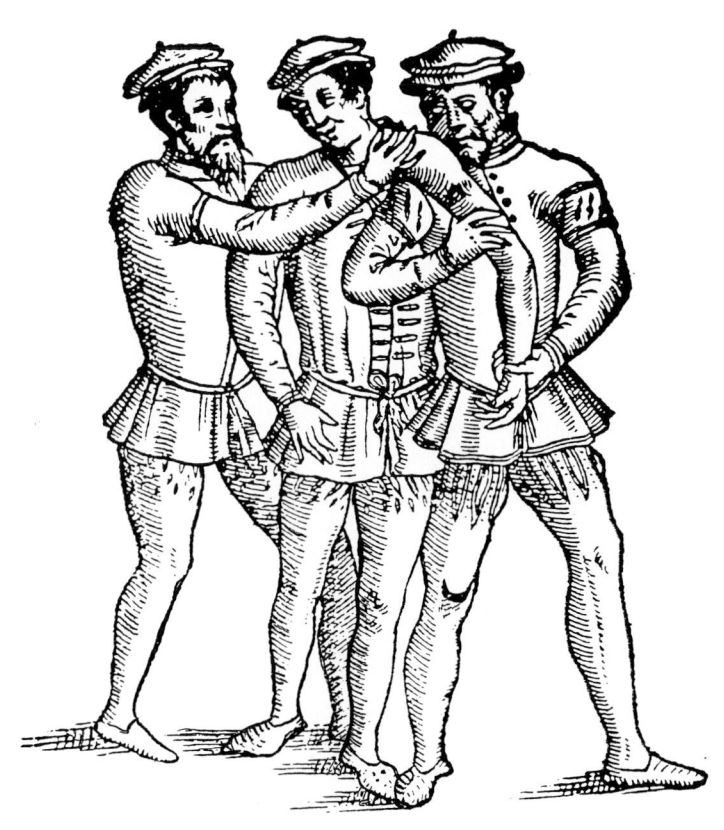

◆ Chapter Sixteen

Injury

He who wishes to be a surgeon should go to war.   Hippocrates

Fractures were the last part of our specialty to be wrenched from the general surgeons, and with good reason. Fractures were common and paid the bills. The transformation could be seen in the content of our journals—in 1940, 15% of papers were about trauma but by 1959 this had risen to 50%.

Causes of Injury

Injuries are traditionally called accidents—as if they are unpredictable. But, of course, that is untrue. When an old lady twists on her osteoporotic hip and breaks it, or when a soldier stands in front of an enemy automatic rifle and is killed, the event is predictable. A change in attitude has given us the means of preventing many injuries: safety guards on machines, seat belts, and bullet-proof vests.

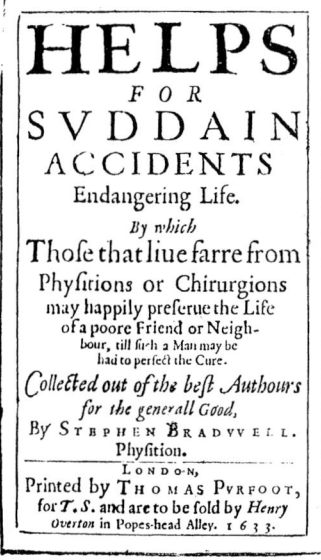

One of the first books on accident prevention and first aid, 1633.

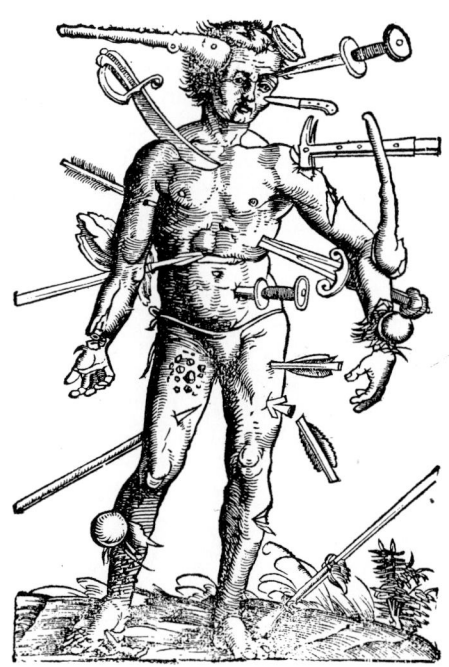

The wound man. Von Gersdorff, 1530.

Injury Prevention

EDITORIAL: THE DANGERS OF THE 'CYCLE'
1896

A whole column of advice is given about avoiding accidents when riding bicycles, including the following: *"Pass horses at a slow speed. Ladies should not attempt to ride in a public thoroughfare until they have absolute control over and confidence in their machine. Persons who let out cycles for hire should be under the control of the police. The hiring out of bicycles to children and roughs bent on what they call a 'spree' should be checked by law."*

What caused the first fracture—did a dinosaur trip in the dark? Museums are full of fossils with united fractures. But many animals with fractures died because they were unable to flee predators. Humans produced fractures in quantity in wars. About 500 years ago gunshot wounds added to their complexity. After 500 years it is surprising that methods of gun control are still an issue. Guns and tobacco are of similar antiquity, and it is hard to know which have been the most harmful.

The Industrial Revolution brought a new wave of injuries. Suddenly, many children and unskilled people were in close proximity to machines in factories. They were undertrained and overworked; the hours were long and many were injured. At this time, F. Engels wrote, in *The Condition of the Working Class in England*, there were so many deformed and maimed that *"it is like living in the midst of an Army just returned from a Campaign."*

In 1883 Lord Ashley in London introduced the 10-hour Bill to regulate child labor. Chadwick proposed that employers should pay the medical expenses of injured children as a deterrent.

With the Industrial Revolution came large industrial projects such as railways and canals. The organization of injury services for projects, such as the Manchester Ship Canal, provided the model for Army Orthopaedic Services in World War I. Later, children's orthopaedic care was based on the Army model—a generic doctor, peripheral clinics, and centralized hospitalization.

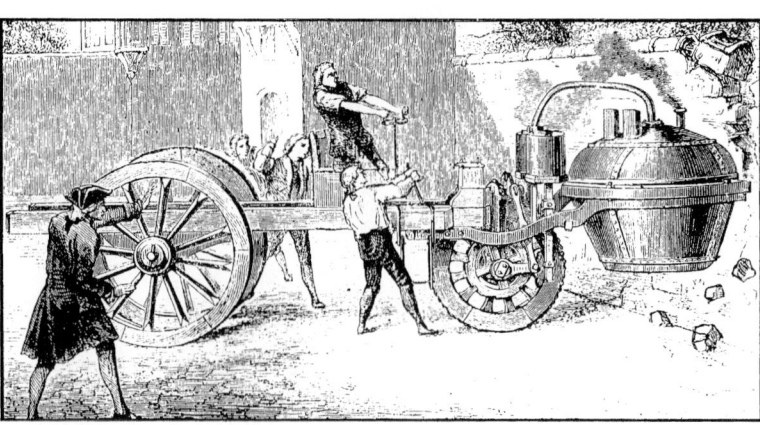

The first automobile accident. This steam-driven colossus was hard to steer and knocks down a wall on its first trip. Cugnot, 1769.

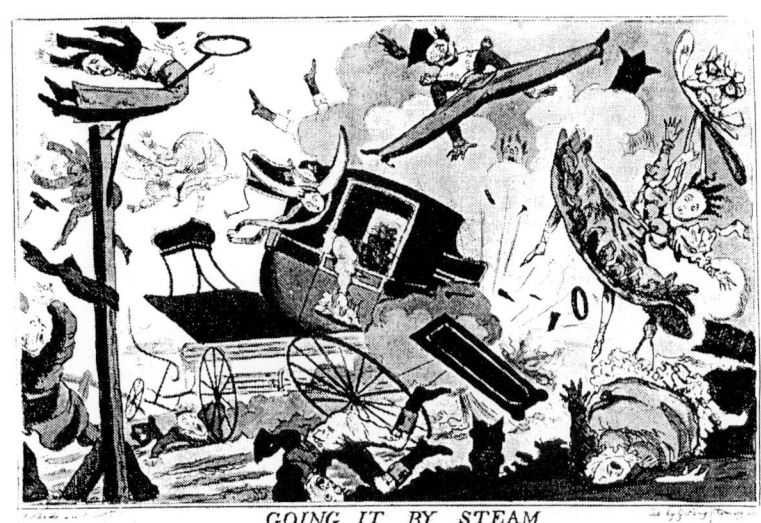

Injury has always been a risk of moving from one place to another. When steam coaches began to transport people, they blew up, providing themes for cartoonists. Robert Seymour, 1829.

Motor Vehicle Accidents

Today, transportation injury—car and pedestrian injuries—provide the most serious trauma. Horses were probably more dangerous than automobiles.

Today's love affair with cars is recent. Initially they were hated.

Ironically, Nicholas-Joseph Cugnot (1725–1804), a French Army captain, who invented the first automobile, was injured by it. He invented a huge, steam-driven tricycle in 1769–1770 to pull guns. It traveled for 20 minutes at 2.25 mph before it had to rest. By 1830 steam-driven buses were traveling between cities at 25

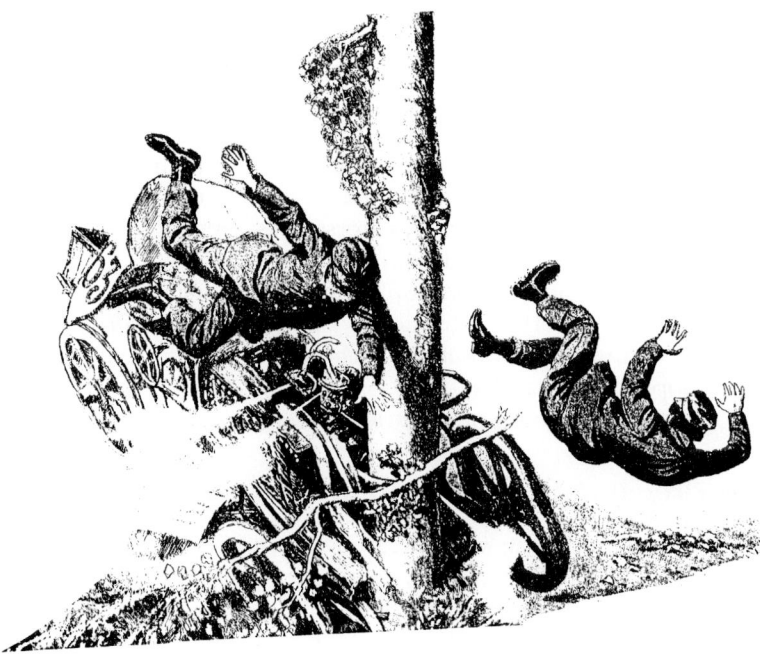

Marcel Renault was killed in a car as he was about to start the 1903 Paris to Madrid race. Seat belts did not come in until 60 years later.

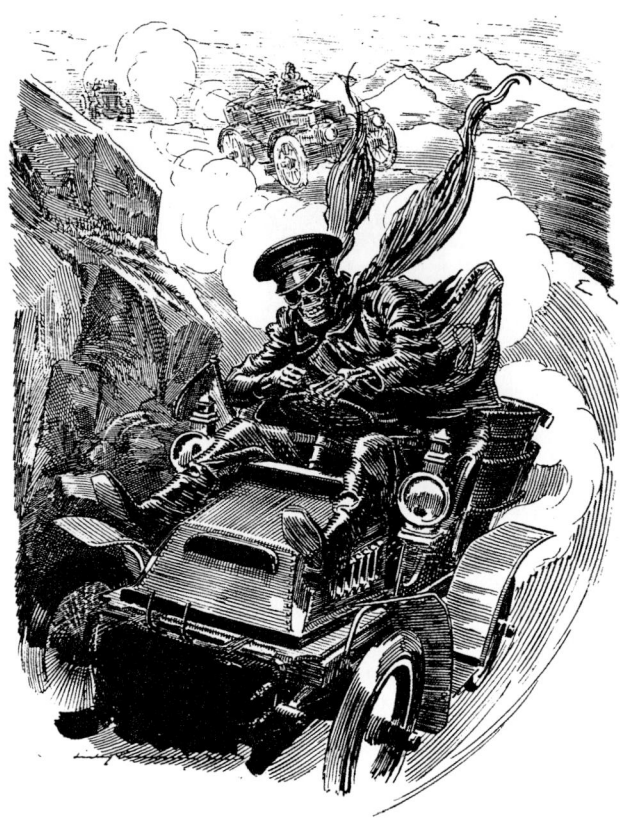

Punch magazine responded to Renault's death with this cartoon, 1903.

mph. They were hated. They were noisy, destroyed the roads, and made horses bolt, causing injuries to riders and overturning carriages. In Britain, Parliament enacted legislation decreeing that a man had to walk in front of a steam-driven vehicle waving a red flag–the Red Flag Law, or Locomotives on Highways Act of 1865. It was not repealed until 1896. In Pennsylvania, the Farmer's Anti-Automotive Society came up with rules that at night automobiles had to stop every mile and release a rocket, then wait for ten minutes before proceeding. If a horse was seen, the automobile had to stop and be covered with a camouflage blanket. In Europe and America automobile development continued, and the first cars were made in the 1890s. Ironically, the first cars in Europe were made at Cannstatt, near Stuttgart, where Jacob Heine had founded an orthopaedic institute in 1829.

Here is an account of an early accident:

The Dreadful Accident to Mr Huskisson

William Huskisson was leader of the House of Commons. On September 15, 1830, he went to open the Manchester and Liverpool Railway. It was a gala occasion. Several trains carried the most famous of the land. They had stopped midway on a double track to take on water, and the passengers were strolling and chatting.

"The Rocket engine, which had to pass the Duke's car to take up its station at the watering place, came slowly up, so silently that it was almost upon the group before they observed it. Mr Holmes, MP, who was standing by the side of Mr Huskisson, desired the gentleman not to stir, but to cling to the side of their own car. Unfortunately Mr Huskisson did not follow this advice. He attempted to get into the car, was hit by the motion of the door as he was mounting the step and was thrown down directly in the path of the Rocket. The wheel went over his left thigh, squeezing it almost to jelly, broke the leg in two places, laid the muscles bare from the ankle, nearly to the hip, and tore out a large piece of flesh, as it left him. Dr Brandreth applied a tourniquet to stop the dreadful effusion of blood. In a few minutes Mr Huskisson fainted away and was removed into the car. The Northumbrian Engine proceeded at a rapid rate to Manchester to procure medical advice. He was carried to Eccles and removed to the house of the Rev Mr Blackburn.

"No operation had been performed, the medical gentlemen deeming it altogether useless to put him to the pain of examining the limb. Mr Huskisson was quite sensible, and so great was his agony, that he wished for a speedy release from his sufferings. He made an addition to his will, received the sacrament and was resigned to his fate."

The main party did not know what to do with their planned celebration—commercial instincts prevailed. Mr. Huskisson died soon.

Shock

Ideas about maintaining circulating blood volume are recent. Blood was thought to contain bad humors and so the less the better. Hence bleeding a patient was frequent. Marshall Hall (1790-1857) was the first to look at the consequences objectively and put an end to the practice.

Marshall Hall was a son of the Industrial Revolution—the period when science came to the traditional arts. Hall, like Hunter, looked upon disease as an experiment devised by nature from which he could understand the physiology of the body. This is what clinical research meant to him.

He was born near Nottingham, where his father ran the family mill. His father discovered the bleaching action of chlorine and used it to bleach cotton; previously this had been achieved by leaving the cotton out in the sun for weeks. His brother remained in the business and made other innovations. Hall graduated from Edinburgh in 1812. In 1814 he made a tour of European centers and walked the 600 miles from Paris to Göttingen with a loaded pistol at the ready to fend off highwaymen and bandits.

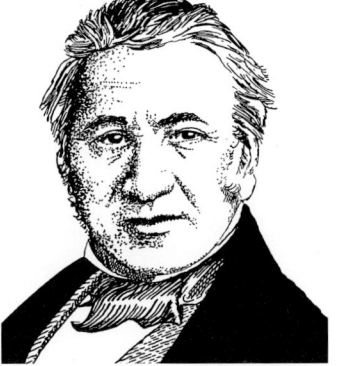

◆ **Marshall Hall**

On his return he set up as a physician in Nottingham at the age of 27, shortly afterward publishing his first book, *Diagnosis,* which was written while he was a student. The president of the Royal College of Physicians wrote to compliment him on this. On Hall's next visit to London he called upon the president. "I hope your father is well," said the President. "I, for one, am much indebted to him for his extraordinary work on diagnosis." Dr. Hall modestly told him that he, not his father, was the author of the work. "Impossible," exclaimed the President, "it would have done credit to the greyest-headed philosopher in our profession." Whereupon he invited Dr. Hall to breakfast with him.

Hall was very struck by the frequence of death in labor associated with abdominal pain and bleeding. He described the features of shock that he observed in these patients and went on to question the value of therapeutic bleeding in a wide range of disorders. His paper produced a great change in the everyday practice of medicine; before it appeared, venesection had been the universal remedy for any serious disease or accident. Hall's teaching that venesection was dangerous has perhaps prevented the loss of as many lives as more positive measures, such as the introduction of antibiotics, have saved.

In 1825, he was elected to the staff of the General Hospital, Nottingham; however, in the following year he took a trip to London, leaving no word about his return. After a while the hospital authorities asked his relations when they were expecting him back. His brother-in-law wrote to him. Hall told him to sell his house and all his belongings as he had decided to remain in London. He bought a house on a site now occupied by the Senate House of the University of London. He never had another hospital appointment. A steady stream of patients came to him as he acquired a name as a wise and kindly physician. "Our mission is to cure the curable," he wrote, "and comfort the incurable."

He married in 1829 and wrote a book on gynecology. The following year he wrote an early infant welfare book, *Letters to a Mother of the Watchful Care of Her Infant.*

At Nottingham he had observed disease and drawn far-reaching conclusions. In London, in a back room in Keppel Street, he began animal experimentation. He wrote about the circulation and was elected to the Royal Society in 1832. In the same year he read a paper before the Royal Society on spinal reflexes. The observation that a decapitated animal could still respond to stimuli led him to realize for the first time that the spinal cord, which had hitherto been looked upon as a cable joining the periphery with the brain, was itself capable of integrating sensory input and motor output. A second paper on the same subject the Royal Society refused to accept. He published it abroad and had nothing to do with the Royal Society again.

Marshall Hall was an intellectual leviathan—he wrote about a decimal pharmacopoeia, the emancipation of slaves, and sewage plans for London; he wrote against flogging; and he introduced artificial respiration. He was a regular traveler and went to the Continent every year, frequently lecturing. In Italy he was often given the best rooms as his Christian name, Marshall, was thought to signify military rank. On the way to America, when everyone was seasick, he wrote a physiologic paper on seasickness.

Paget found him "rather a sharp fellow," which perhaps explains why he followed such a solitary path and, like Hugh Owen Thomas, had no hospital appointment.

ON SOME EFFECTS OF LOSS OF BLOOD
MARSHALL HALL, 1825

"The most familiar of the effects of loss of blood is Syncope. The influence of posture, and the first sensations and appearances of the patient, in this state, appear to denote that the brain is the organ the function of which is first impaired; the respiration suffers as an immediate consequence; and the action of the heart becomes enfeebled as an effect of the defect of stimulus—first from a deficient quantity of blood, and secondly from its deficient arterialisation; the capillary circulation also suffers; and if the state of syncope be long continued the stomach and the bowels become variously affected.

"In ordinary syncope from loss of blood, the patient first experiences a degree of vertigo, to which loss of consciousness succeeds; the respiration is affected in proportion to the degree of insensibility being suspended until the painful sensation produced rouses the patient to draw deep and repeated sighs, and again suspended as before; the beat of the heart and of the pulse is slow and weak; the face and general surface become pale, cool, and bedewed with perspiration; the stomach is apt to be affected with eructation or sickness. On recovery there is perhaps a momentary delirium, yawning, and a return of consciousness; irregular sighing breathing; and a gradual return of the pulse.

"In cases of profuse haemorrhage the state of the patient varies: there is at one moment a greater or lesser degree of syncope, then a degree of recovery. During the syncope the countenance is extremely pallid—there is more or less insensibility—the respiratory movements of the thorax are at one period imperceptible and then there are irregular sighs—the pulse is slow, feeble, or not to be distinguished—the extremities are apt to be cold, and the stomach is frequently affected with sickness.

"In cases of fatal haemorrhage the symptoms gradually and progressively assume a more and more frightful aspect. The countenance does not improve but becomes more and more pale and shrunken; the consciousness sometimes remains until at the last there is some delirium; but everything denotes an impaired state of the brain; the breathing becomes stertorous and at length affected by a terrible gasping; there may be no attempt to vomit; the pulse is extremely feeble or even imperceptible; the animal heat fails and the extremities become colder and colder in spite of every kind of external warmth; the voice may be strong, and there are constant restlessness and jactitation; at length the strength fails, and the patient sinks, gasps and expires."

In 1830 in another article on this subject, Hall wrote:

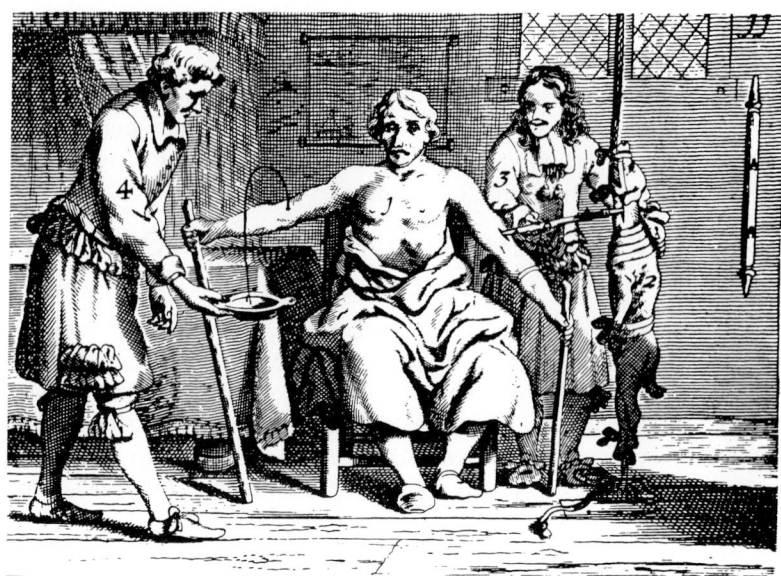

Blood transfusion, 1667. Dog to human transfusion was wisely banned after the doctor was sued.

"When Syncope assumes a dangerous form, the principal remedies are, an attention to the posture of the patient, stimulants, and chiefly brandy, and the transfusion of blood."

In old military textbooks, soldiers fainted and died from hemorrhage. The notion of hypotension had to wait until the sphygmomanometer was invented in the 1890s. John D. Malcolm in the United Kingdom noted the peripheral vasoconstriction in 1893.

There had been attempts at blood transfusion since the time the circulation of the blood was discovered. Dog-to-dog transfusions were tried, and then dog-to-human transfusions, with results so deadly that the doctor, J. B. Denis, was sued in 1667, and transfusion was banned for 150 years. In 1817 James Blundell showed that dogs nearly bled to death could be rescuscitated by transfusion, and interest was reawakened. Saline was used in the 1880s. But it was not until Landsteiner discovered blood groups in 1900, Hektoen in Chicago advocated cross-matching, and Richard Lewisohn at Mount Sinai in New York used citrate to prevent clotting in 1915 that transfusion could make a shaky start in World War I. Marriott invented the slow drip in 1935. Fantus at Cook County Hospital in Chicago started the first blood bank in 1937. Red rubber tubing produced reactions, and I can remember this being replaced by plastic in the 1960s. Now, of course, the emphasis is on self-donated blood, but we still depend on the blood bank for trauma patients.

Fracture Healing

How does a bone heal? The debate is not over yet. But today it does not excite much interest because we have such a decadent variety of plates and nails to apply. But a hundred years ago the subject was the number one research topic. Does bone heal with cells from the periosteum? From osteoblasts in the bone? Or from marrow cells?

The story is an example of experiments adding to confusion rather than providing a scientific answer. One group removed the periosteum and found that bone fragments united—they concluded that periosteum was unimportant. Another group removed the bone and found that bone reformed from the periosteum; they concluded that periosteum was essential. Arthur Keith in *Menders of the Maimed* covers the history in depth.

TIMELINE OF FRACTURE HEALING

1684 Antoine de Heyde in Holland studied fracture healing in frogs and concluded that callus was produced by calcification of the blood extravasated from the broken bone ends.

1736 John Belchier, a surgeon at Guy's Hospital, was given pork by a printer who had fed the pig on madder-soaked bran. The bone was stained red. He did some experiments but seems to have lost interest quickly.

1739-1743 Henri Louis Duhamel used madder to stain bones. He was not a physician but a moneyed French squire who liked to do experiments. He found when bone was broken that the periosteum thickened and produced new bone that was red. The old bone was white. He concluded that periosteum is the mother of bone.

1742 Marie Jean-Pierre Flourens repeats the experiments and reaches the same conclusions.

17?? Haller looks at the epiphyseal ends, sees bone forming around the arteries, and believes that the periosteum plays no direct role.

1840 Syme removed a piece of the shaft of the radius of a young dog and found that it reformed in 6 weeks if the periosteum was intact, but if the periosteum was removed the gap remained. He then lifted the periosteum in another experiment and inserted tinfoil between the periosteum and the bone. After 6 weeks the surface of the tin was covered with new bone. When he repeated this—removing the periosteum—there was no new bone.

1868 Louis Ollier, one of the first surgeon-scientists, carried out many experiments and wrote a book on the regeneration of bone. When he placed periosteum under the skin of rabbits, bone was formed, whereas bone fragments died and were absorbed.

1878 Macewen repeated the experiments and found that bone was not formed by the periosteum—perhaps his flaps were so thin that the periosteum was devascularized. He inserted bone grafts and found that they were not absorbed but formed bone. He concluded that the periosteum was a limiting membrane, preventing bone from entering the muscles. Bone could join directly. Macewen was impressed by a boy who lost his humerus

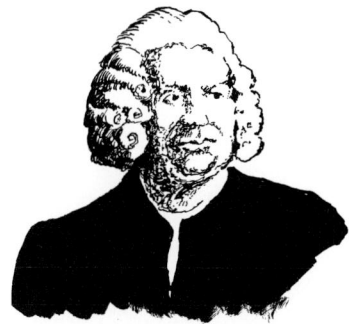

◆ John Belchier

Box continued on following page

> to osteomyelitis and showed no recovery because the periosteum had been killed. Macewen's bone grafts formed a new humerus. Macewen did many experiments, including putting a glass tube in place of a segment of shaft he excised. This excluded the periosteum. The core filled with bone. Today we would regard this as showing that marrow can form bone. For Macewen it confirmed his view that bone forms bone. And periosteum is unimportant.
>
> The conflict about the source of healing bone has been solved by the recent concept of primary and secondary bone healing. Primary healing occurs when there is rigid apposition—the periosteum plays little role. The periosteum produces callus when bone is moving during healing—secondary healing. Soon we will know which gene is switched on and identify the chemical messenger.

One of the first clear accounts of the process of healing was written by Dupuytren.

ON THE FORMATION OF CALLUS; AND ON THE MEANS OF REMEDYING ITS FAULTY OR MISSHAPEN DEPOSIT
BARON DUPUYTREN, 1847

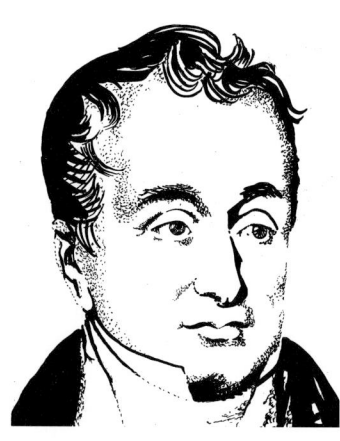

◆ Baron Guillaume Dupuytren (1777–1835)

"There is probably no subject in pathological anatomy which has more largely exercised the sagacity of practical men and the imagination of theorists, without their having recourse to the aid of actual observation or experiment, than the question respecting the formation of callus.

"Convinced by my experiments that Nature never accomplishes the immediate union of a fracture, save by the formation of two successive deposits of callus, I have been induced to name one provisional and the other permanent. The former of these, which is usually perfected in about thirty to forty days, and which comprises the ossification due to the vessels of the periosteum, the filamentous tissue, sometimes even of the muscles, and of the medullary tissue, has not always strength enough (especially in oblique fractures) when the splints and other supports are removed, to resist the power of the muscles, or such passive force as may be applied, even to a moderate extent, to the seat of injury; and the brittleness of this provisional callus is such that the bone more readily yields at the point where it is deposited than at any other part. The second (permanent) callus, formed by the reunion of the surfaces of the fracture, possesses a solidity superior even to that of the bone itself, so that the latter would sooner break at any other point than where the former is deposited. The production and organisation of the permanent callus is never completed under eight, ten, or twelve months, a period which is further marked by the disappearance of the provisional callus, and the renewed continuity of the medullary canal.

"The following are the principal phenomena which may be observed during the time that elapses between the occurrence of the fracture and the complete and exact reunion of the broken bone; their succession is so constant and unvarying, that they may be referred to five different periods.

"The first extends over the eight or ten days which immediately succeed the accident, and presents the following characters: at the moment that the fracture occurs, the periosteum and medullary membrane, the filamentous tissue, and sometimes even the muscles, are torn; blood escapes from the ruptured vessels, and surrounds the fragments, is poured into the medullary canal, and distends the neighbouring filamentous tissue. After a time the vessels retract, and their mouths are closed, the blood ceases to escape, and a mild inflammation is set up in all these parts. The filamentous tissue, reddened by a multitude of small vessels, becomes distended, condensed, and thickened, losing its elasticity, and acquiring a remarkable consistence; irregular prolongations are sent from it into the interstices of the muscles, by which their organisation is altered, and they are made to participate altogether or in part in the changes which are going on; their texture is transformed into one closely allied to the condensed filaments, and they are united and confounded with the periosteum, which, in turn, is also thickened by a network of delicate red vessels distributed over its surface. The medulla being broken through and mingled with blood, at first swells out and hardens, and subsequently becomes of a greyish white colour. The medullary canal is contracted in its diameter by the encroachment of the thickened lining membrane, which assumes a reddish, fleshy or pulpy appearance, resulting from a sort of gelatinous infiltration. The coagulum which results from the primary extravasation is absorbed and disappears. The fragments of the bone are, in short, surrounded by the gorged soft parts, which are converted into a homogeneous tissue of a lardaceous consistence and red colour, but varying in intensity.

"The second period then commences, and comprises the interval between the tenth or twelfth day and the twentieth or twenty-fifth. The gorged condition of the surrounding soft parts diminishes, the muscular tissue resumes its distinctive characteristics, but the filamentous tissue continues condensed. The tumefaction is more concentrated immediately about the fracture, and gradually assumes a more circumscribed character, until it forms a distinct tumour isolated from all surrounding structures, not even excepting the tendons, which play in grooves channeled for them along its surface, or in perfect canals traversing its structure; such is the callus. This tumour is thicker on a level with the fracture than at any other point, and insensibly diminishes in density on either of the fragments. Its tissue is homogeneous, its colour white or whitish, its consistence firm, and its resistance analogous to that of the fibrocartilages, giving out a similar sound when cut with a sharp knife; the cylinder which it forms passes rapidly into a cartilaginous state, and still more quickly into bone, becoming identified with the seat of fracture with the whitish, rosy, red or violet-coloured, viscid, or gelatinous substance as the case may be, which is interposed between the fragments; on the other hand, it is lost in the callus externally. Whilst in this condition it is still possible for the callus to yield opposite the fracture, but crepitus is rarely reproduced.

"The third period extends from the twentieth or twenty-fifth day to the thirtieth, fortieth, or sixtieth, according to the rapidity of the work of reproduction, and the age, constitution, and health of the patient. The conversion into cartilage commences at the centre of the tumour, and proceeds towards its circumference, and ossification speedily succeeds; thus little by little, the whole mass of callus becomes converted into bone. The periosteum, which is abnormally thick, then ceases to present any trace of the solution of continuity to which it had been subjected; and the muscles and tendons become free, though their natural mobility is not quite restored, on account of the induration of the filamentous tissue. If, at this epoch, a section of the callus is made, the fractured ends of the bone are still found moveable on each other; the condition of the intermediate substance not being as yet sensibly changed; and the tissue of the callus presents all the characteristics of the spongy texture of bone.

"The fourth period includes the interval between the fiftieth or sixtieth day and the fifth or sixth month. The substance of the provisional callus becomes condensed, and passes from the condition of a spongy to that of a compact tissue, and the medullary canal is obliterated by osseous matter of greater or less density. The substance intervening between the fragments is reduced to a mere line of a different colour from the bone itself, it gradually assumes more consistence, loses its colour, and ultimately, towards the end of this period, becomes ossified; the definitive, or permanent, callus is then formed.

"The fifth and last period embraces all the time which elapses between the fourth or sixth, and the eighth, tenth, or twelfth months. The temporary callus gradually diminishes in thickness, and at last disappears; the periosteum recovers its natural texture and density, and the muscles and tendons are restored to perfect liberty; the internal deposit of bone disappears, and the canal is insensibly re-established; the medullary membrane is repaired, and the medulla is reproduced. The process of consolidation is then completed."

Special Kinds of Fracture

Children's Fractures

The growth plate has excited much interest since the middle of the 1700s when the structure and function of it were worked out.

P. A. Salmon wrote a thesis in Paris in 1845 on 68 experimental separations of the distal humeral epiphysis achieved by hyperextending the elbow. Growth disturbances were described by several

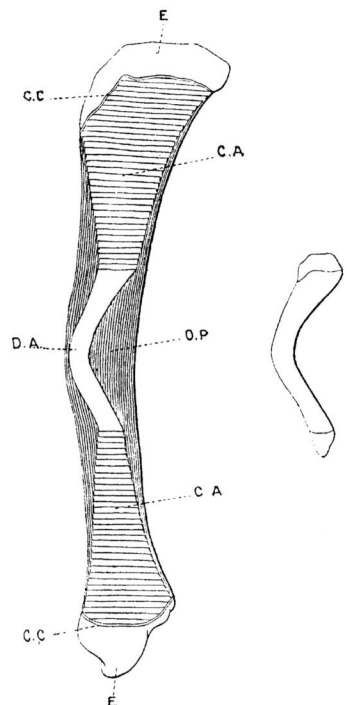

Remodeling of a rachitic bone between infancy and adolescence. This parallels the remodeling after fracture. Ollier, 1885.

investigators. Despite early reports, there remained much controversy—many believed that growth plate injuries did not exist or were very rare, until X-ray made everything clear.

Jean Foucher of Paris seems to have been the first to propose a classification of the injuries in 1863 and did excellent experimental work. He named 3 types: epiphyseal separation, separation with a bony fragment, and a distal metaphyseal fracture.

John Poland proposed a simple classification in 1898; in a book entitled *Traumatic Separation of the Epiphyses*. He understood growth plate injury, growth arrest, and the importance of the perichondrial ring, so that he could write a book of 926 pages—largely by reviewing the writings of others. He describes all kinds of experiments and specimens. Unfortunately he couldn't see the wood for the trees. He does not tell us how to think and make decisions about these injuries and he does not provide advice for choosing what to do. Anyone with something new to say should look at this first.

"Dislocations are among the rarest of accidents in young subjects. A careful examination will reveal the presence of an epiphyseal separation. Moderate traction will usually be sufficient to restore the displaced fragments (but) it is a matter of extreme difficulty to maintain thorough co-aption. In dislocation there is but little tendency for the displacement to recur." (John Poland, p 96)

Aitken and Magill described a classification in 1952. Surprisingly, Blount's book in 1955 on children's fractures makes no

♦ **John Poland (1855–1937)**

He was born outside London and studied at Guy's Hospital, graduating in 1879. He spent 2½ years as a registrar at the North-Eastern Hospital for Children, and this aroused his interest in children's fractures. He wrote 926 pages on traumatic separation of the epiphyses in 1898. Most of the text dates from the era before X-rays, but it includes a few of the first X-ray films. It is a wonderful review of the literature to that time. He worked out the anatomic details as a demonstrator at Guy's Hospital and had his brothers help him with translating some of the literature.

He went on to work at the St. Pancras Hospital (an ex-workhouse infirmary where the current author was an intern and his great-grandfather was a social worker). Later Poland worked at the Miller Hospital in Greenwich and the City Hospitals where he continued to collect cases.

He wrote in the annual report of 1896: "Although the mechanical treatment ... has been carried on ... yet modern methods of surgery have enabled us to relieve more patients more rapidly, and sometimes more thoroughly, by operations. ..."

Despite writing many letters and corresponding with a relative, I have been unable to come up with more information than his obituaries disclose. He wrote an X-ray atlas of the hand in 1898, a history of the Miller Hospital in 1893, and was editor of Chance's book *On the Nature, Causes, Variety and Treatment of Bodily Deformities*. He wrote most of it because E. J. Chance died with only half the manuscript written.

John Poland is often confused with his nephew Alfred Poland, who described Poland's syndrome.

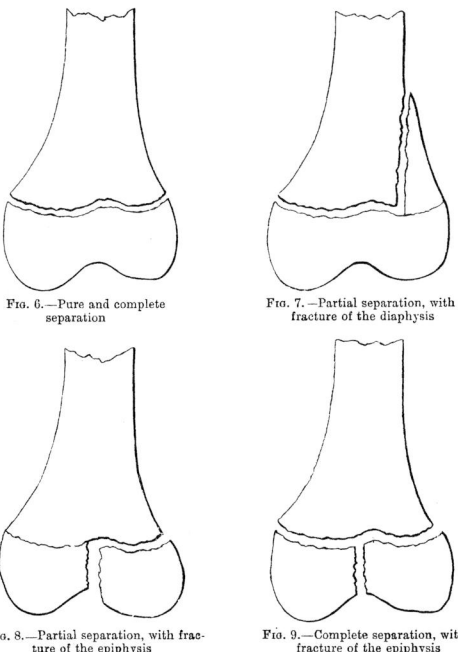

FIG. 6.—Pure and complete separation

FIG. 7.—Partial separation, with fracture of the diaphysis

FIG. 8.—Partial separation, with fracture of the epiphysis

FIG. 9.—Complete separation, with fracture of the epiphysis

John Poland's classification of epiphysial injuries, 1898.

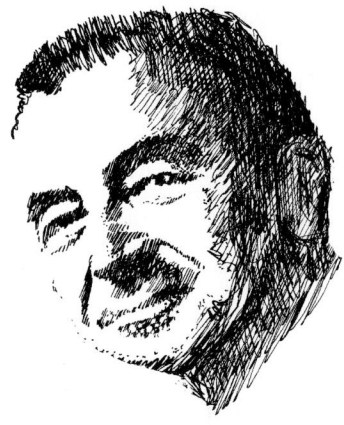

◆ **Robert Harris**
Toronto orthopaedic surgeon. He worked with Ham on fracture healing and focused, with Dr. Salter, on healing after epiphyseal injuries.

◆ **Charles Thurstan Holland (1863–1924)**
Born in Somerset, he studied at University College Hospital, graduating in 1888. He started in general practice in Liverpool and was a keen photographer. In Liverpool he was helping Robert Jones. Through the university physics department they heard of Roentgen's invention and together took the first X-ray film in Britain. Gradually he became one of the leaders on radiology in the country. He was blunt and withering in his conversation. He died lonely.

He gave his name to the Thurstan Holland fragment.

mention of a classification of growth plate injuries and has no specific recommendations. He did not think they had group importance. With the Salter-Harris classification of 1963, these injuries became high profile. Suddenly classification was the guide to treatment and prognosis. Since then new classifications have been proposed by Ogden and H. Petersen.

Nonaccidental injury is centuries old—think of the mutilations done to make convincing beggars. While assault has long been a criminal offense against adults, it is only recently that the law protects children. The first action was taken on behalf of a battered child in New York City in 1870. Mary Ellen was beaten daily by her parents. The police and the District Attorney's office were unable to help. Finally The American Society for Prevention of Cruelty to Animals succeeded on the grounds that Mary was certainly a member of the animal kingdom and was cruelly used.

John Caffey, a radiologist, blew the whistle on the radiographic signs of battering, which had previously been attributed to disease.

A RADIOGRAPHIC NOTE ON INJURIES TO THE DISTAL EPIPHYSES OF THE RADIUS AND ULNA—
THE THURSTAN HOLLAND SIGN, 1929

"A long experience of X-ray work at both large general hospitals and at special hospitals for children has created an impression upon my mind that injuries to bone in childhood and early adolescence are very much more interesting radiographically, as well as clinically, than those which occur during adult life. . . .

"There is a diaphyseal injury, and I believe it occurs in every case in which there is, or has been, a definite displacement of the epiphysis. This injury consists in a piece of the diaphysis, from the edge of the surface in the direction in which the displacement takes place, being torn off and accompanying the epiphysis.

"Now this small fracture of the epiphysis is of importance diagnostically. If you have it present it is positive evidence of epiphyseal injury in those cases in which the epiphysis itself is normally situated at the time it is X-rayed."

He wrote that the fragment "*gives the show away*" if the fracture springs back or is reduced.

I like the way he, as a pioneer of X-rays, uses the word "X-rayed."

TIMELINE OF STRESS FRACTURE
- 1773 Gooch describes cough fracture.
- 1855 Breithaupt, a German military surgeon, describes march fracture.
- 1897 Stechow: first radiograph of march fracture
- 1962 Book by M. Devas: *Stress Fractures* has historical references to every stress fracture

Open Fractures

TIMELINE

- 400 BC — Hippocrates' advice: dress the wound and then at 7 to 10 days reduce the fracture.
- 1561 — Paré describes treatment of his own open fracture.
- 1575 — Paré: the tradition had been to pour boiling oil over gunshot wounds to kill the poisons. This added a burn to the problem. One day Paré ran out of oil and found that open fractures did much better without iatrogenic injury.
- 1676 — Wiseman: reduce the fracture and close the wound. Perhaps the worst possible method of treatment.
- 1756 — Pott: treatment of his own fracture
- circa 1789 — Pierre-Joseph Desault: "I washed the wound, removed all foreign bodies and cut off all disorganised and ragged parts." He coined the word debridement.
- 1832 — William Beaumont: experiments on rabbits
- 1858 — MacLeod—The Crimean War was about the first war to be a media event. Journalists brought home the horror and incompetence, leading to many reforms.
- 1858 — Malgaigne studies statistics and results of operations in hospitals of Paris. Amputation for injury carried a 64% death rate.
- 1861 — Pasteur: particles in the air cause infection
- 1864 — Spencer Wells says that Pasteur might have something.
- 1865 — Lister: asepsis for open fracture
- 1872 — Ollier advocates occlusion and immobilization.
- 1884 — Denis publishes a series of successfully treated cases—not one death using Lister's methods.
- 1897 — Friedrich's experiments: he excises a contused wound as if it were a neoplasm. Thereafter the vitality of tissues is regarded as important.

Box continued on following page

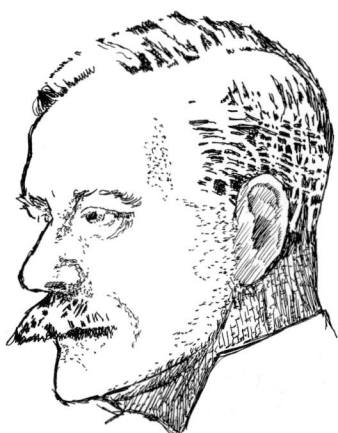

◆ **Paul Leopold Friedrich (1864–1916)**

In animal experiments, he proved the value of debridement.

1915	Carrel/Dakin: irrigation school. Continuous irrigation with antiseptics had been used on a small scale but with Carrel's backing it became the main treatment.
1929	Winnett Orr wrote *Osteomyelitis and Compound Fractures*. Orr noted during World War I that soldiers whose wounds had been cleaned and immobilized in a plaster cast to transport them home were in better shape than those treated conventionally with regular dressings.
1937	Trueta: clean it up and wrap it up, a principle learned from Orr and applied during the Spanish Civil War.
1935	Prontosil: an early form of sulfonamide
1945	Penicillin: the first time an infection can be treated effectively.
1976	Gustilo and Anderson: classification of open fractures

Open Fractures and Gunshot Wounds

Inflicting open fractures was a traditional method of settling human disagreements. The result was usually death. War could be defined as a method of settling disagreement through overwhelming the trauma surgeons. Pirogoff described war as "a traumatic epidemic."

Open fractures carry first the risk of death due to bleeding, then a slower death due to infection. Amputation was common. Nonunion from bone loss or soft tissue damage, stiffness of joints, and malunion was the cause of lifelong disability in other patients.

The ancient Egyptians wrote that an open fracture was "an ailment not to be treated." They knew that their treatment did not affect outcome.

Hippocrates on Open Fractures of the Femur and Humerus

"One should try to escape from such cases, provided one can do so honourably. The hopes of recovery are small and the dangers many. If the physician does not reduce the fractured bones he will be looked on as unskilled, while by reducing them he will bring the patient closer to death than to recovery."

This remained the state of affairs for the next 2000 years. After about 1450, gunshot wounds became an increasingly common cause of open fractures. We can celebrate 500 years of books and papers on the care of gunshot wounds. Organized battles increased the number and severity of open fractures, and horses on the battlefield increased the risk of gas gangrene—these were the worst conditions for attempting treatment.

For centuries the greater part of operative surgery was military surgery. Soldiers were patients in pain with wounds; they were at risk of dying of infection from the wound. Surgery could not make things worse and might help. This was quite different from doing elective surgery.

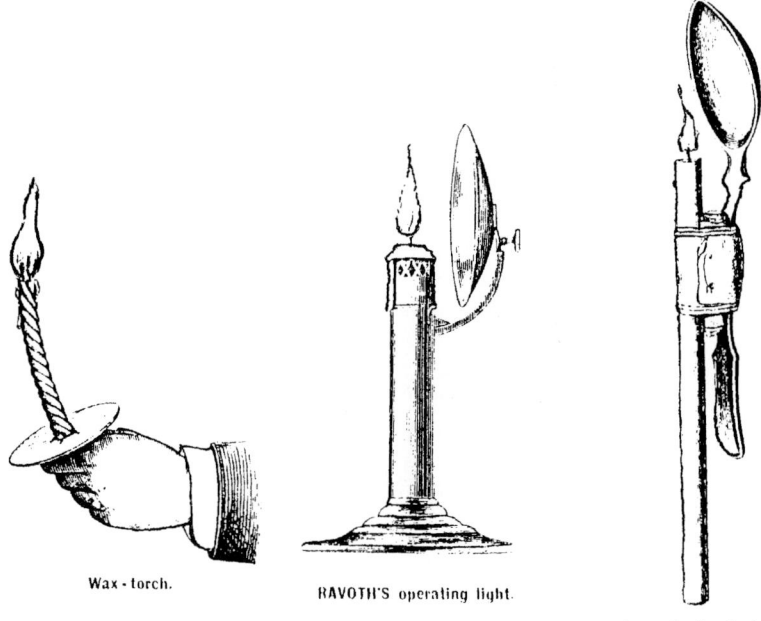

Wax-torch.   RAVOTH'S operating light.   Improvised reflector.

"In war," writes Esmarch in 1884, "the surgeon has frequently to operate at night." Until electric lighting there was little emergency surgery done. Imagine trying to work with no diathermy, an ether anesthetic, in a cloud of carbolic acid and lit by hand-held flares. From *The Surgeon's Handbook*. London: 1884.

In the Crimean War a series of 194 open fractures of the femur was reported. Ninety-six of these patients were treated by amputation, and 47% died. These survival rates were little different in the American Civil War.

Then, about 150 years ago, things changed. Anesthesia made it possible to debride a wound. Asepsis and fracture immobilization reduced the risk of infection. The survival rate improved.

But it was not until the 1930s and 1940s that treatment of infection with sulphonamides and then antibiotics took the terror away from an open fracture.

The Treatment of Open Wounds

The old Greeks used to cauterize wounds, not realizing that dead tissue was the breeding ground of bacteria. Cautery and boiling oil increased the amount of dead tissue and made things worse. Then Paré ran out of boiling oil one day and dressed the wound. He found that there was less pain and better healing. The habit of increasing the damage came to an end. He wrote, "I dressed the wound, God healed it."

Galen, whose word was law for more than 1000 years, believed that the formation of pus was essential for healing—not a helpful concept. The argument ran that visible pus was better than invisible pus. Visible pus could be almost guaranteed by killing the tissues and then applying filthy potions.

With the arrival of gunpowder came the belief that it poisoned wounds; then Leonardo Botallo, an Italian working with the French

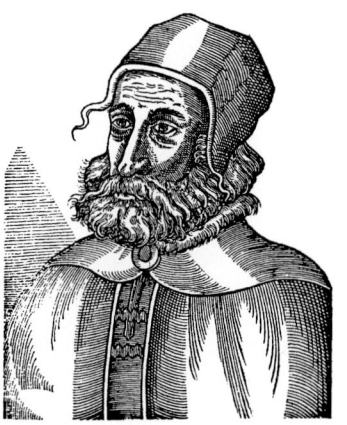

♦ Galen

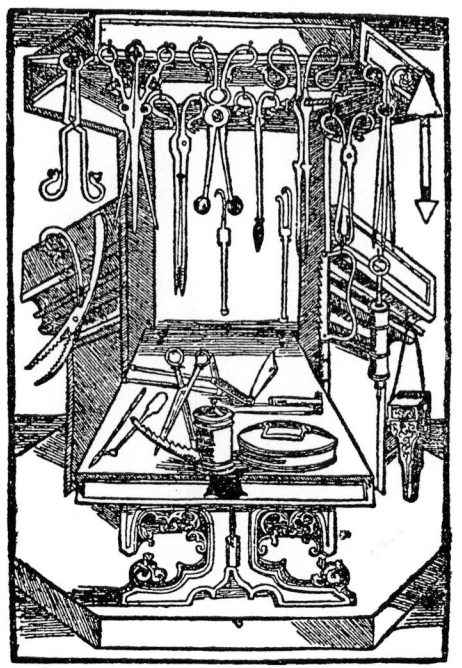

The surgical instruments of the day. There are forceps for removing bullets, stones, and sequestra. The syringe is for enemas. From Hieronymus Brunschwig, *Chirurgia*, 1497.

army, studied the ingredients and found no poison. He concluded, in his book of 1560, that foreign bodies caused harm and must be removed. He included fragments of bone and muscle along with extraneous matter. Few listened. Even today, over 400 years later, this is not always taken seriously.

The term debridement was introduced by Pierre-Joseph Desault to refer to removal of dead tissue. He worked through the French Revolution and his student, Dominique Larrey, put these ideas into practice when he was Napoleon's surgeon.

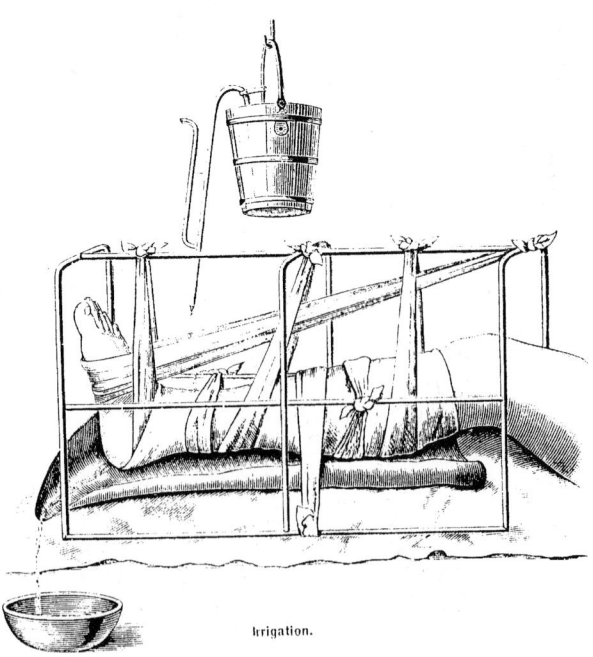

Wound irrigation, 1884. From Esmarch F: The Surgeon's Handbook on the Treatment of Wounded in War (trans by H H Clutton). London: 1884.

Various other ideas have come and gone, such as continuous irrigation, occlusive dressings left undisturbed to stop secondary infection, immobilization to localize infection, and primary closure that favored gas gangrene and was soon abandoned. Debridement and antibiotics have taken the fear out of wounds.

Lister, 1867

"The frequency of disastrous consequences in compound fractures, contrasted with the complete immunity to life or limb in simple fractures, is one of the most striking as well as melancholy facts in surgical practice." So begins Lister's paper on aseptic surgery. He refers to Pasteur's work on particles in the air being responsible for infection and the fact that surgical emphysema due to rib fracture does not become infected because the air is filtered by the lung. He argues that *"all that is requisite is to dress the wound with some material capable of killing these septic germs."*

"In the course of 1864 I was much struck with an account of the remarkable effects produced by carbolic acid upon the sewage of the town of Carlisle, the admixture of a very small proportion not only preventing all odor ... but destroying the enterozoa ..."

He goes on to describe the case of James G., aged 11, with an open fracture of the tibia that healed with carbolic dressings. The article continued in parts published weekly for over a month.

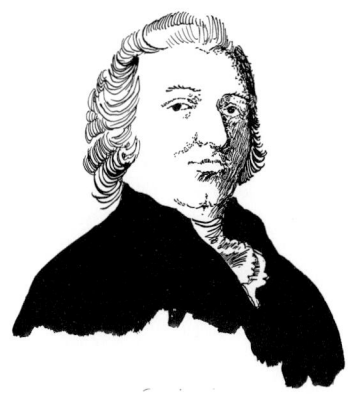

◆ **Pierre-Joseph Desault (1744–1795)**

He was an educator in Paris. Caught up in the French Revolution, he was briefly imprisoned but was then released. King Louis XVII was in prison too and Desault was called in to treat him. Within a few days Desault was dead—whether due to disease or murder has remained a mystery.

War in the Crimea, 1853–1856

The war was fought in the cold of Southern Russia before asepsis and anesthesia. Florence Nightingale was appalled by the conditions, and a public outcry enabled her to invent nursing and test it in this war.

A surgeon at the campaign wrote, *"The depressed condition of the body to which the hardships of the war had reduced the men, made a severe compound fracture of the femur synonymous with death."*

The mortality for amputations for gunshot wounds at this time was well documented—British Army in the Crimea, 1855: 39.8%; Waterloo: 51.3%. The mortality in civilian practice after amputation for injury is little different—Malgaigne, Paris: 64%; University College Hospital, London: Erichsen, 35.8%; Massachusetts Hospital, 33.3%.

◆ **Dominique Larrey (1766–1842)**

He studied in Toulouse and then went to sea with the French Navy as a surgeon. He next joined the Army and became one of the greatest military surgeons working with Napoleon. His care for the wounded was well known. When he was shot and left for dead at the battle of Waterloo, he was taken prisoner by the Prussians. Their general recognized Larrey and gave him safe escort to Belgium and freedom. Larrey did much to invent ambulances. He wrote much.

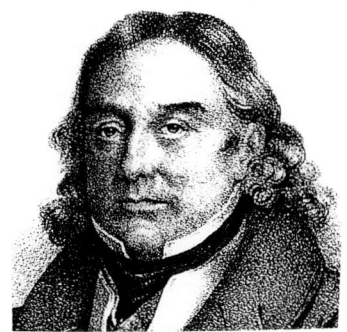

◆ **Dominique Larrey (1766–1842)**

Wounds were not the worst part of the war as these statistics of the French Army at the Crimean War show. Of 145,000 men, 47,800 needed an ambulance during the course of 4 months: 3613 died of gunshot wounds, 112 of frostbite, 639 of scurvy, and nearly 25,000 of cholera and other infectious diseases.

Dislocations

In the days before X-rays, any injury near a joint was regarded as a dislocation. Why, you may ask, did we have to wait until 1814 to have Colles' fracture described for the first time? Until then it had been regarded as a dislocation.

All those pictures of methods of reducing the hip may have been reductions for acetabular fractures. Reduction of late dislocations was common in historical times in Europe and is still common today in Africa because of the difficulty in obtaining medical care.

Compartment Syndrome

Volkmann knew that muscle ischemia and nerve ischemia were the cause of this problem but he did not put an important part of the jigsaw puzzle in place. As you read his account, you will notice that he avoided trying to explain why the muscles died while hand or foot remained alive. Several explanations were suggested but it was not until recently that the correct answer was found from several places at about the same time. In San Diego, the pressure in the tissues of fish was being studied with a manometer—the technology was applied to patients by Mubarak. In Toronto, the effects of raising compartment pressure were studied by Cec Rorabeck and Ian Macnab. In Seattle, Matsen carried out experimental and clinical studies.

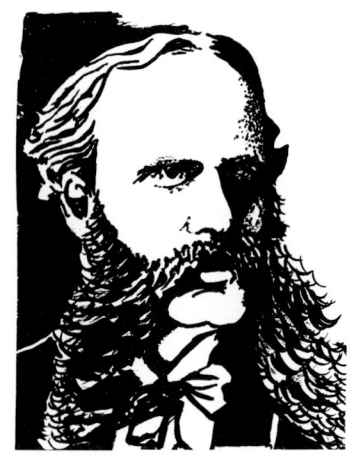

◆ **Richard von Volkmann (1830–1889)**

The whole of Volkmann's life was spent in Halle, Saxony, where his father was professor of anatomy and physiology. He studied at several universities and graduated at the age of 24. Two years later he became deputy professor of surgery and subsequently director. He instituted Lister's antiseptic methods at the hospital; it had previously been subject to so much infection that surgery was almost impossible. He wrote poems and fairy stories, which were very popular, under the pen name Richard Leander, and he also founded a surgical journal.

TIMELINE OF COMPARTMENT SYNDROME

- 1881 Volkmann describes ischemic contracture.
- 1912 Dr. Wilson, who went with Scott to the South Pole, gave a description of an exertional compartment syndrome of the leg.
- 1920 R. Finochetti: ischemic contracture of small muscles of the hand
- 1923 Steindler's book on surgery of the upper extremity discusses tendon lengthening.
- 1926 Jepson: fasciotomy prevents compartment syndrome.
- 1975 Rorabeck and Macnab: experimental animal models produce the syndrome by raising compartment pressure.
- 1975 Whiteside's technique for measuring pressure
- 1978 Wick pressure measurement introduced by Mubarak and Hargens

ISCHEMIC MUSCULAR PARALYSES AND CONTRACTURES
RICHARD VOLKMANN, 1881

"For many years I have been drawing attention to the fact that the paralyses and contractures of the limbs which sometimes follow bandages applied too tightly, do not arise, as was assumed, through paralysis of the nerves by pressure, but through wholesale and swift disintegration of the contractile substance and the resultant reaction and regeneration. The paralysis and contracture should be understood to have their origin in the muscle.

"A series of new discoveries made since has established the correctness of this assertion, and at the same time has allowed us to obtain a more and more precise conception of the occurrences and processes in question. I should like to sum up here my present views as follows:

"(1) The paralyses and contractures following tightly applied bandages, chiefly on the forearm and hand, and less often in the lower extremity, are to be viewed as ischaemic. They arise from the arterial blood supply being interrupted for too long. Venous stasis, though occurring at the same time, does seem to accelerate the onset of the paralysis.

"(2) The paralysis depends on the fact that the primary muscle groups die when deprived of oxygen for too long. The contractile substance coagulates and disintegrates and becomes re-absorbed later. The resultant contracture is therefore most simply described as post-mortem stiffening; the paralysed and contracted limbs always show the same postures as we find in extremities in rigor mortis, if the total musculature of a limb or part of a limb is simultaneously affected.

"(3) It is a feature that paralysis and contracture always appear simultaneously or follow each other closely, whilst in nervous paralysis of the extremities the contracture always develops very gradually and often very late. In the latter cases months and years may elapse before a deformity develops which can no longer be overcome by strong manual force.

"(4) By contrast from the first moment of the appearance of an ischemic contracture there is tremendous resistance to correction of the deformity. The affected muscles completely lose their elasticity and are absolutely rigid at an early stage, so resembling rigor mortis.

"(5) Necrosis of the contractile substance is followed by reactive and regenerative processes of which the latter always remains very incomplete in man; the affected muscles become more unyielding and the contracture increased still further by cicatricial shrinkage.

"(6) Ischaemic paralysis and contractures of identical nature appear not only after the application of unduly tight bandages and the unduly prolonged Esmarch's constriction of the limbs, but also after ligatures, avulsions and contusions of large vessels, but perhaps too after the prolonged exposure to cold. It is possible that some of the so-called rheumatic contractures are of an ischaemic nature.

"(7) Kraske has clearly shewn in his beautiful work that animal muscle cannot withstand the complete occlusion of the arterial blood supply for six hours without a great number of fibres perishing, and that after six hours of complete deprivation the most violent reactionary processes develop, which is a remainder of the so-called auto-digestion. The fact that there have been no unfavourable experiences up till now so far as I know, although the rubber bandages are often left in position for hours at a time, does not count for much, because the great majority of these patients have certainly perished. After the application of tight bandages, however, the ischaemia will almost never be complete. The degree of severity of the sequelae will depend upon the completeness of the ischaemia, and whether many or few fibres were affected by it. If the ischaemia is very considerable, such alarming phenomena appear so quickly that the bandage will be removed; even so, half a day and less is enough to reduce the fingers to permanent and pitiful deformity. If the constriction is less marked and the bandage left in place for a week in spite of complaints of pain, in spite of oedema and cyanosis of fingers and toes, the result is still only a moderate contracture and a moderate loss of muscle fibre. In particular such moderate contractures are frequently observed after Fractura Radii Typica. The residual slight flexion of the fingers yields here, too, only after many months of continuous and energetic treatment.

"(8) The prognosis of ischaemic muscle paralysis and contracture will therefore depend upon the number of fibres which have necrosed or disintegrated. The severest cases affecting the hand and fingers are to be considered absolutely incurable. The prognosis is better in the lower extremity, because here the main symptom, i.e. muscular shortening, can easily be removed by tenotomy. The milder cases are improved and cured only by the most energetic and consistent treatment.

"(9) Anything other than mechanical aids will prove completely useless. For every recent ischaemic contractures one should try to stretch the shortened and stiff muscles by the application of force under chloroform anaesthesia before anything else. In all older cases this is unsuccessful; one would more readily break the bones and rupture the tendons before the muscles would yield."

EXERTIONAL COMPARTMENT SYNDROME

DR. EDWARD WILSON, 1912

Wilson went on Scott's expedition to the South Pole. They had hoped to be the first to reach the South Pole but when they arrived on January 17, 1912, after a terrible journey, they found that Amundsen had beaten them. In poor condition they began their return but never made it.

Wilson wrote in his diary about the pain in his leg, which is probably the first description of this syndrome affecting the anterior compartment.

"Jan 28 1912   We are all on skis.... We are at about 10,130 feet above sea level. We are all pretty hungry.

"Jan 29   We got in a very long march for 9 hours (22 miles) . . . awful for skiing. . . Scott and I were on skis the whole day. I got a nasty bruise on the [tibialis anticus] which gave me great pain all afternoon. . . .

"Jan 30   My left leg exceedingly painful all day so I gave Birdie my ski and hobbled alongside the sledge on foot. The whole of tibialis anticus is swollen and tight, and full of tenosynovitis, and the skin red and odematous over the skin."

His complaints continued for about three weeks. He would have died if he had stopped walking. He and Scott died on March 29, when just 12 miles from the final base.

JEPSON FASCIOTOMY
1926

Copland Hutchison, a naval doctor, is often credited with the first description of compartment syndrome in 1816. He describes fasciotomy—but for erysipelas, not for compartment syndrome.

Here is the first account of fasciotomy for compartment syndrome.

"A method of producing a lesion which appeared similar to that in man having been developed, the next procedure was to determine, if possible, a method of preventing such deformity. A dog in which the incision and ligation (of the femoral vein) had been performed was selected for this experiment. An Esmarch bandage was applied above the knee and left on for eight hours. At the end of this time there was considerable oedema and other signs of a sluggish circulation, and the toes were contracted. Six hours later the wound was opened and the blood and serum were evacuated. Two rubber tubes for drainage were placed deep in the intermuscular space and sutured. The following day, the swelling had gone down markedly, and four days later the dog was walking normally. This was in marked contrast to the condition of the control animals in which drainage had not been instituted. The experiment was repeated often enough to bring out the fact that intrinsic pressure is a factor which must be dealt with in this condition.

"If the intrinsic pressure is relieved within a short time after the formation of the haematoma, the patient will usually recover."

Jepson did this work as a Fellow at the Mayo Clinic, writing a thesis for a Master of Science degree in orthopaedic surgery, in 1926.

Infection

Tetanus

"A convulsion supervening on a wound is deadly."   Hippocrates

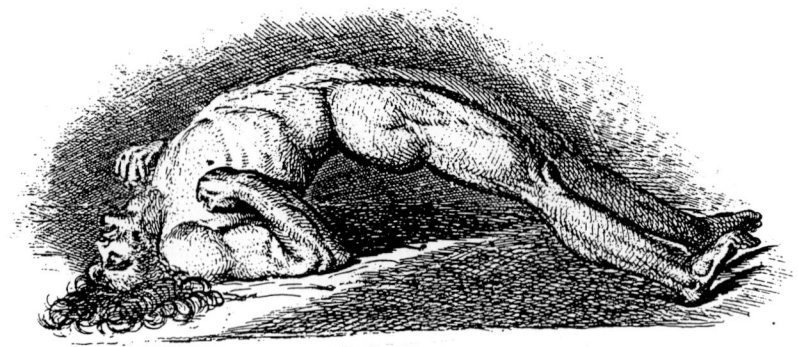

Charles Bell's horrific drawing of tetanus. Bell was a surgeon at the Battle of Waterloo in 1815. "It is impossible to convey to you the picture of human misery continually before my eye . . . While I amputated one man's thigh there lay at one time thirteen all beseeching to be taken next . . . It was a strange thing to feel my clothes stiff with blood, and my arms powerless with the exertion of using the knife."

Areteus (2nd to 3rd Century AD)

"A man, who was struck from behind by a sharp dart, had a wound that did not look serious because it did not go deep. But later, after the point was extracted, the patient was seized with backward bending convulsions—like those of opisthotonus. His jaws were locked, and any fluid that he attempted to swallow was returned through his nostrils. He died on the second day."

Tetanus was common in wounded soldiers and was usually fatal. The antitoxin was developed by Behring in 1892 and toxoid by Gaston Ramon in 1927.

TIMELINE OF GAS GANGRENE

- 1853 Classic descriptions of the disease by Maisonneuve
- 1864 Pirogoff describes it vividly.
- 1871 Bottini in 1871 noted that it was infective in origin.
- 1891 William Welch, professor of pathology at Johns Hopkins, isolated the organism in 1891. He was doing an autopsy on a patient with areas of skin breakdown and noted the crepitus under the skin. The veins were full of gas and when he nicked a vein, holding a match close, the escaping gas produced a small explosion and burned with a blue flame. The tissues and veins were full of bacteria. The Society of American Bacteriologists decreed that it should be called *Clostridium welchii* after its discoverer. The Library at Baltimore is named after him.

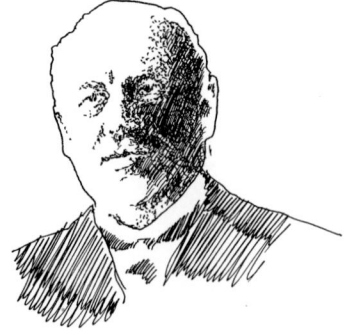

◆ William Welch

Books on Fractures

3000 BC   Edwin Smith papyrus, Egypt
400 BC   Hippocrates of Cos, Greece
600 BC   Susruta, India
30   Celsus. He was not a physician but a writer and collector of information—like a data banker. He collected everything known at the time and gave his name to the signs of inflammation.
c200   Galen, surgeon to the gladiators in Turkey and Rome
c600   Paul of Aegina, Greece
c1000   Albucasis, Arab Spain
1275   William of Salicet
1296   Lanfranc of France
          Henri de Monville
1363   Guy de Chauliac of France
1465   Le premier manuscript, Persia
1497   Hieronymus Braunschweig, Strasbourg—good illustrations
1543   Vesalius
1544   Guido Guidi (Vidius), illustrations of the ancients
1575   Ambroise Paré, first book in French—a huge amount of new information
1676   Richard Wiseman, England
1718   Lorenz Heister, Germany
1723   Jean-Louis Petit, Paris
1733   William Cheselden, London, osteology
1751   Joseph-Guichard Duverny, Paris
1765   Percivall Pott, London
1775   John Jones, first American fracture book
1813—1816 Giovanni Monteggia, Milan
1813   John Syng Dorsey, Philadelphia
1822   Astley Cooper, London, dissections and experiments
1823   Joseph Wattman, Austria, mechanical models to practice reduction of dislocations
1828   Adolph Leopold Richter, Prussia, atlas
1830   Samuel D. Gross, Philadelphia
1847   Baron Guillaume, Dupuytren, France
1847   Robert William Smith, Dublin
1847   Joseph Francis Malgaigne, Paris, statistics
1852   Antonius Mathijsen, Holland, plaster bandages
1860   Frank Hastings Hamilton, United States
1862   Ernst Julius Gurlt, Germany
1886   Hugh Owen Thomas, Liverpool, rest—prolonged, enforced, and uninterrupted
1895   Just Lucas-Championière, Paris, massage and mobilization
1896   Theodor Kocher, Bern
1898   John Poland, London, growth plate injuries
1900   Charles L. Scudder, Boston
1905   Lewis Atterbury Stimson, New York
1905   Arbuthnot Lane, London, operative treatment

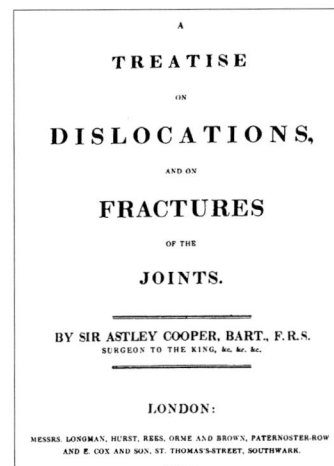

Title page of Astley Cooper's classic on fractures, 1822. This was one of the first academic books on fractures.

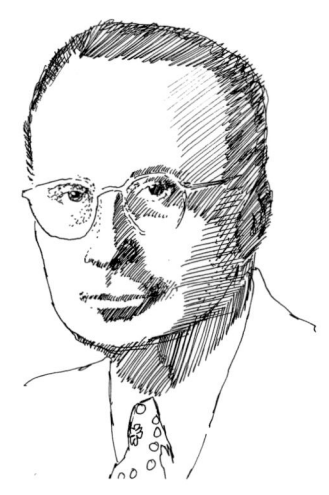

◆ Walter P. Blount

◆ Walter P. Blount

He was born in 1900 in Oak Park, Illinois, the son of a surgeon mother. He was a classmate of Ernest Hemingway. He graduated from Rush Medical College in 1925 and studied orthopaedics in Madison, Wisconsin, then toured orthopaedic centers in Europe and wrote a travelogue in 1929. He settled in Milwaukee and opened a practice there. In 1958 he became clinical professor and head of the department of orthopaedic surgery at Marquette. He received many honors and played a leading role in important organizations.

He wrote two books, *Fractures in Children* in 1954 and *The Milwaukee Brace* in 1979. He introduced drill osteotomy for children's deformities and was known for hip osteotomies in the days before joint replacement. He described Blount's disease in 1937 and devised epiphyseal stapling for the control of bone growth in 1949.

1907	Albin Lambotte, Belgium
1910	Fredric J. Cotton, Boston
1915	Jean Tanton, Paris
1916	Hey Groves, Bristol
1916	Kellogg Speed, Chicago
1922	A. W. Tubby, London
1929	Lorenz Bohler, Vienna
1934	J. Albert Key, St. Louis
1940	Reginald Watson-Jones, Liverpool
1949	Danis, Belgium, compression fixation
1950	Walter Blount, Milwaukee, children's fractures
1950	John Charnley, Manchester
1961	Maurice Müller, M. Allgower, H. Willenegger, *Technik der operativen Frakturenbehandlung*, Switzerland. Translated 1963—The AO Manual.

References

Chapter references are located in Chapter 26.

◆ Chapter Seventeen

Lower Limb Fractures

"Thomas leg splint: a neolithic masterpiece of tapes and granny knots." Novelist Anthony Burgess

Famous Patients

Talleyrand. At the age of 4, he fell off a chest of drawers and injured his foot. He went into the church because he was not fit for the Army. He became a bishop and after the Terror became Napoleon's chamberlain.

John Charnley was rock climbing in 1935 with friends in the Lake District. One, named Roberts, fell. "When they reached the top, John Charnley (who had the merit of being small and who had just become a doctor) was lowered to the ledge where Roberts was lying with a fractured femur. Charnley managed to apply a Thomas splint and they were both pulled up to the top of the crag. By now night had fallen and it was impossible to carry the injured man down the mountain. Charnley stayed with him, but Roberts, who was severely shocked, died during the night (Waugh, 1990). Charnley's first interest was fractures.

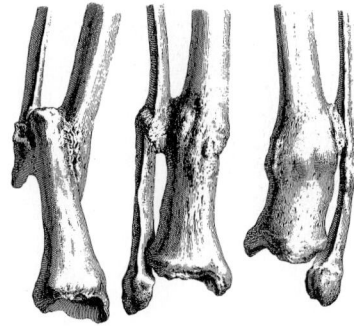

William Cheselden: Fracture callus, in *Osteographia*, 1733. This book with its many lovely engravings was an academic triumph and a financial disaster.

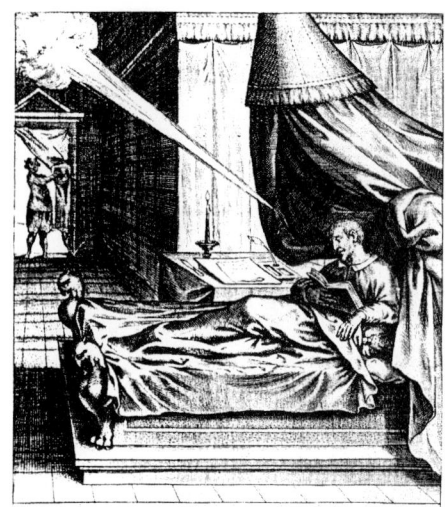

Ignatius recovering from an open fracture of the tibia. He is reading a holy book and being inspired to become a religious leader.

St. Ignatius of Loyola (1491–1556). The founder of the Jesuits was a wild youth—"given over to the vanities of the world." In 1521 he was in the Spanish Army defending Pamplona against the French when "a shot hit him in the leg, breaking it completely: since the ball passed through both legs, the other was also badly damaged," he writes in his third-person autobiography.

"When he fell the defenders of the fortress surrendered immediately. The French treated the wounded man well. After he had been in Pamplona for 12 or 15 days, they carried him on a litter to his own country where he was very ill. All the doctors and surgeons who were summoned decided that the leg ought to be broken again and the bones reset. This butchery was done again:

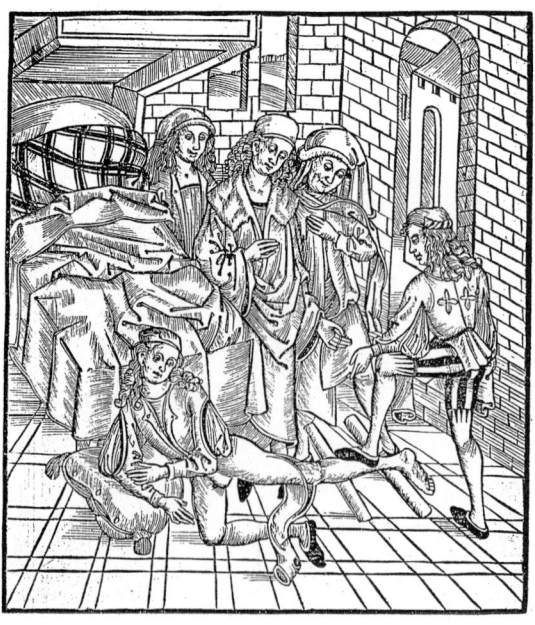

Hieronymus Brunschwig of Strasburg; Osteoclasis for a malunited fracture. *Book of Surgery*, 1497. Presumably this is what Ignatius is describing.

he never spoke a word nor showed any sign of pain other than to clench his fists. Yet he continued to get worse, not being able to eat and showing the other indications that are usually the signs of death. He received the sacraments. The doctors said that if he did not feel better by midnight he could consider himself dead. Our Lord willed that he should begin to improve and some days later he was out of danger of death.

"As his bones knit together, one bone below the knee remained on top of the other, shortening his leg. The bone protruded so much that it was an ugly sight. He was unable to abide it and he thought it would deform him; he asked the surgeons if it could be cut away. After the flesh and excess bone were cut away, means were taken so that the leg would not be so short: many ointments were applied to it, and, as it was stretched out continually with instruments, he suffered martyrdom for many days. In everything else he was perfectly healthy except that he could not stand on the leg and had to stay in bed. As he was much given to reading books of chivalry, he asked for some to pass the time. None of those he usually read could be found so they gave him a Life of Christ and a Book on the lives of the Saints."

He had a vision, changed his way of life, and later founded the Order of Jesuits, which has been very successful in spreading the power of the church around the world.

Ronald Reagan was playing a charity baseball game in 1947. He suffered a comminuted fracture of the femur and spent 2 months in traction.

TIMELINE OF LOWER LIMB FRACTURES

Pelvis
- 1832 Malgaigne fracture
- 1964 Judet and Latournel classification of acetabular fractures
- 1980 Tile-Pennal classification of pelvic fractures finally published

Hip
- 1681 Gerrit Borst—fracture of the neck of the femur
- 1869 Bigelow ligament and dislocation of the hip
- 1932 Johannson nail

Shaft of Femur
- 1857 Buck's traction
- 1875 Thomas' splint
- 1880 Bryant's traction
- 1903 Balkan beam—an overhead traction frame clamped to the bed
- 1924 Hamilton Russell traction
- 1940 Küntscher intramedullary nail
- 1970 Ender nails
- 1985 Grosse Kempf locked nails

Box continued on following page

Knee
1877 Lister wires a fractured patella.

Tibia
1555 Paré sustains an open fracture of the tibia and lives.
1557 Paré ruptures his tendo Achillis.
1832 Malgaigne's external fixator for the tibia.
1856 Abraham Lincoln defends two doctors for malpractice.
1947 Hansen Street intramedullary nail

Ankle
1768 Pott
1819 Dupuytren's fracture

Fractures of the Pelvis and Acetabulum

Joseph-François Malgaigne (1806–1865)

The son of an Army surgeon, he was born in Charmes Moselle. He graduated as a health officer at Nancy, aged 19, and did some writing. His writing ability complemented his surgical career. He went to work as a secretary for a historian for a time before further medical studies in Paris. Broke, he joined the army. Upon demobilization he organized a volunteer hospital for the Poles after the defeat by the Russians and finally wrote his degree.

In 1835 he became surgeon for a group of hospitals in Paris.

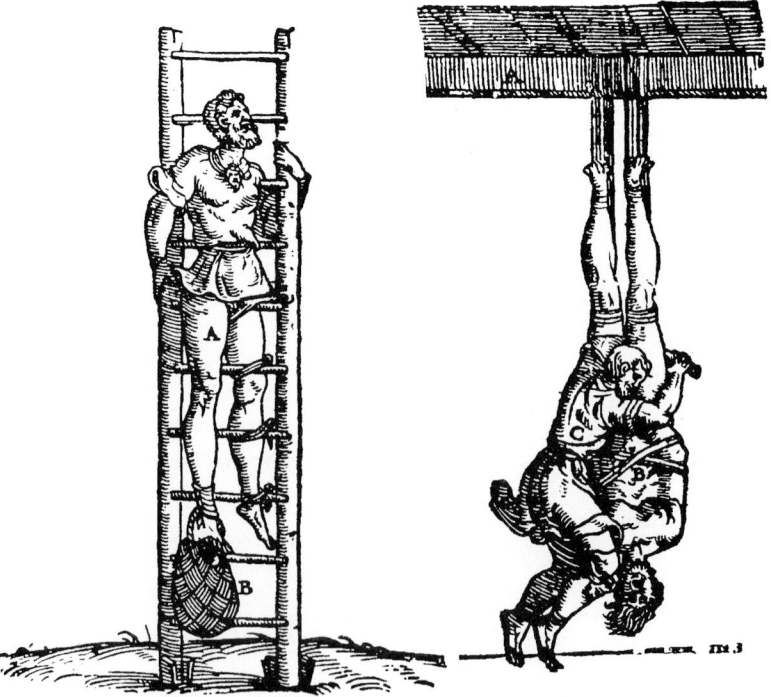

Reduction of a dislocated hip. From Guido Guidi, 1544.

He came to the attention of Guérin, who edited the *Gazette Medicale de Paris*, and became an associate editor. He became a clever writer: *"The work of Dr. X contains many things both new and good. Unfortunately the good things are not new and the new things are not good."*

He fell out with Guérin over myotomy for scoliosis and wrote a critical editorial in a journal he founded in 1840. This ended in a lawsuit. The case revolved around the right to publish results of tests that showed that a method of treatment was ineffective, despite support by eminent surgeons. Malgaigne gave the final speech in his own defense, and the case against him was thrown out.

His *Traite des fractures et des luxations* of 1847 (English translation in 1859) included an analysis of 2328 fractures and an atlas. It was very comprehensive. He was a staunch advocate of statistics in medicine.

He wrote a monograph on the history of fractures.

His *Manuel de médicine opératoire (Manual of Operative Surgery)*, published in 1834, was translated into four languages. He wrote a history of surgery and a biography of Paré and edited Paré's works.

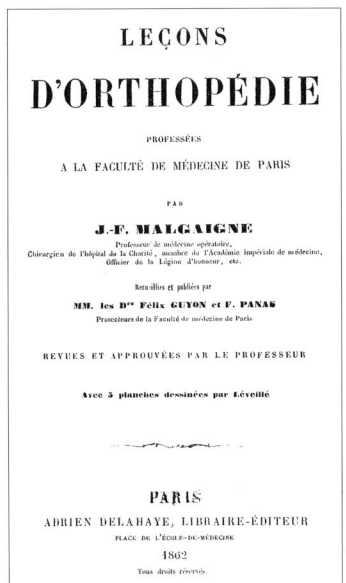

Galen (131–201 AD) must have found reducing a hip dislocation very difficult because he had these alternatives. From the *Opera* of Galen. English translation, 1625.

MALGAIGNE'S VERTICAL SHEAR FRACTURE

1847

"I shall describe a form of multiple fracture of the pelvis, distinguished from all others by a species of regularity, and meriting, besides, special attention in the triple aspect of diagnosis, prognosis and treatment. It is a combination of two vertical fractures, separating at one side of the pelvis a middle fragment comprising the hip joint: according as this fragment is carried upwards or inwards so the femur follows its movements, and hence results in changes in the length and direction of the limb which have often mislead practitioners.

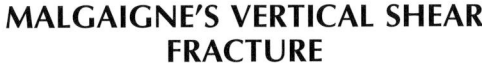

Title page of Malgaigne's book.

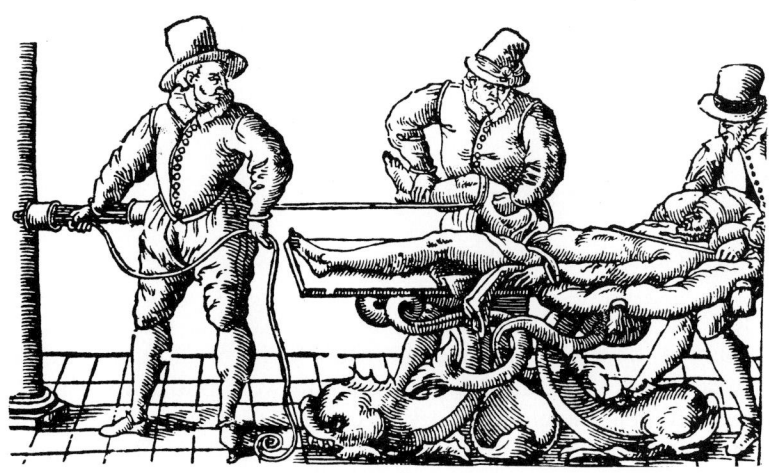

Reduction of a dislocated hip. Paré; English translation, 1678.

"Of these two fractures, the anterior is almost constantly seated in the horizontal and descending ramus of the pubis, separating this bone from the ilium and the ischium: the posterior is always back of the cotyloid cavity, and generally in the ilium: once however it was seen by Richerand in the sacrum. Lastly instead of a fracture, we may have here a separation of the sacro-iliac symphysis.

"The prognosis is rendered serious mainly by injury inflicted on the viscera."

He advised traction.

A HIP INJURY DURING THE CIVIL WAR
1865

Before X-rays, fracture-dislocations were thought to be dislocations. Whatever the injury, this account shows how tough life was during the Civil War.

"June 12th, 1865. Voluntary Dislocation of the Hip. Dr. Hodges showed some photographs of a man who was able to partially dislocate his hip at will with the following account of the case:

" 'John B. Parker, Private, Co. H, 1,18th N. Y. Vols., on the march from Bermuda Hundred to Drury's Bluff, May 13th, 1864, while skirmishing up a hill, sprang back suddenly, to avoid the gun of a comrade in advance. His left foot became entangled, and his weight dislocated his hip. He felt the injury, and supposed the joint was out. Some comrades pulled it in. He immediately resumed his skirmishing, and marched seven miles, from 10 till 6 P.M. He laid down at night, and went on duty the next day, sharp-shooting, crawling all day.

" 'He continued this kind of work five days, and returned to camp, when he was immediately put on entrenchments, and worked two days and nights. Afterwards he went on picket, and entered the hospital May 28th.

" 'He is able at any time to luxate the hip-joint, and does it by pressing the foot on the floor, to fix it firmly. He then contracts the adductors, throwing out the pelvis, when the head leaves the socket and goes on the dorsum.' "

Fractures of the Femur

A fracture of the shaft of the femur is easily treated in the Third World today with a pin, a piece of string, and a brick—Perkins' method. Yet in the past, veritable Cadillacs of equipment have been produced for this injury. If all the cord used to treat fractures of the femur in traction were put end to end, it would encircle the globe. Today, of course, it is rare to find anyone under 40 who can set up traction; every fracture comes to operation. More of this in Chapter 20, but meanwhile here are some examples of fracture beds.

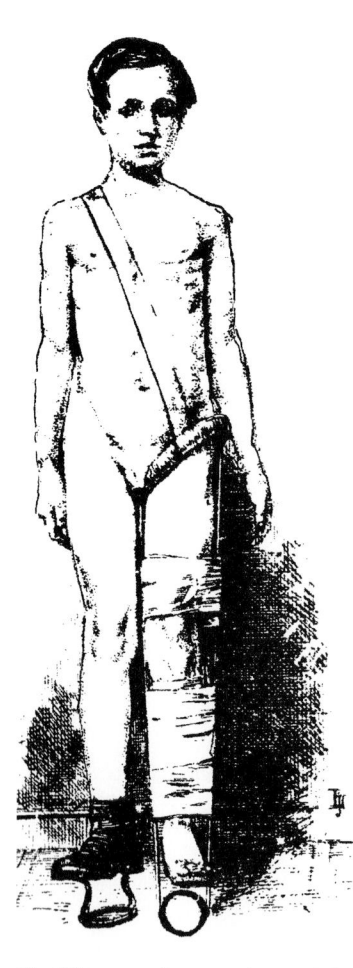

The Thomas splint was designed for the treatment of tuberculosis of the knee joint. Much used for femoral fractures, it is seen here as it was intended to be used. From Thomas HO: Hip, Knee and Ankle. Self-published in 1876.

Chapter 17 ◆ Lower Limb Fractures   379

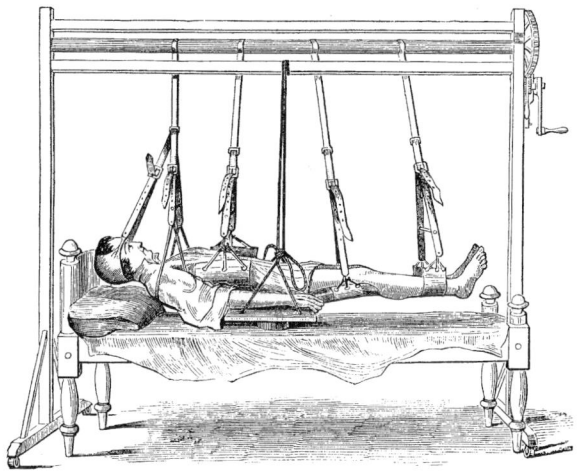

Another system of fracture care that takes into account toileting needs. From Hamilton FH: [An important] Treatise on Fractures and Dislocations, 1860.

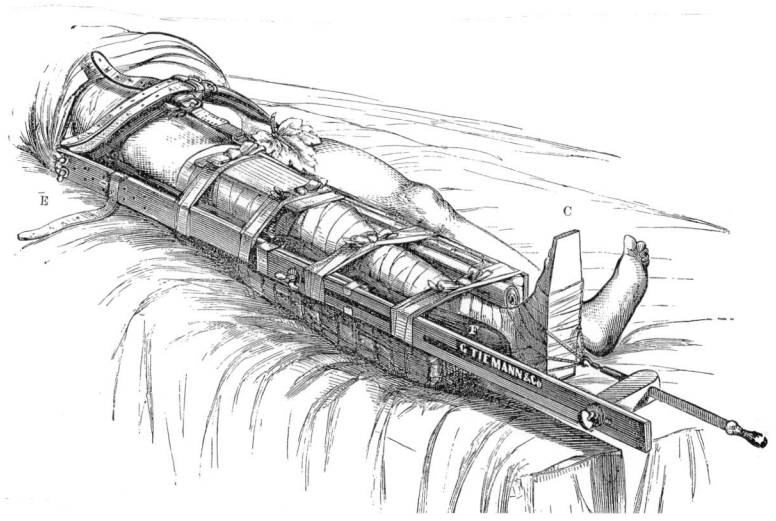

The belt, buckle, bow, and fig leaf treatment of a fractured shaft of femur. From Hamilton FH: [An important] Treatise on Fractures and Dislocations, 1860.

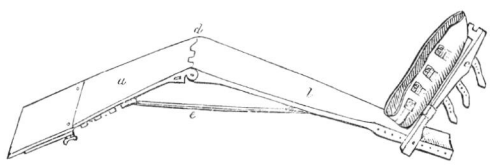

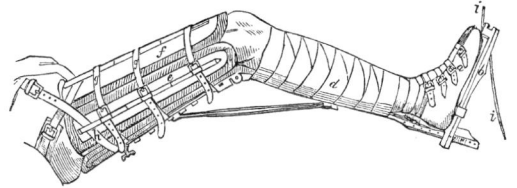

Amesbury's splint for fractures of the femur, *circa* 1831. From Hamilton FH: [An important] Treatise on Fractures and Dislocations, 1860.

Fractures of the Patella

AN ADDRESS ON THE TREATMENT OF FRACTURE OF THE PATELLA
JOSEPH LISTER, 1883

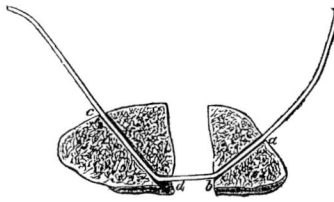

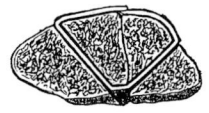

Lister: Wiring a fractured patella, 1883. From Br Med J 1883, 2, 855.

In 1873, Lister wired an un-united fracture of the olecranon with success. *"The third case ... had consulted no fewer than eighteen surgeons . . .* (There is nothing new about what is known to health care providers as overdoctoring—in fact, it took 18 opinions before the correct treatment was available.) In 1877, an old houseman of his wired a fracture of the patella. Lister did one soon afterward and presented seven cases in 1883.

The illustration shows what he did:

"I was on the lookout for a fracture of the patella (to treat on the same principle as a fracture of the olecranon). In October 1877, a patient with a transverse fracture of the patella was admitted under my care in King's College Hospital. He was a man forty years of age, who, while riding on horseback, had his horse stumble and fall. He was thrown over the horse's head, falling on his right knee. He could not rise, and was brought to the hospital. In the first instance, I attempted with this patient to bring the upper fragment down, so that it would be in contact with the lower [using traction. The fracture remained separated]. I suggested to the patient the operation of cutting down and applying the wire suture. This, however, he would not consent to, and preferred returning home to be under the care of his ordinary medical attendant. Eight days later, or fourteen days after the accident, he was readmitted, expressing a wish to be operated upon. On October 26th, I accordingly proceeded to operate, making a vertical incision, about two inches in length over the patella, exposing the fragments which were then about one inch apart. My inability to bring down the upper fragment into contact with the lower became explained, there were found between the fragments extremely firm coagula. The clots having been completely cleared I applied a common bradawl in the midline of the patella, drilling each fragment obliquely so as to bring out the drill on the broken surface a little distance from the cartilage. Pretty stout silver wire was then passed through the drilled openings, and the fragments thus strung upon it were pushed firmly home, and so brought accurately into apposition. Before they were brought together, however, an arrangement was made for the drainage of the joint. The ends of the wire were now twisted together. The wound was closed with sutures.

"Antiseptic treatment was applied throughout ... The wounds healed without suppuration. At the end of eight weeks the wire was removed. At the end of ten weeks the patient was allowed to get up, and, though passive motion had been employed, he could move the limb freely through an angle of about thirty degrees. Two days later he was discharged and, unfortunately, nothing has been heard of him since. I saw him on a cart a few days after he was dismissed. This, I believe, is the first instance of

a recent fracture of the patella being treated by wire suture aseptically applied.

"Before I made the incision I remarked to those who were assembled in the theatre that I considered no man justified in performing such an operation, unless he could say with a clear conscience that he considered himself morally certain of avoiding the entrance of any septic mischief into the wound.

"Disasters happen. Gentlemen with whom things go wrong invariably say that everything has been perfectly done—a thing which, for my part, I am always loth to say."

Fractures of the Tibia

AMBROISE PARÉ
1561

He describes the management of open fractures using his own experience.

"This happened to me the fourth day of the month of May, 1561. [I went with other barber surgeons] to visit some patients in the village of Les Bons Hommes near Paris.

"The misfortune befell me in the manner which follows: Wishing to pass across the water and trying to make my hackney enter a boat, I struck her on the crupper with a riding crop, stimulated by which the animal gave me such a kick that she broke entirely the two bones of my left leg at four inches above the juncture of the foot. Having received the blow and fearing that the horse might kick again, I stepped back one pace, and suddenly fell to the ground; the already fractured bones came out, and broke the flesh, the hose, and the boot, whence I felt such pain that it is not possible for a man (at least according to my judgment) to endure greater without death. My bones thus broken and my foot bent upward, I feared greatly that my leg had to be cut off to save my life.

"I was quickly carried into the boat to cross to the other side in order to have me treated. But its shaking almost made me die, because the ends of the broken bones rubbed against the flesh, and those who were carrying me could not give it fit posture. From the boat I was carried into a house of the village with greater pain than I had endured in the boat, for one held my body, another my leg, the other my foot, and in walking one lifted to the left, the other lowered to the right. Finally, however, they placed me on a bed to regain my breath a little, where, while my dressing was being made, I had my whole body wiped dry, because I was in a general sweat. If I had been thrown in the water, I would not have been wetter. This done, I was treated with a medicament such as we were able to practice in the said place which we compounded of white of egg, wheat flour, oven soot, with fresh melted butter.

"Above all, I prayed M. Richard Hubert not to spare me any more than if I had been the greatest stranger in the world as far

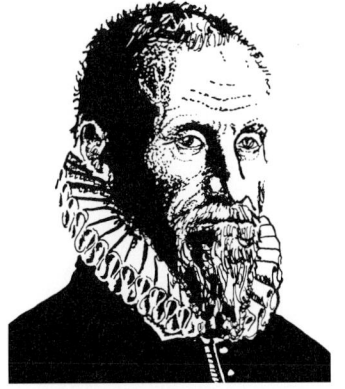

◆ **Ambroise Paré (Father of French Surgery) (1510–1590)**

He was born in Bourg Hersent in the old French province of Maine, where his father was a valet and barber. Several of his near relatives were in similar medical occupations. He studied with his brother Jean, in 1532 was apprenticed to a Parisian barber-surgeon, then worked for four years at the Hôtel Dieu in Paris. He became a master barber-surgeon in 1541, and subsequently worked partly in Paris and partly as an army surgeon. He was surgeon to four kings of France.

In 1575 he published a superb, monumental work on surgery. The first part is devoted to anatomy and physiology and the second to surgery, which includes descriptions of many surgical instruments; he reintroduced the ligation of vessels, and described prostheses for amputation.

He was one of the few Huguenots spared at the Massacre of St. Bartholomew.

as he was concerned, and that in reducing the fracture he put in oblivion the friendship that he bore me. Further, I admonished him, although he knew his art perfectly, to put my foot strongly in a straight line, and that if the wound were not sufficient in size, that he should increase it with a razor in order to more easily to put the bones back in their natural position. Also, that he should search diligently in the wound with his fingers, rather than with another instrument (for the sense of feeling is more certain than any other instrument), in order to take out the fragments and pieces of bones which could be separated from their whole, and especially that he should express and make issue forth the blood which was in great abundance around the wound."

The leg was then splinted as shown and various ointments applied.

"I was two months and more before callus was made, during which time I remained on my back. It was yet another month before I could even press my foot on the ground without a crutch. Yet I have been entirely cured without limping in any fashion. On this, I will make an end to my treatise on fractures and shall pray God that He will guard from such an accident all those who read this history and to send me to death rather than fall again."

POTT AND AN OPEN FRACTURE OF THE TIBIA
1756

His son-in-law gives this account of the famous injury which led Pott to start writing:

"In the year 1756, an accident befell Mr. Pott. As he was riding in Kent Street, Southwark, he was thrown from his horse, and suffered a compound fracture of the leg, the bone being forced through the integuments. Conscious of the dangers attendant on fractures of this nature, and thoroughly aware how much they may be increased by rough treatment, or improper position, he would not suffer himself to be moved until he had made the necessary dispositions. He sent to Westminster, then the nearest place, for two chairmen, to bring their poles; and patiently lay on the cold pavement, it being the middle of January, till they arrived. In this situation he purchased a door, to which he made them nail their poles. When all was ready, he caused himself to be laid on it, and was carried through Southwark, over London bridge, to Watling-street near St. Paul's, where he had lived for some time—a tremendous distance in such a state! I cannot forbear remarking that on such occasions a coach is too frequently employed, the jolting motion of which, with the unavoidable awkwardness of position and the difficulty of getting in and out, cause a great, and often a fatal, aggravation of the mischief. At a consultation of surgeons, the case was thought so desperate as to require immediate amputation. Mr. Pott, con-

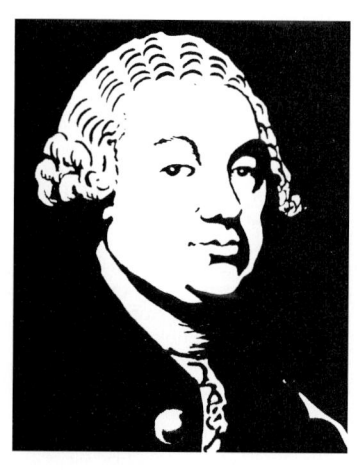

◆ Percivall Pott

vinced that no one could be a proper judge in his own case, submitted to their opinion; and the instruments were actually got ready, when Mr. Nourse, who had been prevented from coming sooner, fortunately entered the room. After examining the limb, he conceived there was a possibility of preserving it: an attempt to save it was acquiesced in, and succeeded. This case, which Mr. Pott sometimes referred to, was a strong instance of the great advantage of preventing the insinuation of air into the wound of a compound fracture; and it probably would not have ended so happily, if the bone had not made its exit, or external opening, at a distance from the fracture, so that, when it was returned into the proper place, a sort of valve was formed, which excluded air. Thus no bad symptom ensued, but the wound healed, in some measure, by the first intention. The appearance of Mr. Pott as an author was an immediate effect of this accident. During the leisure of his necessary confinement, he planned, and partly executed his treatise upon ruptures, which was completed by the latter end of the year."

The site of the fracture is not mentioned, but as the fracture was at a distance from the skin wound it is more likely to have been a fracture of the shaft of the tibia than a Pott's fracture.

ABRAHAM LINCOLN DEFENDS DOCTORS ACCUSED OF MALPRACTICE FOR THE CARE OF A FRACTURE OF THE TIBIA

1856

In 1856, four years before he was elected President, Lincoln was still working as a lawyer.

The suit for malpractice that was filed in the McLean County Circuit Court had as defendants Drs. Crothers and Rodgers. The plaintiff was Samuel Fleming. The most interesting feature of the action was the presence of Abraham Lincoln as attorney for the defendants. Both of the physicians knew Lincoln well. The nurse who had taken care of Lincoln's children had also served the children of Dr. Crothers, and there were other bonds of friendship.

As the records show, Mr. Fleming fractured a leg and engaged the two defendents to set the bone. The break was a bad one, and the knitting process slow—when completed it was seen, as is said to be the case with elderly patients, that the limb was a trifle shorter than it was before. Holding that the two surgeons had not given the fracture proper attention, Fleming sued them for malpractice. Lincoln was sent for and agreed to take the case. He was then living in Springfield and came up to Bloomington on several occasions to be coached upon the subject of broken bones. The two surgeons, both distinguished in their profession, used a chicken bone to explain the different conditions in bones of young people and those of advanced age. In the former case the bone has a springy, wiry condition less apt to break and a tendency to knit quickly. In the case of old people the bone is more brittle while the lime and other qualities impair the knitting qualities. The physical characteristics of bones were explained to Lincoln in minute detail, and when the coaching was completed he knew about as much about the subject as the physicians themselves.

When the suit finally came to trial, Lincoln argued the case using the chicken bone and other illustrations. He concluded a brilliant argument by saying: "Mr. Fleming, instead of bringing suit against these surgeons for not giving your bone proper attention, you should go on your knees and thank God and them that you have your leg. Most other practitioners with such a break would have insisted upon amputation. In your case, they exercised their skill and ability to preserve it and did so. The slight defect that finally resulted, through Nature's methods of aiding the work of the surgeons, is nothing compared to the loss of the limb altogether."

The President-to-be threw his whole soul into the defense, and the jury promptly brought in a verdict for the defendents and threw the costs, reaching a large figure, onto the plaintiff.

Malpractice was unknown until the early 1800s. When surgeons stopped amputating for open fracture and started to save limbs the public started to sue for deformity. There were many court actions, and book chapters that deal with this. The first monograph was published in 1860.

Pseudarthrosis of the Tibia

UN-UNITED FRACTURES IN CHILDREN
PAGET, 1891

"The general course of events begins with a fracture produced by what may seem like an inadequate cause, proceeds though a series of vain attempts to obtain reunion, and ends with amputation of the limb....

"When she was 4 days old it was observed that her right leg was bent to an obtuse angle just below its middle; it may have been so at or before birth. The bones were entire, but when she was 3 years old a bone setter broke them, made the leg straight, and so fixed it and kept it straight for some long time. But the fracture was not repaired, and all means employed to obtain union completely failed."

The leg could be bent in all directions and was amputated.

Ankle Fractures

Today most ankle fractures that are likely to give future problems are fixed internally and become asymptomatic. But in the past ankle fractures were a source of lifelong disability because joint incongruity was uncorrected.

These fractures were another example of doctors not knowing exactly what they were treating, having ineffective methods of treatment available, and not having any means to monitor position.

During the centuries up to 1800, ankles were repositioned to minimize obvious deformity, and the patient lay down with a

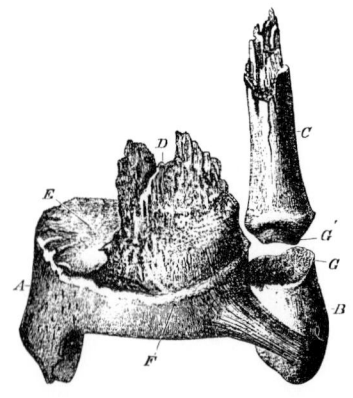

The pathology of an epiphyseal separation of the ankle. Anger: 1865, from Poland J: *Traumatic Separation of Epiphyes*, London: 1898.

splint until the pain settled. For the next hundred years much experimentation was done to try to relate the mechanism of injury to the fractures produced. One might think that this would be a simple exercise, but even today it remains controversial. Both Dupuytren and Maisonneuve in France compared the fractures that could be produced in cadavers with the fractures in patients. Maisonneuve's name is attached to the fracture he produced by externally rotating the foot—a diastasis of the ankle with a proximal fracture of the fibula—commonly missed unless a film of the whole leg is ordered.

The coming of X-rays and internal fixation about the same time transformed the means of diagnosis, treatment, and monitoring of fractures.

When Lauge was preparing his classification of ankle fractures, he wrote a 60-page history of ankle fractures, providing all the references and comments in an easily obtained journal for future aspiring authors.

Pott's Fracture

Some years after Pott had suffered a compound fracture of the tibia, he wrote this account. Judging from his son-in-law's description of the injury, it is unlikely that he suffered the fracture that bears his name.

REMARKS ON FRACTURES AND DISLOCATIONS
PERCIVALL POTT, 1769

"There is a case which, according to the general manner of treating it, gives infinite pain and trouble both to the patient and surgeon, and very frequently ends in the lameness and disappointment of the former, and the disgrace and concern of the latter—I mean the fracture of the fibula attended with a dislocation of the tibia.

"Whoever will take a view of the leg of a skeleton, will see that although the fibula be a very small and slender bone, and very inconsiderable in strength, when compared with the tibia, yet the support of the lower joint of that limb (the ancle), depends so much on this slender bone, that without it the body would not be upheld, nor locomotion performed, without hazard of dislocation every moment. The lower extremity of this bone, which descends considerably below the end of the tibia, is by strong and inelastic ligaments firmly connected with the last-named bone, and with the astragalus, or that bone of the tarsus which is principally concerned in forming the joint of the ancle.

"If the tibia only be broken, and no act of violence, indiscretion, or inadvertence be committed, either on the part of the patient or of those who conduct him, the limb most commonly preserves its figure and length; the same thing generally happens if the fibula only be broken, in all that part of it which is superior

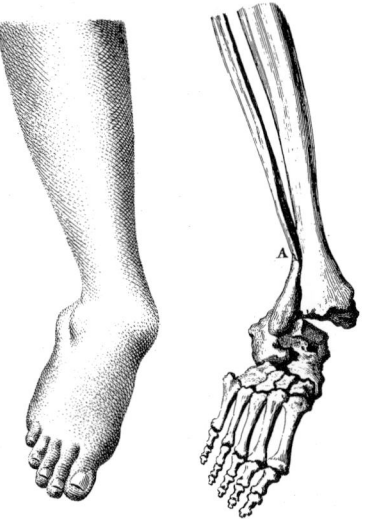

Pott's fracture.

to letter A in the annexed figure, or in any part of it between its upper extremity, and within two or three inches of its lower one.

"When, by leaping or jumping, the fibula breaks in the weak part; that is, within two or three inches of its lower extremity, the inferior fractured end of the fibula falls inward toward the tibia, that extremity of the bone which forms the outer ancle is turned somewhat outward and upward, and the tibia having lost its proper support, and not being of itself capable of steadily preserving its true perpendicular bearing, is forced off from the astragalus inwards, by which means the weak bursal, or common ligament of the joint, is violently stretched, if not torn, and the strong ones, which fasten the tibia to the astragalus and os calces, are always lacerated; thus producing at the same time a perfect fracture and partial dislocation, to which is sometimes added a wound in the integuments, made by the bone at the inner ancle. By this means and indeed as a necessary consequence, all the tendons which pass behind or under, or are attached to the extremities of the tibia and fibula, or os calces, have their natural direction and disposition so altered, that instead of performing their appointed actions, they all contribute to the distortion of the foot, and that by turning it outward and upward.

"When this accident is accompanied, as it sometimes is, with a wound of the integuments of the inner ancle, and that made by the protrusion of the bone, it not infrequently ends in a fatal gangrene, unless prevented by timely amputation, though I have several times seen it do very well without. But in its most simple state, unaccompanied with any wound, it is extremely troublesome to put to rights, still more so to keep it in order, and unless managed with address and skill, is very frequently productive both of lameness and deformity ever after."

DUPUYTREN'S FRACTURE
1819

Baron Dupuytren gave a lecture on fractures and dislocations of the ankle, describing the varieties that he had observed, and, in an appendix, provided a statistical analysis of their frequency and outcome.

"Dislocation of the foot outwards and upwards. This form of displacement is so rare that I have only seen it once in nearly two hundred cases of fractured fibula which have fallen under my observation in the last fifteen years. It involves not only fracture of the fibula, but also laceration of the strong tibio-peroneal ligaments, which generally resist a force to which the osseous tissue itself yields. The following is the remarkable case to which I refer.

◆ CASE XVI
"Fracture of the fibula and rupture of ligaments, with dislocation of the foot upwards and outwards. C. N. Guillemain, a joiner, aged 54, of sanguine temperament, was coming half-drunk out of a pot-house, for the purpose of making water, when, reeling along in a hurried manner, he came to an

inclined and slippery piece of ground, where he fell, his right leg being extended outwards from the body, the weight of which it had to sustain together with the superadded momentum of the fall. Being unable to walk, he was immediately conveyed to the Hotel-Dieu. This occurred in the winter of 1816.

"When admitted, the presence of the usual signs indicating fractured fibula low down were readily detected; but what most attracted attention was the shortness of the leg, together with the almost doubled interval comprised between the malleoli, and the prolongation of the tibia downwards to a level with the sole of the foot: the astragalus and outer malleolus, with the whole of the foot, were drawn up on the outer side of the tibia, two inches above their normal position. All these signs left no doubt that the ligaments connecting the tibia and fibula were torn through, and that the foot was dislocated outwards and upwards, carrying with it the outer malleolus.

"The swelling, tension, and pain momentarily increasing, it was necessary at once to reduce the parts; and this was satisfactorily accomplished after the patient had been bled. The foot and leg then resumed their natural form and direction and my apparatus for fractured fibula was forthwith applied, and an evaporating lotion laid over the joint.

"On the following day the apparatus was removed with a view to re-apply it, and in consequence of an involuntary contraction of the muscles, the parts were again thrown out of place: the reduction was more readily affected this time by distracting the attention of the patient, and the apparatus was again adjusted: a second bleeding was ordered, and low diet prescribed.

"On the third day the tension, swelling, and pain had nearly subsided; and from this time, strange to say, considering the serious mischief which must have existed, the case proceeded as if it had been one of simple fracture; so that on the thirty-sixth day the patient began to walk with crutches, and there was not the slightest irregularity in the form of the injured limb. He speedily regained his strength; and when seen six months afterwards, he retained only the recollection of the accident, without any of the consequences which it originally threatened".

Fractures of the Foot

Albert H. Freiberg (1868–1940)

Freiberg spent all his life in his birthplace, Cincinnati, apart from a period of study in Germany and Austria. He established himself as an orthopaedic surgeon in the city and played an important part in the establishment of orthopaedic facilities there. His influence on the development of American orthopaedics was felt for two reasons: first, he was an active medical author, one of the leaders of thought—he has been called the philosopher of

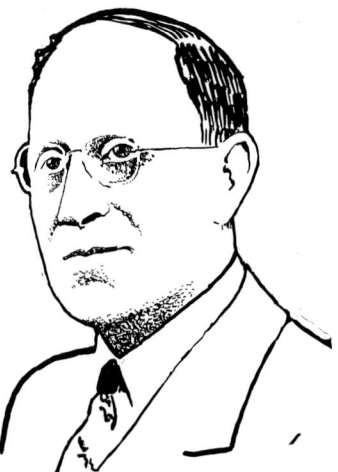

◆ Albert H. Freiberg

orthopaedic surgery. The second reason for his eminence was his conmitteemanship; an able, kindly speaker, he had the ability to turn discussions.

He is best remembered for being the first to describe flattening of the head of the second metatarsal. It is interesting to note that he considered that it was an injury. Since then opinion has swung toward osteochondritis and back again; most people would now agree that Freiberg was right.

In 1910–1911 he was president of the American Orthopaedic Association. Freiberg spent World War I at the Walter Reed Hospital.

INFRACTION OF THE SECOND METATARSAL BONE: A TYPICAL INJURY
ALBERT H. FREIBERG, 1914

"I have often found thickening of such degree in the second metatarso-phalangeal joint that I have sought for organic change in the radiogram; always without finding it, however, until I encountered Case 1 of the series which I am now reporting. In this case I felt justified in the diagnosis of infraction of the distal end of the second metatarsal, a condition which I have thus far failed to find described in literature.

"During the past few years I have encountered six cases of infraction of the distal end of the second metatarsal bone. I feel justified in speaking of it as a typical injury because in each of my six cases not only was the same bone end involved, but the conditions under which the patients presented themselves were very similar, as was also the character of the trauma which produced the lesion.

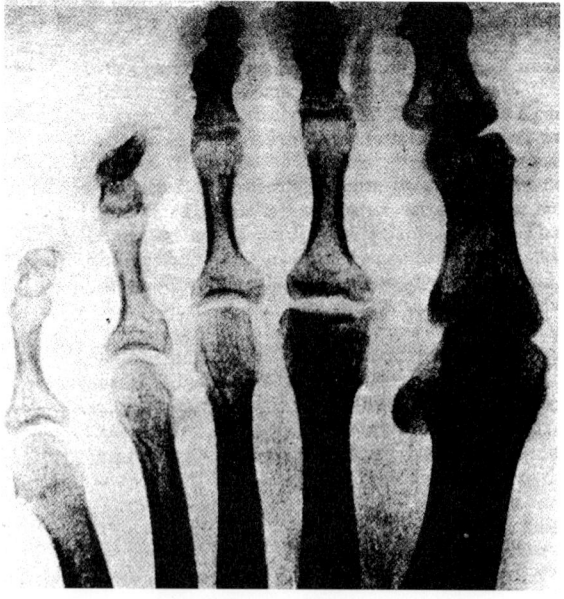

Freiberg's infraction. This girl of 16 years injured her foot at tennis 6 months earlier and suffered an infraction of the second metatarsal head and a small loose body. 1914.

"Ten years ago the first patient in whom I recognized this lesion was referred to me by Dr. E. W. Mitchell, of Cincinnati. The patient was a girl of sixteen. She had been suffering from pain in the ball of the foot for about six months. The pain was precisely like that which we so often encounter in the metatarso-phalangeal region in connection with static incompetence of the foot. At the time I examined the patient she complained of pain in weightbearing only. In attempting any unusual exertion, as in walking considerable distances, she was compelled to limp and the pain became severe.

"The patient was quite sure that the condition dated from and was due to a game of tennis in which she "stubbed" her foot. The pain was severe at the time; it was considered a sprain and she was able to be about the next day.

"My examination disclosed a well formed and apparently strong foot. The metatarso-phalangeal articulation of the second toe was thickened, on palpation, and very tender to pressure. Passive movement of this joint was very painful and accomplished by slight grating. The X-ray showed quite clearly that the distal end of the second metatarsal had been crushed in, causing the articular surface to lose its curved outline. There was apparently a small loose body in the joint about two mm. in diameter.

"The treatment consisted in applying a felt pad to the plantar surface of the foot by means of adhesive plaster, so that its anterior end was placed just back of the injured joint. In this case I also had a steel plate inserted between the layers of the sole of the boot in order to deprive the foot of the motion in the metatarso-phalangeal joints, in walking. I have not done this in my later cases.

"The patient was able to walk painlessly without the pad within six weeks and has had no further trouble with this foot.

"Three of my six cases have shown loose bodies in the radiogram, and grating upon examination. In two of these three cases I was unable to give definite relief by mechanical support alone and, therefore, removed the loose bodies by means of an arthrotomy from the dorsal surface of the foot. This resulted in entire relief from discomfort and pain.

"It is a curious fact that in two of the six cases, no injury whatever could be recalled by the patients in spite of careful questioning on my part. In one of these cases operative removal of small corpora libera was necessary. I have no doubt of the traumatic origin of these three cases.

"Two of my cases were women below middle age, but the remaining four were girls under eighteen years of age.

"The cases with loose bodies will require arthrotomy as a rule.

"Not a little interest attaches to the mechanism by which this injury to the foot takes place. Under normal circumstances the second metatarsal bone is slightly longer than the first. In the presence of a diminished power of toe flexion and especially of the great toe, it is apparent that forcible impact of the ball of the foot against the ground not sufficiently guarded by the flexor *power of the toes will cause the distal end of the second metatarsal to bear the brunt of the blow. It seems likely to me that we have here the explanation of the mechanism of this injury."*

The Ambulatory Treatment of Fractures

For many years patients lay in bed until a fracture of the femur or tibia had united. Then Erichsen advised nonweight-bearing casts in 1878, Krause in Germany in 1891 started weight bearing, and the practice was adopted in Brooklyn in 1893. An editorial in 1896 describes this break with a thousand-year tradition.

"It is evident that most fractures of the lower extremity may be safely treated by apparatus which will early permit the injured limb to be actively used in locomotion. As a result the tedium and disadvantage of prolonged detention from the activities of life may be avoided, the amount of muscular atrophy and joint stiffness incident to disuse of the limb may be much lessened, and the restoration of the full function of the limb after consolidation may be expedited, a more vigorous state of nutrition in the injured parts will be maintained, and the possibilities of delayed or non-union will be lessened: in the aged and in alcoholics the ability to early get the patients up and about will tend to prevent the development of the hypostatic congestions and the nervous disturbances to be feared in such patients; and finally, the beds of hospitals, which otherwise would be encumbered by

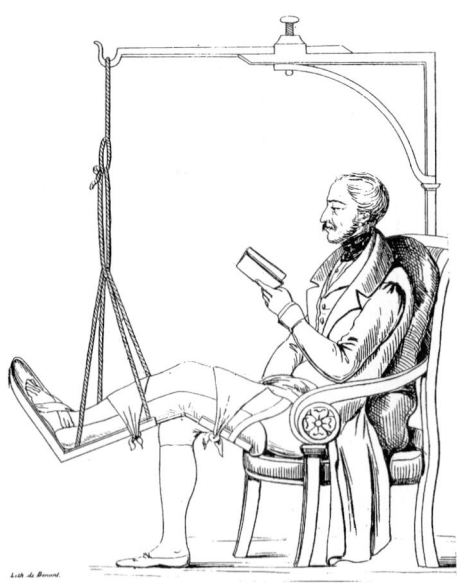

For years all lower limb fractures were treated by putting the patient to bed with a splint. This is one of the earlier attempts at mobilizing the patient. From M Mayor, Paris: 1835.

such patients for many weeks, may be emptied after a few days, and opportunity for the reception of new patients made."

The ambulatory treatment was carried a step further to become the functional treatment. Ernst Dehne in El Paso was an early vocal advocate. But the enthusiasm and good results of Augusto Sarmiento of Miami influenced everyone. He allowed the joints above and below the fracture to move and expected the limb to be used.

"Fracture bracing is predicated on the belief that immobilization of the joints above and below the fracture is not necessary for fracture healing. It proposes also that the soft tissues of the injured extremity play a major role in providing the necessary to allow uninterrupted osteogenesis." A series of animal experiments showed that both immobilization and plating resulted in less callus and less strength than in functionally treated fractures.

"By instrumenting fracture braces on patients with fresh over-riding fractures of the tibia and fibula, it was shown that the soft tissues of the lower leg bear over 80% of the loads placed on the limb. The fracture brace supports only 17% of actual loads. The brace, therefore, is not the major load bearing structure.

"The brace encapsulates the soft tissues of the extremity so that extrusion of the water-like tissues cannot occur. Cineradiography tests conducted on patients with fresh fractures of the tibia indicate that motion at the fracture site occurs quite readily even with low levels of load. These displacements, however, are recoverable as demonstrated by the fact that the fragments returned to their initial position once loads on the limb were relaxed. The fragments move but return to their initial position without allowing progressive deformity to occur."

The brace was applied as soon as the acute symptoms subside and was abandoned if an acceptable reduction and alignment could not be maintained.

THE WALKING CAST FOR A FRACTURE OF THE TIBIA

1891 Fedor Krause put on a cast with little padding and a cast shoe.
1897 Paul Reclus used the proximal flare to take most of the weight.
1929 Lorenz Bohler in Vienna popularized the skintight cast—directly on the skin, hairs and all. This allowed the leg to rest while the rest of the body was active. Others found this hard to replicate.
1930 Winnett Orr: pins and plaster
1950 Ernst Dehne promoted aggressive early weight bearing to avoid nonunion.
1967 Augusto Sarmiento applied prosthetic principles and came up with the patellar tendon-bearing cast, avoiding knee stiffness.

RUPTURE OF THE TENDO ACHILLIES: AN AFFECT OF THE LARGE TENDON OF THE HEEL

PARÉ, 1575

" ... It oft times is rent or torn by a small occasion without any sign of injury or solution of continuity apparent on the outside as by a little jump, the slipping aside of the foot, the too nimble getting on horseback, or the slipping of the foot out of the stirrup in mounting into the saddle. When this chance happens, it will give a crack like a coachman's whip; above the head where the tendon is broken the depressed cavity may be felt with your finger; there is great pain in the part and the party is not able to go. This mischance may be amended by long lying and resting in bed and repelling medicines applied to the part ... neither must we hereon promise to ourselves or the patient certain or absolute health. But on the contrary at the beginning of the disease we must foretell that it will never be so cured, and that some relics may remain ..."

RUPTURE OF THE TENDO ACHILLES

JOHN HUNTER, 1766

"On Thursday morning at four o'clock the 20th February 1766 I broke my Tendo Achilles. I was jumping and lighting upon my toes without allowing my heels to come to the ground, by which means I supported the whole weight of my body upon the gastrocnemei and solei muscles—these two joined was too much for the tendon, which gave way at once, by which means my heel came to the ground. The snap (or report) made by the breaking of the tendon was heard all over the room. I stood still without being able to make another spring; and the sensation it gave me was as if something had struck the calf of my leg; and that the noise was the body which had struck me falling on the floor, and I looked down to see what it was, but saw nothing. I walked to a chair but could not throw myself forwards on my toes on that foot, the calf of the leg was extremely painful and was in the state of a cramp. I endeavoured to take off the cramp by bending the foot, but found that that motion had no effect upon the contraction of the muscles of the calf of the leg and upon further examination I found that the Tendo Achilles was broken.

"I bound it up at first with the foot extended, and the knee a little bent; with the ends of the Tendon about half an inch distant. This bandage remained for five days. In shifting the bandage I had an opportunity of examining the parts but they were a good deal swelled, so that I could not now tell whether the ends of the tendon were closed together or not. I examined the parts every day, and when the swelling from the inflammation abated, which was in less than a fortnight, the parts were so smooth that I could not find any inequality; the only swelling that remained was of the oedematous kind, which only swelled at night and was down in the morning.

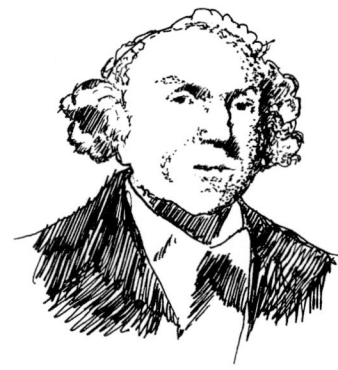

◆ **John Hunter (1728–1793)**

Hunter grew up in Scotland under the shadow of his jealous surgeon-brother. He was a student and surgeon at St. George's and spent time as an Army surgeon. What singled him out was his research. He did this at home and on a research farm in Earl's Court. He transplanted tissues, looked at bone and tendon healing, and so on. As a surgeon-scientist he saw everything as a research question, and he inspired many followers—including Dr. Physick, the Father of surgery in Philadelphia. If you visit London you should go to Hunter's Museum at the Royal College of Surgeons; though blitzed during World War II, it is still huge and contains specimens selected to illustrate principles and laws of nature.

"About this time I found that the left leg began to swell, which I suppose was owing to my confinement. I then took the bark three or four times every day and took a ride in a chaise into the country, on the 14th day, and found that neither of the legs swelled so much that day as they had done before.

"It continued much the same for about three weeks after the accident, when my foot slipt upon a wet floor, which made me pitch upon the toe of that foot; which gave me great pain at the time, and which continued for a considerable time. Whether the parts were torn asunder or not I could not tell, the inflammation from this accident was more than the former; was now in a good deal of pain upon the least motion of the parts; and the swelling was more considerable than before.

"In about a fortnight after this last accident, the parts became again easy, and the swelling abated. I now began to walk again; for this purpose I got an old shoe raised in the heel about an inch, with a strap behind to buckle to a laced bandage round the Calf; and this was principally when I went to bed that I wore it, which was to avoid the consequence that might arise from any involuntary motions in those muscles in my sleep.

"When I first began to walk I did not use or move the joint of the Ankle, therefore was obliged to turn my toe almost quite out to allow of my body being thrown forwards for the motion of the other leg; by this means I avoided being thrown upon my toes of that foot; to support which I should have been obliged to have acted with my Gastrocnemius and Soleus muscles. For about eight weeks the small of the leg was in the morning almost as small as the other, and then I could find a thickness in the tendon for above two inches in length.

"The shoe for such cases should be either an old one, or one made on purpose for the case of putting it off and on. If an old one, then the heel should be principally raised on the inside."

References

Chapter references are located in Chapter 26.

◆ Chapter Eighteen

Upper Limb Fractures

The surgeon ought to be very cautious in delivering his prognostic concerning fractures. He should avoid being too hasty in promising a quick, easy, and certain cure, lest his art should be overcome by accidental disorders, and he should be accused of Knavery or Ignorance.
Heister (1683-1758)

The creative genius that went into designing strange-looking splints and gravity-defying traction for fractures of the lower limb overlooked the upper limb. Hippocrates used ladders to reduce old dislocations, and Thomas used a wrench for wrist fractures but no exotic kinds of immobilization. Hence, there are more words than pictures in this chapter.

Famous Patients

Andrew Jackson (1767-1845), 7th United States President. At the City Hotel, Nashville, on September 4th, 1813, Jackson pulled a pistol on Tom Benton and before he could fire Tom's brother shot him in the left shoulder. He bled through two mattresses, and the doctors advised amputation. The General said, as people do today, "I'll keep my arm." He was governor of Mississippi

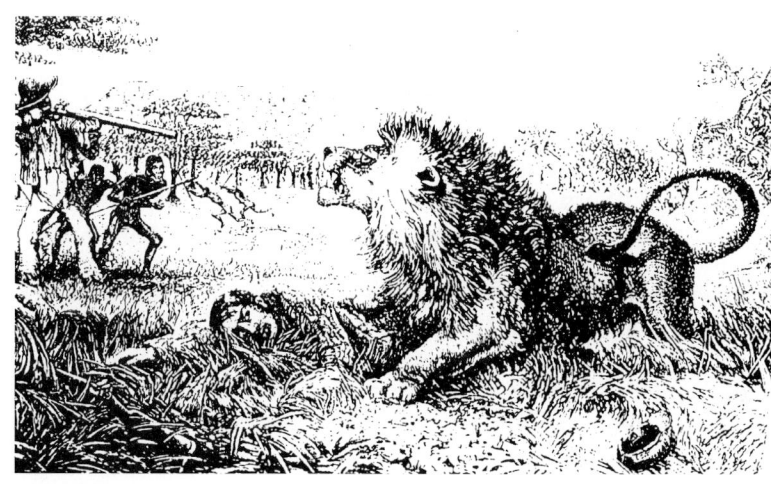

David Livingston nearly died when he was attacked by a lion in 1843 during his exploration of Africa. He suffered an arm wound or fracture. Reproduced with permission from King M: The Story of Medicine and Disease in Malawi. Blantyre, 1988.

Territory at the time and before he recovered he was campaigning again. The arm never healed; a sequestrum was discharged the next year which he sent to his wife, and 19 years later a surgeon took the bullet out without an anesthetic.

Sir Robert Peel, British Prime Minister, was thrown by a horse in 1850 and sustained a fracture of the clavicle from which he died the next day. His care was criticized, leading *The Lancet* to write an editorial:

"As soon as surgical aid was procured, it was found that there was a comminuted fracture of the left clavicle, with considerable swelling from the first, which, together with the excruciating pain of the whole shoulder, rendered a minute examination extremely difficult. A swelling as large as the hand might cover subsequently formed below the fractured clavicle, which pulsated to the touch synchronously with the action of the heart. When examined carefully by the eye, it was found that the movement of this tumour corresponded with the contractions of the auricle, and was, in some respects, similar to the pulsations observed in the veins of the neck in very thin persons, and in certain forms of venous regurgitation. It was evident from these signs, that some vein beneath the clavicle, probably the subclavian, had been wounded by the broken bone at the time of the fall; and that the subclavicular swelling consisted of blood effused from the wounded vessel. It was also evident that the swelling was in this way connected with the heart, forming what might be called a diffused false venous aneurism. This was all that could be ascertained positively. Sir Robert Peel was well known to be of a gouty habit, and he was at all times extremely sensitive to physical pain. His sufferings during the whole of his brief illness were of the most agonizing kind. This might have arisen from the laceration of some of the nerves converging beneath the collarbone, to form the axillary plexus; a complication which, as is well known, sometimes occurs from severe fractures in this situation. After death, one or two of the ribs on the left side were found to be fractured, which had not been detected during life. The injuries we have referred to would have been sufficient to cause death in such a subject; but there may possibly have been further injury, or disease, resulting from the accident, within the chest."

No autopsy was done at the request of the family. *The Lancet* had another editorial the next week defending the doctors who were criticized for not intervening in some way.

King William of William and Mary. Today people die in motor vehicle accidents. In the 18th century it was horses. King William was riding in Hampton Court in 1702 when the horse put its foot in a hole and fell. The king landed on his right shoulder, broke his collarbone, and died of complications 2 weeks later.

Wilhelm II. Victoria Louise, daughter of Queen Victoria, delivered a child after a breech presentation in 1859. The baby boy sustained a fracture of the left humerus and a brachial plexus palsy. He became Kaiser Bill—German leader during World War I.

Stalin had a supracondylar fracture that left him with some stiffness and features of Volkmann's contracture. Every time I set one of these fractures I hope I am not going to produce another Stalin.

TIMELINE OF UPPER LIMB INJURIES

3rd century BC	Hippocrates writes about many fractures, including reduction of a dislocated shoulder and recurrent dislocation.
1814	Monteggia fracture
1814	Colles fracture
1822	First description of Galeazzi fracture
1843	Rodrigues' posterior sternoclavicular joint dislocation
1850	Sir Robert Peel dies of a fractured clavicle.
1870	Kocher's maneuver
1882	Bennett's thumb fracture
1910	Rolando's thumb fracture
1934	Galeazzi fracture described by Galeazzi
1937	Matte bone graft for scaphoid
1948	Swenson pins for supracondylar fracture

Shoulder Dislocation

REDUCTION OF A DISLOCATED SHOULDER

HIPPOCRATES, 3RD CENTURY BC

"In all dislocations, reduction is to be effected if possible immediately, while still warm, but otherwise, as quickly as it can be done; for reduction will be a much quicker and easier process for the operator, and a much less painful one to the patient, if effected before swelling comes on.

"Those who attempt reduction with the heel operate in a manner which is an approach to the natural. The patient must be on the ground on his back, while the person who is to effect the reduction is seated upon the ground on the side of the dislocation; then the operator, seizing with his hand the affected arm, is to pull it, while with his heel in the armpit he pushes in the contrary direction, the right heel being placed in the right armpit, and the left heel in the left armpit. But a round bag of suitable size must be placed in the hollow of the armpit; the most convenient are very small and hard balls, formed from several pieces of leather sewn together. For without something of this kind the heel cannot reach to the head of the humerus, since, when the arm is stretched, the armpit becomes hollow, the tendons on both sides of the armpit making countercontraction so as to oppose the reduction. But another person should be seated on the other side of the patient to hold the sound shoulder, so that the body may not be dragged along when the arm of the affected side is pulled and then, when the ball is placed in the

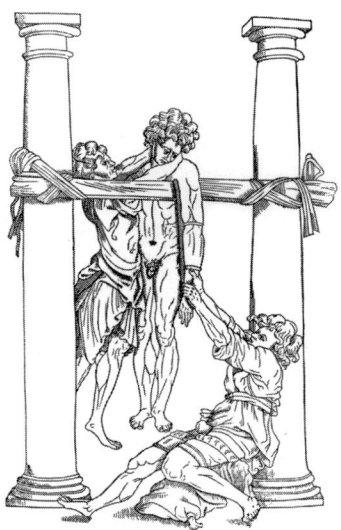

Vidus Vidius: Reduction of a dislocated shoulder, 1544. This must have been a very old dislocation to have required this amount of force. The risk of rupturing the brachial artery and injuring the brachial plexus could not have been explained to the patient before he signed an informed consent.

armpit, a supple piece of thong sufficiently broad is placed around it, and some person taking hold of its two ends is to seat himself above the patient's head to make counter extension, while at the same time he pushes with his foot against the bone at the top of the shoulder. The bag should be placed as much inside as possible, upon the ribs, and not upon the head of the humerus."

Theodor Kocher (1841–1917)

Kocher was one of the most brilliant surgeons of his day, who combined a mastery of basic principles, an enquiring mind, and superb operating technique, which was recognized by the award of the Nobel Prize for Medicine in 1909.

He was born in Berne and studied in Berlin, London, Paris, and Vienna, graduating from Berne in 1865. He became professor of surgery there in 1872. During the whole of his life he maintained an interest in surgical anatomy and surgical approaches; most days he would work out approaches on cadavers. This had two orthopaedic consequences: he devised a rational technique for relaxing the muscles around the shoulder and easing a dislocated shoulder into position. One day he was in the audience watching Billroth and his firm trying to reduce a shoulder dislocation without success. Kocher asked if he could try his newly reasoned method. He succeeded, and later published his technique in 1870.

The other consequence of his study of surgical approaches was a remarkable book, which was translated into English, describing a tremendous variety of incisions, many of which remain classic. It is well worth consulting.

One feels that Kocher used orthopaedics only to sharpen his wits for his main interest—thyroid disease, to which he contributed so much. In addition, he wrote widely and deeply on many topics, and invented surgical instruments as he needed them, without thinking it anything but commonplace. When he died, Moynihan wrote an epitaph worth bearing in mind: he had a "freedom from prejudice for his own intellectual progeny."

♦ Theodor Kocher

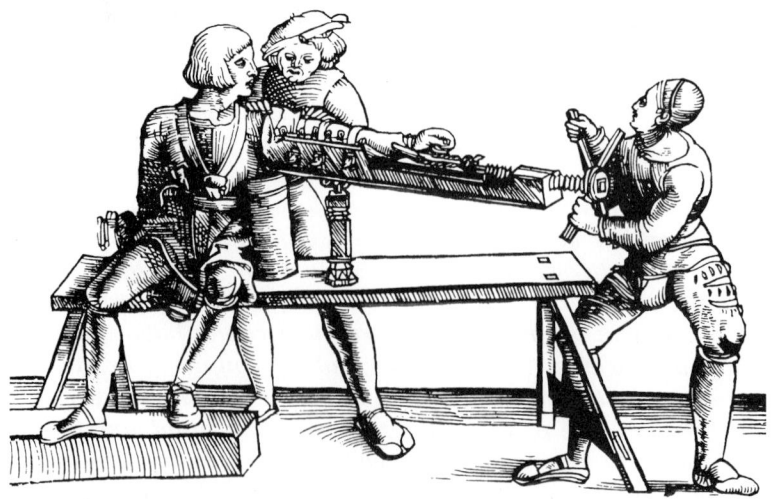

Hans von Gersdorff: Traction for a dislocated shoulder, 1517. Today we treat acute dislocations the same day, and reduction is easy. But in the past, there was delay—hence these machines. Some of the so-called dislocations may have been fracture-dislocations and incapable of stable reduction.

KOCHER'S METHOD OF REDUCTION OF A DISLOCATED SHOULDER
1870

"Bend the arm at the elbow, press it against the body, rotate outwards till a resistance is felt, lift the externally rotated upper arm in the sagittal plane as far as possible forwards, and finally turn inwards slowly."

This is taken from a long, closely reasoned article confusingly illustrated by six engravings, some of which are printed upside down.

Kocher worked out his technique on cadavers. He aimed at bringing the greater tuberosity of the humerus into contact with the glenoid rim to act as a fulcrum. This was achieved by flexing the externally rotated shoulder, which also relaxed the upper anterior part of the capsule that would otherwise form a tense cord. When the arm is internally rotated, the head pivots on the fulcrum and slips into the glenoid.

Kocher claimed these advantages of the method—it was painless because movements were not forced, and it did not require either anesthesia or assistants. It was only suitable for subcoracoid dislocations with three provisos: that capsular damage was not so extensive that the bone surfaces were not held apposed, that neither the glenoid rim, nor the greater tuberosity, were fractured, which would also prevent them from pivoting one on the other.

Posterior Dislocation of the Shoulder

Astley Cooper was one of the first to describe this. He encountered two cases in 38 years. His description shows the change in the style of medical writing. There is a big change between what he believed was important and what seems important today when we are reading it. The history is full of information that we would regard as inconsequential, and it is not in the style of a textbook.

"The gentleman, to whom the dislocation of the head of the humerus upon the dorsum scapulae occurred, was Mr. Collinson, who was about 36 years of age, 6 feet high, and unusually muscular. The injury occurred in the neighbourhood of Windsor, in consequence of his horse falling with him, by which he was thrown over the animal's head. He applied to a surgeon at Windsor, but the character of the injury was not detected. He returned in a post-chaise to his own house when Mr Hacon and myself saw him. The shoulder had lost its usual roundness; the arm could be moved considerably either upwards or downwards; but the motion, either in the anterior or posterior direction, was very limited. On raising the arm to a right angle with the side, the direction of the limb was obviously behind the glenoid cavity, and by placing the hand over the dorsum scapulae, and then rotating the arm, the head of the bone was felt to obey the rotating motion."

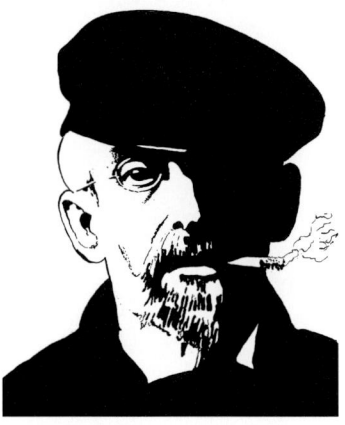

◆ Hugh Owen Thomas (1834–1891)

This short, quick man, seen around the streets of Liverpool always wearing a black coat buttoned up to the neck and a second-mate's discharge cap and smoking a cigarette, came from a line of Anglesey bonesetters. His father was a successful bonesetter in Liverpool and sent all his sons to medical school. After a brief period working with his father, he became a general practitioner on his own. He never had a hospital appointment and made a point of treating his patients at home. Perhaps with managed care we will all be doing this in the future. His special interests were lithopaxy, the management of the acute abdomen, and orthopaedics. His ideas became accepted despite his unconventional background and his intolerance of others.

He was an advocate of enforced, prolonged, and uninterrupted rest for the treatment of tuberculous joints. His armentarium of splints was superbly designed to achieve this and remain widely used: he devised the cervical collar, metatarsal bar, heel wedges, and the knee splint that is now called a Thomas splint. He was able to fit a patient at a few moments' notice.

Robert Jones, his nephew, was brought up by Thomas and assisted him for a while; later Jones popularized Thomas' ideas and added his own, establishing the "Liverpool School" of orthopaedics.

Thomas published a number of books written in a polemic style that gives a good idea of his character and ideas. For example, "The crying evil of our art is the fact that much of our surgery is too mechanical, our medical practice too chemical: and there is a hankering to interfere, which thwarts the inherent tendency to recovery possessed by all persons not actually dying."

He reduced the dislocation by traction. It snapped back and functioned well.

The second case happened during an anatomy lecture at Guy's Hospital. All the class rushed out to watch the lecturer reduce the dislocation.

Pulled Elbow

Toddlers, yanked along by adults, cry over this common injury, which is so easily treated by a manipulation. Attempts to explain this phenomenon began in 1671 with Fournier suggesting that the radius moved distally.

Duverney in 1751 wrote about it in his book *Maladies des Os*. He pointed out that it occurred in small children who had the wrist pulled. The child opposed supination, and he believed that it was due to the radial head being pulled through the orbicular ligament. Pingaudin in 1878 confirmed this in cadavers. Since then there have been so many cadaver studies and speculations that Poland could spend six pages reviewing the papers written before the invention of X-rays. Here is one of them.

PULLED ELBOW
HUGH OWEN THOMAS, 1883

"This accident is invariably the result of applying traction and pronation by grasping the hand of the infant.

"The mother or servant by whose agency the accident occurred often brings the child for advice, and informs the surgeon that she only pulled him by the hand, which caused him to stumble whilst still held by the hand, and since then the arm had been disabled, and that the infant complained if any attempt were made to flex the elbow.

"On examination, the surgeon finds that the arm lies dependent, slightly flexed, and pronated, and that the child dreads being touched. If the arm be forcibly flexed and manipulated, it may or may not be instantly relieved—but this is not what the surgeon ought to do. There is a method which—if followed—is painless to the child, is immediately effectual, and favourably impresses any observers. We will here suppose that it is the right elbow. The surgeon must very gently grasp the child's hand with the thumb and index finger of his own right hand, planting his thumbs in the palmar base of the child's thumb while the index finger hooks round the ulnar edge and back of the child's hand, then placing the olecranon point of the child's elbow in the cupped palm of the surgeon's left hand, let him supinate the arm, and at the same time fully extend it, using the cupped palm of the left hand as a fulcrum; and now the surgeon in nearly every case will feel a click of some part slipping into place, and then let him instantly flex the elbow and fix it in a sling.

"The procedure is painless and the relief instant, and in nearly every case the little patient, after this operation, expresses a desire to use the elbow."

Wrist Fractures

Fractures close to a joint were thought to be dislocations for 2000 years, and so fractures of the distal radius were thought to be dislocations of the wrist—something almost unknown. Then, in the last century, dissections and clinical studies revealed several kinds of wrist fracture—Colles', Smith's, and Barton's. With the arrival of X-rays, the individual patient stood a chance of having the nature of the injury recognized in all its subtlety and knowing whether the deformity had been corrected.

Wrist fractures in children were known often to be epiphyseal separations and residual deformity was corrected.

ON FRACTURE OF THE CARPAL EXTREMITY OF THE RADIUS

ABRAHAM COLLES, 1814

"The injury to which I wish to direct the attention of surgeons has not, as far as I know, been described by any other author; indeed the form of the carpal extremity would rather induce us to question its being liable to fracture. The absence of crepitus, and of the other common symptoms of fracture, together with the swelling which instantly arises in this, as in other injuries of the wrist, render the difficulty of ascertaining the real nature of the case very considerable.

"This fracture takes place about an inch and a half above the carpal extremity of the radius, and exhibits the following appearances: The posterior surface of the limb presents a considerable deformity; for a depression is seen in the fore-arm, about an inch and a half above the end of this bone, while a considerable swelling occupies the wrist and metacarpus. Indeed the carpus and base of the metacarpus appear to be thrown backwards so much as on first view to excite a suspicion that the carpus had been dislocated forward.

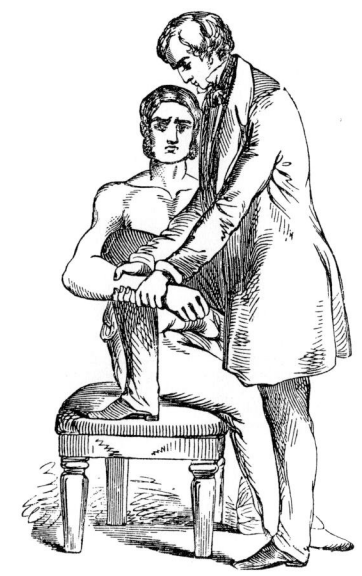

Reduction of a dislocated elbow by means of a knee in the bend of the elbow. From Hamilton FH: [An important] Treatise on Fractures and Dislocations, 1860.

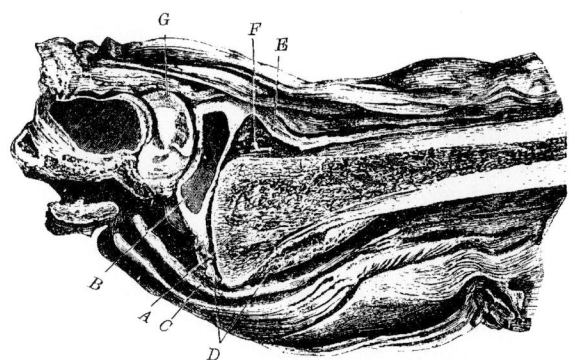

John Poland made this dissection in 1883. A 12 year old boy was sliding down the bannister of a warehouse when he overbalanced and fell to his death from the third floor. The pathology of a type II separation of the distal radius can be seen. The posterior stripping and the anterior tear of the periosteum are shown.

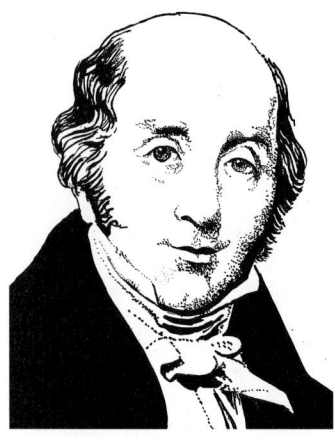

◆ **Abraham Colles (1773–1843)**

Colles was born near Kilkenny, Ireland. The story goes that while he was at school, a flood swept through the local doctor's house, carrying away his possessions. One of his anatomy books landed near the Colles' home. Abraham found it, and on returning it to the doctor, he was made a present of the book. This is thought to have turned his mind toward medicine.

He trained at Dublin and then went to Edinburgh for postgraduate study. After obtaining the degree of M.D. in 1797, he walked from Edinburgh to London. The following year he settled in surgical practice in Dublin, and was elected President of the Royal College of Surgeons of Ireland at the age of 29. He wrote a book on surgical anatomy in 1811 and a paper on clubfoot in 1818. His paper on radial fractures was published in 1814, followed in 1837 by a book on venereal disease and the use of mercury. An early riser, he ran one of the most lucrative practices in Dublin.

"As an operator he has many equals, and some superiors; but in advice, from long experience and a peculiar tact in discovering the hidden causes of disease, he has scarcely a rival." So wrote a contemporary.

Teachers often complain that today's doctors cannot write plain English. The long-winded, chaotic description shows that we are better than some 19th century writers. If we had to learn orthopaedics from books written by Colles, we would lose the power of logical and orderly thought.

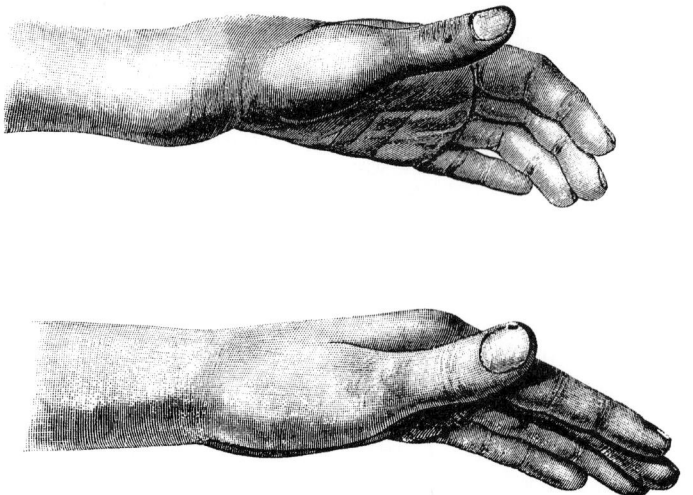

Fracture remodeling, 1896. John Poland started to look after this boy about six weeks after injury. The lower picture shows the appearance two years later.

"On observing the anterior surface of the limb, we observe a considerable fullness, as if caused by the flexor tendons being thrown forwards. This fullness extends upwards to about one third of the length of the fore-arm, and terminated below at the upper edge of the annular ligament of the wrist. The extremity of the ulna is seen projecting towards the palm and inner edge of the limb; the degree, however, which this projection takes is different in different instances.

"If the surgeon proceeds to investigate the nature of this injury he will find that the end of the ulna admits of being readily moved backwards and forwards.

"On the posterior surface he will discover, by the touch, that the swelling on the wrist and metacarpus is not caused entirely by the effusion among the soft parts; he will perceive that the ends of the metacarpal and second row of carpal bones form no small part of it. This, strengthening the suspicion which the first view of the case had excited, leads him to examine, in a more particular manner, the anterior part of the joint; but the want of that solid resistance which a dislocation of the carpus forwards must occasion forces him to abandon this notion, and leaves him in a state of perplexing uncertainty as to the real nature of the injury. He will, therefore, endeavour to gain some information by examining the bones of the forearm. The facility with which (as was noticed) the ulna can be moved backwards and forwards does not furnish him with any useful hint. When he moves his fingers along the anterior surface of the radius he finds it more full and prominent than is natural; a similar examination of the posterior surface of this bone induces him to think that a depression is felt about an inch and a half above its carpal extremity. He now expects to find satisfactory proofs of a fracture of the radius at this spot. For this purpose he attempts to move

the broken pieces of bone in opposite directions; but, although the patient is by this examination excited by considerable pain, yet neither crepitus nor a yielding of the bone at the seat of the fracture, nor any other positive evidence of the existence of such an injury, is thereby obtained. The patient complains of severe pain as often as an attempt is made to give to the limb the motions of pronation and supination.

"If the surgeon lock his hand in that of the patient and make extension, even with considerable force, he restores the limb to its natural form, but the distortion of the limb instantly returns on the extension being removed. Should the facility with which a moderate extension restores the limb to its form induce the practitioner to treat this as a case of sprain, he will find, after a lapse of time sufficient for the removal of similar swellings, the deformity undiminished. Or, should he mistake the case for a dislocation of the wrist, and attempt to retain the parts in situ by tight bandages and splints, the pain caused by the pressure on the back of the wrist will force him to unbend them in a few hours; and if they be applied more loosely, he will find, at the expiration of a few weeks, that the deformity still exhibits in its fullest extent, and that it is now no longer to be removed by making extension of the limb. By such mistakes the patient is doomed to endure for many months considerable lameness and stiffness of the limb, accompanied by severe pains on attempting to bend the hand and fingers. One consolation only remains, that the limb at some remote period will again enjoy perfect freedom in all its motions, and be completely exempt from pain; the deformity, however, will remain undiminished throughout life.

"The unfavourable result of some of the first cases of this description which came under my care forced me to investigate with peculiar anxiety the nature of the injury. But while the absence of crepitus and of the other usual symptoms of fracture render the diagnosis extremely difficult, a recollection of the superior strength and thickness of this part of the radius, joined to the mobility of its articulation with the carpus and ulna, rather inclined me to question the possibility of a fracture taking place at this part of the bone. At last, after many unsuccessful trials, I hit upon the following simple method of examination by which I was enabled to ascertain that the symptoms above enumerated actually rose from a fracture seated about one and half inches above the carpal extremity of the radius.

"Let the surgeon apply the fingers of one hand to the seat of the suspected fracture, and, locking the other hand in that of the patient, make a moderate extension until he observes the limb restored to its natural form. As soon as this is effected let him move the patient's hand backwards and forwards, and he will at every such attempt be sensible of yielding of the fractured ends of the bone, and this to such a degree as must remove all doubt from his mind.

"The nature of this injury, once ascertained, will be a very easy matter to explain the different phenomena attendant on it, and to point out a method of treatment which will prove completely successful. The hard swelling which appears on the back of the hand is caused by the carpal surface of the radius being directed slightly backwards instead of looking directly downwards. The carpus and metacarpus, retaining their connections with this bone, must follow it in its derangements and cause the convexity above alluded to. This change of direction in the articulating surface of the radius is caused by the tendons of the exterior surface of the thumb, which pass along the posterior surface of the radius in sheaths firmly connected with the inferior extremity of this bone. The broken extremity of the radius being thus drawn backwards causes the ulna to appear prominent towards the palmar surface, while it is probably thrown more towards the inner or ulnar side of the limb by the upper end of the fragment of the radius pressing against it in that direction. The separation of these two bones from each other is facilitated by a previous rupture of their capsular ligament, an event which may be readily occasioned by the violence of the injury. An effusion in the sheaths of the flexor tendons will account for that swelling which occupies the limb anteriorly.

"It is obvious that in the treatment of this fracture our attention should be principally directed to guard against the carpal end of the radius being drawn backwards. For this purpose, while assistants hold the limb in a middle state between pronation and supination, let a thick and firm compress be applied transversely on the anterior surface of the limb, at the seat of the fracture, taking care that it shall not press on the ulna; let this be bound on firmly with a roller and then let a tin splint, formed to the shape of the arm, be applied to both its anterior and posterior surfaces. In cases where the end of the ulna is much displaced, I have laid a very narrow wooden splint along the naked side of the bone. This latter splint, I now think, should be used in every instance, as, by pressing the extremity of the ulna against the side of the radius, it will tend to oppose the displacement of the fractured end of this bone. It is scarcely necessary to observe that the two principal splints should be much more narrow at the wrist than those in general use, and should also extend to the roots of the fingers, spreading out so as to give a firm support to the hand. The cases treated on this plan have all recovered without the smallest defect or deformity of the limb, in the ordinary time for the care of fractures.

"I cannot conclude these observations without remarking that were my opinion to be drawn from those cases only which have occurred to me, I should consider this as by far the most common injury to which the wrist or carpal extremities are exposed. During the last three years I have not met a single instance of Desault's dislocation of the inferior end of the radius, while I have had opportunities of seeing a vast number of the fracture of the lower end of this bone."

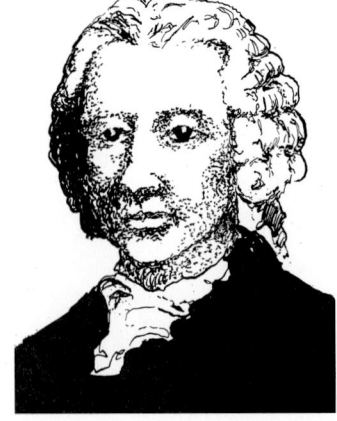

◆ Claude Poutreau (1725–1775)

◆ Claude Poutreau (1725–1775)

Chief Surgeon at Hôtel Dieu, Lyon, France. He described fractures of the distal radius in 1783 and realized that they were not dislocations. For the French they are Poutreau-Colles fractures.

Smith's Fracture

FRACTURE OF THE LOWER EXTREMITY OF THE RADIUS, WITH DISPLACEMENT OF THE LOWER FRAGMENT FORWARDS
ROBERT WILLIAM SMITH, 1847

"This is an injury of exceedingly rare occurrence, and one which presents characters closely resembling those of dislocation of the carpus forwards. It generally occurs in consequence of a fall upon the back of the hand, and the situation of the fracture is from half an inch to an inch above the articulation; it is accompanied by great deformity, the principal features of which are a dorsal and a palmar tumour, and a striking projection of the head of the ulna at the posterior and inner part of the forearm; the dorsal tumour occupies the entire breadth of the forearm; but is most conspicuous internally, where it is constituted by the lower extremity of the ulna displaced backwards; from this point, the inferior outline of the tumour passes obliquely upwards and outwards, corresponding in the latter direction to the lower end of the superior fragment of the radius. Immediately below the dorsal swelling there is a well-marked sulcus, deepest internally below the head of the ulna, directed nearly transversely, but ascending a little as it approaches the radial border of the fore-arm.

"The palmar is less remarkable than the dorsal tumour; formed principally by the lower fragment of the radius, it is obscured by the thick mass of flexor tendons which cross the front of the carpus, but towards the ulnar border of the limb there is a considerable projection, which marks the situation of the pisiform bone, passing down to its attachment into which, can be seen the tendon of the flexor carpi ulnaris thrown forwards in strong relief. The transverse diameter of the fore-arm is not much altered, but the anteroposterior is considerably increased, and the radial border of the limb becomes concave at its lowest part.

"In the case from which the preceding drawings was made, the patient, in endeavouring to save himself from being run over by a car, fell with great violence upon the back of his hand; the lower end of the radius was broken and driven forwards along with the carpus, and the head of the ulna was displaced backwards.

"I cannot speak with accuracy as to the anatomical characters of the injury, having never had an opportunity of examining after death the skeleton of the fore-arm, in those who had during life met with this accident; nor is there any preparation shewing the exact relative position of the fragments, in any of the pathological collections in Dublin; but still I feel satisfied that the injury, the external characters of which have just been described, is a fracture of the lower end of the radius, with displacement of the lower fragment carrying the carpus forwards, and of the head of the ulna backwards, and that it has not unfrequently been mistaken for dislocation of the carpus forwards and of the bones of the fore-arm backwards.

"The facility, however, with which the deformity can be removed, its ability to recur when the extending force ceases to act, the production of crepitus when the limb is extended, and a motion of rotation given to the hand, and our being able to feel the irregular margin of the upper fragment of the radius posteriorly, are sufficient to enable us to distinguish this accident from luxation of the bones of the wrist forwards."

BARTON'S FRACTURE
1838

"The accidents which are to be the principal subject of my remarks, usually pass either for sprains or dislocations of the wrist. Between these two injuries there is too great a dissimilarity to admit of an excuse for the surgeon who mistakes the one for the other; but he may confound with these and it is a common fault to do so, **a subluxation of the wrist, consequent to fracture through the articular surface of the carpal extremity of the radius**, although to this accident belong appearances exclusively its own.

"It is to the peculiar injury that I wish to draw attention. This accident must not be confounded with those which are also of frequent occurrence, namely, fractures of the radius, or of the radius and ulna, just above, and not involving the joint."

BENNETT'S FRACTURE: FRACTURES OF THE METACARPAL BONES
E. H. BENNETT, 1882

"The specimens I submit are united fractures of the third and fifth metacarpals of the same right hand, one of the shaft and one of the base of the fifth, both from right hands, and five of the first, all from the right side.

"These are the entire number of these fractures which I have collected.

"Of greater interest is the fact that in each of the five examples of fracture of the metacarpal bone of the thumb, allowing for shades of difference such as must always exist, the type and character of the fracture is the same—a form and type of fracture not hitherto described in these bones; and if this series be of any value as representing the ordinary injuries, the commonest fracture, certainly the most common of thumb. All have the lines of fracture marked by changes on the articular surface which corresponds to trapezium. The fracture passes obliquely (a b in illustration) through the base of the bone, detaching the greater part of the articular facette with that piece of bone supporting it, which projects into the palm. The amount of displacement in this and all the specimens is trivial, and from clinical observation of the injury it is evident that the fragment displaced is not the smaller, as one might infer from an examination of the isolated specimens of united fractures, but the larger—in fact, to the extent that the irregularity of the surface indicates that the meta-

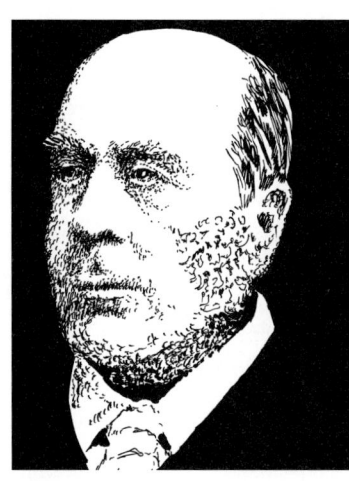

◆ **Edward Hallaran Bennett (1837–1907)**

The son of the Recorder of Cork, Bennett studied at Trinity College, Dublin. Soon after qualifying he established himself as an anatomist at the University and built up a wonderful collection of specimens of bone pathology, upon which he drew to write his papers on metacarpal fractures, in which he mentioned the fracture dislocation of the thumb that bears his name.

In 1873 he succeeded Smith as professor of surgery at Trinity College. He was a stimulating teacher, the model of honor and uprightness, who never did a crooked thing and was blunt but not unkind. He became president of the Royal College of Surgeons of Ireland.

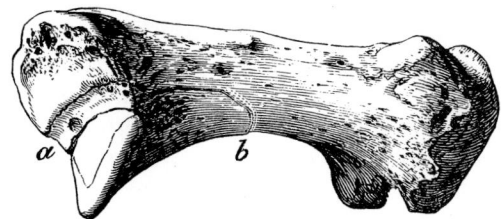

Bennett's fracture

carpal bone of the thumb undergoes subluxation backwards. In all these specimens the dorsal surface of the bone is free from any implication in the fracture, and this fact, combined with the small amount of displacement which occurs, renders the fracture one extremely liable to escape detection. The importance of a correct diagnosis of this injury is illustrated by a case which I have had for nearly two years under observation.

"A girl, aged twenty, was thrown from an outside car and fell to the ground, saving herself from graver injury by putting forward her arm; she struck the ball of the thumb against the ground; and at once suffered extreme pain in it. Next morning I saw her at Sir P. Dun's Hospital, when at first sight no injury was apparent beyond the swelling of a bruised and sprained thumb. In handling the ball of the thumb I felt osseus crepitus, and, having my attention so arrested, I was not long in establishing the diagnosis of this injury, for the dorsal surface of the metacarpal was entire; it projected backwards at the articulation with the carpus, and by reducing it into place crepitus could easily be elicited. So trivial an injury does this appear to be, and the specimens show so little deformity, except in some the sign of arthritis consequent on it, I might fairly be asked what importance attaches to the correct diagnosis. All will admit that a correct diagnosis even in trivial injuries is desirable, but in this case the diagnosis is essential to a correct prognosis, and here lies the importance of the injury. Seeing the value of the movement of the thumb, no injury of it is to be lightly regarded, and this fracture, though it unites readily by bone and with almost inappreciable deformity renders the thumb for many months lame and useless. In the case I have reported, even now, nearly two years after the accident occurring in a young and healthy subject, the hand fails to grasp or lift with certainty any body requiring a wide gape of the thumb—for instance, to lift a tumbler full of water from the table, and this in a case where every care was taken to keep the parts in place and at rest for a proper time."

MONTEGGIA FRACTURE

1814

"I unhappily remember the case of a girl who, after a fall, seemed to me to have sustained a fracture of the ulna in its upper third. It might have been that some commotion of the dislocated bone misled me at the beginning of treatment, or else it might have been that there really was a fracture of the ulna

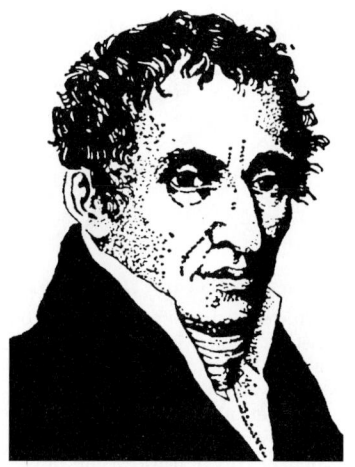

◆ **Giovanni Battista Monteggia (1762–1815)**

Monteggia was born at Lake Maggiore and studied at Milan. At first he was a surgical pathologist; while performing an autopsy on a woman who had died of syphilis, he had the misfortune to cut his finger and infected himself with the disease. Later he became a successful general surgeon and pleased one patient so much that he was given an annuity to keep his library up-to-date.

When he became professor of surgery at Milan, he published his lectures, which are remarkable for the wide acquaintance with the work of his contemporaries. He is particularly remembered for his description of a fracture dislocation of the forearm that he described in the same year that Colles described his fracture.

with a dislocation of the radius, as I undoubtedly found in another case. The fact is that at the end of the month, when the bandage was removed and all the swelling had disappeared (which, however, in simple dislocation of the radius is usually slight), I found that on extending the forearm the head of the radius jumped outwards, forming a hard ugly prominence on the anterior surface of the elbow, showing in an extremely obvious way that this was a true anterior dislocation of the head of the radius. When compressed it went back into place, but left to itself it came out again, especially on extension of the forearm. I applied compresses and a new bandage to hold it in, but it would not stay in place."

CONCERNING A PARTICULAR SYNDROME OF INJURY OF THE FOREARM BONES

R. GALEAZZI 1934

"We have observed, with relative frequency, a fracture of the diaphysis of the radius at the junction of the middle and lower thirds combined with luxation of the ulnar head. In this form of trauma we have a repetition of the Monteggia syndrome: i.e. one bone remains uninjured while the other is fractured.

"The consequent shortening of the radius is probably one of the important causes of the subluxation or dislocation of the distal radioulnar joint, as occurs in the proximal joint in fractures of the ulna.

"The angulation of the radial fracture is sometimes lateral and sometimes posterior; and the luxation of the ulnar head may be anterior, dorsal or medial, all with more or less equal frequency though medial displacement is perhaps most common. Fracture of the ulnar styloid with displacement of the distal fragment towards the radius is fairly common.

"As for the relative incidence of the present syndrome and that of Monteggia—my material shows that the distal syndrome is much more common: in 300 cases of forearm fractures that I have collected, the Monteggia injury accounted for 2% of the cases, whereas the injury that I am describing accounted for 6%.

"Both the proximal and distal syndromes may follow direct or indirect injuries. I, myself, have encountered more cases of the present syndrome than that of Monteggia, arising from indirect injury, such as a fall on the palm of the hand with the arm abducted."

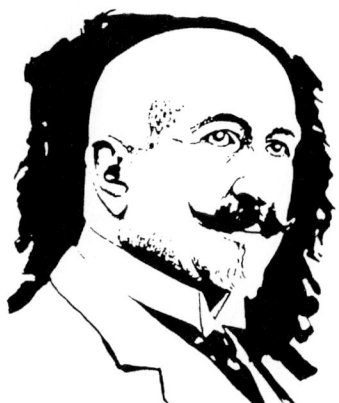

◆ **Riccardo Galeazzi (1866–1952)**
Fractures of the forearm should be superbly treated in Milan; Monteggia was there and then Galeazzi, who between them described upper and lower dislocations that may accompany fractures of one bone only. Galeazzi was director of the orthopaedic clinic for 35 years; he built up the unit and established ancillary centers. He was a prolific writer on many topics; for example, he reviewed 12,000 cases of congenital dislocation of the hip.

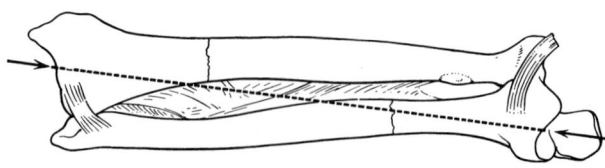

Galeazzi fracture dislocation

Galeazzi then describes with great formality and at considerable length the mechanical forces responsible for the two injuries. He points out that the axis of the forearm passes through the humeroulnar joint at the upper end and through the radiocarpal joint at the lower end. Both these joints are formed by the strongest ends of the bones. The other ends of the bones are weakly linked to the humerus above and to the carpus below. In a fall on the hand, the compression force on the forearm bones may cause a fracture of one of them at the point of maximal bowing, for example at the junction of the middle and the lower third of the radius. If the force continues to operate, either the ulnar will fracture or the distal arm will pivot at the fracture site, putting a strain on the inferior radioulnar ligament. If this ruptures, dislocation of the head of the ulna follows.

"When the fracture is due to direct violence then muscle shortening produces overlapping. Again the distal arm pivots and the ligament may rupture."

Galeazzi mentions that the dislocation may develop slowly during the course of treatment for what initially appears to be a solitary fracture.

He discusses treatment and we return to his words for an account of this.

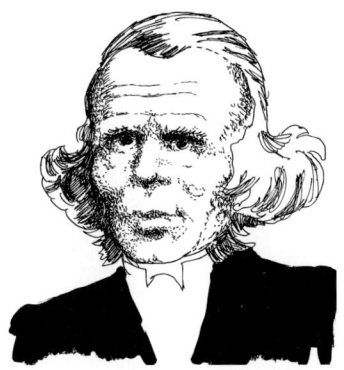

◆ **Alfred Velpeau (1795–1867)**

He was the son of a village blacksmith and was training to follow his father when he was drawn to become a surgeon. Not, as some have claimed, because the skills of a blacksmith have a lot in common with those of an orthopaedic surgeon. He settled in Paris and wrote books on operative surgery. He is remembered for his bandage that hugs the arm to the chest.

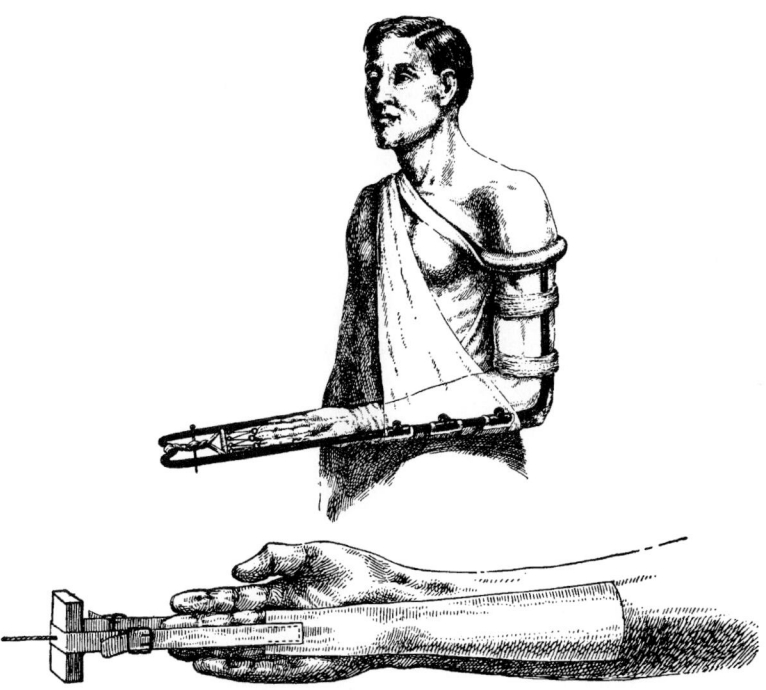

A recommended treatment for forearm fractures in 1922 in Scudder's book. Traction was applied by a glove. This is little different from mediaeval methods, and one could imagine that the only moving part in the forearm and the hand after a month or two would be at the fracture site. From Scudder, The Treatment of Fractures, 9th ed, Philadelphia, WB Saunders: 1922.

"In my experience traction has always yielded the best results. The distal fragment of the radius is usually pronated by pronator quadratus and displaced towards the ulna by abductor pollicis bowstringing across it.

"In my experience, energetic traction on the thumb with the hand in supination has always permitted immediate reduction of the fracture, then by deviating the hand radially the dislocated ulnar head is reduced without further manipulation. Only if the diastasis of the inferior radioulnar joint is very severe, because the ligaments have suffered total rupture, does the dislocation tend to recur; it is then necessary to transfix both bones with threads after reduction."

Many eponymous conditions were described by an earlier unknown. Here is an earlier account of the Galeazzi fracture-dislocation.

RICKMAN GODLEE
1883

"A case of fracture of the radius and dislocation forwards of the ulna at the wrist, in which the lower end of the latter was removed to effect reduction."

The fracture occurred in a 20-year-old in a gymnasium. The fracture dislocation was irreducible.

"An incision was made over the lower end of the ulna, and a hook passed under the tendon of flexor carpi ulnaris, which had slipped behind the bone, but the bones could not be replaced until first the styloid process, and then the lower end of the ulna had been sawn off. The wound was treated aseptically, and healed. In ten days, it was placed in a plaster-of-Paris apparatus, and, in about six weeks, passive movement was commenced. The limb is now almost as useful as the other, and could be employed for gymnastic exercises."

Mr. Godlee presented this paper at a meeting; other cases were presented; the injuries came to amputation, and the patients died after operation.

References

Chapter references are located in Chapter 26.

◆ Chapter Nineteen

Spine Fractures and Traumatic Paraplegia

"All power of motion and feeling below my chest are gone. I can live but a short time."   Lord Nelson

Famous Patients

THE PROFESSIONAL REPORT ON THE DEATH OF NELSON BY HIS SURGEON
WILLIAM BEATTY, 1805

"About the middle of the action with the combined Fleets on the 21st of October last, the late illustrious Commander in Chief Lord Nelson was mortally wounded in the left breast by a musket-ball, supposed to be fired from the mizzen-top of La Redoubtable, French ship of the line. His Lordship was in the act of turning on the quarter-deck with his face towards the Enemy, when he re-

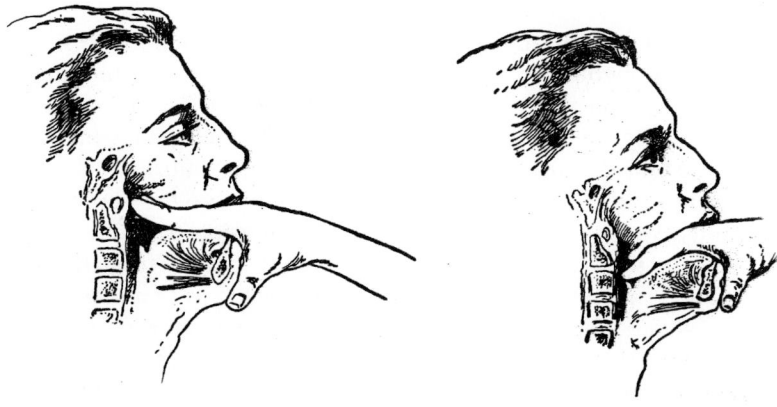

The diagnosis of spine fractures has come a long way since this was recommended for the diagnosis of cervical spine fractures. Roberts and Kelly, 1921.

ceived his wound: he instantly fell; and was carried to the cockpit, where he lived about two hours. On being brought below, he complained of acute pain about the sixth or seventh dorsal vertebra, and of privation of sense and motion of the body and inferior extremities. His respiration was short and difficult; pulse weak, small, and irregular. He frequently declared his back was shot through, that he felt every instant a gush of blood within his breast, and that he had sensations which indicated to him the approach of death."

Course and Site of the Ball, as Ascertained Since Death

"The ball struck the fore part of his Lordship's epaulette, and entered the left shoulder immediately before the acromion, which was slightly fractured. It then descended obliquely into the thorax, fracturing the second and third ribs: and after penetrating the left lobe of the lungs, and dividing in its passage a large branch of the pulmonary artery, it entered the left side of the spine between the sixth and seventh dorsal vertebrae, fracturing the left transverse process of the sixth dorsal vertebra, wounding the medulla spinalis . . ."

Nelson knew that he had a spinal cord injury and would die. Nelson had learned all about paraplegia after one of his crew had suffered a similar injury.

President Garfield was shot in the back on July 2, 1881, in Washington, D.C., and sustained a bullet wound of the 1st lumbar vertebra. He developed infection and septicemia and died of a ruptured traumatic aneurysm of the nearby splenic artery. The full account in the *Journal of the American Medical Association* shows how far trauma care has come. When his surgeon arrived he said, "Mr. President, are you badly hurt?" The President answered, "I'm afraid I am." The wound was explored with a finger and the only resuscitation used was half an ounce of brandy and some smelling salts. This is a far cry from modern advanced life support protocol.

Spine Fractures

To begin with, most spine fractures were thought to result in paraplegia; then came X-rays, which showed fractures without cord injury. Attempts were made to describe the variety of injury. At first the films were poor, and most surgeons classified fractures into flexion, extension, rotation, and shearing injuries. Posterior ligamentous disruption and anterior wedging were the commonest features. Watson Jones advocated hyperextension to reduce them in 1934. Then came Nicoll, who classified them into stable and unstable fractures in 1949, and this was a guide to treatment. Olof Percy added burst fractures in 1957. Seat belt injuries were described in 1969 by Smith and Kaufer, very soon after seat belts became popular. Francis Denis, from Montreal, described the three-column classification of spinal fractures in 1983. With modern methods of imaging, a lot of the guesswork has gone.

Chance Fracture

NOTE ON A TYPE OF FLEXION FRACTURE OF THE SPINE
G. Q. CHANCE, DERBY, 1948

"When flexion of the spine exceeds normal limits something has to give way. This is usually the vertebral body, which assumes the characteristic wedging in varying degrees.

"Occasionally the body, for some reason, is relatively incompressible, so the posterior arch system is disrupted. The commonest types of posterior disruption are

"1. The ligamentous rupture with dislocation of the apophyseal joints.
2. Fractures of the articular processes.
3. Combinations of these.

"The fracture which I illustrate is a true flexion fracture, though of a rarer type. It consists of a horizontal splitting of the spine and neural arch, ending in an upward curve which usually reaches the upper surface of the body just in front of the neural foramen. In good radiographs its recognition is easy.

In my three cases there has been very little wedging of the vertebral body, no dislocation of the apophyseal joints, nor has there been any cord damage. I cannot think of any anatomical explanation of the peculiar site and direction of the fracture. The importance of the recognition of this fracture lies in the fact that its treatment and prognosis are constant and clear. As there is no major ligamentous damage, the upper half of the fractured neural arch is firmly fixed to the normal arch of the vertebra above, and similarly the lower half is fixed to the vertebra below. The outline of these halves, in a horizontal plane, is therefore still undisturbed, so that a simple hyperextension of the spine must inevitably bring the two halves into perfect anatomical apposition, and give a near 100 per cent prognosis."

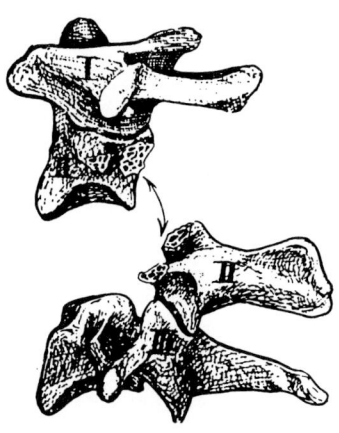

Wood-Jones: Hangman's fracture, 1913. C. Schneider and associates introduced the term hangman's fracture in 1965. From Wood-Jones J: The ideal lesion produced by judicial hanging. Lancet 1913, 1, 53.

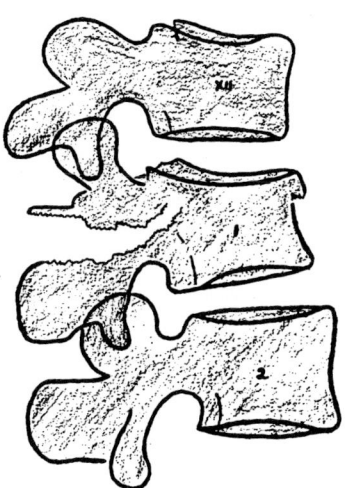

Flexion distraction injury of the spine. From Chance GQ: Br J Radiol: 1948, 21, 452.

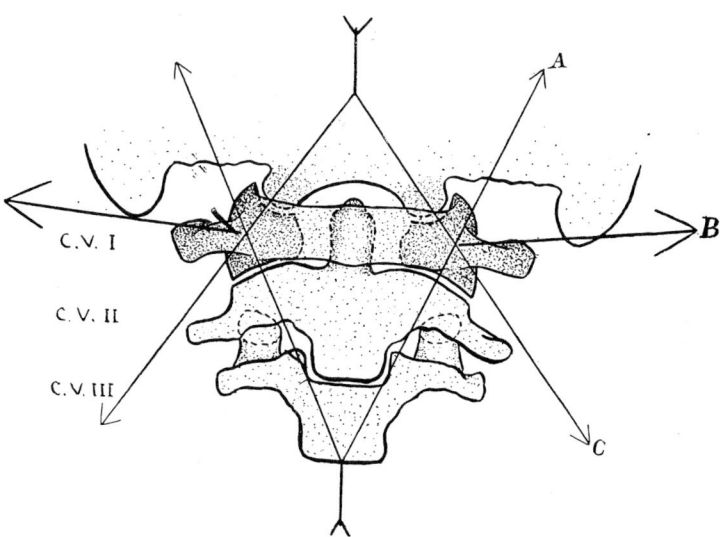

Jefferson fracture, 1920. The transmission of forces through the outwardly facing facets tend to burst C1.

Spinal Cord Injury

A disease not to treat.   Edwin Smith papyrus, 2800 BC

His case is hopeless, so do not concern yourself with his treatment.   Albucasis on traumatic paraplegia, 1000 AD

Experimental Studies

Galen wrote in 177 AD, "*Exposure of the spinal cord, and the effects produced by section of the cord at various levels.*" He began: "*The animal which you vivisect . . .*" and went on to describe tying the animal down and exposing the cord exactly as we do today. He told us to transect the cord low down and note loss of movement and sensibility of the legs, and then make higher and higher transections until breathing stopped.

Charles-Édouard Brown-Séquard (1817–1894). A wandering neurologist, who was professor at Harvard, Virginia, Geneva, and Paris and consultant in London. (Immigration departments today would have had a lot of fun with him.) His experimental work on hemisection of the cord began with a thesis in 1846 and papers in 1850–1851. This was the era of discoveries about the spinal cord.

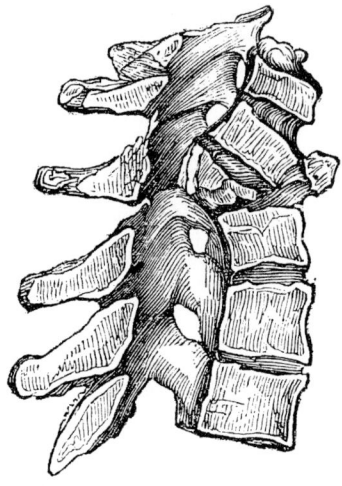

Burst fracture of the upper thoracic spine, 1838. "John Bright, aetat 19, on the 1st of October, climbed a walnut tree, for the purpose of picking the fruit, when he had attained a very considerable height slipped, and was precipitated to the ground. He was soon afterwards found, in a cold and pulseless condition, with his lower extremities numb and motionless." From Marshall Hall: Lancet, 1838, p 38.

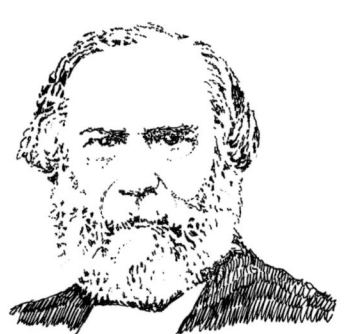

◆ Charles-Édouard Brown-Séquard

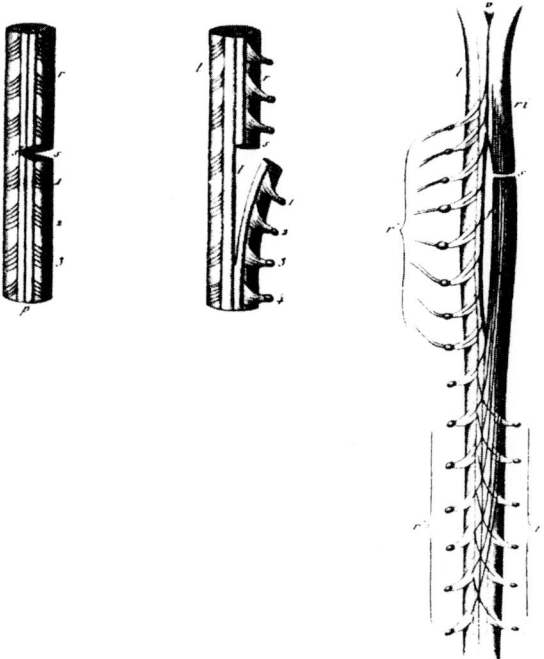

Brown-Séquard's experiment on hemisection of the cord, 1846.

Natural History

From the beginning of time, death from paraplegia was well known and led to a defeatist attitude. However, there have always been arguments about whether to carry out a closed reduction for what was always believed to be a dislocation. Until the days of X-rays, any injury in the vicinity of a joint was supposed to be a dislocation and therefore stable upon reduction—quite different from the view today. Most cord injuries are due to fractures that are very unstable.

The results of paraplegia in World War I were 80% mortality in the first 3 years, and in World War II this fell to about 7%. This means that the earlier descriptions are interesting for their clinical detail and that it is only recently that management has become effective and available. The emphasis has changed from cure to care.

Treatment

Manipulative Reduction

Traction was used by Hippocrates in 400 BC. Straps around the waist and straps in the axillae were attached to winches to pull seriously on the spine. It was a forerunner of the rack. Pictures of spinal deformities being treated by reduction using a ladder are dramatic. The patient was tied upside down by the ankles to the top of a vertical ladder. The ladder was then dropped, jerking the spine. It is hard to imagine that many patients were benefited. Various kinds of forceful manipulation continued until the last century. Malgaigne, for instance, used hyperextension to reduce a

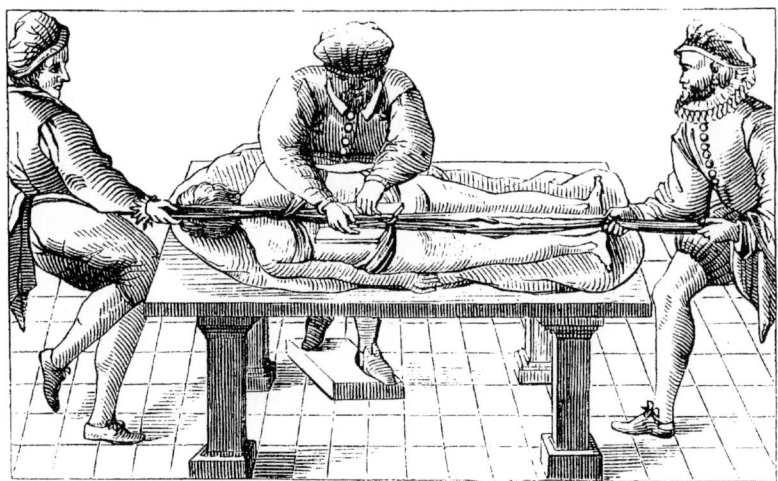

Hippocrates and almost everyone else has used traction. From J Bishop, 1852.

dislocation in 1847. There are still some fractures that are immobilized in extension.

What was the cause of the deformities that led to this drastic treatment? The ancients thought they were dealing with dislocations. They did not have X-rays, which would have told them that dislocations are rare. Perhaps they were late wedge fractures and tuberculous spines.

Hippocrates wrote that manual reduction was not possible—a surgeon would need to put a hand inside the body to do it.

Skull Traction

Various gentle halters were in use for the treatment of tuberculosis and scoliosis, but use of heavy traction for fracture dislocations of the neck is recent. In the days before refrigeration, tongs were used for delivering ice to the home—these were modified to be attached to the skull by Crutchfield in 1933. Then in the late 1950s the halo was developed at Rancho los Amigos in California by J. Perry, R. Snelson, and Verne Nickel. It was modeled after the crown used for maxillofacial fracture by dentists.

Homer Stryker of Kalamazoo developed the Stryker frame in the 1930s.

Operative Decompression

Laminectomy for traumatic paraplegia has an ancient history and a simple appeal, despite the fact that it has only a small place in treatment. The Babylonians did it occasionally. Paul of Aegina (625–690) tells us how to do laminectomy for paraplegia in his fracture book. The question about laminectomy was kept going by the occasional success in an otherwise fatal condition. It was batted around for centuries and can still produce a heated discussion. Today magnetic resonance imaging and computed tomography help define the cases needing decompression and whether it should be anterior or posterior. Old timers had none of this and operated under primitive conditions—poor lighting, no electrocautery, and no aseptic technique—and no control of kidney infection or embolism afterward. No wonder they had difficulty working out the indications with so many confounding variables. In the past, even patients with incomplete lesions, who had improved power and sensation after operation, usually died of renal damage and infection. There is a list of reports of 19th century operations in *Clinical Orthopaedics and Related Research*, 1989, 189, 3–11.

In 1814 Henry Cline in London, and in 1829 Alban Smith of Kentucky, used laminectomy.

"*Results of cases must be the true criteria by which the most plausible theories are to be tested*" wrote Robert M'Donnell about laminectomy for the spine in Dublin in the 1860s.

BENJAMIN BRODIE
1836

"*If the whole or nearly the whole of a vertebra be driven forwards, the depression of the posterior part of it will occasion a diminution of the size of the spinal canal, but the removal of any portion of the vertebra which is accessible to an operation, will be of little avail, as the irregularity of the anterior part of the canal, made by the displacement of the body, must be the same after, as it was before, the operation."*

Stabilization

Further damage to the cord can be prevented by stabilizing unstable fractures with rods and fusion.

Berthold Ernest Hadra (1842–1903)

Hadra was born in Silesia. He came to the United States in 1869, settling first in Houston, Texas, then moving to Austin in 1872 where he remained engaged in a thriving practice. He finally settled in Galveston, where he was professor and author of a book on gynecology. He is remembered for wiring the cervical spine. In 1891 he operated on a fracture dislocation of a cervical spine in a child showing progressive cord deterioration, using wires wrapped around the spinous processes to stabilize the vertebral levels. The concept of vertebral stabilization was highly original and the first recorded in surgical literature. He later applied the procedure to vertebrae involved in Potts' disease.

He reported these cases in the Medical Times and Register and later that year presented his material to the American Orthopaedic Association. This presentation appeared in their Transactions (1891, 4, 206) and thereby came to the attention of European orthopedic surgeons who, like Fritz Lange of Munich, modified but continued the use of spinal wiring until the advent of Russell Hibbs' spine fusion operation in 1911.

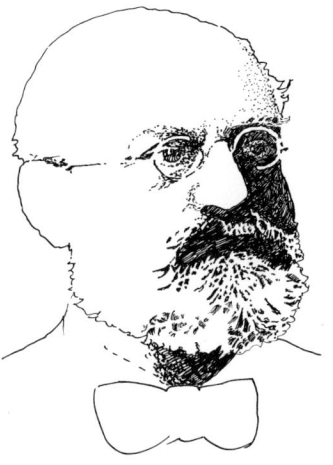

◆ Berthold Ernest Hadra

WIRING OF THE VERTEBRAE AS A MEANS OF IMMOBILIZATION IN FRACTURE AND POTT'S DISEASE

B. E. HADRA, 1891

"Present surgical interference in fractures of the spine consists in the removal of loose bones and in resection of parts of the arch, in order to free the spinal canal. The latter is done when grave symptoms indicate pressure upon the cord, or morbid changes of it or of the dura mater. Thus, mostly older cases will be submitted to resection. It is my purpose to propose to you a means of adaptation and retention of the broken ends before such damage is done, or before vicious consolidation has taken place.

"The present apparatus of immobilization by position, extension, splints, braces, dressings, etc., is evidently sufficient only in the lightest and most tractable cases, which, unfortunately, constitute only a very small percentage. Aside from the enormous inconvenience, all these helps are ineffective when the broken ends are thoroughly separated. I remember two cases of dorsal fracture where I had the patients encased in plaster of Paris from the axilla down to the thigh. I know they were not benefited, but

were made most unhappy by the treatment. It is simply impossible to keep the loosened vertebrae from gliding upon each other as long as no fixation can be had all around. Obviously, though, the contents of the thoracic and abdominal cavities cannot be immobilized. Still, absolute apposition is here more a necessity than in other fractures, because, aside from giving the broken bones a chance to properly consolidate, it must be the main aim to protect the cord and the spinal nerves against pressure, twisting, and also against changes due to irritation and to extension of morbid processes from the surrounding tissues. What do we do in other cases to keep the parts well adapted? We do the most natural thing in the world; we fix them to each other by direct means—clamps, nails, wires, sutures, and so on. Now, there is no good reason why vertebral fractures should not enjoy similar advantages. There is no danger in cutting down on the vertebral column, as all operators testify, as long, of course, as the cord and the nerves remain undisturbed; and even they stand a good deal more interference than is generally conceded. It is, then, a question of feasibility and efficacy. Theoretically there should be no doubt about it. Still, practical evidence alone will satisfy nowadays. The literature—at least that at my command—offers only one case where direct fixation of broken vertebrae was planned and executed, and I think this case deserves the fullest attention. It is that of Dr. W. T. Wilkins, a short history of which is given by Prof. Keen in the "Reference Hand-book of Medical Science." It reads thus:*

> " 'I find reported a case of a child born with a hunch on its back, the mother having been severely injured the day before its birth. On operation, on the day after birth, the last dorsal and the first lumbar vertebra were found separated a half-inch, and a hernia protruded through the fissure. The spinal cord was pushed to one side. The hernia was reduced, the two vertebrae held together by a figure of 8 carbolized silk ligature, passing through the intervertebral notches of the two vertebrae, above and below, and the child was practically well in a few days.'
>
> "It was my lot to test the problem in a case which was operated on last December, and I regret that I, at that time, did not know anything of Dr. Wilkins' case. I fastened together the spinous processes of the sixth and seventh cervical vertebrae by silver-wire loops, in a case of fracture which had been acquired nearly a year before. The patient is still at the John Scaly Hospital, and I must confess is not perfectly well yet, though the efficacy of the operation has been fully demonstrated. To give a short history of the case, it may be stated that a man of thirty years of age, working as waiter in a restaurant, fell to the floor, striking with great force on his buttocks. Immediately after, he felt intense pain in his neck, and was unable to move it. On examination, the sixth cervical vertebra was found pushed forward and turned around its vertical axis to the right, whilst the spinous process of the seventh vertebra appeared unusually prominent. Patient could not open his mouth more than an inch, from what cause

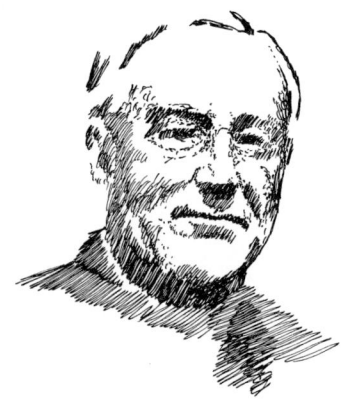

◆ **W. E. Gallie (1882–1959)**
Professor and Dean at the University of Toronto. He was best known for the use of autogenous fascia lata grafts as a living suture for hernias, ligaments, and repair of recurrent dislocations. He was a very inventive man and is mentioned here because he introduced wire fusion of C1–C2 in 1936.

I could never understand. Exsection was made by the head, and as the parts seemingly returned to their normal position, the neck was put in a firm cravatte. Patient, from reasons of no medical interest, left the St. Mary's Hospital a few days after his admission, and returned to his former occupation, wearing constantly his apparatus, getting along well enough with an occasional hypodermic injection of morphine. But once, when he imprudently bent his neck in a rapid and forcible way, the cravatte having been left away, he fainted, and when recovered could not stand upright. His head and neck were turned to the right and kept perfectly stiff; right hand became numb, right arm weak; girdle pains around his upper abdomen; bladder not fully under control; slight priapism. In such condition he came to the John Scaly Hospital on November 1st, 1890, ten months after the first accident. His face flushed up on the slightest provocation; his mouth could not be opened over an inch; the left upper portion of the trapezius muscle was hard and protruding, forming a tumor; his right hand colder than the left; extreme hypesthesia on the right side; head was rolled around to the right, and the vertebrae in same position as on the first observation; muscles, though, reacted alike on both sides of the body to either current. Patient was put under chloroform, not being able to stand any manipulation without an anesthetic. Head and upper portion of neck very movable, and crepitation distinctly heard. Reduction was easy, and the stiff cravatte was applied again. In spite of frequent adjustment and modification of the retaining apparatus, patient grew steadily worse. Pains in back, arms and around abdomen became unbearable, and walking impossible. He was in such a pitiful condition, that he insisted upon any operation which would give the faintest hope of relief. I finally consented to cut down on the place of injury, which I did on the 22 of December. My plan was to remove loose bones, if present; to sever the posterior ligaments, if they should be thickened and contracted; and finally, to wire the spinous processes, in order to steady the vertebral column.

"*From the improvement setting in every time the bones were well adjusted, I inferred that there was no serious change within the vertebral canal, nor in the cord itself. I therefore did not consider the opening of the canal called for. Not finding loose bones, I severed the ligamentum nuchae and the interspinous ligaments transversely in several places, so as to expose the spinous processes fully, and also in order to remove the interference of the perhaps thickened and contracted ligaments which could have acted as an impediment to the replacement and retention of the dislocated parts, exactly as in other fractures or dislocations. I am satisfied that this part of the operation was not only unnecessary, but that it caused all the following inflammatory symptoms, as a good deal of lacerating was unavoidable. The main aim of the operation, the wiring of the sixth and seventh spinous process was done with silver wire, carrying it four to five times around in a figure of 8. The wound which extended from the occiput down to the first dorsal vertebrae was then closed, a small drainage tube inserted right over the place of wiring and the stiff cravatte reapplied. Patient did not improve for several days, but then gradually got better. After some weeks I thought that the wire had become loose, because he began to exhibit some of his former symptoms. He was put under chloroform again, the wire removed, and a new one fixed on. On this occasion it was easily seen that the lower end of the fractured spine slipped away from the upper for about one and a half inches to the right. From now on improvement went on more rapidly. Patient was able three weeks ago, that is twelve weeks after the operation, to move his head in a normal way in every direction, without pain. He could open his mouth fully, walk as well as anybody else; no headache; no trouble with bladder or bowels. The right arm remained somewhat weaker, but was otherwise normal in all its functions and of normal sensation. The favorable condition though made me, I fear, too careless. I allowed him to be without the bandage occasionally, and removed the wire, as it kept a fistulous ulcer from closing. He became worse again, and has now considerable pain in his right arm and shoulder. The spinous process of the sixth cervical vertebra is very tender on pressure, and requires further attention, as the probable cause of the new trouble. Otherwise patient is well, and can make use of his neck without any difficulty.*

"*This is my case, which shows that the operation is feasible and effective. But I would be a poor surgeon if I had felt satisfied with my method and the course of my case. Further experiments on the cadaver, and further reflection has led me to believe that the proposed wiring is one of the most promising, and at the same time simplest surgical procedures, provided that it be so modified as I will describe it hereafter. Of course, it is intended only for the readjustment and retention of the broken bones, therefore, in some cases, it may fill all the indications; in others, it will simply be an addition to other operations.*

"*But before proceeding I show you here a vertebral column, on which two adjoining spinous processes have been wired together in the three portions of the spine. Of course, more than two may be joined if necessary. You see how firmly the vertebrae hold together, and how resistant they become. In fact, common forces, as experienced in human life, are hardly able to undo the fixation of the two lumbar vertebrae. Of course, this method is possible only when the spinous processes are not fractured themselves. If so, one would have to resort to the wiring of the transverse processes, as shown also on the model.*

"*The operation consists then of the following simple acts. A good long skin incision, the center of which should be over the seat of fracture; next the muscles on either side of the spinous processes should be lifted up and drawn aside with blunt instruments, but not more than to allow one to feel the contours of the bones. Then a stout curved needle, armed with wire, is carried through the interspace between the spinous process of the broken vertebra, and that of the next upper one, as deep as possible; brought out, entered again into the next inferior interspace; brought out on the other side; entered there again into the next lower interspace; carried around the spinous process of the verte-*

bra, below the fracture, and again carried through the middle interspace, and meeting the wire where it entered, well twisted together to a knot. In short, a figure of eight loop is carried around the spinous processes of the broken vertebra and that of the next lower one, which may be repeated as often as seems advisable. In the lumbar portion of the spine simple loops will suffice, as the processes are almost horizontal. Then the wound is closed with or without drainage. Under certain circumstances three or even more vertebrae may be fixed together.

"All this can be done in a few minutes. The operation is nearly bloodless; involves no great laceration of tissues, and can be made thoroughly aseptic. The wires are well secured in their position by the ligaments, which remain undisturbed.

"More difficult is the wiring of the transverse processes. Here the muscles have to be lifted and drawn aside much more extensively. In order to avoid impeding nerves in the loops, I think it would be best to do it as shown on the model; that is, first to surround one process, and then carry the thread to the next one, and again tie it here by a loop, so as to have only one wire in the interspace.

"I cannot resist the temptation to connect my device also with the treatment of Pott's disease. Here, too, the indication in cases where the abscess or carious bones do not call for other surgical attempts, is mainly to steady the vertebral column in order to protect the cord, to prevent the diseased bones from rubbing on each other, and, finally, to make the outcome, in regard to disfigurement, as favorable as possible."

The Modern Era

The Change of Emphasis from Cure to Rehabilitation

Spinal cord injuries were treated in general hospitals until death from renal infection and bed sores put the victim out of misery. Then during World War II a decision was made to set up hospital spinal injuries units. Many thought that these would be dumping grounds. But two events made these units a success story. First, antibiotics had become available to treat renal infections, and second, Ludwig Guttmann was available to be put in charge of the unit at Stoke Mandeville, just outside London. His obsession about patient rolling prevented bedsores. He kept the patients alive and then went on to make them fit and motivated through sports. He himself was overweight and and would not have run for a bus. But his most lasting achievement has been the Para-Olympics (or Special Olympics). He put paraplegics back to work—something that had not been possible before for people who were legally 100% disabled.

Sporadic attempts to fix spinal fractures were made during the 1950s. They were hampered by poor design and Guttmann's denunciations—he showed slides of plates shining through the skin of the back. He was really denouncing poor fixation. But Harrington started a whole new era of implants, and now most fractures are stabilized so that the patient can be up quickly and avoid recumbent disease.

Sir Ludwig Guttmann

He was born in Upper Silesia in 1899. During World War I, he worked as an orderly in a hospital for coalminers. Spinal cord injuries were common due to roof falls, and he was impressed when a young miner died in 5 weeks from a spinal cord injury. He went to Breslau to study, training and working as a neurosurgeon until he was fired in 1933 during the anti-Jewish purges. In 1939 he found a job doing research at Oxford and was asked to start a Spinal Cord Injuries unit at Stoke Mandeville in 1944. He became known for his care of paraplegia and to a greater extent for wheelchair sports as a method of rehabilitation. In the autumn of 1944 some wheelchair patients were chasing a puck around, and this gave Guttmann the idea of wheelchair sports to alleviate the boredom and depression. He started with polo, but this was too rough. The first Games were held with 16 competitors in 1948.

He wrote a textbook of spinal cord injuries in 1973.

Guttmann feared that the spinal units in Britain would become "*merely an accumulation of doomed cripples,*" and his chief object for patients "*was to give them a purpose in life.*"

Sport is of even greater significance for the wellbeing of the severely disabled than the able bodied.   Ludwig Guttmann

The first duty of a paraplegic is to cheer up his visitors.   Rev. Albert Bull, a patient at Stoke Mandeville

References

Chapter references are located in Chapter 26.

◆ Chapter Twenty

Fracture Treatment

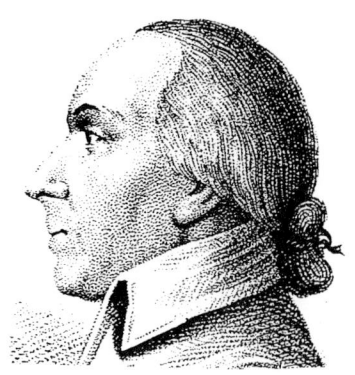

◆ **John Jones (1729–1791)**
Born in New York, he studied in Philadelphia, Paris, London, and Edinburgh. He set up a practice in New York and started a medical school, becoming the professor of surgery. The war of 1776 disrupted his life, leading him to write a simple book for army surgeons—the first textbook of surgery written in the United States.

A broken bone cannot *be too soon put to rights.*   Percivall Pott

When a bone is broken and separated, it has no power of restoring itself to its natural situation.   John Jones, first American fracture textbook, 1776

To put the fragments of a fractured bone into their proper situation, which is called setting the fracture, is one thing: and keeping them there, during the uniting process, is another.   Joseph Amesbury, fracture book, London, 1831

Introduction

The arrival of X-rays changed the fracture scene. Surgeons for the first time could see what they were dealing with. They could tell whether the fracture healed in a good position. The game was up for bonesetters (see later). It was not just a coincidence that the discovery of X-rays and the development of open reduction and internal fixation occurred at about the same time.

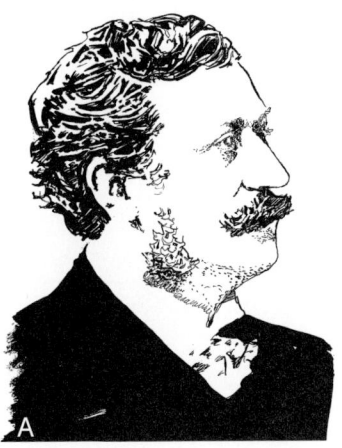

◆ **Carl Beck**
Wrote the first book on fractures based on their x-ray appearances, in 1900.

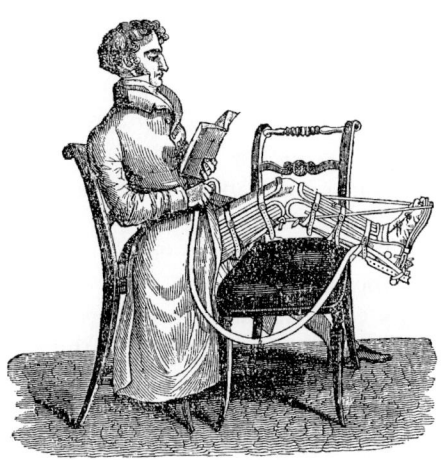

Ambulatory treatment of fractures of the leg.
From Amesbury J: London: Longman, 1831.

423

Fractures had always been common in the working population, and they had important economic implications. For the first time the economic difference between a well-treated fracture and a poorly treated fracture could be measured. And various commissions offered guidelines. Fracture clinics were started, modeled on factory production lines.

Realization that many fractures healed in poor position led many surgeons to think of operating and using internal fixation. Patients could, as they still do, look at the fracture and tell whether it was reduced. In 1912 Robert Jones wrote, *"Patients who call upon me are often armed with X-ray prints, which they authoritatively expound. Anything but a faultless end to end apposition imparts a war-like spirit."*

The British Medical Association organized a committee on the treatment of simple fractures in 1910-1912. A team examined 2940 patients and in a remarkably modern report concluded that *"the most certain way to obtain a good functional result is to secure a good anatomical result. In order to secure the most satisfactory results from operative treatment, it should be resorted to as soon after the accident as possible."* And the most contentious conclusion of all: *"In nearly all age groups, operative cases show a higher percentage of good results than non-operative cases (79.5% vs 70.4%)."*

And this was at a time when the methods of internal fixation were poor! Someone described them as homeopathic plates.

First Aid

When the surgeon Percivall Pott broke his leg in the middle of London in 1756 he could not phone for an ambulance. He had to buy a door and hire bearers to carry him home. Injured soldiers had to make their own way back from the battlefield. Gradually society realized that care of a fracture at the scene of injury is important—both to relieve pain and to prevent further injury—particularly on the battlefield.

Larrey, Napoleon's surgeon, was the first to organize an ambulance service in the French Army at the beginning of the 19th century. The British took it up in the Crimean War in 1858. Jean Henri Durant, a Swiss banker, saw the suffering at the Battle of Solferino in 1859. He wrote *Un Souvenir de Solferino* in 1862 to suggest the formation of permanent societies to aid the wounded. This led to the Geneva Convention in 1864 and the formation of the Red Cross and its humanitarian goals, such as protecting the wounded from further attack.

Esmarch was a German battle surgeon who wrote one of the first books on first aid in 1869 and founded the Samaritan's School to teach first aid throughout Germany.

In England, the St. John's Ambulance for civilians was started in 1878. First aid was taught, and a civilian ambulance association began. From this time horses, bicycles, and real ambulances transported the injured.

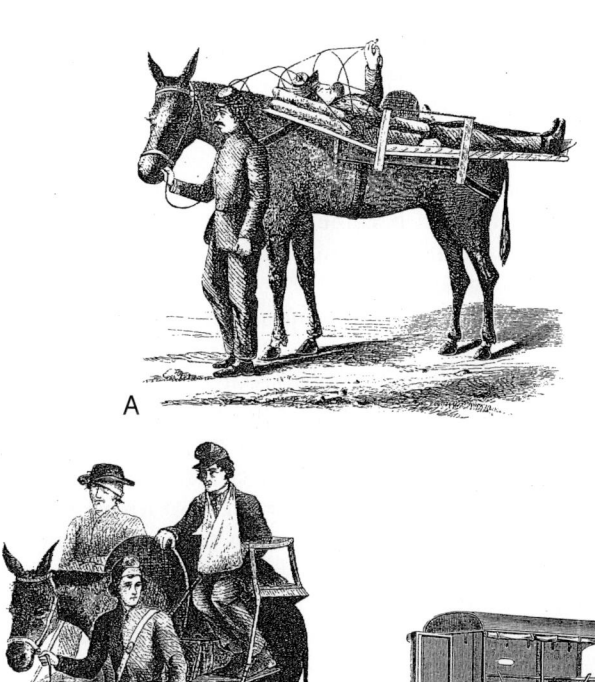
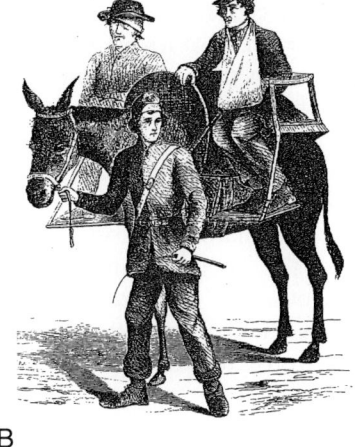
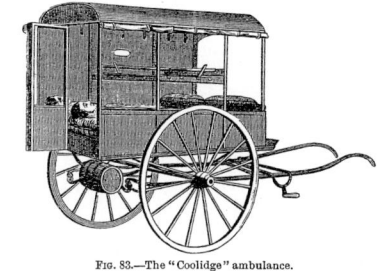

FIG. 83.—The "Coolidge" ambulance.

The Army was the first to use ambulances and they were multipurpose. These are examples from the Civil War.

Philosophy of Fracture Treatment

Fracture treatment has always generated controversy. There are so many therapeutic possibilities. But argument becomes less as our methods improve and fractures are categorized in more and more detail and results are collected. Years ago, when surgeons asked, "What is the best way to treat a fracture of the shaft of the femur?" there were many different answers. But today the question is focused down. The treatment of a closed transverse fracture of the midshaft in a head-injured 25-year-old has only one option. Controversy is less—partly because of better methods but also because of better thinking and training.

Today, fracture care has become a specialty. When I was in training I was advised that fracture care was only for surgeons who could not cultivate an elective practice. Those days are gone.

Recent advances may have been made in the wrong direction.   Lancet, 1942, 2, 439

Every fracture is potentially a deformity.   Robert Jones, Am J Orthop Surg 1913, 11, 314

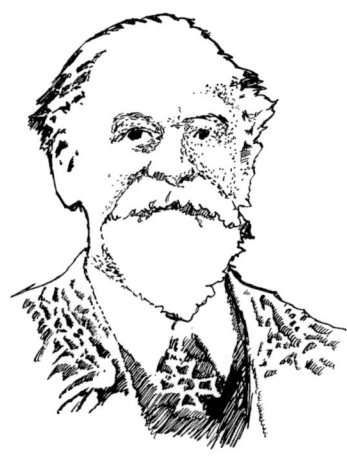

◆ Just Lucas-Championnière (1843–1913)

He studied in Paris and then visited Lister as an elective student, bringing aseptic surgery to France and writing a book on the aseptic technique. He is best known for advocating movement for fracture healing in a book published in 1905. His views are expressed in English in J. B. Mennell's 1911 book, *Fractures Treated by Mobilisation*.

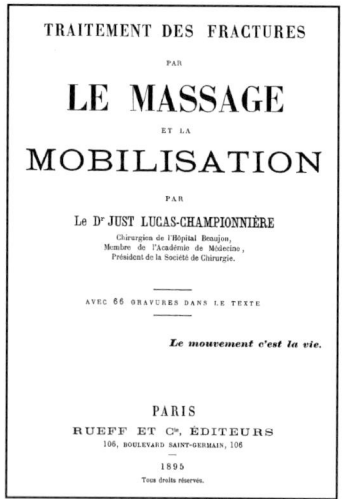

Title page of Lucas-Championnière's book.

(1) Rest Versus Motion

Movement is life.   Aristotle

Some diaphyseal fractures will heal straight only if they are immobilized. Immobilization became synonymous with orthopaedics. Nothing could be more immobile than a tree tied to a stake—the symbol of orthopaedics.

The ideas about the care of chronic infections spilled over to fracture care. John Hilton's book *Rest and Pain*, 1862, was written about chronic infections of joints. Rest secured a fibrous or bony ankylosis—the nearest thing to a cure in the days before antibiotics, when infection killed. His motto was "Pain the monitor and rest the cure." Hugh Owen Thomas had similar views. He believed that rest should be *complete, prolonged, enforced, and uninterrupted*. He went to the extent of putting his seal on the splint so that he would know whether it had been disturbed.

Lucas-Championnière challenged the view that immobilization was essential. He wanted to avoid atrophy and stiffness, later described by the AO* school as plaster disease. Some fractures came to be treated by early movement, culminating in R. B. Salter's continuous passive motion machines. The focus changed from treating established stiffness with physiotherapy and exercise systems to avoiding it. Only recently has the battle between the movers and the resters been resolved by rigid early fixation and early movement.

Immobilization does not favour the formation of callus, movement does.   Just Lucas-Championnière, 1910

The object of early passive movement in recent fractures is the very simple one of preventing adhesions. Steady fixation of the fracture itself should be insured, either by grasp of the hand or by appropriate splints or apparatus. Voluntary movement by the patient is in itself better than passive movement.   Sir William Bennett, 1910

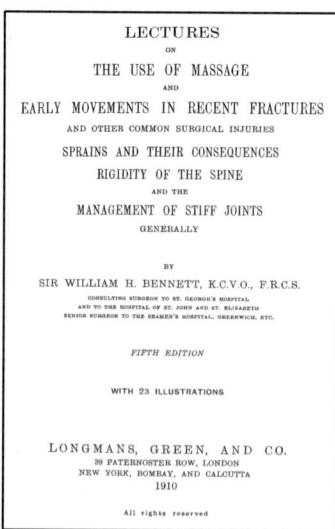

Title page of Bennett's book.

* Arbeitsgemeinschaft für Osteosynthesefragen.

Let anyone place a normal limb in splints for 20 hours a day and see what it is like at the end of a month. The result will be a useless limb.   J. W. Dowden, 1924

(2) Open Versus Closed Reduction

Initial attempts at open reduction with internal fixation (ORIF) about 150 years ago were on subcutaneous bones with easily diagnosed fractures, such as of the patella. But ORIF came into its own only after the aseptic technique and anesthesia made surgery safe, after X-rays made it possible to define the fracture, and after metallurgists gave us an inert metal.

Closed Reduction

In the early days, bonesetters used to care for fractures. They were not doctors—these were the days when doctors were few. Real doctors prescribed nostrums and turned up their noses at anything as gross as fractures. Before aseptic surgery, patients had to accept the best that manipulation could offer.

Bonesetters. Old-time bonesetters often kept their methods secret, much as many manufacturers do today. Their skills were handed down from father to son. One such family was the Thomases of Anglesea, Wales. The father of Hugh Owen Thomas set and splinted bones. One of his patients died and an inquest was held. Thomas was held liable but said that the patient had tampered with the immobilization. As a result of this experience, his son used a signet ring and when he had completed a dressing he applied a drop of wax and imprinted it with his seal to be sure it remained intact. I have often thought of doing this. In the United Kingdom there were many bonesetters, and some became famous, such as Joshua Ward, who reduced the dislocated thumb of King George II. Some became infamous, such as Mrs. Sally Mapp, the Bonesetter of Epsom, a town not far from London. Crazy Sally did not cure everyone, as appears from this advertisement:

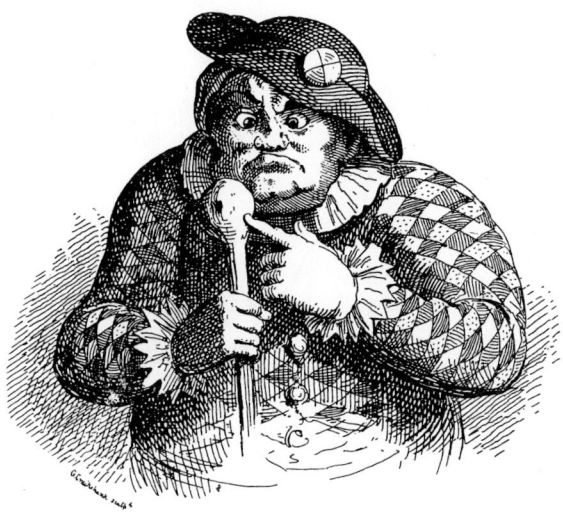

Mrs. Sarah Mapp. From a print after G. Cruickshank in the British Museum.

"Grubb Street Journal, Sept. 1, 1736

"Whereas it has been reported that I found great benefit from a certain female bone-setter's performance, this is to give notice that any person afflicted with lameness (who are willing to know what good or harm others may receive, before they venture on desperate measures themselves) will be welcome any morning to see the dressing on my leg, which was sound before the operation, and they will then be able to judge of the performance, and to whom I owe my present unhappy confinement to my bed and chair.

"Thomas Barber, Tallow Chandler
"Saffron Hill"

We should all be grateful that newspapers no longer accept advertisements of this nature.

In Japan, a system of fracture and dislocation care started in the second half of the 17th century, called Seikotsu-Jutsu. These surgeons did nothing but handle fractures and were called Seiko-suka. They were guided by three books: *Seikotsu Han* by Ken Ninomiya, *Seikotsu Shinsho* by Bunken Koumu, and *Seikotsu Yoketsu* by Gento Yoshiwara.

More Conventional Closed Reduction

The principles of closed reduction were best described by Charnley:

"Contrary to popular ideas, the operative treatment of fractures is much simpler than is the non-operative. At operation the fracture lies open for all to see, and the mechanical procedures which may be needed are obvious in the extreme. Far from

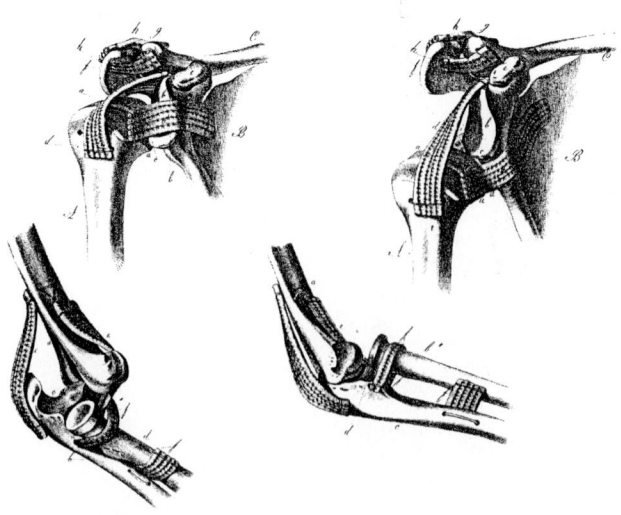

Joseph Wattmann, 1823, made these models to teach the reduction of dislocations. A covering could be used to hide the works.

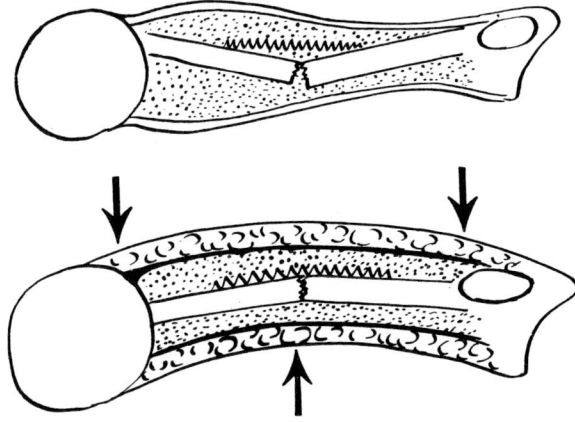

Showing that a skin-tight plaster, beautifully molded to the external shape of a limb, is capable of allowing redisplacement to occur because it does not exert a three-point action. On the other hand, a padded plaster is capable of preventing redisplacement, provided that it is molded into the correct three-point forces. From Charnley J: The Closed Treatment of Common Fractures, 3rd ed. Edinburgh: Livingstone, reprint 1970. Used with permission.

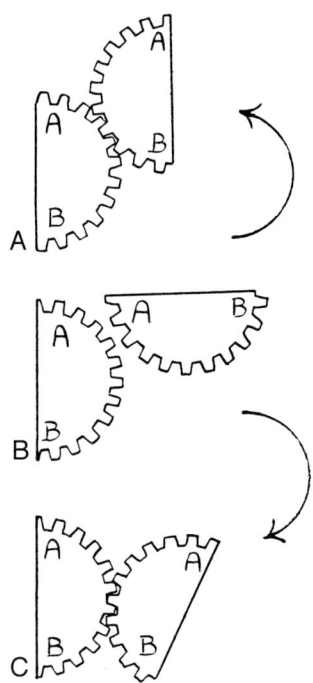

Mechanical analogy in reducing a Colles' fracture. (A) Fracture in displaced position (teeth incorrectly meshed). (B) Fracture distracted and backward angulation increased in order to mesh the dorsal teeth correctly. (C) Flexion will now bring the volar cortices correctly into register. From Charnley J: The Closed Treatment of Common Fractures, 3rd ed. Edinburgh: Livingstone, reprint 1970. Used with permission.

being a crude and uncertain art, the manipulative treatment of fractures can be resolved into something of a science.

"Manual reduction of a case would appear not unlike the assembling of a jigsaw puzzle in the dark. The solution of the difficulty emerges only when the supreme importance of the soft tissues is appreciated. The importance of the soft tissues is often forgotten because these are not seen on an X-Ray. Bone fragments are to be regarded as of secondary importance to damaged and undamaged soft parts: the mere fracture of a bone does not determine the displacements of its fragments. . . . The action of soft tissues [is] in guiding displaced fragments back to their normal position.

"The mechanism of the soft tissue 'hinge'—The intact fibrous tissues on the concave side of the original deformity prevent over-reduction unless the force is so great that it ruptures them [pp. 46–47].

"Fractures with potential stability against shortening—If a short oblique fracture is reduced by manipulation and is then slightly angulated in the direction of over-correction, the intact soft tissue hinge will be put into slight tension. Tension in the soft-tissue hinge can be maintained by applying a plaster moulded to over-correct the original angulation.

"A curved plaster is necessary to make a straight limb. The 'three point' plaster exerts pressure at certain precisely determined points on the skeleton and none at others."

There is a paradox that Charnley described both bonesetting and hip replacement—they seem to be at opposite poles of the orthopaedic personality.

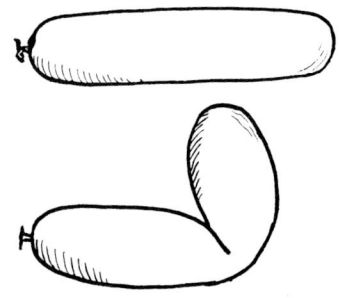

Mechanical analogy of *kinking* a distended balloon to show the disastrous results of forcibly flexing the tensely swollen elbow of a supracondylar fracture. From Charnley J: The Closed Treatment of Common Fractures, 3rd ed. Edinburgh: Livingstone, reprint 1970. Used with permission.

Positions for Splinting Limbs

Paré, in the 16th century, was one of the first to draw attention to the ill effects resulting from splinting limbs, or allowing them to remain, in a bad position. By choice, limbs should be splinted in a functional position.

"Vicious posture increases ill symptoms.

"When the wound is in the wrist or joints of the fingers either internally or externally, the hand must be kept half shut continually moving a ball therein. For if the fingers be held straight stretched forth, after it is cicatrized, they will be unapt to take up or hold anything, which is their proper faculty. But if after it is healed it remains half shut, no great inconvenience will follow thereon: for so may he use his hand diverse ways to his sword, pike, bridle, or in anything else."

FUNCTION OF SPLINTS
POTT, 1769

"The true and proper use of splints is, to preserve steadiness in the whole limb, without compressing the fracture at all. By the former they become very assistant to the curative intention; by the latter they are very capable of causing pain and other inconveniences; at the same time that they cannot, in the nature of things, contribute to the steadiness of the limb.

"In order to be of any real use at all, splints should, in the case of a broken leg, reach above the knee and below the ankle.

"By this they become really serviceable; but a short splint, which only extends a little above and a little below the fracture, and does not take in the two joints, is an absurdity and, what is worse, it is a mischievous absurdity."

Plaster of Paris Bandages

Bandaging should be done quickly, without pain, with ease and with elegance. Hippocrates

In the days of Hippocrates, bandages that set hard were used for nasal fractures. Initially, wheat glues were used and later, wax and resins. Rhazes, an Arabian physician of the 9th century, wrote: *"But if thou make thine apparatus with lime and white of egg, it will be much handsomer and will not need to be removed until the healing is complete."*

In the 18th century, Cheselden in England was a keen advocate of egg white bandages for fractures and the correction of club feet, but in Arabia, plaster was used. Mr. Eton, the British Consul in Bassora, wrote in 1798:

"I saw in the Eastern parts of the Empire a method of setting bones practised, which appears to be worthy of the attention of surgeons in Europe. It is by enclosing the broken limb, after the

◆ **William Cheselden (1688–1752)**
While waiting for his surgical practice to improve, he lectured on anatomy and wrote a book on anatomy in 1714 that went through new editions long after his death. Later he produced one of the best illustrated books on bones - *Osteographia*, 1733. Pictures of fractures were included. As a child, he was treated for an elbow fracture by a bonesetter with egg white and flour bandages. He used this for clubfeet. He tenotomized torticollis. He taught Belchier and J. Hunter.

bones are put in their places, in a case of plaster of Paris (gypsum) which takes exactly the form of the limb, without any pressure, and in a few minutes the mass is solid and strong. . . . This substance may be easily cut with a knife, and removed, and replaced with another. If, when the swelling subsides, the cavity is too large for the limb, a hole or holes being left, liquid gypsum plaster may be poured in, which will perfectly fill up the void, and exactly fit the limb. A hole may be made at first by placing an oiled cork or bit of wood against any part where it is required, and when the plaster is set, it is to be removed. There is nothing in gypsum injurious, if it be free from lime; it will soon become very dry and light, and the limb may be bathed with spirits, which will penetrate through the covering. I saw a case of a most terrible compound fracture of the leg and thigh, by the fall of a cannon, cured in this manner. The person was seated on the ground, and the plaster case extended from below the heel to the upper part of his thigh, whence a bandage, fastened into the plaster, went round his body."

In India, too, similar methods were used. Sir George Ballingall wrote in *Outline of Military Surgery* in 1852:

"The practice of enveloping fractured limbs in splints and bandages, without undoing them, for weeks together, is akin to that followed by the natives of India of enclosing fractured limbs in moulds of clay. Of the successful result of this practice I remember a remarkable instance in the case of a little boy who was brought into my tent one morning, having been run over by a waggon on the line of march, and having sustained a severe compound fracture of the leg. I was preparing to amputate this boy's limb when the parents came in and carried him away to a potter in an adjoining village, who enveloped the leg in clay, and I believe finally cured the patient."

In Europe Hubenthal seems to have used plaster of Paris in 1816; it was mixed with ground-up blotting paper. Twelve years later Koyle and Kluge introduced a plaster box to the Charité Hospital, Berlin. The injured limb was laid in a wooden box into which plaster was poured. But while these developments were going on, egg white remained the favorite bonding agent. Louis Seutin, senior medical officer of the Belgian Army, inaugurated a period of starch bandages in 1834 and realized that it was better if patients with fractures of the leg could be ambulatory.

Another Army surgeon—Mathijsen, in the Dutch Army—introduced plaster bandages in 1852. The technique was popularized by its extensive use in the Crimean War.

The Russian surgical genius Nikolai Pirogoff began to cast fractures in plaster bandages, independently of Mathijsen, about the same time. He used them in the Seige of Sebastopol. In America, Samuel St. John of New York was a strong advocate of plaster because, he taught, the splint should be fitted to the limb, and not the limb to the splint. He introduced the padding of

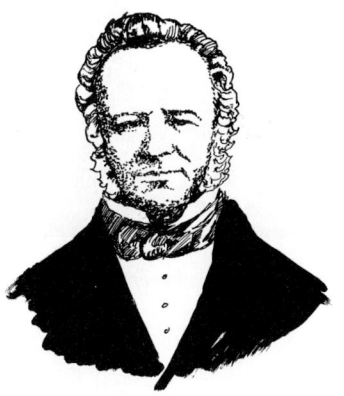

◆ **Louis Jean Seutin (1793–1865)**
Chief Surgeon to the Belgian Army. He was at the Battle of Waterloo. He married an heiress and renounced private practice. In 1835 he came across a goat with a broken leg next to a linen-starching shop. Eureka, the starch bandage was reinvented! He wrote a book about this bandage in 1840 and went on lecture tours to promote it. He was awarded medals for his great gift to humanity and became a Baron.

plasters with cotton wadding and, like Mathijsen, split the plaster while it was wet.

But voices were raised against plaster immobilization of fractures—Hugh Owen Thomas wrote that *"it did not allow frequent inspection, was much labour at first, and little afterwards, and provided no opportunity for the display of skill."* He thought that compression and covering up an injured limb reduced its vitality. A splint allowed the position to be improved as the fracture softened. About the same time, a man with ideas diametrically opposed to those of Thomas, Lucas-Champonnière, was questioning the tenets of fracture treatment. He was concerned with movement after the fracture had healed. *"The return of the limb to the maximum possible muscular strength, and the maximum joint mobility is a hundred times more important than the exact form of the skeleton."* Callus formation was encouraged by regulated movement that kept the joints moving. Further, if the limb were left free, the bone remained strong and was less likely to refracture.

The Crimean War spread the word about plaster fixation, but it was during World War I, when radiology was used for the first time on a large scale for the treatment of fractures, that the use of plaster became popular.

Antonius Mathijsen (1805–1878)

Mathijsen was born in Brudel, a small village in North Brabant, Holland, of a medical family, and trained as a military surgeon at Brussels and Utrecht. In 1831 he was involved in a 10-day campaign in Belgium and was decorated.

Mathijsen wrote a short paper on plaster splints in 1852 and a monograph in 1854. The idea caught on rapidly—in 1858 he devised plaster shears and was widely honored for his inventiveness. A monument was erected in 1948 at Brudel to commemorate him, and his portrait appeared on a Dutch stamp.

THE INVENTION OF PLASTER APPLIANCES
MATHIJSEN, 1852

"At the end of 1851, when I was stationed at Harlem (N. Holland), I made my first attempt to use plaster for surgical treatment. The bandages which I made at that time consisted of a layer of dry plaster in powder form spread evenly between two compresses. The wounded limb was placed on this; the bandage was then well wetted and wound around the limb. In this way the wounded limb was given a solid shell; however, when one wanted to strip off this casing to examine the injured parts, the bed of plaster broke, and the bandage lost its shape and strength.

"Soon I succeeded in introducing an improved modification to this poultice-like bandage. Immediately after having wet the bandage, I marked out a groove along it, parallel to the limb, using the edge of a spatula; in this way the plaster could be

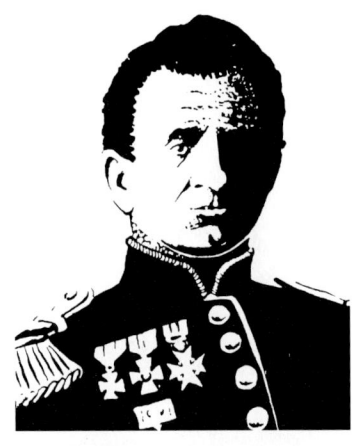

◆ Antonius Mathijsen (1805–1878)

hinged and one could even separate the slabs without running the risk of breaking or damaging the plaster.

"As I realised that my methods had resulted in success I continued my experiments assiduously for, although the groove allowed the bandage to be removed fairly easily, it was still far from what it should be to compete with other methods of treatment; it was too heavy and was not firm enough.

"To overcome these problems, I looked for a substance which could be mixed with the plaster to give it more firmness, render it less easily breakable and thus obtain a strong appliance. However, my search proved fruitless.

"Then I struck upon the idea of spreading the plaster in thin layers between three or four compresses and rubbing it into the closely woven weft of the pieces of material. The result was just what I wanted: the appliances made from these plastered pieces of material were light, firm, and elastic, and thus I realised my aim.

"Soon I also tried using plaster with pieces of cotton and partly worn linen which worked perfectly—in this way I obtained cottonplaster. From the original large sheet I cut off pieces in various sized strips, with which I very easily made various types of bandage. These bandages satisfied me on all counts, and I can confidently attribute them with the following properties and advantages:

(1) Simplicity: To make up plaster bandages one only needs some cotton or woollen material, some plaster, and water, and one can dispense with splints and other similar things.

(2) Easy Application: The strips of bandage can be put on in the easiest way: one winds the plastered pieces around the affected part like ordinary bandages; they shape themselves, so to speak, and one immediately obtains a solid shell which encases the affected part exactly.

(3) Instant Setting: This is a quality which no other appliance possesses, and this gives a particular advantage to plaster bandage. To justify this statement, one has only to consider fracture cases which involve fretful children, agitated or delirious patients, and above all, injuries on the battlefield. This instant-setting property of plaster would allow the evacuation of battlefield casualties by any means of transport, without exposing them to the appalling dangers and suffering with which they are threatened today.

(4) Plaster bandages can be applied without assistance.

(5) Plaster bandages can be applied in a few minutes.

(6) Complete Fixation: This bandage can be made so firm that it resists heavy knocks.

(7) Removability: The plaster appliance can be applied straight away as a bivalve. One can easily change the fixed bandage into a removable one, by cutting with large scissors.

(8) It has exact retention, because the plaster bandage encases the parts with the same strength all over; the parts rest on as wide a surface as possible—for this reason the injured part is well supported and does not become tired.

(9) The plaster bandage maintains extension and counter-extension from the time of application. Because of this one does not need any other temporary appliances, as one does with other fixed apparatus.

(10) Porosity: This property allows cutaneous perspiration to evaporate through the plaster shell, and also allows any other fluid secreted beneath the bandage to come through the plaster and thus give warning of unexpected complications.

(11) The plaster appliance resists all types of liquid action: neither urine, pus nor water harm[s] its firmness or strength in any way.

(12) Plaster can be easily removed: to do so, one wets the bandage with water and unrolls it like an ordinary bandage—in a few minutes one can remove or re-apply the plaster bandage.

(13) Price: no other appliance is as cheap.

(14) Appearance: the plaster appliance excels in its regular and beautiful appearance.

"From all the properties that I have just mentioned one can conclude a priori *that not only can these bandages be applied in cases of fractures of the limbs and trunk, but also in cases of those infirmities known as orthopaedic maladies, and in general in all cases in which M. Seutin has used his starch bandages; also, this technique has the advantage that dressings can be greatly simplified: splints, cradles, etc., can be abandoned; there is also the advantage of having fewer objects to carry about, which is of the greatest importance, particularly in battlefield surgery.*

"It is obvious that one could also use these bandages very advantageously in veterinary surgery."

THE THOMAS SPLINT

HUGH OWEN THOMAS

Robert Jones' Views on Thomas Splints, 1925

"The Great War afforded the most convincing proof of the mishandling of complicated, and even of simple, fractures. Fractures of the femur serve as a notable example. The splint with which we are all so familiar, invented by Thomas, was barely known, and yet it was the type of splint which ultimately saved the situation. In 1916 the mortality from these fractures amounted to 80 per cent, a large proportion of the deaths occurring on their way to or at Casualty Clearing Stations. Later, when the Thomas Splint was applied almost exclusively, and as near to the firing line as possible, the mortality in 1918 was reduced to 20 per cent."

It is ironic that on one of the few occasions Hugh Owen Thomas left his practice, he went to offer this splint to the French Army in the 1870s, and that it was refused.

THE KNEE APPLIANCE
HUGH OWEN THOMAS, 1875

"The upper crescent is formed of an iron ring three-eighths of an inch thick, varying according to the age and weight of the patient. The ring is nearly ovoid in shape and is covered with boiler felt and basil leather; from its upper and lower portions two iron rods pass down to the lower end of the machine, where may be noticed a small staple for retention purposes, only used for the reduction of flexion.

"The ovoid ring should join the inner stem, forming an angle of 55 degrees, which when correctly padded becomes reduced to 45 degrees. This arrangement of the splint will be the most acceptable for wearing. The staple can be cut off at a subsequent stage and replaced by a patten, which is welded on in its place, for the use of the patient in locomotion."

This was designed for the treatment of tuberculous knees in order to achieve "prolonged, uninterrupted, and enforced rest" in the extended position so that the infection could settle and leave an undeformed joint. He also used it for femoral shaft fractures, and to mobilize amputations before a prosthesis could be fitted. The basic splint had several variations. He put wheels on the lower end to make it more comfortable in bed rather than sling it up. The lower end had a patten for walking, and he developed one with the ring in two halves (inner and outer) for use when the knee was very swollen.

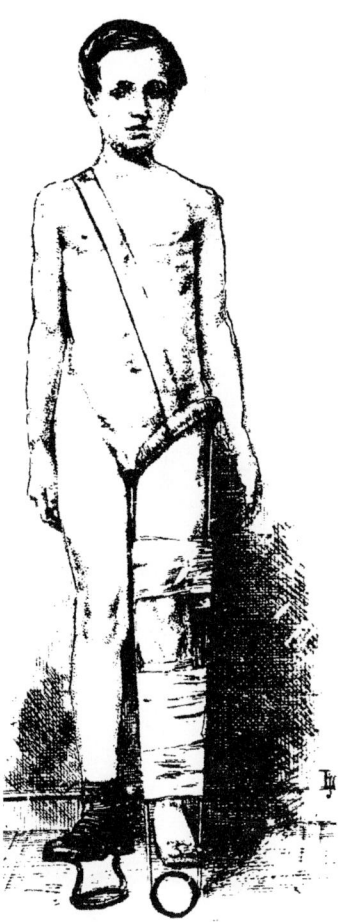

The Thomas splint. From Thomas HO: Hip, Knee, and Ankle. Self-published, 1876.

Traction

Since the earliest days traction has been used to reduce dislocations. Hippocrates used his heel, ladders, poles, and a sort of rack known as the scamnum of Hippocrates. His successors vied with one another to produce ever more fearsome equipment with more pulleys, longer levers, and stronger ropes. These were for short, sharp pulls. This sort of equipment was quite unsuited for prolonged traction as it damaged the skin and impaired the circulation. Anesthesia has largely abolished the need for brute force; but there are fracture tables to remind us of those rack and pinion days.

It is not surprising that continuous traction is of recent origin. In the past, unreduced simple fractures and circumferential bandages used to produce a toll of ulcers, gangrene, and erysipelas, without adding the hazard of badly applied continuous traction. A method of applying continuous traction without these complications proved difficult to find. Fractures of the femur were the first to be treated by continuous traction as the undamaged shin provided some sort of purchase. In the 18th century several surgeons, such as Pott and Petit, began to use inclined planes. They had the first realization that gravity could be used to maintain the position. Much later, in 1839, John Haddy James of Exeter (1788–1869)

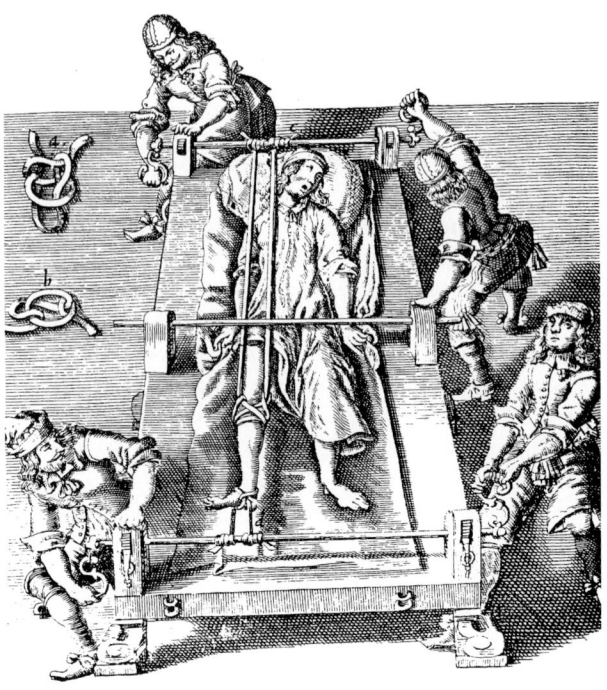

Hippocrates' scamnum, from Sculetus' 17th century book. Hippocrates suggests that every practitioner with an interest in fractures should invest in this equipment. It is hard to believe that it did more good than harm.

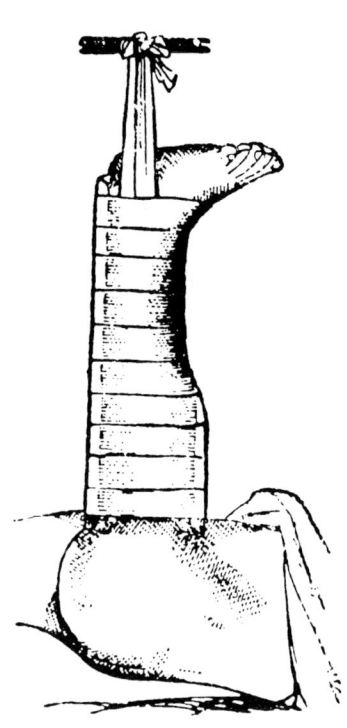

Bryant's traction, 1872.

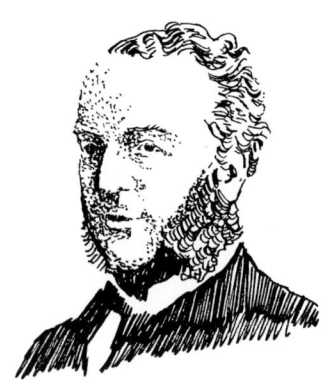

◆ Thomas Bryant

described continuous traction using a weight suspended over a pulley. He bandaged the leg to a wooden splint that rested on rollers; a string from the splint passed over a pulley to a weight. As he did not tip the bed, the patient was fixed to the headboard by a harness, to prevent him from being pulled out of bed feet first by the weight.

Josse, of Amiens, had solved the problem differently two years before. He lashed the patient's foot to the raised end of the bed.

It was some 26 years before the two ideas were amalgamated. Straight leg traction was popularized in the American Civil War. At

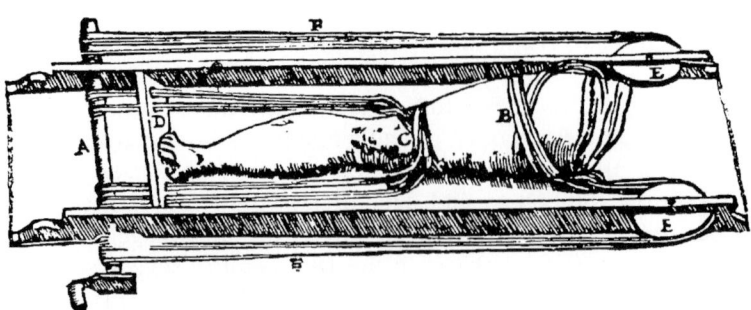

Galen's glossocomium, for fractures of the femur, dates from the 1st century. This wood engraving is from a 1625 edition of one of his books.

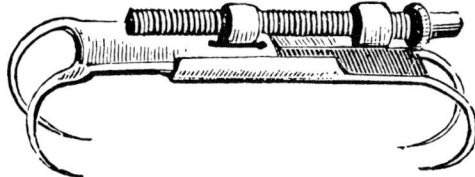

Malgaigne's claw for fractures of the patella. The fracture was held together without the need to open it—safe in the days before aseptic surgery, 1847.

the beginning of this war, in 1860, Gurdon Buck described a simple form of traction, easily applied in wartime conditions. His description follows later, from which it will be seen that the meaning of Buck's traction was changed through the years.

It was another war, the Balkan war, that saw the introduction, by a Dutch ambulance unit, of the Balkan beam—an overhead system clamped to the bed—in 1903. About this time the standard of conservative treatment received a stimulus to improve; X-rays and internal fixation were becoming available. A poor position was less easily tolerated, and the search began for more sophisticated forms of traction. Codivilla tried applying traction to a below-knee plaster but found that it produced skin necrosis. Skeletal traction was introduced. It had its antecedents in the ice tongs that Malgaigne used to hold a fractured patella together, more than 50 years before. Martin Kirschner (1879-1942), a surgeon at Heidelberg, used thin wires in 1909; he inserted them at first both above and below the fracture line and, with the aid of a distraction apparatus, prevented overlapping. Fritz Steinmann (1872-1932), a surgeon at Berne, introduced thicker pins and stirrups in 1911. He introduced the sites at which this form of traction is applied—femoral condyle, tibial tubercle, and calcaneum.

At its inception, opponents to skeletal traction maintained that it was a "compromise between inefficient closed operation and a hazardous open operation."

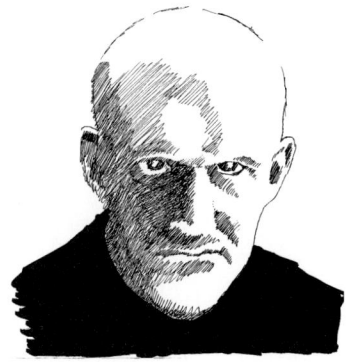

◆ Martin Kirschner

> *There are many methods of applying traction. But the best thing for any physician who practices in a large city, is to have prepared a proper wooden machine, with all the mechanical powers applicable in cases of fractures and dislocation.* Hippocrates on fractures

Gurdon Buck (1807–1877)

Buck was a general surgeon in New York. He described a form of extension for fractures of the femoral shaft just before the American Civil War. It proved popular in the war and preserved his name for posterity. Genealogists have established that the Gurdon family came to England with William the Conqueror, and another stem came to America with the Pilgrim Fathers. Gurdon Buck's father ran a shipping business in New York. Buck studied medicine, and graduated in 1830. After a period as a house physi-

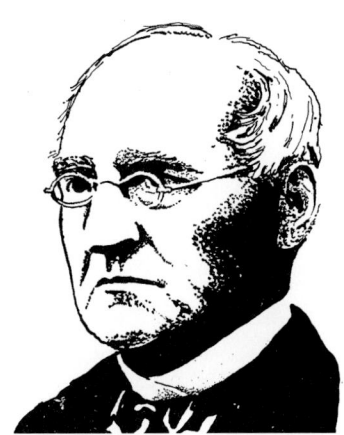

◆ Gurdon Buck

cian at New York Hospital, he went to Europe to study surgery, spending two years visiting Paris, Vienna, and Berlin.

In 1837 he was visiting surgeon to the New York Hospital. His particular field of interest was plastic surgery—the Civil War left an aftermath of facial injuries that he repaired with rotation and pedicle flaps; secondary defects were left to heal by themselves. A year before he died, he published a classic, entitled *Reparative Surgery*, which is filled with striking illustrations. In addition he was a good anatomist, describing Buck's fascia of the perineum.

BUCK'S EXTENSION
1860

[Dr. Gurdon Buck read an interesting paper upon a new treatment for fractures of the femur, of which the following is an abstract:]

"The appliances to the limb itself for the purpose of making extension are the same as have been in use in our hospitals for several years past, and are as follows: A roller bandage is commenced at the toes in the usual way, and continued to the ankles, where it is temporarily arrested. A band of adhesive plaster two and a half to three inches broad, and long enough to allow the middle of it to form a loop below the sole of the foot, and the ends to extend above the condyles of the femur, is then applied on either side, in immediate contact with the limb, from the ankle upwards. Over this the bandage is continued as high up as the plaster. A thin block of wood of the width of the plaster, and long enough to prevent pressure over the ankle, is inserted into the loop, and serves for the attachment of the extending cord, which is fastened to an elastic rubber band (such as is used for door springs) that passes round the block. By this arrangement elasticity is combined with the extension. The limb is now prepared to be put under extension. The arrangement for the pulley is very simple. A strip of inch board three inches wide is fastened upright to the foot of the bedstead, and perforated at the height of four or five inches above the level of the mattress. Through this hole the extending cord is to be passed, and on the further side of the strap a screw pulley should be inserted at the proper level over which the cord, with the weight attached, is to play, The footboard of the bedstead, if there is one, may be perforated at the proper level, and the screw pulley inserted in the further side of it, so as to answer equally well. To allow the application of lotions to the thigh during the first few days of treatment, the ends of the adhesive bands should stop short at the condyles of the femur, and be turned down. They may afterwards be replaced upon the thigh and the bandages continued over them, preparatory to the application of the coaptation splints, which should be added at this stage of the treatment. The coaptation splints, which may be of the ordinary sort, should be secured by those elastic bands, like suspender webbing fitted with buckles; these have the advantage of keeping up uniform concentric pressure as the limb diminishes from the subsidence of swelling. Counter-extension must be maintained by the usual perineum band lengthened out

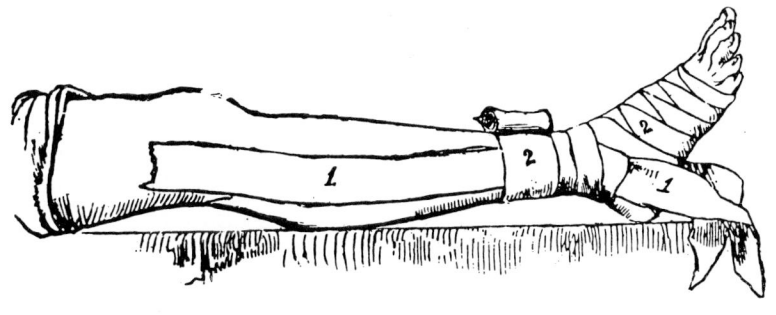

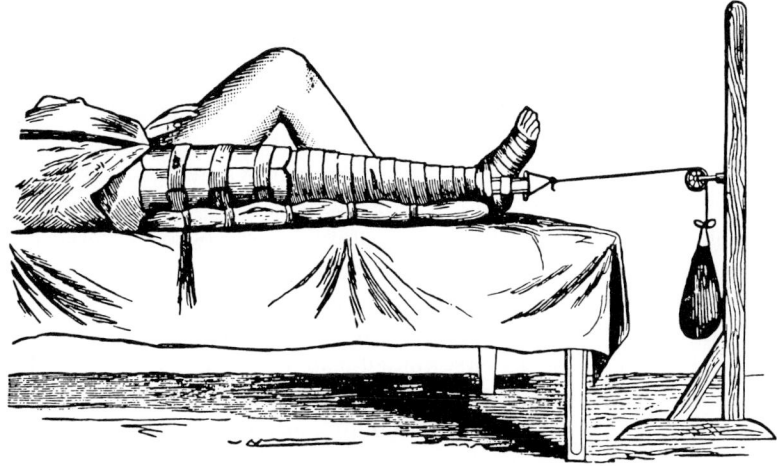

Buck's extension, 1883.

in the direction of the long axis of the body, and fastened to the head of the bedstead. India rubber tubing of three quarters of an inch calibre, stuffed with a skein of cotton lamp wick, makes an excellent perineum strap. A piece of two feet long with a ring fastened at each end answers this purpose admirably. A thin, wedge-shaped hair cushion, to raise the heel above the mattress, and a bag filled with bran or sand to place on the outside of the foot to prevent rotation outwards, complete the appliances requisite to carry out this method of treatment. There need be no delay in its application. The sooner after the occurrence of the injury, the limb is put up, the better. The contraction of the muscles is thus antagonised from the outset, and the rough ends of the fragments are prevented from fretting the soft parts."

[The author then gave twenty-one cases in detail where this treatment was employed; and the results, as shown by actual measurement, are equal to any that have hitherto been obtained. Dr. Buck claims for the apparatus the following advantages:]

"I. It maintains uninterrupted and efficient extension without producing intolerable pain, excoriations, sloughing, and tedious sores.

II. It diminishes very materially the suffering of the patient and the irksomeness of long confinement to one position. There is no inconvenience attending the evacuation of the bowels.

III. It is cheap and easy of application.

IV. It is not liable to become deranged, thus rendering it unnecessary for as frequent visits on the part of the surgeon as when the ordinary apparatus is applied. The author considers it very necessary to apply coaptation splints, for reasons already given."

Robert Hamilton Russell (1860–1933)

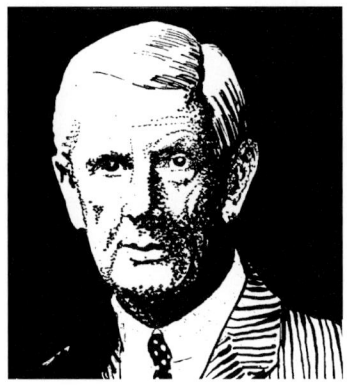

◆ Hamilton Russell

Russell was born in Kent and was Lister's house surgeon. He emigrated to Melbourne in 1890. He brought antiseptic surgery with him and did much to establish a high standard of general surgery in Australia. In particular he founded the College of Surgeons of Australasia and was its first Director-General.

He is remembered for devising a very useful system of traction; though now used to relieve the painful spasm of an irritable hip from any cause, it was designed for something different. Percivall Pott used to teach that the deformity of long bone fractures was maintained by muscle pull and that the muscles must be relaxed for reduction to be stable. Russell had the same approach—his traction was designed to circumvent undesirable muscle spasm in fractures of the femur. It is not much used today as it requires constant vigilance.

In the Outback he sustained a Colles' fracture and as there was no medical help near he promptly reduced it himself and continued to treat it.

He was killed in a motor accident.

In a previous book I included the complete article. At that time, patients in traction distinguished the orthopaedic ward from other wards in a hospital. Coping with traction made it necessary for nurses to take special diplomas in orthopaedic nursing. Today traction is a rare sight, and this paper is on its way out and has been greatly shortened.

FRACTURE OF THE FEMUR: A CLINICAL STUDY

R. HAMILTON RUSSELL, 1924

"Let us suppose a patient with fracture of the middle of the femoral shaft just admitted to hospital. The thigh is shortened. Why? The shortening is caused by the tonic contraction of certain long muscles that are attached above to the pelvic bone, and traverse the entire length of the thigh to be inserted into the tibia and fibula. Of these there are two opposing sets, consisting (in the main) of the hamstrings and the rectus femoris.

"The numerous muscles that are attached to the femur itself play little if any part in the production of shortening.

"The house surgeon's duty will be to take the measurements at least every morning and evening, and to inspect and adjust

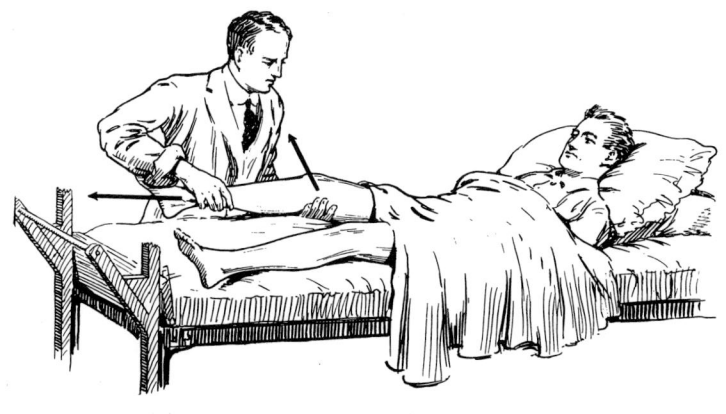

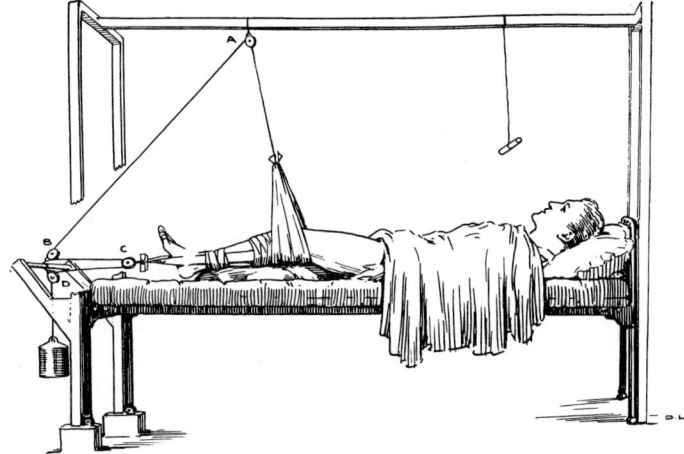

Hamilton Russell traction for fracture of the shaft of the femur.

the pillows beneath the thigh and the leg so that there may be no backward sagging at the seat of fracture and the heel shall not be in contact with the bed. It is very little to require of him; but while it is very little and very easy, yet it is absolutely indispensable and must be faithfully given. The apparatus is far from being 'fool-proof' and cannot and will not look after itself.

"One more word as to the significance of comfort. Comfort is the first essential in the treatment of a fracture. No apparatus that is not perfectly comfortable can be a good apparatus, for the muscles will never be at rest, but will always be striving to achieve a position of greater comfort. Moreover, there is, I am convinced, a direct relationship between comfort and rapid union, and an equally direct relationship between discomfort and delayed union, feeble union, and non-union. Explain this how we may, I have no doubt whatever about the clinical fact as a matter of bedside observation. Therefore let us never be content with any means, no matter how ingenious, and complicated, and satisfying to our theoretical preconceptions, that is not perfectly comfortable."

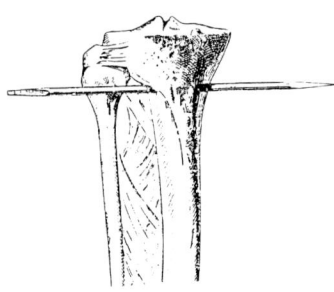

Steinmann traction, 1912.

A NEW TRACTION METHOD IN THE TREATMENT OF FRACTURES
DR. FR. STEINMANN OF BERN, 1907

"*The employers' liability act and roentgenray photography have shown us how bad the results of fracture treatment still are in general. When we think that according to Hoffa, two thirds of disability compensation is accounted for by fractures, we can judge what improvement in the national economy even the least improvements in this treatment represents. The most frequent causes of trouble after fractures are severe contractions and stiffness of the involved joints, then muscle atrophy, hypertrophic callus, decubitus, gangrene and so forth. Various methods have been attempted in fracture therapy, from the purely anatomic (open suture) to the purely functional (Lucas-Championnière). The essence of successful fracture therapy lies in the correct combination of both. The fragments must be well reduced and reduction maintained; but the function of the uninjured neighboring muscles and joints on the contrary must be immediately exercised (early motion, massage). Extension best meets this requirement.*

"*Bardenheuer gained considerable competence with traction and obtained the best results of modern times. Next to the development of transverse and rotational traction, one of his chief innovations is the introduction of the use of sufficient weight to overcome the displacement, that is, much greater weight than was formerly employed (e.g., 30 Kg. for femoral shaft fractures). The high weight must be applied from the first day. Along with this, gymnastic measures should be instituted early. The Bardenheuer adhesive plaster bandages served these demands better than all others. But these too have their drawbacks. The technic is not easy; for it, one needs continual control, which in reality can hardly be conducted properly in a hospital, and in rural circumstances it is impossible. To use traction of 15 to 30 Kg. by means of adhesive plaster bandages without pressure or damage is an art. We see eczema, decubitus and even gangrene appear with adhesive plaster traction. I myself have seen a case of the last in a hospital which led to amputation. Bardenheuer would certainly object that such a case could be traced back to a defect in technic or control. It merely proves to me that adhesive plaster traction is not simple enough to make such an occurrence impossible.*

"*I believe that the procedure that I now present as nail traction is a method which does not possess all these disadvantages. Let us take, for example, a femoral shaft fracture. My management of this is as follows. I take 2 very pointed, slender, nickel-plated steel nails from 6 to 8 cm. long with a broad head, sterilize them by boiling, and strike them with a hammer through opposite sides at the lower end of the femur through the disinfected skin and the soft tissues into the condyles. As place of entry I sometimes choose the upper edge of the condyle and direct the point obliquely downward toward the opposite epicondyle. At entering, the nail is held with a sterilized pair of pliers. From the* head of the nail projecting about 1 cm. out of the skin, a suitable weight can be attached by cord, or better by wire, on the usual traction apparatus. The traction is set up in a few minutes.

"The insertion of the nail is in itself bearable without local anesthesia, as I have proved in the fixation of a chronic clavicular luxation. In fractures, because of anticipated shock, usually I have given a short anesthesia, less often in fractures of the leg, or at times omitted it here unless the patient had complained of unbearable pain. Perhaps, a satisfactory fixation of the outer fragments or the construction of an apparatus to drive the nail more slowly would make the anesthesia unnecessary. But the latter (anesthesia) has the advantage that the patient sees nothing and is not disturbed by the idea of a nail driven through the bone.

"The method is still new and certainly capable of many improvements. I believe that a useful procedure is presented, and it seems to me that whoever has seen it work on a femoral fracture would agree."

Open Reduction and Internal Fixation

Although wiring fractures is ancient, ORIF became practical only after aseptic technique and anesthesia made surgery safe. Little was done until the discovery of X-rays because it was essential to define the fracture to be sure that the primitive implants were capable of holding the fracture. Corrosion was soon a problem—ORIF started before the concept of stainless steel—later metallurgy delivered an inert metal.

Sir William Arbuthnot Lane (1856–1938)

Arbuthnot Lane was a superb technician, and this was to some extent his downfall in his later years—operating became safe and enabled him to perform hundreds of colectomies for constipation.

He was born at Inverness, the son of an army surgeon, and began to study at Guy's Hospital at the age of 16. For the first six years after qualifying, apart from a period as a ship's surgeon, he studied in the dissecting room, trying to relate occupation to skeletal form. Conan Doyle is said to have had him in mind to some extent when he created Sherlock Holmes. He paid great attention to the effects of fractures on joint form. The deleterious effect of malunion on the joint and the earning capacity of the patient led him to undertake internal fixation of fractures. In 1892 he originated the "no touch" technique, which was used for so many years, to make surgery safe. After screwing a few fractures of the tibia with success, he proceeded to fix with screws all those he came across in order to show other surgeons that it could be done and that it was safe. The metal he used was ordinary steel, which became corroded—fortunately the film of rust that formed

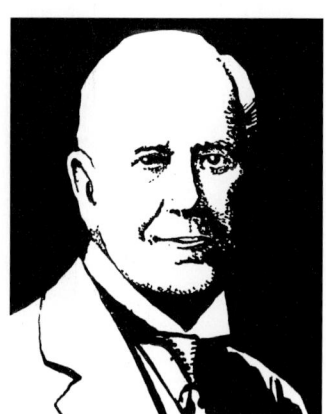

◆ Sir William Arbuthnot Lane (1856–1938)

acted to some extent as an insulator, preventing gross oxidation. If dissimilar metals are used this film does not form, and a severe electrolyte reaction occurs, leading to destruction of the metal and inflammation of the tissues. In 1905 he started to use plates. Though internal fixation had been used sporadically for almost a century before in the form of bronze and silver wire, it was Arbuthnot Lane who made internal fixation a practical procedure, and he wrote a book about his methods.

He was always a general surgeon; he was one of the first to open the mastoid antrum for an infected mastoid and to resect part of a rib for empyema. The enthusiasm he brought to colonic surgery was his chief claim to fame. It was his opinion that diseases such as tuberculosis of bone, rheumatoid arthritis, and many other conditions were largely due to constipation, and he treated them by ileocolectomy. He removed colons wholesale; he introduced liquid paraffin to the pharmocopeia. Finally he realized he could not cope with the therapeutic problem he had set for himself and started a program of health education. He initiated columns in newspapers, public lectures, and the New Health Society. He resigned from the Medical Register before embarking on this so that he could not be accused of unethical conduct. He raised money to found the first Chair of Dietetics, and improved the distribution of fruit and vegetables.

He did the first open cardiac massage when a patient whose abdomen he was operating on had a cardiac arrest. The heart started again, and the patient recovered. Though the things he was most devoted to seem to have been the triumph of technique over reason, he started a new era of fracture treatment.

A METHOD OF TREATING SIMPLE OBLIQUE FRACTURES OF THE TIBIA AND FIBULA MORE EFFICIENT THAN THOSE IN COMMON USE

W. ARBUTHNOT LANE, M.S., 1894

"My experience of the usual methods of treating simple oblique fractures of the tibia and fibula in certain classes of labouring men, by manipulation of the fragments and the subsequent retention of the limb in some form of splint, is that the results so obtained are but too frequently unsatisfactory in the extreme.

"I do not allude to the presence of any considerable shortening or deformity, for with moderate skill and care such conditions can be generally avoided, though in some cases deformity and shortening are noticeable features. In this paper I will confine myself solely to the consideration of the physical capacity of the man to perform his accustomed heavy work after he has sustained an oblique fracture of both bones of the leg, or in other words of his relative financial value as a machine, both before and after the accident, and I have no hesitation whatever in asserting that, under the methods of treatment at present adopted, not only is the man totally incapacitated from earning a living for an unnecessarily long period, but in a considerable

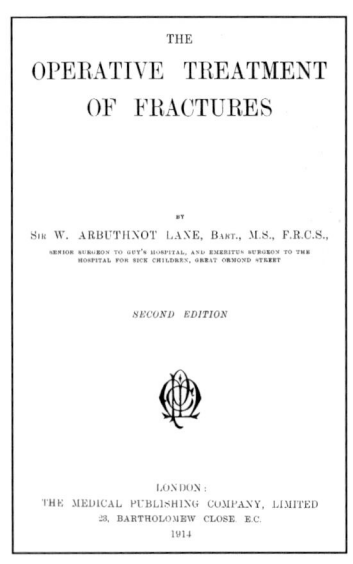

Title page of Lane's book.

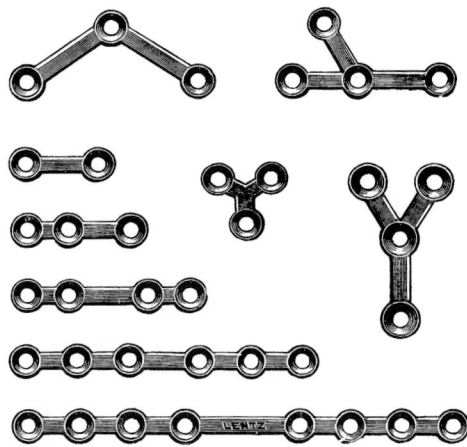

Lane's plates, 1907.

proportion of cases he is unable subsequently to perform such heavy work as he was able to do before the injury, so that he is obliged to follow some less remunerative pursuit, if indeed he has not to depend solely on charity. In fact, his machinery is financially depreciated by the accident, occasionally to the extent of at least 70 to 80 per cent of its original value.

"*If what I state is true, the form of treatment of such fractures which is universally adopted in our hospitals is simply disastrous, and can only be perpetuated because we are unaware of the financial loss or even ruin which our very imperfect surgical methods entail on our unfortunate patients. Though the shortening and deformity are usually trifling, the somewhat complicated displacement of the ends of the fragments on one another is sufficient to completely alter, and often irretrievably damage, the machinery of the lower extremity. The deviation of the axes of the lower fragments of the tibia and fibula from the directions they originally occupied when in continuity with the upper portions of the respective bones causes pressure to be transmitted through the joints of the ankle and foot, of the knee, and to some extent even of the hip, in such an abnormal manner that the individual experiences not only a feeling of insecurity in these joints, which is especially marked in the foot and ankle, but he also suffers from progressively increasing pain and discomfort.*

"*This means that the anatomy of the several joints which are called upon to perform a function other than that they were accustomed to carry out must alter in consequence of, and in proportion to, the degree in which the directions of the lines of pressure which is transmitted through the joints are [sic] changed.*

"*Under these altered circumstances the joints are unable to carry out their physiological functions with the same accuracy and perfection that they did previous to the accident, and this inability is a progressive one, and is accompanied by pain and discomfort which increases rapidly, and is most marked in those who sustain such fractures when past middle age.*

"*Even if there is only a small proportion of truth in what I assert—and in my opinion my experience justifies me in making* the assertion—it is obvious folly to continue our present methods of treatment, especially as more effectual means are ready to hand.

"Why should we hesitate for one moment to bring common sense mechanical principles to bear in the case of simple fractures of the tibia and fibula, when most surgeons of the present day would not dream of doing otherwise in the case of fracture of the patella with separation of fragments? May I ask this question: are we able by operative measures to treat oblique fractures of the tibia and fibula so that there shall be no alteration from the normal in the lines of pressure through the several joints? In other words, can we restore the bones to their original form? This can certainly be done, and at a minimum risk to the patient, by freely exposing the fragments at the seat of fracture, by bringing the surfaces into accurate apposition, and retaining them permanently in that position.

"Such operative measures offer to the patient the following advantages:

(a) They at once relieve him from the pain of any movement of the fragments upon one another.

(b) They free him from the tension and discomfort due to the extensive extravasation of blood between and into the tissues.

(c) They shorten the duration of the period during which he is incapacitated from work, since union is practically by first intention, and consequently very rapid and perfect.

(d) Lastly, and by far the most important, they leave his skeletal mechanics in the condition in which they were before he sustained the injury.

"The two questions which now arise are: Is much difficulty experienced in bringing the surfaces into accurate apposition? and What is the best method of retaining them in that apposition?

"In answer to the first question, it is often very difficult, even when the tibial fracture is freely exposed, to bring the surfaces into apposition by means of manipulation of the limb and of the broken ends, but in every case in which I have used screw pressure I have succeeded in doing so. At the same time it is obvious that even though by these means the surgeon may fail in obtaining perfectly accurate apposition, he will get union with very much less displacement than with the ordinary methods, and consequently, a correspondingly better result.

"Now as regards the best means of fixation of the fragments: in my earlier cases I used silver wire, but soon gave it up, as it was open to two great objections. Firstly, as it is necessary to fasten its ends, it could only be passed in certain directions with safety, and to secure it satisfactorily one was at times obliged to incise the parts very freely. Secondly, one frequently found that no amount of traction upon the ends of the wires would retain the surfaces in accurate apposition after the grip of the lion forceps was relaxed.

"Therefore I decided to treat the bones as one would the broken leg of a table or chair. The surfaces were brought into accurate apposition, and kept in their normal relationship by

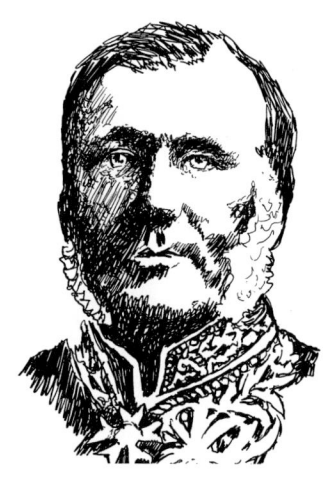

◆ **Laurent Jean Baptiste Bérenger-Féraud (1832–1900)**

The son of a naval surgeon, he became surgeon-in-chief of the French Navy. While a student in Toulon he saw patients with open fractures treated by wiring and made this the subject of his thesis. He had two careers—one as an army surgeon in which he treated fractures and wrote the first book on open reduction, *Immobilisation Directe*, in 1870. His other career was as a naval surgeon interested in tropical disease; he described blackwater fever.

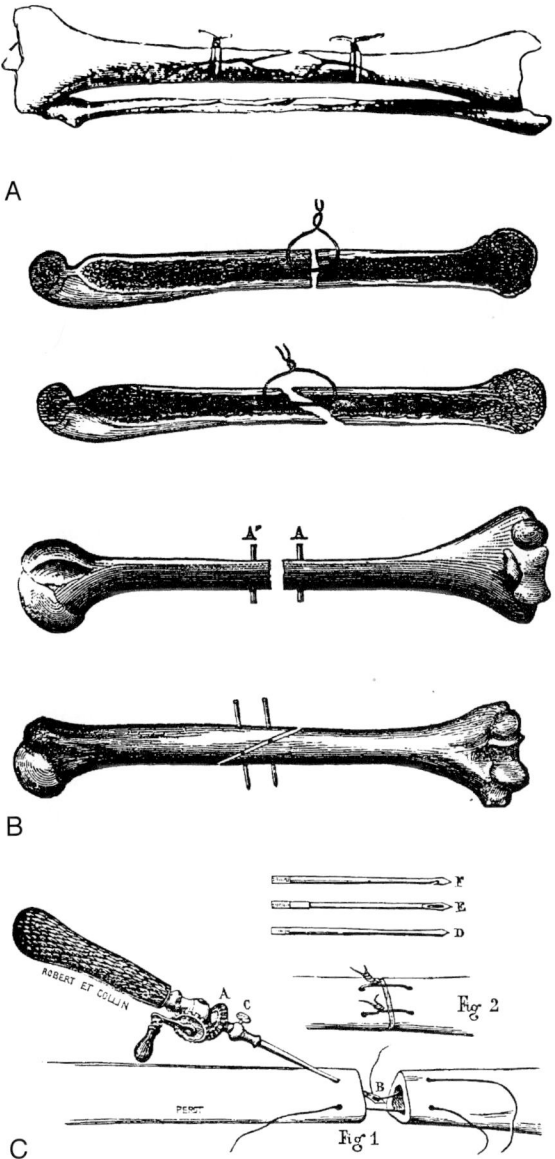

(A) Cerclage for fracture fixation. From Bérenger-Féraud, 1870. (B) and (C), Methods of bone sutures. From Bérenger-Féraud, 1871.

lion forceps. Holes were drilled above and below the forceps, and screws were driven in. The screws could be passed in any direction, and they retained the surfaces in an apposition more accurate and more forcible than I fancy can be attained by any other mechanical arrangement.

"As far as I know, they cause no subsequent trouble; should they do so they can be removed through an incision equal to the diameter of the head of the screw.

"Although I have limited myself to the consideration of the difficulties experienced in establishing exact continuity of the fragments in oblique fractures of the tibia and fibula, yet occa-

sionally in a transverse fracture of the tibia it may be absolutely necessary to expose the broken ends before they can be brought into accurate apposition. As instances of this mode of treatment I am bringing three cases before the Society, as they were all done during the same take-in week, and represent the more simple and effectual means of approximation of the surfaces by screw pressure.

"If the conclusions at which I have arrived are correct, it is obvious that any surgeon who resorts to the treatment of oblique fractures of both tibia and fibula, in Labourers, by manipulation and splinting, without having previously explained to the patient the consequent disadvantages under which he will very possibly labour, and urged on him the importance of operative interference, is acting unjustly to his patient.

"In the case of compound fractures of these bones it is equally advisable to procure perfect union, but for obvious reasons the surgeon is unable to offer the patient the same certainty of a successful result as he can when operating on a recent fracture.

"I.D.M., aet. 34, admitted under my care December 17, 1893. He fell with his leg twisted under him. The tibia was found to be fractured obliquely about two inches above the malleolus, and the fibula was broken about its centre. The lower fragment was displaced behind and outside the upper. Small fragments were felt. No amount of manipulation or traction served to bring the fragments into anything like accurate apposition. His permission for an operation not being obtained, a splint with a foot-piece everted at an angle equal to its fellow was applied.

"On January 8, 1894, as no callus could be felt, and as there was definite deformity, operative measures were urged on him, and he consented.

"The fracture in the tibia was exposed by an incision 4½ inches long, when its direction was seen to be very oblique, running downwards, outwards, and backwards. Several small fragments of bone and muscle intervened between the ends of the bone.

"Another effort to reduce the fragments by manipulation and traction was made, and the result was observed through the incision, when it was quite obvious that it could not have been effectual in this case in producing anything like apposition. The fragments of bone and muscle which intervened were removed, and after much difficulty the broken surfaces were brought into accurate apposition by means of lion forceps, and two screws were inserted. The temperature on one occasion after the operation rose to 99.2."

Lane then described two further similar cases.

"In none of these cases was there ever any sign of pus.
"I am very much indebted to Mr. F. J. Steward, who obtained for me the details of forty cases of fracture of both bones of the

leg taken indiscriminately from those treated in Guy's Hospital, and from various infirmaries. He started his investigations in an attitude antagonistic to the conclusions at which I had arrived, and this fact therefore renders his observations all the more reliable and valuable. From a consideration of the cases he collected he obtained the following deductions, which fully bear out the statements I have made in the early part of this paper."

Deductions From Cases

"In 40 cases of fractures of the tibia and fibula below the middle of the leg in men following various occupations, 19, or 48 per cent. suffered financially, owing either to inability to follow their former occupation or to earn as much as was earned at their original occupation; 15, or 38 per cent., suffered pain at the seat of injury; and 6, or 15 per cent., had pain in the ankle; and 4 of them had pain in the knee-joint; 12, or 30 per cent., suffered from insecurity in the limb, in nearly every case this insecurity being referred to the ankle-joint. In several of these cases the pain and insecurity in the ankle-joint was not noticed till a period varying from one to ten years had elapsed after the injury was received, showing that slow changes took place in the ankle-joint in consequence of the alteration in the mechanical arrangements of the limb produced by the fracture.

"In 23 cases of similar fractures in men following occupations, which necessitated heavy work and lifting of weights, 13, or 56 per cent., suffered financially owing to inability to do such heavy work; 12, or 52 per cent., had pain either at the seat of fracture or in the ankle- or knee-joint or in both; and 9, or 39 per cent., suffered from more or less insecurity in the whole limb, this last being in all cases the cause of the inability to follow their former laborious occupations."

He writes that, in 1892, "I made it my habitual practice to operate on all cases of simple fractures of the long bones in which I was not able to obtain accurate apposition of the fragments when the restoration of the bone to its normal form was of mechanical importance to the individual." Ironically, he shows many children's fractures that would not be treated by internal fixation today.

OSTEOSYNTHESIS, 1949
ROBERT DANIS (1880–1962)

"In order to be completely satisfactory, internal fixation must fulfill the following three requirements. (1) Enablement of immediate, active movement of muscles in the affected region and of the adjacent joints. (2) Complete restoration of the original shape of the bone. (3) Direct union of the bone fragments without the formation of visible callus."

1. Early Active Remobilization

"If the adjacent joints are immobilized with a cast following internal fixation, the main benefit of the operation is lost. Even

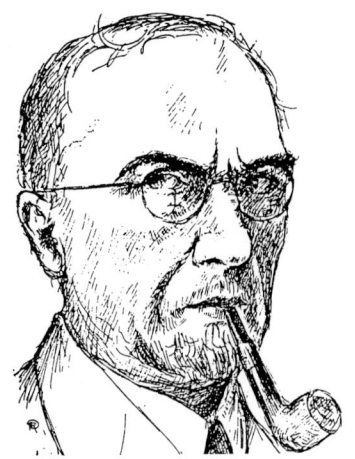

◆ Robert Danis (1880–1962)

a walking cast is associated with appreciable atrophy of muscles and tendons as well as vascular disturbances and skin changes. These may severely prolong convalescence and may even leave permanent stigmata."

Intramedullary Fixation

The problem at first was getting inside the bone. Operations were done through small incisions, with limited exposure, for fear of infection. Before antibiotics this was a much greater calamity than it is now. So the first attempt, made with short pegs, was quickly followed by thin pins. Fixation was insecure compared with a plate, and the principle did not become accepted until rigid, reamed intramedullary nailing became available.

The Use of Intramedullary Pegs

Various pegs had been tried from the days of the Mayans, who used sticks. Hey Groves published the results of his experimental work in 1916. He used short pegs in a small number of animals and people with good results. The fracture was always opened. Metal pegs were better in animals than a variety of absorbable materials. They were never more than an ingenious first concept.

One problem was that stainless steel had not been invented, and surgeons were trying to put in as little reactive metal as possible. These short pegs did not give enough mechanical stability. Hey Groves concluded:

"Bone left to natural repair will heal by granulation. Bones firmly and accurately fixed will heal by first intention. Bones weakly joined by a method which allows more and more movement between them will not join at all, or their junction will be long delayed."

Rush Rods

Lowry Rush was a gynecologist who helped his brother, Leslie, a general surgeon, with fracture surgery in Meridian, Mississippi. In 1936 they held an unstable Monteggia fracture with a Steinmann pin down the ulna. They were pleased with the position but not with the pin. This led to the development of the Rush rod, which enjoyed some popularity prior to the use of reamed nails. The Rush rods were loose in the canal and never held the bones very securely.

"We have been able to develop a pin so versatile that we have found it applicable to practically all of the long bones of the body and we now believe that it is indicated in a large variety of fractures.

"This work has been motivated by a desire to eliminate the need for plaster casts in fracture treatment. The aim has been to develop a type of internal fixation which would splint a broken bone while leaving the extremity free for function, permitting the patient to be ambulatory."

Kuntscher Nailing

Gerhard Kuntscher in 1940 pointed out that if hip nailing works well, nailing of other bones should too. He tries it out on human femurs and finds the canal large enough for the nail to pass without reaming. Because the nail does not fill the canal, he argues that the endosteal contribution to healing is unimpeded. From the start he practiced closed nailing, and if he could not achieve this he went on to casts or traction.

"The use of intramedullary nailing in dogs after breaking their thigh with an osteoclast gave suprisingly good results. Eight days after nailing the animals could stand by themselves.

"The method was used for 11 human femur fractures as well as fractures of the tibia and humerus. The first eight proximal femur fractures were opened and the greater trochanter was exposed. A hole was bored and a guide wire inserted. The nail was driven down. The upper fragment gripped the nail to aim it down the distal fragment. Subsequent nails were inserted percutaneously using a spike to find the starting point."

Patients were up quickly and required little specialized care. Callus was abundant and formed quickly. Kuntscher developed his nail in Germany during World War II so that reports were few. There was a story in *Time Magazine*, 1942: Soldiers returned with the *K* nail and no cast. After World War II the nails became public knowledge and many surgeons produced their own pattern. General acceptance seemed likely until Watson Jones wrote a damning article that held back further development for 20 years. He did the same thing for hip hemiarthroplasty until he needed a prosthesis himself after a subcapital fracture.

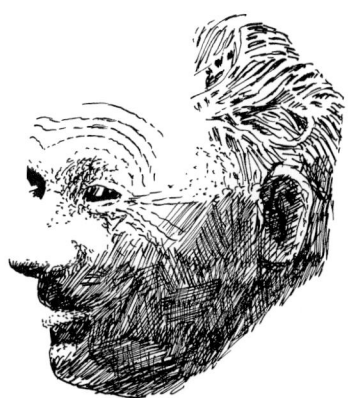

◆ **Gerhard Kuntscher (1900–1972)**
Born in Saxony, he graduated with the highest marks from Würzburg in 1926. This was the university where x-rays were discovered and where there is an X-ray Museum. After spending a time in radiology, he joined the university clinic in Kiel in 1930. He presented a paper on intramedullary nailing in 1940. During World War II he was on the eastern front. Knowledge of his intramedullary nailing came to the Allies at the end of the war; they found it hard to believe and mocked the infected cases. Following the war, he went to Schleswig Hesterberg and then to Hamburg, where he wrote *The Practice of Intramedullary Nailing.*

Compression and Bone Healing

Does compression promote healing by improving fracture stability or by affecting bone cells favorably? George Eggers looked at this before AO in 1949.

He did experiments on the skulls of rats, compressing skull flaps with wire. He concluded, *"The presence of the contact-compression factor favorably influences purposeful osteogenesis and fracture union.*

"Excessive pressure causes necrosis of the compressed bone, and lack of pressure fails to stimulate osteogenesis. The most advantageous compression force on the fracture surfaces appar-

ently is midway between the extremes, and probably is exerted by the physiological forces of the musculature. . . ."

He designed a slotted sliding plate that allowed the muscles to keep the bone ends in contact even if there was absorption of the bone ends. Unfortunately, they allowed the fracture to wobble, and his plates failed.

George W. Bagby from Spokane, Washington, described a self-compression plate in 1956, when he was at the Mayo Clinic. The design was later adopted for the dynamic compression plate. Bagby had tested these plates in animals and concluded:

"There was no evidence that osteogenesis was either stimulated or retarded by compression, but that compression minimized the fracture gap and held the fracture fragments rigidly. These factors resulting from compression led to earlier union."

INTERNAL FIXATION OF FRACTURES: EVOLUTION OF CONCEPTS
MARTIN ALLGOWER AND PHILLIP G. SPIEGEL

"In 1958, some 15 Swiss general and orthopedic surgeons met and discussed the status of the poor results obtained with both nonoperative and operative methods of fracture treatment in their country. This nucleus later developed into the group called ASIF (Association for the Study of Internal Fixation) or AO (ArbeitsgemeinSchaft für Osteosynthesefragen). The meeting was initiated by Maurice E. Muller who had spent some time with Danis and was impressed by his compression fixation of fractures, the avoidance of external immobilization, and the early pain-free active immobilization of the injured extremity.

"Out of this meeting, four principles seemed clearly instrumental for obtaining optimal results and were accepted as working hypotheses. (1) Anatomical reduction. (2) Rigid internal fixation. (3) Atraumatic technique on soft-tissue as well as on bone. (4) Early pain-free active mobilization during the first 10 postoperative days."

The figures from the Swiss Workman's Compensation Board provided the evidence for the poor results. The AO group invented new equipment, which was generally derided by the godfathers of British, American, and Austrian orthopaedics. The Swiss persisted and would not sell their system until the purchaser had taken a course so that it was used properly.

The enormous success of the AO system is a story in itself.

External Fixators

External fixators got off to a slow start because pin track infection could be fatal until the advent of antibiotics.

Jean-François Malgaigne described a "point" in 1840 to hold a fracture of the tibia in position and in 1843 a clamp to approximate fractures of the patella.

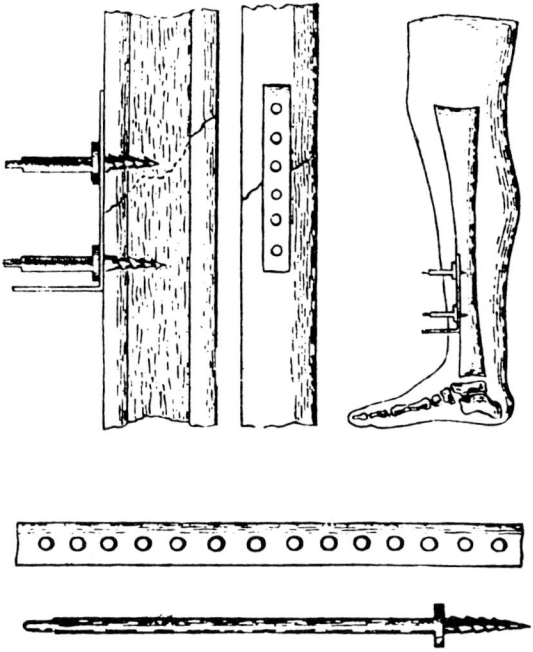

Hansmann's plates had screws that protruded through the skin to facilitate removal. 1886.

A fracture of the olecranon was held together with a tangle of screws and string by Rigaud in Strasbourg in 1850, and in 1870 Beranger-Feraud used screws and a wooden bar.

A NEW APPARATUS FOR THE FIXATION OF BONES

CLAYTON PARKHILL, 1897

"We believe that the time has come when a more accurate fixation of the bones, both after resection for cases of pseudarthrosis and for malunion, and also for fractures with a tendency to displacement, particularly if they be compound, should be used."

He devised the clamp for a young man with an old gunshot wound of the humerus.

"The destruction of tissue was so great that but a quarter of an inch of the shaft remained attached to the head of the bone. I knew of no method in use which would fix this upper fragment."

He describes success in 9 cases.

"Case 1. Pseudarthrosis of the right humerus as a result of a gunshot-fracture eleven months previous. An open infected wound communicated with the upper fragment. On November 22d, 1894, this wound was scraped out, removing all the infected tissue. It healed kindly, and on January 3, 1895, the

◆ **Clayton Parkhill (1860–1902)**
Born in Pennsylvania, he practiced in Denver and became professor of surgery and dean of the medical school at University of Colorado. He worked as a medical officer in the war with Spain in 1898. Soon afterward he developed acute appendicitis, refused operation, and died.

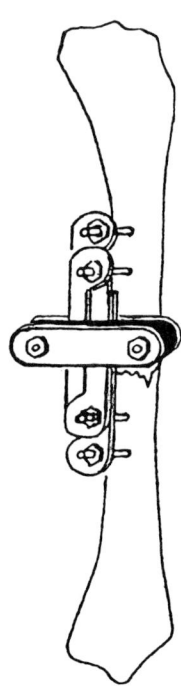

Clayton Parkhill's external fixator, 1897.

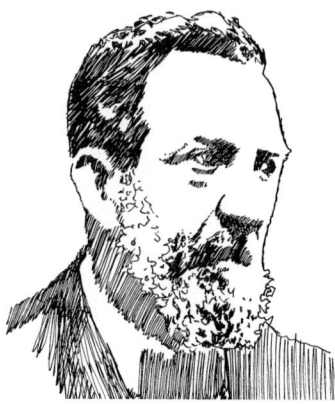

◆ **Albin Lambote (1866–1956)**
Belgian general surgeon with a special interest in fractures, making violins, and drawing and painting. He coined the term osteosynthesis in his book in 1907. Early movement was expected after fracture fixation. He made prototypes of tools and plates in his workshop.

clamp was used for uniting the fragments. The bones were found separated by a distance of two inches. The upper fragment had a length of one and a half inches, including the head, and was very soft. Transverse resection. The wound was closed about the clamp without drainage. The extremity, including the chest, was inclosed in a plaster-of-Paris dressing. No reaction. The dressing was removed February 9, 1895, when the wound was entirely healed. No infection. The clamp screws were lifted out without force. The sutures were removed. A dressing and cast applied. This was removed at the end of four weeks. Perfect union was observed."

"We claim for this instrument: first, that it may be easily and accurately adjusted, and prevents both longitudinal and lateral movements between the fragments: second, that nothing is left in the tissues which might reduce their vitality and lead to pain or infection: third, that no secondary operation is necessary; fourth, that no operation has ever before given 100 percent of cures."

For gunshot fractures, the value of external fixation became obvious. Borchgrevink developed them for the Balkan war, Lambret made some, and Hey Groves describes his apparatus in 1914. Pins and plaster was a cheap alternative.

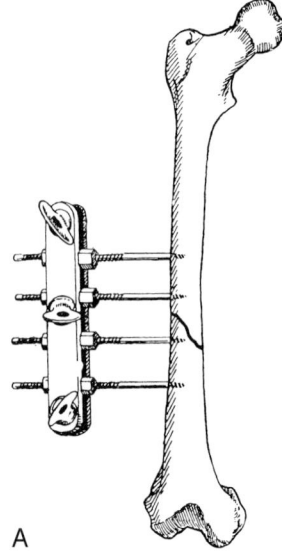

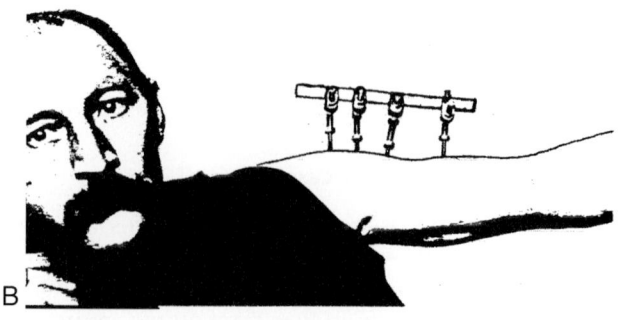

(A) Lambotte's external fixator, 1907. (B) The fixator in use.

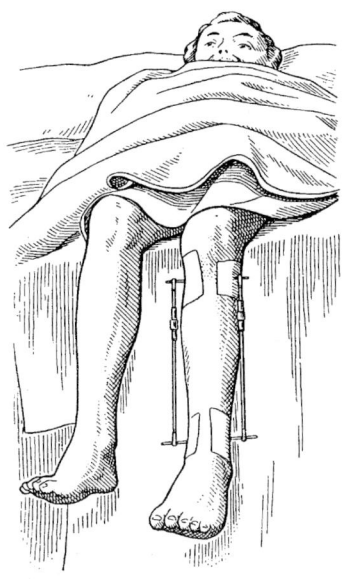

Lambret's extension apparatus from Steinmann's book, 1912.

Roger Anderson, 1934

"Our criteria of end results have been altered with the change in the medico-legal aspect of cases. Functional restoration is now insufficient. The present public also demands a practically normal reposition of the fracture fragments, as demonstrable on the final X-Ray films." He devised a *"veritable fracture robot."* This was a frame with pins above and below.

The Stader Reduction Splint, 1937

In 1931, Stader, working in the field of veterinary surgery, was impressed with the inadequate methods then in vogue for treating fractures of the shafts of the long bones of dogs. Plaster encasements were not tolerated by the canines, who frequently destroyed them by constant biting and tearing.

He began to use half pins joined by a metal bar. By 1942, he had treated 1200 dogs.

"In 1937 the other two authors of this paper had the opportunity of seeing the application of the Stader splint in a police dog with a fractured shaft of femur. The ease of application, the prompt and accurate reduction obtained, and the simplicity of the instrument made a distinct impression.

"It was then decided to have a larger model of the splint manufactured for use in the human."

The first patient was treated at the Bellevue Hospital in New York City. The patient was walking on the fractured tibia without crutches after 3 weeks, and the fracture was united in 11 weeks.

The versatility and subtlety of transfixion apparatus were elevated to a high level by Ilizarov, who was sent as a general practitioner to the wastes of Siberia, where bad results from fractures

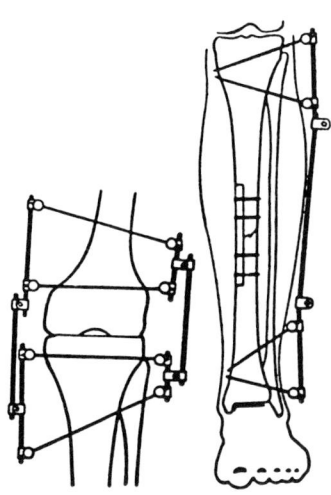

Roger Anderson's external fixator, 1942.

were commonplace. In 1950, with limited resources, necessity proved to be the mother of invention. A nearby factory produced rings, and he had a lot of wire. Slowly he started to operate but was officially ignored until a famous athlete came to him with an un-united fracture. On went a frame and within 2 years the patient was winning medals at the Olympics. Ilizarov was recognized, and a huge hospital was built for him in Kurgan. His methods of distraction osteogenesis swept the world.

The Treatment of Un-united Fractures

All kinds of abuse have been heaped on nonunions of fractures. They have been splinted, hammered, infected, magnetized, prayed over, and electrified, and all kinds of materials have been implanted. Today the chief standbys are bone grafting and rigid fixation.

Bone Grafting

Experimentalists trying to understand how bone works have studied bone grafting for 150 years. Bone has been taken from one site and put in another, and all kinds of interpretations have been put on the results—leading to more heat than light about the role of periosteum, osteocyte survival, bone induction, and the effect of load bearing. Ollier, Flourens, and Macewen kept up a lively controversy in the 19th century.

Some surgeons are gardeners by nature and used living grafts. Others are carpenters, who work with dead tissues to produce mechanical stability. Bone banks have been used by Ollier (1858), Macewen (1870), Lexer (1909), and Wilson (1947).

Title page of Béranger-Féraud's 1871 book.

Carpentered Cortical Grafts

Albee used his newly developed power saw to make elaborate joints and bridge defects with cortical grafts. Most of the bone died. He pioneered a tightly carpentered fit to allow the vessels to grow across.

Fred Albee, 1917

"Callus . . . may well be compared to the cabinet maker's glue, which will not hold unless the wood is exactly fitted and coapted. It will not bridge space. The surgeon must execute cabinet bone work in order to approximate 100 per cent of successful results, and this can be accomplished only by employing the inlay method with the author's bone mill." He developed a huge practice of bone graft surgery.

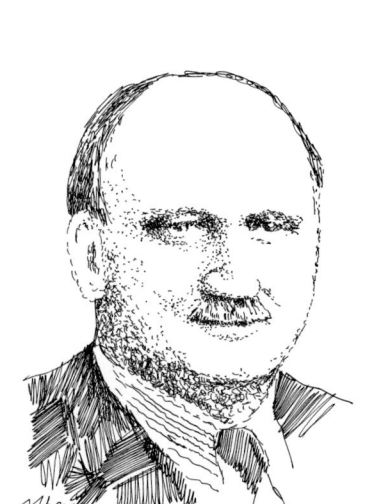

◆ Fred Albee

W. E. Gallie, 1931

"There are still a few who fancy that when a piece of bone is transplanted from one place in the body to another it will continue to live, as does a transplant of fascia or skin. This is an idea which must be eradicated if we are to reduce the percentage of failures. . . . The successful grafting of bone calls for a fair degree of craftsmanship."

Cancellous Bone Grafting

Rainsford Mowlem was a plastic surgeon in London and looked at bone grafting in the same light as split skin grafting. In 1944 he described 75 cases of success from creating iliac grafts measuring $1 \times 0.2 \times 0.5$ cm.

"On biological grounds it was thought that fragmentation of the graft might be expected to provide a much greater surface area through which the transplanted bone cells would become accessible, first to serum and secondly to the ingress of newly formed capillaries, and that the chances of their survival would thereby be enhanced. Once survival is ensured, fusion of the fragments can be expected to be rapid . . . It is unlikely to occur in cortical bone."

Corticoperiosteal Grafts

Petaling the cortex and raising the periosteum has Phemister's name erroneously attached. In fact Phemister described a full thickness grafting through an incision away from an infected fracture.

SPLINT GRAFTS IN THE TREATMENT OF DELAYED AND NONUNION OF FRACTURES

D. B. PHEMISTER, 1931

"In some cases of non-union of infected fractures, the infection persists along only one side of the bone. A whole thickness splint graft may be inserted along the opposite side soon after the infection has healed, thereby saving much time, since any other type of graft would necessitate entrance of the recently infected field and could not be done safely until several months later."

Henri Delangenière described free osteoperiosteal grafts in 1920. *"The grafts are usually obtained by removing from the tibia thin layers of bone with the periosteum."* He reported 237 cases with mostly good results—many were for craniofacial surgery.

THE FREE VASCULARIZED BONE GRAFT; A CLINICAL EXTENSION OF MICROVASCULAR TECHNIQUES

G. I. TAYLOR, G. D. H. MILLER, AND F. J. HAM, 1975

A living graft of bone relocated on a pedicle has been done since 1918, and then Alfred W. Farmer of Toronto transferred bone on a cross-leg pedicle graft. But it was in Melbourne, Australia, in 1974 that Ian Taylor and colleagues treated two patients facing amputation because of loss of more than 12 cm of tibia after an open fracture. They removed the fibula on a vascular pedicle and re-anastomosed it on the other leg. The anastomosis remained patent on their second case, who showed early callus—but there the story stops.

"*Union,*" they wrote, "*should theoretically be quicker, as the reconstructed tibia is comparable to a bone with a double fracture.*

"*The disadvantages are as follows. It is a long procedure, 12 hours and 10 hours respectively. There is some donor site morbidity. Patency of the anastomosis cannot be reassessed for possible revision in the immediate postoperative phase. A major vessel must be sacrificed in both limbs.*"

Since then surgical times are shorter and the indications increased.

History recounts that a limb transplant was conducted by Saints Cosmas and Damien. Part of the leg of a deceased person of color was attached to a white limb.

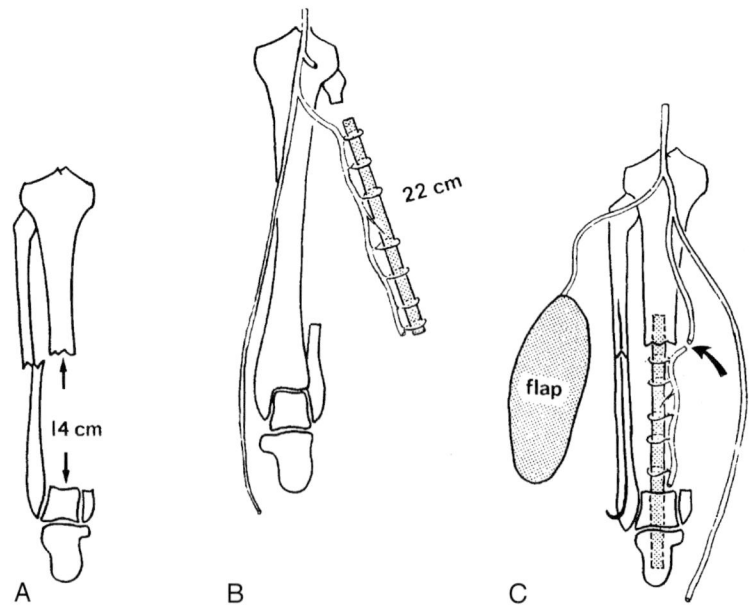

Free vascularized bone graft. From Taylor GI, Miller GDH, Ham FJ: The free vascularized bone graft. Plast Reconstr Surg 1975, 55, 533-544, Fig. 6. Used with permission.

Feelings of Patients

Joseph Amesbury, 1831

> "It is not easy for gentlemen, who have not observed the feelings of patients and their friends against a surgeon, under whose care a fracture badly united was placed, to form an estimate of their usual inveteracy. They sometimes think they can never injure his reputation sufficiently; and though the surgeon, in many instances, is not at all deserving of blame, they usually load him with epithets of ignorance, neglect, and presumption. If we examine a little into this feeling, we shall find that it is nothing more than what might naturally be expected. Patients know nothing scientifically of the nature of fractures, or of the means made use of in their cure, consequently they judge of the surgeon's ability according to the results of his cases. If the case of an individual terminate well, he conceives that the surgeon has done his duty: but if the limb be deformed, the patient will immediately say that the fracture was badly set, and he gets confirmed in this opinion by the observations of his friends, who seldom fail to find out cases to substantiate their belief."

◆ **Joseph Amesbury (1795–1864)**
Author of a more complete book on fractures in 1831.

TIMELINE OF PLASTER AND OTHER CASTING MATERIALS

From the beginning of time, sticks and mud and cloth have been used to stop fractures from moving about. We have knowledge only of recent events.

- 400 BC Hippocrates describes splints.
- 970 In Persia, Abu Mansur Muwaffak advises coating fractures with plaster.
- 1740 In Britain, as a child Cheselden has a fracture treated by a bonesetter with bandages dipped in egg white and starch. When Cheselden becomes a surgeon, he introduces the method for his patients. The bandages take a day to harden.
- 1799 A visiting diplomat reports that he saw a Turkish patient treated by holding the injured limb in a box that was then filled with plaster. He tried to interest European doctors in the method. The cast was big and heavy and prevented ambulation.
- 1814 Pieter Hendriks uses plaster bandages but without propaganda so that the idea does not catch on.
- 1824 Dominique Larrey, Napoleon's surgeon, uses egg white and lead powder.
- 1835 Louis Seutin: starch bandages
- 1852 Antonius Mathijsen introduces plaster bandages in a medical book and has a friend who popularizes it. Pirogoff in Russia introduces plaster bandages independently at the same time. Soon, large numbers of people are putting plaster into bandages. Until the 1950s, it was a job for medical students on emergency call. Then machines led to commercial manufacture. New materials were developed—first celluloid, which used to explode, and now fiberglass.

Box continued on following page

1903 Hoffa's belief that "the plaster bandage will remain the essence of orthopaedics for all time" seems to be going the way of all predictions.

Plaster did not enjoy universal popularity. Complete casts on fresh fractures can produce dreadful complications, and this led some influential leaders to ban casts. Thomas and Jones in Britain and Knight, founder of the first residency program in the United States, would have nothing to do with plaster, and Knight fired one member of his staff for promoting its use.

THE RISE AND FALL OF TRACTION FOR FRACTURES

Traction for fractures lasted for about 200 years. During its heyday it was the symbol of an orthopaedic ward, and it was one of the main reasons for the evolution of an orthopaedic nurse as somebody different. Now traction is dead—a victim of economics.

Two problems held back the development of traction: (1) connecting the limb to a weight without causing a skin slough, and (2) pulling in two directions at once.

circa 400 BC Hippocrates used traction to secure reduction and then used bandages and splints to hold a fracture of the femur.

circa 1350 Guy de Chauliac of Montpellier used egg white bandages, traction, weights, and pulleys.

1564 Paré: rope and windlass traction

circa 1700 Petit in France used an inclined plane to solve the problem of pulling in opposite directions. The limb was raised on a splint, and the patient's weight provided countertraction.

circa 1800 Robert Chessher used a double-incline plane. A splint like a letter A was placed under the knee. Lifting up the splint put traction on the femur, and tapes could put traction on the tibia.

1828 J. H. James: adhesive tape; also Joseph K. Swift of Philadelphia and Samuel D. Gross

1831 Nathan Smith: inclined plane

1831 John Hodgen of St. Louis develops a system of tapes fixed to the end of a splint, which is used during the Civil War.

1856 Henry Gassett Davis, United States: elastic material for traction

1860 Thomas splint, originally designed for the treatment of a tuberculous knee, is popularized during World War I for femoral shaft fractures.

1861 Gurdon Buck: straight leg traction

1872 Tom Bryant of London uses overhead traction for small children, whose fractures had been somewhat neglected

1900 Walter Hermann Heinecke of Erlangen used tongs in the os calcis to pull on a fracture of the tibia.

1903 The Balkan beam was developed during the Balkan War and provided great versatility in the placement of slings, pulleys, and weights. For a long time it was the symbol of an orthopaedic ward. Rows of these lined the long, 30-bed wards where patients spent 3 to 4

Susruta was the Hippocrates of Sanskrit. He lived in India, somewhere between 600 BC and 600 AD. The designs of his instruments incorporated the symbols of gods. His clinical descriptions are as baffling to me as mine would be to him.

months waiting for their fracture to unite. On a recent visit to the Caribbean, the wards were seen still full of Balkan beams—each had a bird or two perched on it, adding a new hazard for the patient below.

1903 Alessandro Codivilla of Bologna uses a pin in the os calcis for traction and stumbles on the notion of leg lengthening.

1907 Fritz Steinmann of Bern introduces a thick pin inserted into the supracondylar region.

1912 Joseph Ransohoff uses ice tongs for the femur; they were popular during World War I because they were easy to make and simple to apply.

1914 Rudolf Klapp of Berlin used a thin wire—inserted through a hollow tube—for os calcis traction.

1920 Erich Herzberg invented the traction bow to tension the wire so that it did not bend.

1921 Hamilton Russell of Australia solves the problem of keeping the hip and knee flexed with use of split traction.

1927 Fritz Kirschner used a wire thick enough to be drilled using a guide, but thin enough to need tensioning. Kirschner wires are never used for traction today but have become invaluable for open and percutaneous fixation.

1950 Perkins traction: just a Steinmann pin and a split bed allowed immediate exercising, speeding union and avoiding stiffness.

1951 Nangle's Jangles: this was a whole book on traction—it included sections on how to make a plaster bed. It was the high point of traction techniques.

1996 Due to the economic changes it is hard to find a young surgeon who has seen traction used. All interest in traction is lost.

1998 Gustilo: *Traction is a thing of the past.*

◆ **Jean Louis Petit (1674–1750)**
Parisian surgeon who invented splints, named the tourniquet, and wrote a treatise on diseases of bone in 1723.

THE TIMELINE OF WIRES, SCREWS, AND PLATES

1775 Icart reports in Journal Français de Chirurgie that two Toulouse surgeons, Lapoyde and Sicre, used a brass wire for a fracture—no other reference.

1861 Samuel Cooper in San Francisco successfully treats a fresh fracture of the patella with wire, using alcohol for asepsis.

1862 Gurlt described principles of screws, nails, and wires.

Box continued on following page

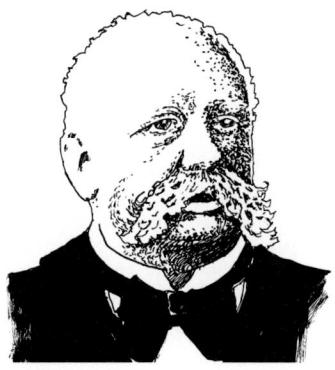

◆ **Ernst Julius Gurlt (1825–1899)**
Professor of surgery at Berlin. He published a 3-volume work on the history of surgery and, in 1860, one of the classic texts on fractures.

462 *Chapter 20* ◆ Fracture Treatment

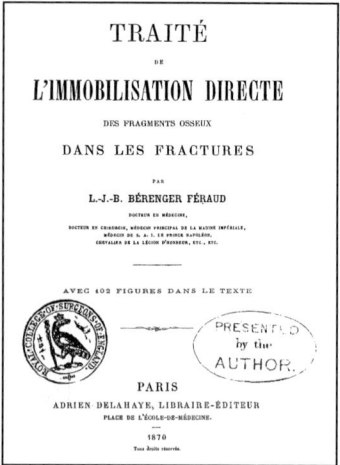

Title page of Béranger-Féraud's 1870 book

◆ **Themistocles Gluck (1853–1942)**

He studied in Leipzig, became professor of surgery in Bucharest and later in Berlin. He fixed fractures with nickel-plated plates, used synthetic tendons, made joint replacements of ivory, used intramedullary pegs. He was a man before his time.

The evolution of plates. From Bagby GW: Compression bone plating. J Bone Jt Surg Am 1977, 59A. 625, Figs. 1-5. Used with permission.

1864 L. J. B. Berenger-Feraud, French naval surgeon, writes synopsis on Immobilisation Directe which he expands into a book in 1870. It is mostly a review of known methods of treating ununited fractures.
1865 Lister begins treating compound fractures operatively.
1877 Lister treats a closed fracture of the patella by wiring, having established the principles of aseptic surgery. In 1883 he published a series, and a few years later wiring became the treatment of choice. With minor improvements, it still is!
1885 Themistocles Gluck: nickel-plated plates
1886 Hansmann plate with screws. The screws had the screwdriver welded to them so that the handle protruded through the skin. The screw could be removed without reopening the wound. The plate had a handle at right angles so that it protruded through the skin. When the screws were removed, the plate could be taken out too! No need for another anesthetic.

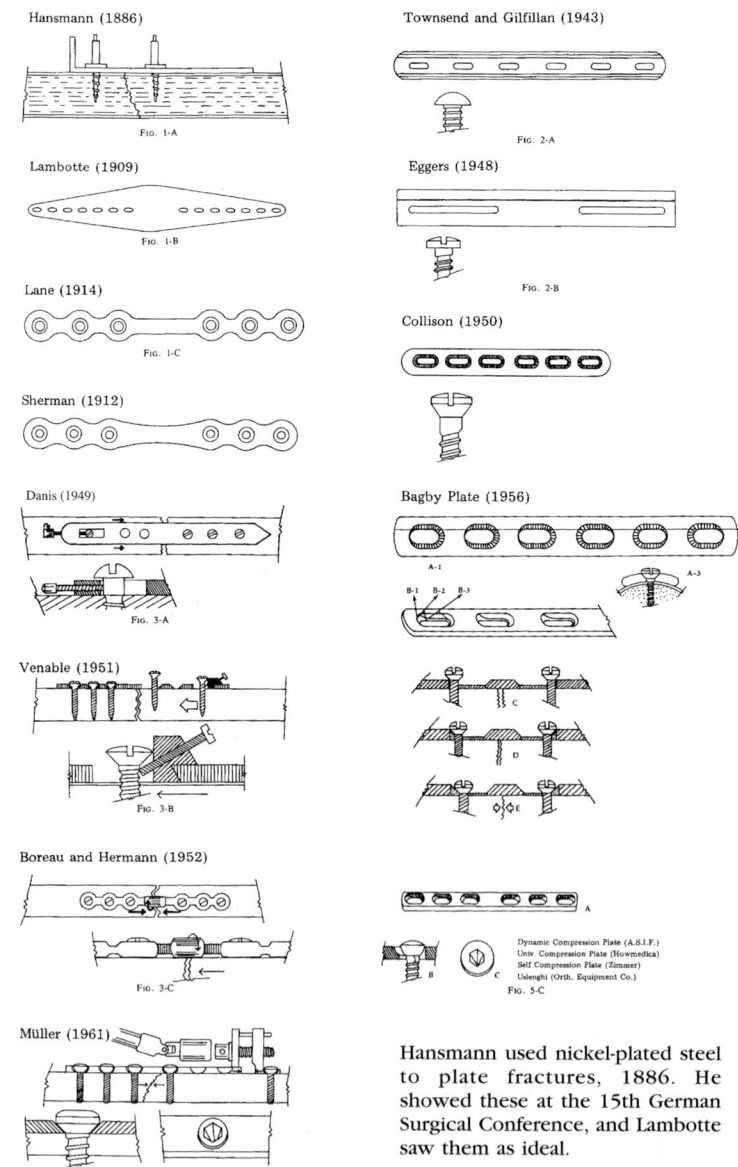

Hansmann used nickel-plated steel to plate fractures, 1886. He showed these at the 15th German Surgical Conference, and Lambotte saw them as ideal.

1893 Nicholas Senn gives the Presidential Address at the American Surgical Society on the direct fixation of compound and ununited fractures. He used absorbable bone, intramedullary tubes, and extraperiosteal tubes into which the bone was plugged.

1893 Bircher: ivory H clamp for metaphyseal fractures

1900 Scudder writes a paper, *The open or operative treatment of fresh fractures: is it ever justified?* He reviews 153 lower limb fractures treated at Massachussetts General Hospital and concludes that nonoperative treatment resulted in unsatisfactory results in 81% of hip fractures, 69% of adult femur fractures, and 60% of closed tibial fractures. This was a strong argument for more operative treatment.

1901 Alberto Jacoel: staples

1905 W. Arbuthnot Lane: book on *The Operative Treatment of Fractures*. He began operating on fractures in 1892, wrote about screw fixation in 1894, and invents his plate in 1907. A second edition of the book was published in 1914.

1907 Albin Lambotte writes a book on his experiences operating on fresh fractures—coining the word osteosynthesis. He began this in 1890 when he was appointed general surgeon at Stuyvenberg, Belgium. He made his own plates as well as 182 violins.

1910 The British Medical Association strikes a committee to look into fracture care. In 1912, it reports that operative cases show a higher percentage of good results than nonoperative cases.

1912 The American Surgical Association strikes a committee to prepare a statement on the relative value of operative and nonoperative treatment and on the value of radiography to determine the choice of treatment. The report did not appear for nine years!

Box continued on following page

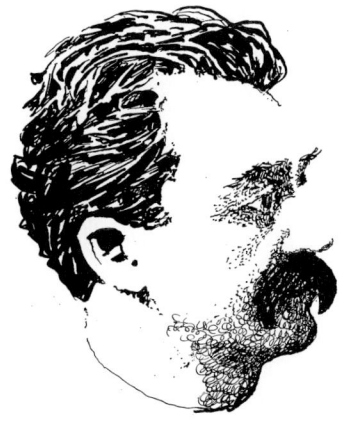

◆ **Nicholas Senn (1844–1908)**

As an infant, he was brought from Switzerland to Wisconsin; he studied in Chicago, and became professor at Rush Medical College. He served in the Spanish-American War and was president of the American Medical Association. He was a great experimenter but lacked the courage to put his discoveries into practice because they offended customary wisdom.

Title page of Lambotte's book.

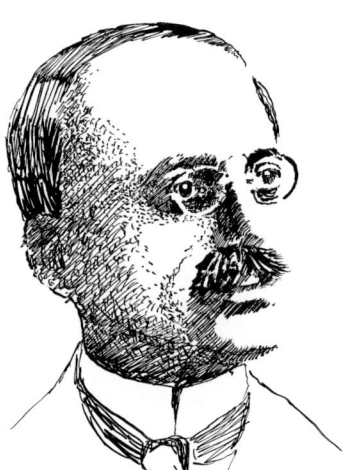

◆ **Charles Locke Scudder (1860–1949)**

After studying at Harvard and Yale, he went to work at the Massachusetts General Hospital and stayed for 56 years. He was a general surgeon who wrote a fracture text in 1900 and kept producing new editions for 38 years.

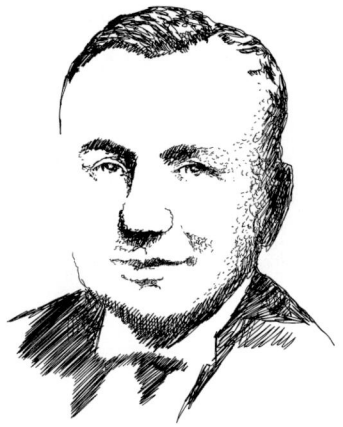

◆ **William O'Neill Sherman (1880–1979)**

He popularized plates in the United States. He was surgeon to a Pittsburgh steel company and was able to use better alloys. He introduced the self-tapping screws which seemed like a good idea at the time, but using a tap to cut the thread gives a better hold. The Sherman plate of 1912 was the gold standard for 50 years.

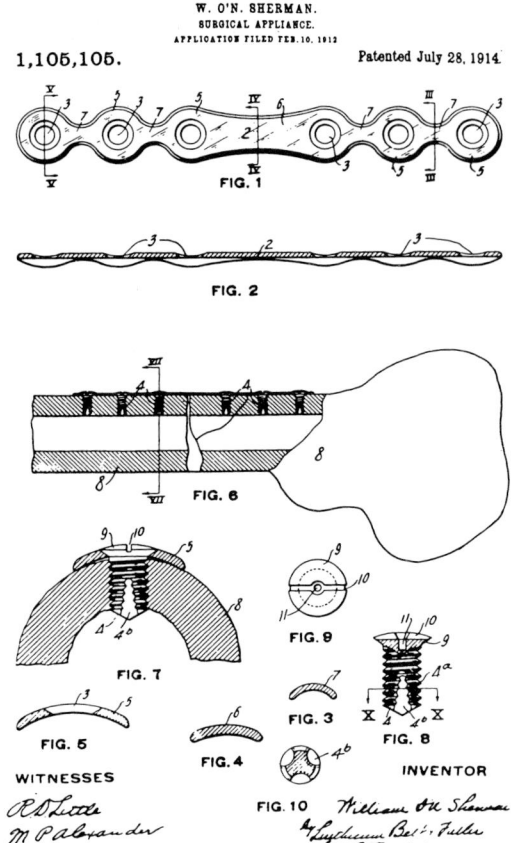

Sherman's plate and self-tapping screw, 1912.

1912 William O'N. Sherman: plates and self-tapping screws. He was surgeon to a steel company in Pittsburgh and sought better alloys and better-engineered designs. These plates did not break and corrode like Lane's plates and remained the standard for 50 years until the AO plates were introduced.

1916 Fredrick W. Parham and E. Denegre Martin: cerclage band. There had been many attempts with wire and muffs but the Parham band represented the apogee. Unfortunately, it does not provide enough fixation and caused bone ischemia.

1916 Ernest W. Hey Groves, a surgeon in Bristol, publishes *On Modern Methods of Treating Fractures*, based on much experimental work. He illustrates plates, intramedullary rods, and external fixators.

1924 Zierold studies metal corrosion in dogs.

1926 Stainless steel was introduced.

1936 G. Mengaux and D. Odiette review the work on cytotoxicity of metal on fracture healing.

1947 Venable and Stuck review electrolytic reactions of implanted metal.

THE COMPRESSION IDEA

1914 Henry S. MacLean uses a plate with oval holes to permit approximation after bone absorption at the fracture site.

1932 Key uses "positive pressure" to secure arthrodesis of the knee, and the same principle is used by Charnley in 1948.

1933 Tension band principle is proposed by Fredrick Pauwels.

1943 E. Townsend and C. Gilfillian produce a plate with oval holes to permit manual compression.

1947 Danis' book, *Theory and Practice of Osteosynthesis*. Paris: Masson.

1949 George W. N. Eggers reports experiments on compressing osteotomies in a rat skull. These experiments are the basis for his slotted plate—muscles compress the fracture site and the slightly loose screws permit the fracture to close.

1949 Danis' coapteurs plates: the end hole has a set screw to secure compression.

1950 In his book, Collison publishes a plate with oval holes.

1950 AO group formed—Müller, Algower, Willenegger

1951 Charles S. Venable uses an inboard compressor on a plate.

1952 Zachary B. Freidenberg and George French show that 12 to 18 pounds is the optimal interfragmentary pressure and that 30 pounds causes bone necrosis in an animal fracture model.

1952 "Sir Reginald Watson Jones, with all the eloquence of which he is a master, devotes a chapter to an ardent denounciation of the use of mechanical compression in osseous union." (Charnley in *Compression Arthrodesis*, page 71)

1953 John Charnley publishes a book, *Compression Arthrodesis*, that explores the whole idea of compression.

1956 George W. Bagby of the Mayo Clinic modifies the Collison plate by adding a slot so that it is self-compressing—virtually a dynamic compression plate.

1961 Maurice Mueller describes outboard compressor.

1963 *AO Manual* published

1964 B. G. Weber: tension band used for cancellous fractures

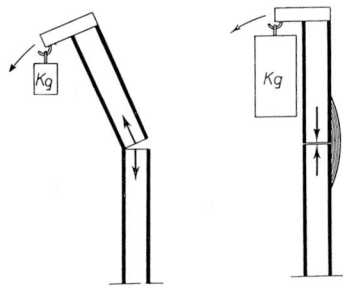

Pauwels' principle of the tension band. From Pauwels F: Der Schenkelhalsbruch: ein mechanisches problem. Stuttgart: Ferdinand Enke, 1935.

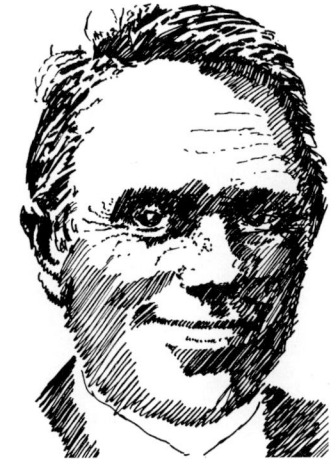

◆ **Maurice Müller**
The mainspring of the AO group.

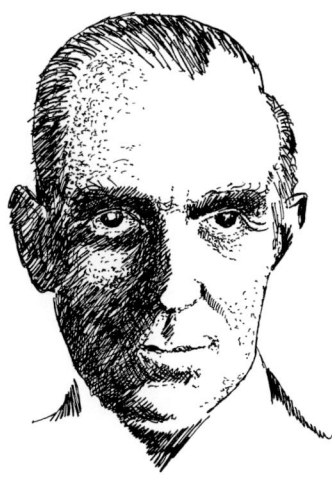

◆ **Sir Reginald Watson Jones (1902–1972)**

Though no relation of Robert Jones, he was both his student and voice after Robert Jones had passed away. He started to lecture on fractures and turned his notes into a fracture text that was published, by good fortune, at the beginning of World War II. It served as the guiding hand for all the military surgeons. It went through several editions, continuing a nonoperative approach, until it lost out to the *AO Manual*. Reggie was a charming man with tremendous style.

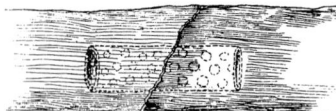

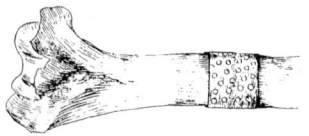

Nicholas Senn used cuffs and intramedullary plugs to hold fractures.

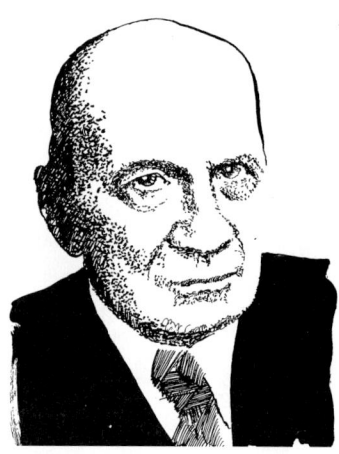

◆ **Georg Schone**
Used intramedullary nail for ulna, 1913.

INTRAMEDULLARY NAILS

Initially short pegs were used; long thin pins followed. Next were reamed heavy nails, which came to be locked.

1500 Aztecs used sticks in the bony canal!
1890 Themistocles Gluck: intramedullary ivory rod
1893 Senn: short pegs
1893 Bircher: short pegs
1913 Georg Schone: closed pinning under x-ray control—4 mm silver rods for forearm fractures
1916 Hey Groves: short pegs and later long rods for femoral shaft fractures. Poor metal prevented him from being as successful as Kuntscher.
1925 Lambotte: pins for metacarpal fractures
1933 Muller-Meernach: open nailing
1936 Leslie and Lowry Rush introduce a system of intramedullary pins with a sled end and a prebent dynamic shape. Multiple rods were used for metaphyseal fractures.
1940 Lambrinudi: intramedullary Kirschner wires for forearm fractures
1940 Kuntscher and Maatz start intramedullary nailing, and it remains unknown outside the German Army until the war is over.
1942 Maatz starts reaming.
1945 The Western world learns of K nails, and they become popular and imitated.
1950 Dana Street: nail for the tibia
1952 Otto Lottes: nail for tibia
1955 Rush book on techniques using thin nails and three-point fixation principle.
1961 Hackethal: multiple thin pins
1970 Enders: retrograde nails for trochanteric fractures
1980 Locked nails

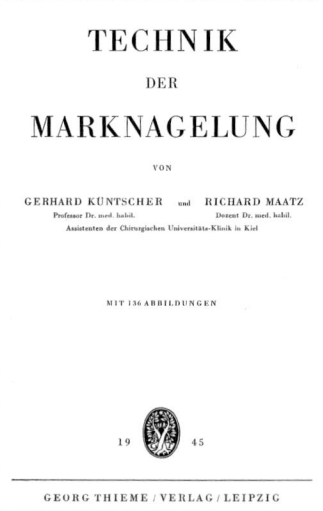

Title page of book by Küntscher and Maatz.

EXTERNAL FIXATORS

These really came into use only after antibiotics solved the problem of pin track infection.

- 300 BC Hippocrates uses rings at knee and ankle and sticks to hold the alignment
- 1536 Paracelsus uses ring and rod system.
- 1833 Malgaigne: hooks for fractured patella and olecranon
- 1850 Philippe Rigaud uses external fixation for patella. Two screws are tied together.
- 1840 Malgaigne: spike and strap for fracture of the tibia
- 1886 Langenbeck uses screws above and below the fracture united by a rod.
- 1897 Clayton Parkhill of Denver inserts screws into the bone, bolted through holes in a plate.
- 1907 Albin Lambotte of Belgium uses a monolateral system that looks like the AO fixator.
- 1912 Lilienthal inserted gimlets and joined them with plaster bandage.
- 1913 Hey Groves carried out experiments with cats and showed that external fixators are good for comminuted fractures and open fractures. However well suited they were for military surgery, they were too fiddly for front line surgeons to use.
- 1919 Freeman writes a series of papers, 1909 to 1919.
- 1927 Abbott modifies external fixators for leg lengthening.
- 1927 Conn introduces stainless steel pins, which reduce some of the pin problems.
- 1934 Henri Judet uses pins in both cortices.
- 1937 Otto Stader, a veterinarian, produces a splint with universal joints for animals and is persuaded to allow its use for people.
- 1938 Raoul Hoffmann of Switzerland produces a frame that allows the fracture to be mechanically manipulated and reduced.
- 1942 Roger Anderson advocates castless ambulatory treatment of fractures, using a versatile linkage system. It had the distinction of being banned in World War II as being too elaborate.
- 1950 A survey by the Committee on Fractures and Traumatic Surgery of the American Academy of Orthopaedic Surgery concludes that the complications of external fixation frequently exceed any advantages. Any surgeon contemplating using an external fixator should have special training from a colleague who has applied at least 200.
- 1950 Ilizarov, working in Siberia, develops the ring system for fractures and deformities. It becomes known in the West only in the late 1970s.
- 1980 Giovanni de Bastiani in Verona produces the Orthofix.

TIMELINE OF BONE REPAIR

1739 Duhamel in France feeds madder to pigs and studies bone repair after fracture. Bone formed under the periosteum. Albrecht von Haller, a Swiss (1708-1777), repeats the experiments and concludes that the periosteum has no role in bone

Box continued on following page

formation. It is an investing membrane, and the arteries form bone. This argument continued for nearly 200 years, and it is hard to know why different results were reached. Perhaps infection and ischemia confused observers.

1842 Flourens' book on experiments relating to the the development of bone—supporting the role of periosteum in bone formation

1868 The era of the animal experimenters contiues with the publication of Ollier's book on bone regeneration and the supporting periosteal osteogenesis.

1878 Macewen of Glasgow begins years of experiments, denying periosteal osteogenesis and culminating in replacing a whole child's humerus destroyed by osteomyelitis in 1878. He publishes a book, *The Growth of Bone*, in 1912, which reviews 34 years of work.

1908 Auxhausen shows that grafted bone cells remain alive.

1919 Lexer reviews his and others' results.

♦ **Celsus (25 BC–50 AD)**

A Roman writer of encyclopedias. He was not a doctor but a collector of information. All his work was lost until his volume on medicine was found in 1443. It was one of the first printed books. Best known for the signs of Celsus: rubor, tumor, calor, and dolor.

NONUNION AND BONE DEFECTS

30 Celsus: stretch the limb and let the ends rub together so that "the whole thing is like a fresh fracture."

1682 Job von Meekren in Holland treats a skull defect with a piece of dog bone. The Church makes him remove it.

1770 Charles White of Manchester exposes the fracture, scrapes the periosteum, and applies antimony with success.

1783 White has several successes with infected un-united fractures of the humerus.

1802 Philip Syng Physick uses a nonabsorbable suture in the fracture nonunion to excite inflammation.

1805 Alexis Boyer, Napoleon's surgeon, describes splints, rubbing, and resection.

1812 Birch at St. Thomas' Hospital, London, uses electricity.

1818 Joseph White in New York uses multiple drilling of the callus with success.

1826 John Rhea Barton exposes the bone and applies caustics.

1827 J. Kearney Rodgers of New York exposes bone and holds the ends together with silver wire.

1841 Edward Hartshorne of Philadelphia writes a thesis on pseudarthrosis and is one of the first to use the term.

1855 Henry H. Smith of Philadelphia uses a brace and encourages function.

187? H. O. Thomas put a venous tourniquet around the limb to produce chronic venous congestion and made a religion of giving the patient a little hammer to hit the nonunion—*"percussion, damming, and dependency."*

1875 Volkmann: ivory peg as an irritant and as fixation

1889 Nicholas Senn: decalcified bone as graft

1911 Hibbs uses cancellous grafts for spinal fusion. Several years passed before it was realized that cancellous grafts brought in living cells.

1911 Albee used the carpenter's approach. He cut dovetails and other kinds of fancy joints, using the patient's cortical bone and a power saw. In 8 years he reported 3000 cases. He initiated the era of using thick grafts that functioned as fixation.
1920 Delangenière: osteoperiosteal grafts. A sliver of bone the thickness of a 10 cent piece, together with the overlying periosteum, is taken and used to replace bone defects.
1931 Gallie grafts all kinds of tissue.
1932 Matti: scaphoid grafting
1934 Ghormley uses local cancellous grafts for lumbosacral fusion
1934 Phemister: cancellous grafts
1934 Svante Orell: processed bone—os purum and os novum
1942 Inclan of Havana starts world's first bone bank
1944 Plastic surgeon Rainsford Mowlem popularizes cancellous bone grafting for war injuries.
195? Ilizarov uses the stress tension principle to transport bone into a defect, but the technique remains unknown in the West for 20 years.
1957 Maatz: animal bone is processed to make it less antigenic and is sold as Kiel bone.
195? Urist begins the search for the chemical messenger for bone formation.
196? The Naval Bone Bank at Bethesda sets the standard, and many banks follow.
1963 The AO group divide nonunion into hypertrophic, requiring compression fixation, and atrophic, requiring grafting.
1977 Taylor: microvascular transfer of living fibula
1978 Bassett: electricity to stimulate bone formation remains a contentious issue.

Biographies

Galen (AD 130-200). Galen was born in Turkey, which was then under Roman control, and studied in various parts of the Middle East before becoming Physician to the Gladiators in Pergamon, Turkey. He moved to Rome, where he became a leading doctor and retired at the age of about 60 to write—and these writings stamped his ideas on the world. He believed in the four humors and had carried out just enough dissection and physiologic study for succeeding generations to hold his writings as sacred as gospel—Galen was to be believed and not questioned. Through no fault of his, his ideas were a barricade against new information for more than 1000 years.

Guy de Chauliac (1300-1368). He studied in Paris, Montpellier, and Prague and collected a big library. Starting as an itinerant surgeon, he settled in Avignon to work for the Popes. He wrote *The Large Book of Surgery* in 1363, in which fracture treatment was described. He was an inventor of traction with weights and pulleys for fractures of the shaft of the femur. At our hospital we have only just given this up—it took over 600 years. Some physicians are still using it.

Guido Guidi (1500-1569). Florentine surgeon who took the long-lost works of Hippocrates to Paris and produced an edition in Latin in 1544 with some of the best early illustrations of fracture reduction. It is not clear whether he wrote a book of his own.

Richard Wiseman (1622-1676). A British surgeon who spent the period of the English civil war in exile in Europe as an Army surgeon. When the King returned, Wiseman became his physician. His book, *Severall Chirurgical Treatises*, of 1676 contained descriptions of tuberculous joints, fractures, and gunshot wounds.

Lorenz Heister (1683-1758). Nuremberg surgeon. His book on fractures was written in German in 1719 but was translated into most languages, and it has excellent illustrations.

John Hunter (1728-1793). An early surgeon scientist. He was born near Glasgow and after doing badly at school went to London to help his brother teach anatomy. He studied surgery and joined the Army, working in Portugal. This formed the basis of his book *A Treatise on the Blood, Inflammation and Gunshot Wounds* in 1794. He subsequently worked at St. George's Hospital. The Hyde Park site is now a hotel. His claim to fame was his use of observation and scientific reasoning, his experiments on transplantation and bone growth, and his museum at the Royal College of Surgeons, London, which illustrated his discoveries. He died at a stormy staff meeting in the hospital board room. A warning to all.

Pierre-Joseph Desault (1744-1795). Chief surgeon at Hôtel Dieu in Paris. He founded the first surgical journal, Journal de Chirurgie, and invented debridement of fractures. He had a huge surgical practice and pioneered bedside teaching. He operated in an amphitheater seating 300. During the French Revolution he was carted to prison by citizen students for his teaching.

Sir Astley Cooper (1768-1845). London surgeon. He spent time studying in Paris during the Revolution. Author of a treatise on dislocations and fractures in 1822. This is a fine atlas and includes some experimental studies. Used catgut before Lister. Avoided amputation for open fractures by immobilizing the limb.

Philip Syng Physick (1768-1837). Born in the United States, he studied with Hunter in London and was offered a job. He returned to America to become the first professor of surgery at Philadelphia. He operated on un-united fractures by putting a suture in the fracture site. He invented a splint for fracture of the shaft of the femur. His lectures were published as the first surgical text for students by his nephew, John Syng Dorsey, in 1813. The father of American Surgery.

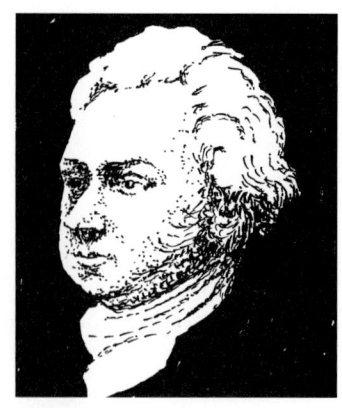

◆ Sir Astley Cooper

William Gibson (1788-1868). Reflections on surgery, published in 1824, had a lot to say about fractures. Early United States surgeon.

Joseph Wattmann (1789-1866). Professor of surgery in Vienna. He invented teaching mannikins for practicing reduction of fractures, which are described in a book published in 1823.

Adolph Leopold Richter (1798-1876). Prussian Army surgeon who published an illustrated book on fracture splints and apparatus in 1828.

Samuel D. Gross (1805-1884). Early Philadelphia surgeon. Wrote the first American orthopaedic textbook at the age of 25.

John Hilton (1805-1878). Surgeon at Guy's Hospital, London. He is best known for writing *On the Influence of Mechanical and Physiological Rest in the Treatment of Accidents and Surgical Disease and the Diagnostic Value of Pain*—abbreviated to *On Rest and Pain* in a book title of 1877. He explained why hip pain is referred to the knee. He was an advocate of rest.

Joseph François Malgaigne (1806-1865). He was the son of a poor French country doctor and worked as a secretary to help pay for education. He became a general surgeon and medical writer. In 1847 appeared a text on fractures and dislocations in a two-volume atlas, with statistical analysis of a huge number of fractures. He edited the works of Paré and wrote about the history of fractures. He founded a surgical journal. Malgaigne criticized Guérin's work and was sued for libel. Malgaigne established the freedom of scientific criticism in court. He invented hooks to approximate a fracture of the patella and a point for the tibia. He described ischemic contracture before Volkmann, the nature of gas in gas gangrene, and vertical fracture of the pelvis.

Frank Hastings Hamilton (1813-1886). United States surgeon. Born in Vermont, student at New York and Pennsylvania, he became professor at Buffalo. He joined the Union Army and worked at Bellevue Hospital in New York City. He collected information on the results of treatment to use in medicolegal cases. In 1855 he published statistics on deformities after fractures and published the first comprehensive fracture book in English in 1860.

Lewis Atterbury Simpson (1844-1917). He was born in New Jersey and worked as a stockbroker. His wife was diabetic and he started to study medicine, graduating from Bellevue in 1875. He wrote a treatise on fractures in 1883.

Fred Cotton (1869-1938) started helping Scudder but then wrote his own book with his own drawings in 1910. He is remembered for the Cotton-Loder position of extreme flexion for a Colles' fracture. Some thought this was a term derived from the textile industry.

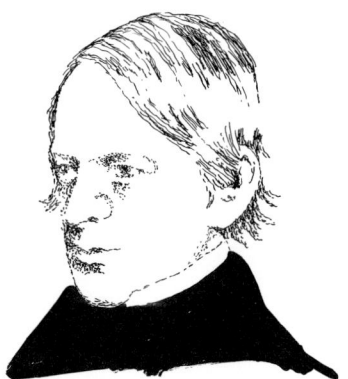
◆ Joseph Wattman

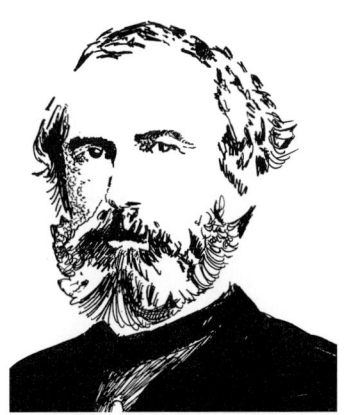
◆ Frank Hastings Hamilton

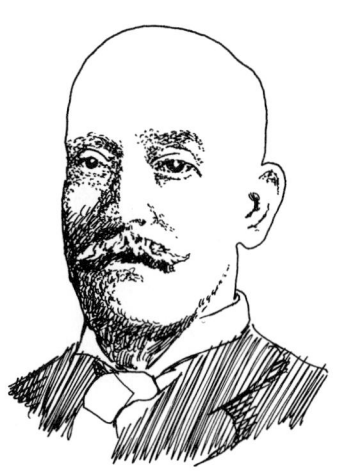
◆ Lewis Atterbury Simpson

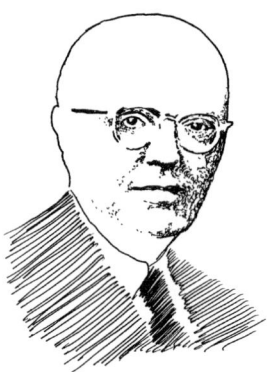

◆ H. Winnett Orr

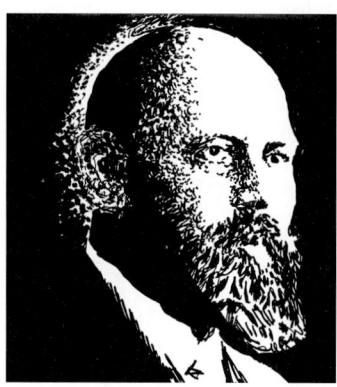

◆ Lorenz Bohler

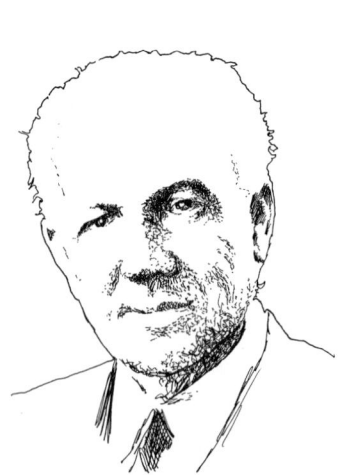

◆ Joseph Trueta

H. Winnett Orr (1877–1956). He graduated from the University of Nebraska and, after a time in general practice, trained in orthopaedics. He went to Europe in World War I and started to treat open fractures by debridement followed by immobilization and infrequent dressings in the Thomas tradition.

Lorenz Bohler (1885–1973). While he was a student at Vienna, trauma wards were opened, which impressed him. During a short visit to the Mayo Clinic in 1914 he saw the value of organization and set up an army hospital for fractures during World War I, which showed superior results. He, like Robert Jones, saw the similarity between military and industrial injuries. In 1925, Austrian insurance companies founded an Accident Hospital in Vienna, and Bohler led this for 30 years. He influenced everyone in his generation and wrote the book on fractures, which was published in 1929 and went through many editions and translations. Hey Groves translated it into English. Dr. Bohler "demonstrated that the proper treatment of fractures is not only a scientific problem or a philanthropic duty, but also a business proposition. In other words, it pays to treat fractures well." The hospital was run on authoritarian lines. He developed the Bohler-Braun splint for treatment of lower limb fractures. He used skintight casts. His organizing ability was his strength. He tried to make it respectable to be a fracture surgeon, but didn't quite succeed in his lifetime.

Alberto Inclan (1888–1965). Professor at Havana, who started the first bone bank.

Joseph Trueta (1897–1977). He was born in Barcelona and became chief surgeon and professor there when the Spanish Civil War broke out and he found himself on the losing side. He cared for many injured soldiers and developed a closed plaster treatment of open fractures. He escaped to Britain and climbed to the top again because of his clinical and research skills. He became professor at Oxford, drawing students from around the world. Peace returned to Catalonia in time for him to retire there.

◆
◆
◆ PART THREE

The Story of Sports Medicine

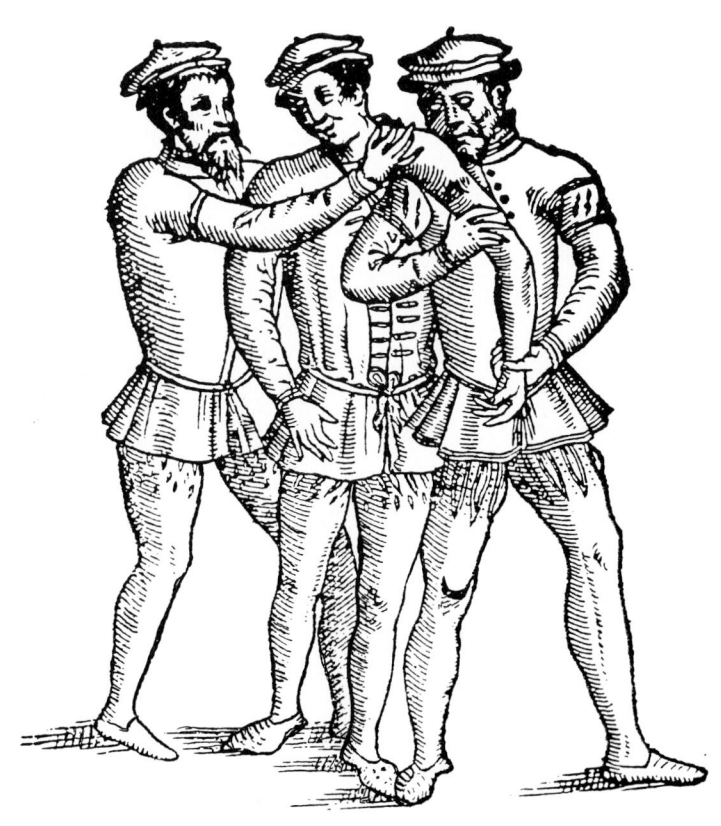

◆ Chapter Twenty-one

Sports and Medicine

We are growing more skilled in the arts of leisure. We expect our doctors to become more skilled in fixing the consequences of leisure injuries.

There was once a time when injuries were either ignored or treated by amputation; patients gave thanks for surviving. Today, the expectation is for a quick return to the previous level of activity. In particular, this is true for injured highly paid professional athletes who are not earning their keep until they play again. Hence the need and financial support for sports medicine doctors. The need is not just from professional players—the overweight arthritic weekend Olympian playing out a fantasy wants to share the same "jock doc" as a baseball great.

In former times the human need for muscular activity was fulfilled by work or the use of survival skills. Today we have to find it in sports. Injury used to be work related or transportation related, but now leisure injury or sports injury is important.

Sports medicine is divided into three parts:

1. *Sports medicine and physiology*—concerned with physical fitness and with exercise physiology. The ancient Greeks started the idea of the sound mind in a fit body. Now it is very scientific.
2. *Sports surgery*—about injuries and their prevention. Galen was surgeon to the gladiators.
3. *Sports rehabilitation*—the benefits of sports as a means to recovery from illness. Ludwig Guttman of Stoke Mandeville Hospital, England, started the Para-Olympics for paraplegics, and the Special Olympics movement now includes those with all kinds of disabilities.

Sports Style

The idea of sports has changed over the years, and today it includes everything from a boy kicking a ball around unobserved to a professional player with the eyes of the world on him.

Each era has had characteristic features.

Greek. This style included running, jumping, and wrestling, without team sports. War was stopped to allow organized sports and to allow athletes to cross enemy lines to reach the site of the Olympics. The men were naked, and women were not allowed to participate or watch.

Roman. Sports had become a spectator occupation, with battles to the death between gladiators, men, and wild animals, and then there were the chariot races. The Victor Ludorum (winner of the games) was a survivor.

As surgeon to the gladiators, Galen could be considered the first sports medicine doctor. He may have taken the job just because human dissection was prohibited, and these bloodthirsty games gave him the opportunity to examine the interior of the human body.

Medieval. Peasants worked and prayed and fought. The nobles had leisure for falconry, the chase, and jousting. These would have been lean times for a sports doctor.

Victorian. Sports were promoted to encourage the team spirit—putting others ahead of self. Individual sports were not a feature of this time. Team sports were a way of maximizing the mental, emotional, and physical effort that a person could put into a task without much risk. If a person would do this for his team, he would do it for his community and country. "The Battle of Waterloo was won on the playing fields of Eton," so the saying goes. From this time nationalism affects sports.

20th Century Communism. Sports broke down traditional society. Power used to come from land ownership and social class. With the new order, sports heroes took precedence over everyone except the politicians. The role of sports doctors was often clandestine—using performance-enhancing methods, such as steroids or blood transfusion.

Professional Sports. Sports has returned to its Roman roots as spectator activity. Team owners are anxious to keep the players fit, because they want a return on their investment. Hence the emergence of elite patients who will support a lucrative practice.

Fitness Movement. There was a time when work meant hard physical effort, but now it generally means sedentary occupations. We all tend to get stiff and do not feel the glow of a recently exercised muscle, and then as the years pass we get fat. The response has been leisure exercise. Streets are filled with joggers. The windows of health clubs frame silhouettes of men and women wrestling with machines. Now "fitness injuries" occur in large numbers. Every town has a sports medicine clinic where middle-aged citizens can compare their injuries with those of the stars. Their income and their fame may not be the same, but they are brothers in symptoms. Type A personalities get overuse problems for which they want relief. Now that most fitness enthusiasts have health insurance, the provision of care for them is attractive.

Para-Olympic (Special Olympic) Movement. Wheelchair sports have done wonders for paraplegics. It makes them fit and is a boost to morale. And it was all started by a man who wouldn't run for a bus—Ludwig Guttman.

TIMELINE OF SPORTS MEDICINE BEFORE 1900

- 160 Galen, surgeon to the gladiators in Turkey. *"I regard the mode of living of athletes as a regime far more favorable to illness than to health."*
- 1400 Vittorino da Feltre (1378-1446) founds a school for children that has sports and physical education.
- 1553 Christobal Mendez of Spain writes the first printed book on exercise, *The Book of Bodily Exercise*, reprinted in English in 1960.
- 1569 *Six Books on the Art of Gymnastics* by Geronimo Mercuriale (1530-1606). This professor of medicine at Padua publishes a book on physical education. It has lovely woodcuts depicting various sports. The emphasis is on health rather than injury.
- 1582 Laurent Joubert (1529-1583), professor of medicine at Montpellier, introduces lectures on therapeutic gymnastics into the medical course.
- 1680 Borelli, *On the Movement of Animals*, a book on biomechanics
- 1813 Pehr Henrik Ling founds the Royal Central Institute of Gymnastics in Sweden for remedial gymnastics.
- 1879 Zander exercise machines.
- 1888 Fernand Lagrange, *Physiology of Bodily Exercise*, New York. An early work on exercise physiology; many follow.

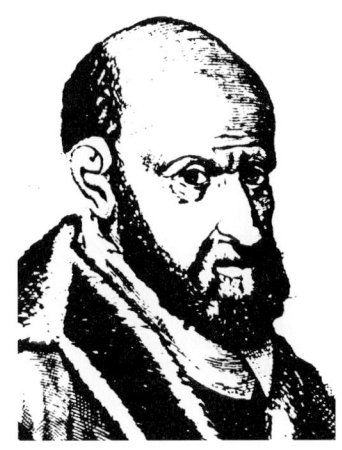

◆ Galen

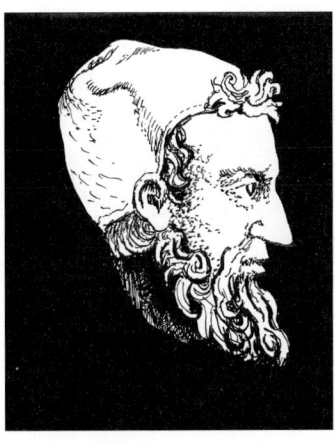

◆ **Geronimo Mercuriale (1530–1606)**

Professor of medicine at Padua, Bologna, and Pisa. He translated Hippocrates, wrote texts on dermatology, pediatrics, the ear, and the gymnastic arts (1569). He promoted the Greek ideal of health through exercise, and his book remained in print for more than 100 years.

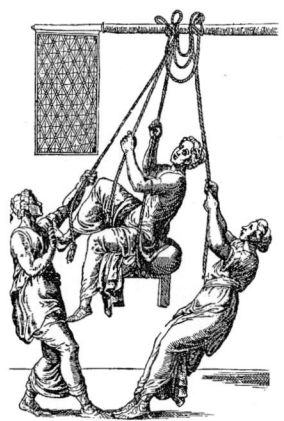

◆ **Geronimo Mercuriale, 1569.**
Six books on the art of gymnastics. Exercise for men and women.

TIMELINE OF SPORTS MEDICINE AFTER 1900

1904 Arthur Mallwitz uses the term sports physician.
1909 Robert Tait McKenzie (professor of physical education and physical therapy at the University of Pennsylvania) writes *Exercise in Education and Medicine*. He graduated in Medicine from McGill in 1892 and was a sculptor.
1910 *Hygiene of Sports* in two volumes by Siegfried Weissbein of Berlin
1912 First sports physician Congress in Oberhof/Thuringen
1913 Congress on physical therapy for sports in Paris
1914 "Die Sportverletzungen" by G. Van Saar in *Encyclopaedia of Surgery* by Van Bruns
1917 *The Trainer's Bible* by Samuel Bilik included care of injuries.
1923 F. A. Bainbridge publishes *Physiology of Muscular Exercise*, University of London.
1924 German Association of Physicians for the Promotion of Physical Culture publishes first sports medicine journal.
1928 Meeting during the Winter Olympics in St. Moritz plans the first meeting of the Federation International Medico-sportive et Scientifique to be held during the Summer Olympics in Amsterdam. Meetings are held subsequently with each Olympic Games.
1930 F. J. Kirby publishes *Baseball Pitcher's Elbow*.
1931 Charles B. Heald: *Injuries and Sport; A General Guide for the Practitioner*, London
1933 *Foundations of Sports Medicine* by F. Herxheimer in German
1938 Augustus Thorndike (Harvard team physician) writes *Athletic Injuries: Prevention, Diagnosis and Treatment*
1949 National Athletic Trainers Association established
1954 American College of Sports Medicine founded with 45 members; by 1992 there are 13,155 members. The organization has been more interested in physical education and exercise physiology than in orthopaedics.
1954-1977 American Medical Association Committee on Sports
1961 *Journal of Sports Medicine* founded
1962 American Academy of Orthopaedic Surgeons Committee on Sports Medicine
1962 Don O'Donaghue: *Treatment of Injuries to Athletes*, Philadelphia
1972 *American Journal of Sports Medicine* founded

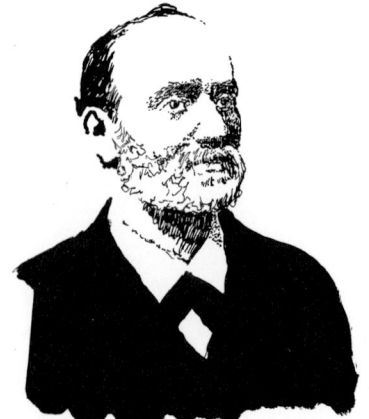

Jonas Zander (1835–1920), Stockholm

He built exercise machines in 1862 which live on today as rowing and stepping machines. Some were electrically powered machines for passive motion, and others were for active exercise against resistance. He opened Medico-Mechanical Institutes in many cities, with more than 70 different machines.

◆ **Jonas Zander (1835–1920)**
A native of Stockholm, he was a founder of health clubs. His machines were popular for rehabilitation during World War I.

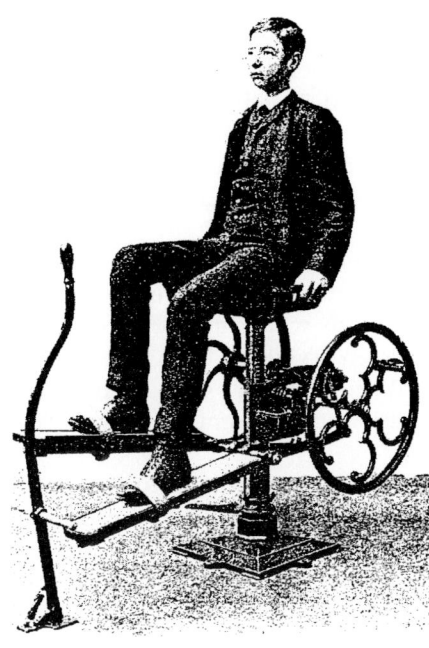

Zander's machines provided exercise and were the first robot therapists. This is Dr. Zander's velocipede. From Lavertin A: Dr. Zander's Medico-mechanical Gymnastics. Stockholm, 1893.

History of Team Games

Mayan Ball Courts. Today's sportsmen do it to get fit and to win. The aim here was to avoid losing and becoming a human sacrifice. Sports did not catch on as a popular activity at this time.

Rackets. Played against a wall, rackets started in many lands. In Britain it was a popular jail sport. Squash is the private school version.

Polo. Played on horseback, polo began in Persia before 500 BC. There were international matches in the 11th century.

Cricket. This began in the 1500s, and there were County matches in England from 1719; the Marylebone Cricket Club was founded in 1787. Test cricket (international competition) began in 1877.

Lawn Tennis. This evolved from royal tennis. Henry the Eighth built a court for himself in 1529. Wimbledon has been going since 1877.

Football. The compulsion to kick a stone is irresistible, and the rudiments go back to our beginnings. The Greeks did it. The Brits did it so wildly (as they do today) that there were Royal Proclamations against it in 1314, 1349, 1447, 1449, 1572, and 1581. Accidents were common, and the serfs spent time playing football when they should have been practicing archery to fight the enemy. The Football Association was formed in 1863 and produced soccer. Rugger began when William Webb Ellis "with a fine disregard for the rules of football . . . first took the ball in his arms and ran with it" in 1823.

Australian Football. 1860s.

American Football. Goes back to 1873 when Columbia, Princeton, Yale, and Harvard agreed on some rules.

Baseball. A blend of rounders and cricket. Players ran from stake to stake, but injuries in the 1840s led to the use of sandbags called bases. The rules gradually evolved. The first game was played under one set of rules in Cooperstown, New York, in 1839, and the first game under other rules in 1846 at Hoboken, New Jersey. A Professional Baseball Players organization began in 1871. The World Series began in 1903.

Basketball. This game was invented in 1891 by a Canadian clergyman and later physician, James Naismith, at the YMCA in Springfield, Massachusetts, as a vigorous winter indoor sport.

Golf. Golf began with Scotsmen trying to hit a ball farther than each other until the Royal and Ancient Golf Club at St. Andrews, founded in 1754, established the current objectives. The British Open began in 1860.

Hockey. This is an ancient stick game that took to the ice in 1853 when British soldiers stationed in Canada made the best of the weather conditions.

The Olympian Games

These athletic contests began in 776 BC as a tribute to the god Zeus. There were footraces, wrestling, boxing, horse racing, pentathlon (running, long jump, javelin, discus, wrestling), and races in armor. The men were naked and women were not allowed—especially in the audience. The Games were abolished in 394. There were other Greek games. The Romans favored games of a more violent nature—battles to the death. In 1896 a Frenchman, Baron Pierre de Coubertin, initiated the Olympic Games on the Greek model.

Baseball Injury

FOREIGN BODIES IN THE ELBOW JOINT ("BASEBALL PITCHER'S ELBOW")
F. J. KIRBY, BALTIMORE, 1930

"This type of injury, giving rise to a foreign body in the elbow joint, I have designated 'the baseball pitcher's elbow.' The cases I have seen all occurred in strong young men, who were pitchers on the baseball teams in their respective colleges. In each case, the injury which later led to the formation of the foreign body in the elbow joint occurred while the patient was pitching during a game of ball.

"Frequently a pitcher, during the wind-up, . . . extends the forearm rapidly and fully and the head of the radius is brought backward suddenly and with great force against the condyle of the humerus. The result is that a small piece of cartilage and bone from the head of the radius is chipped off—a chisel fracture of the head of the radius. This small, broken-off piece of bone and cartilage remains about the joint and by constant irritation it is likely to increase somewhat in size.

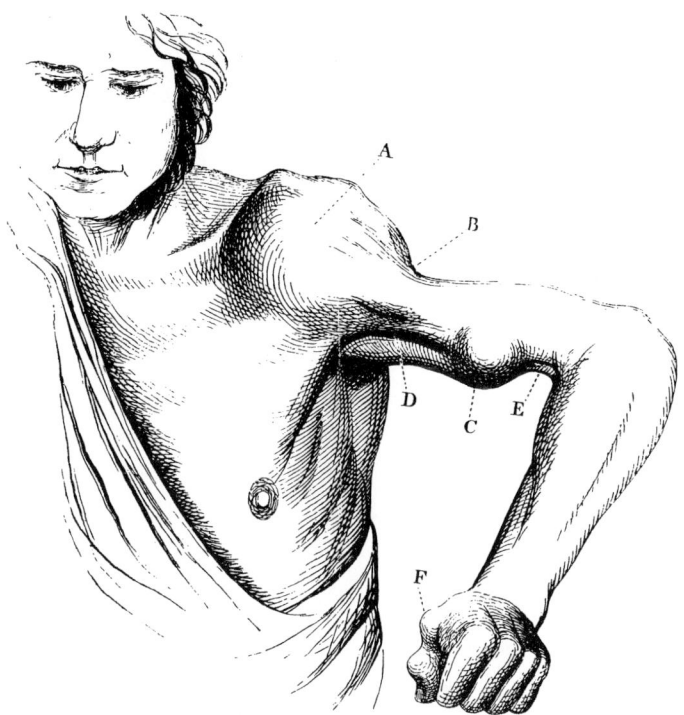

Rupture of the long head of the biceps. From Adams, 1883.

"The treatment consisted of opening the elbow joint over the head of the radius and removing the foreign body, and then closing the wound.

"The lesion (fracture) occurs on the posterior inner surface of the head of the radius. The bodies varied in size, from one the size of a coffee bean to two as large as almonds, and oval. They consisted of cartilage and, when sectioned, were found to contain bone in the center.

"The patients all did well after removal of the foreign body and secured a fully useful joint, with an arm and forearm as strong as before injury."

Biomechanics

Giovanni Borelli (1608-1679) saw the muscles and bones as levers and studied the motion of birds in flight. The illustrations in his book *On the movement of animals* (1680-1681) provided the basis for scientific study. A contemporary, Marcello Malpighi, wrote that *"the mechanisms of our bodies are composed of strings, thread, beams, levers, cloth, flowing fluid, cisterns, ducts, filters, sieves and other similar mechanisms."* This was the era when the body was beginning to be seen in mechanical terms. The body *"is a machine that winds its own springs,"* wrote Julien de la Mettrie in 1748.

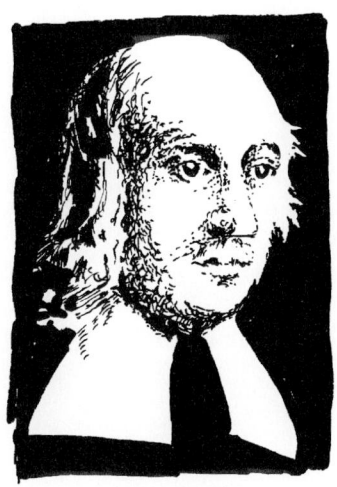

◆ **Giovanni Borelli (1608–1679)**

The study of motion took a leap forward with Eadweard Muybridge in California in 1870 when he took slow-motion photographs. Étienne-Jules Marey (1830–1904) in France made objective measurement of motion, and the German Army looked at the work done in marching.

References

Chapter references are located in Chapter 26.

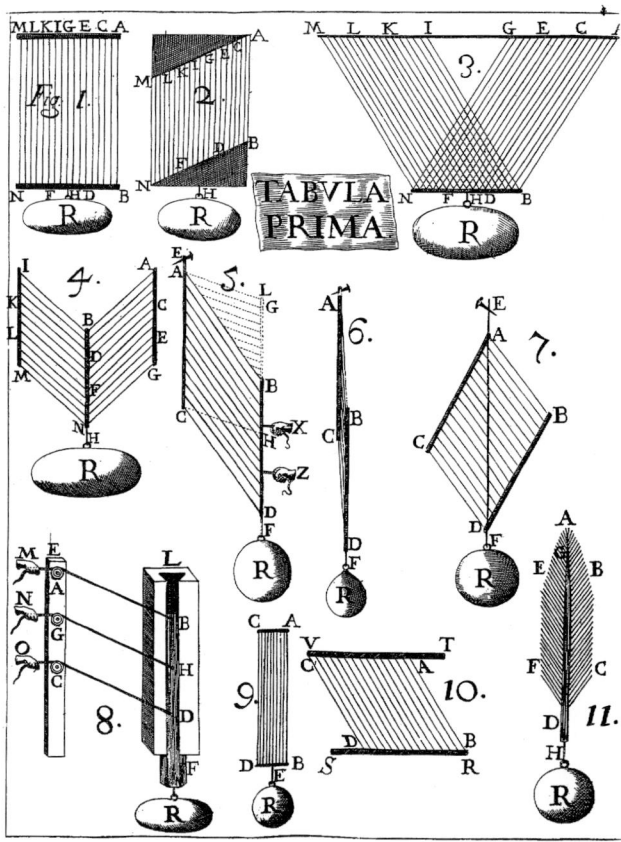

Figures 21 ◆ 8, 21 ◆ 9, 21 ◆ 10, 21 ◆ 11, 21 ◆ 12, 21 ◆ 13.
Borelli's studies of the body as a machine made of levers, 1680.
Figure continued on pages 483, 484, and 485

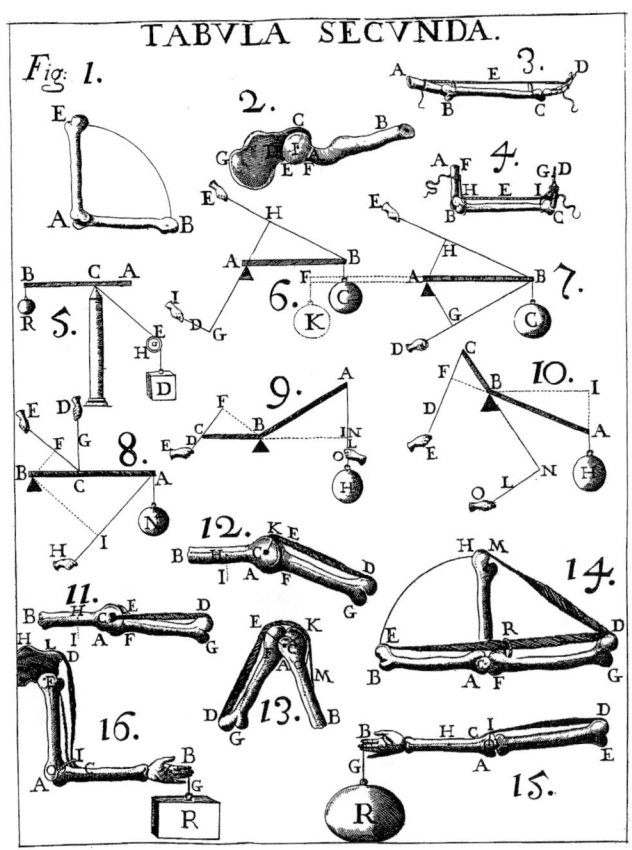

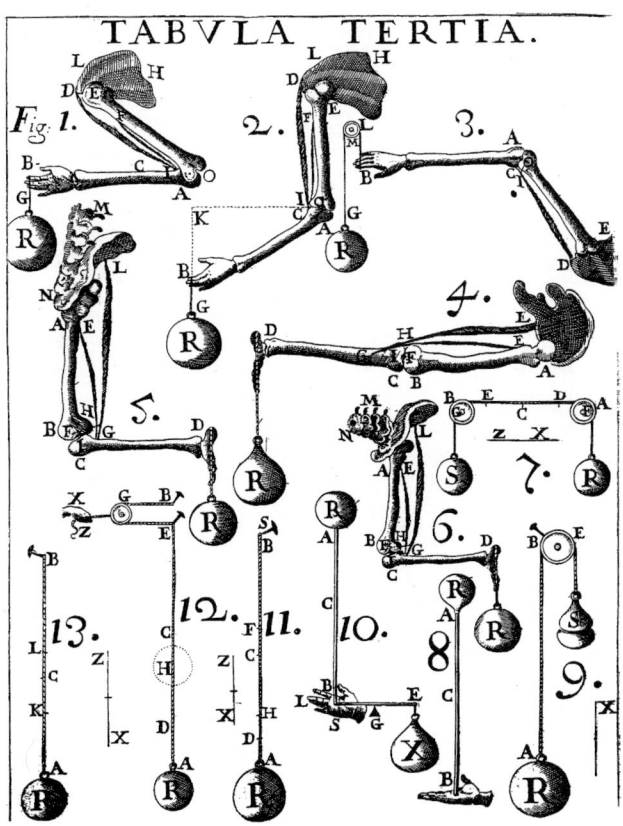

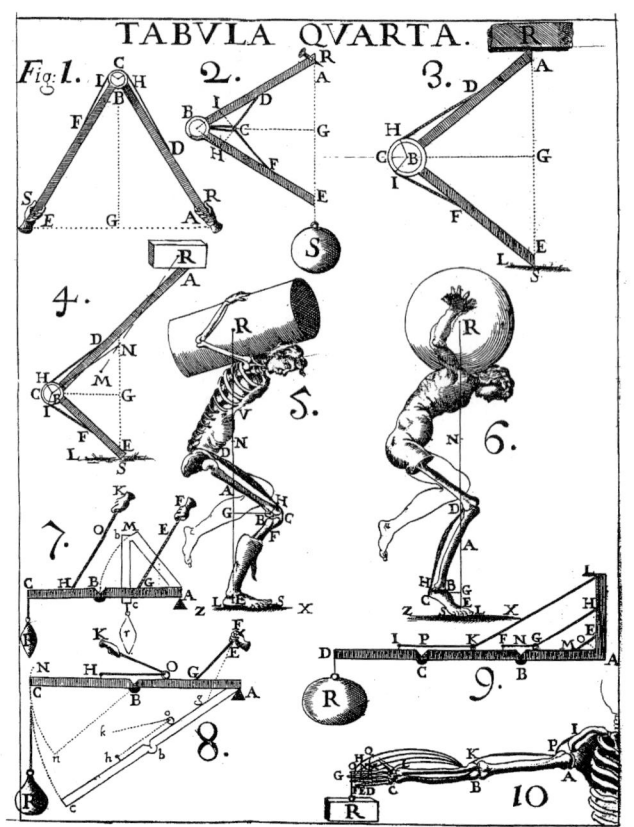
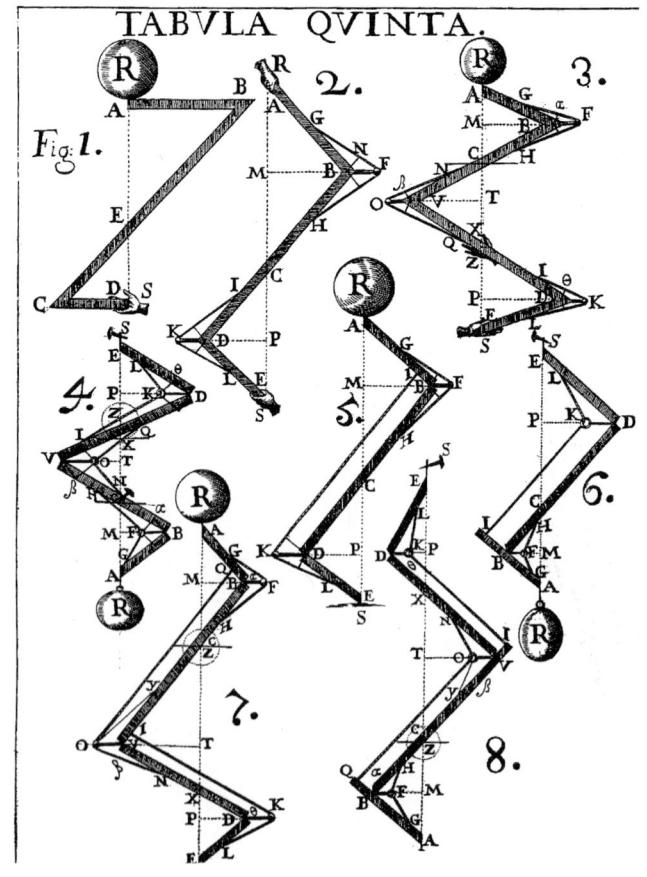

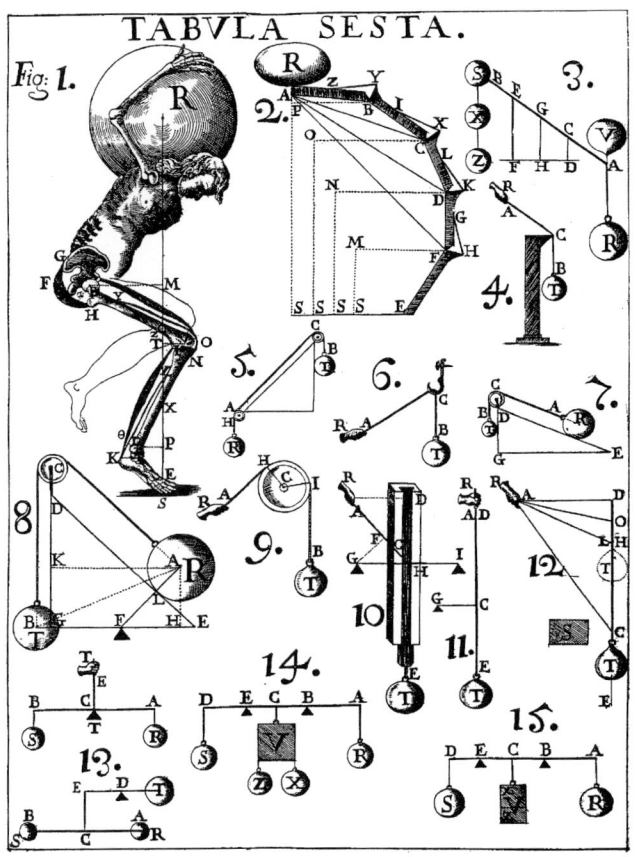

◆ Chapter Twenty-two

Knee

The knee is a joint of great subtlety. The finer points are still being discovered. Arthroscopy and magnetic resonance imaging bring information to the clinic that used to be available only in the laboratory, in operating rooms, and post mortem.

In earlier times, only the gross problems of the knee received attention. There has been a gradual move toward the subtle. The old focus was on infection and rachitic deformity, then locking, and now instability. In the past people did not live long enough to develop arthritis and want a joint replacement as they do now.

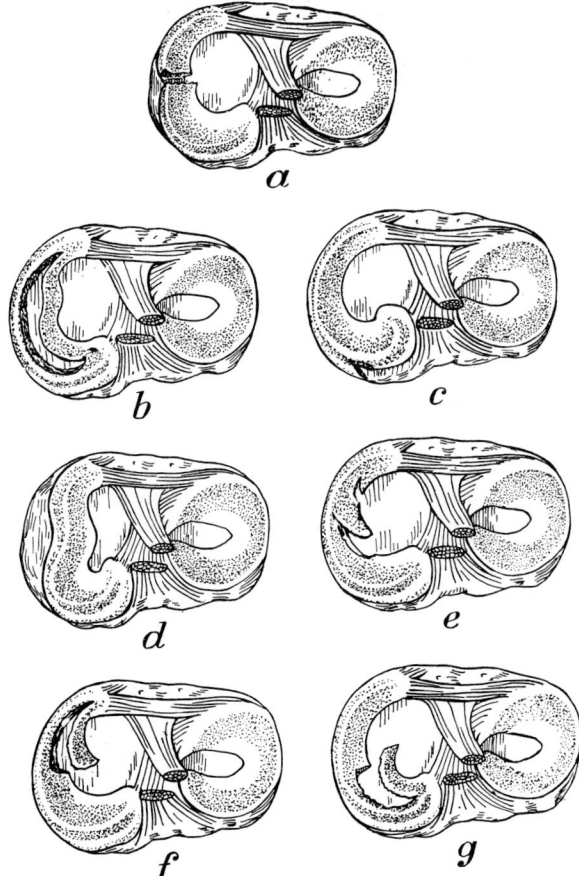

Types of cartilage tear. From McMurray TP: A Practice of Orthopaedic Surgery, 3rd ed. London: E. Arnold, 1949, Fig 18. Used with permission.

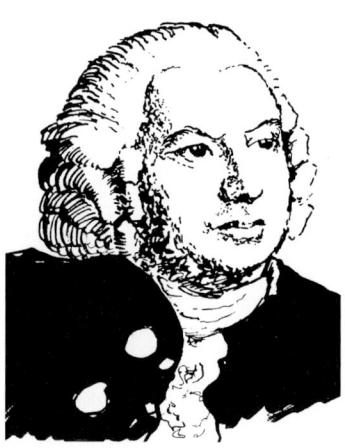

◆ William Bromfeild

TIMELINE OF MENISCI

1773 William Bromfeild, London surgeon, writes an early account of meniscal locking. *"I have seen a temporary lameness happen from one of the semilunar cartilages within the joint having flipped out of its situation; the knee immediately became swelled and very painful . . . The assistant having hold of the leg and sometimes lightly extending and at other times gently bending it while I was examining the joint of the knee, the cartilage flipped into its place and the patient soon became easy."*

1803 William Hey coins the phrase "internal derangement of the knee."

1834 John Reid: pathology of meniscal tears. He described a peripheral detachment.

1845 Amedee Bonnet: In his book on diseases of joints he describes producing experimental injuries in cadavers. A varus force in the young separates an epiphysis; in the young adult the lateral and cruciate ligaments are torn. In elderly people, the bone fractures. Rotation produced sliding of the medial femoral condyle behind the posterior horn, but he did not produce a tear.

1885 Thomas Annandale writes about an operation for displaced semilunar cartilage.

1928 McMurray sign of torn meniscus

1936 Don King shows that an experimental peripheral detachment of the meniscus in a dog will heal.

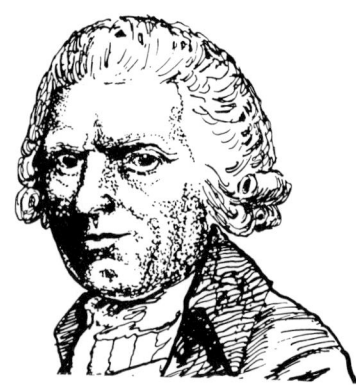

◆ William Hey

William Hey (1736–1819)

William Hey was the founder of surgery at Leeds, England, and initiated the construction of a hospital there. His life story was written by his pupil, John Pearson; it is a most remarkable work, describing his lofty ideals and religious fervor, so much so that it resembles a book about a saint, destined for Sunday reading by a Victorian family. Many consultants would envy this devotion from a pupil.

Hey was born in Pudsey near Leeds, and his father was a drysalter (a dealer in the ingredients for manufacturing cloth). At the age of 14 he was apprenticed to a surgeon and apothecary and nearly died of an overdose of opium while studying its effects. In 1757 he went to St. George's Hospital, and when he qualified set up in practice in Leeds. He was a busy general surgeon and accoucheur and a friend of Joseph Priestly, the physicist, who proposed him as Fellow of the Royal Society in 1775. Hey was always a fervent churchman: he preached to Wesley and wrote tracts. During his time as Mayor and Magistrate at Leeds he enforced the Sunday observance laws very strictly. The local inhabitants retaliated by burning an effigy of him.

He wrote a small book on surgery that includes several chapters on orthopaedics. He described subacute osteomyelitis of the tibia before Brodie and advocated deroofing the lesion. His interest in the knee may be due to the fact that he banged his knee getting out of a bath in 1773 and remained lame all his days. However, he coined the phrase "internal derangement of the knee," and described meniscus injuries. He wrote about loose bodies and introduced tarsometatarsal amputation.

He died in 1819, and his son succeeded him as surgeon at Leeds Infirmary, where his statue still graces the entrance.

INTERNAL DERANGEMENT OF THE KNEE
WILLIAM HEY, 1803

"The joint of the knee is so firmly supported on all sides by tendinous ligamentous substances that the bones of the thigh and leg are very rarely separated from each other, so as to form a dislocation, in the common sense of the term. Great violence must take place, and a considerable laceration must happen, before the tibia can be completely separated from the os femoris. Yet this joint is not unfrequently affected with an internal derangement of its component parts; and that sometimes in consequence of trifling accidents. The disease is, indeed, now and then removed, as suddenly as it is produced, by the natural motions of the joint, without surgical assistance; but it may remain for weeks or months; and will then become a serious misfortune, as it causes a considerable degree of lameness. I am not acquainted with any author who has described either the disease or the remedy; I shall, therefore, give such a description as my own experience has furnished me with, and such as will suffice to distinguish a complaint, which, when recent, admits of an easy method of cure.

"This disorder may happen either with, or without, contusion. In the latter case it is readily distinguished. In the former, the symptoms are equivocal, till the effects of the contusion are removed. When no contusion has happened, or the effects of it are removed, the joint, with respect to its shape, appears to be uninjured. If there is any difference from its usual appearance, it is, that the ligament of the patella appears rather more relaxed than in the sound limb. The leg is readily bent or extended by the hands of the surgeon, and without pain to the patient; at most, the degree of uneasiness caused by this flexion and extension is trifling. But the patient himself cannot freely bend, nor perfectly extend, the limb in walking; he is compelled to walk with an invariable and small degree of flexion. Though the patient is obliged to keep the leg thus stiff in walking; yet in sitting down the affected joint will move like the other.

"The complaint which I have described may be brought on, I apprehend, by any such alteration in the state of the joint, as will prevent the condyles of the os femoris from moving truly in the hollow formed by the semilunar cartilages and articular depressions of the tibia. An unequal tension of the lateral, or cross ligaments, of the joint, or some slight derangement of the semilunar cartilages, may probably be sufficient to bring on the complaint. When the disorder is the effect of contusion, it is most likely that the lateral ligament on one side of the joint may be rendered somewhat more rigid than usual; and hereby prevent

Written in a charming old world style, this account shows the difficulties confronting the doctor who looks for first descriptions. Hey's description may be the first about a locked knee, but much of the information is irrelevant, some is misleading (e.g., the relaxed patella ligament), important features are omitted, and the interpretation is off key.

that equable motion of the condyles of the os femoris, which is necessary for walking with firmness.

"The method of cure, which I am about to propose, must not be used while there is any inflammatory affection, or swelling of the joint; but only when these effects of contusion are removed. The following cases will further illustrate the nature of this complaint; and point out the method which I have hitherto found successful in removing it.

◆ CASE

In 1784, the Honourable Miss Harriet Ingram (now Mrs. Ashton), as she was playing with a child, and making a considerable exertion, in stretching herself forwards, and stooping to take hold of the child, while she rested upon one leg, brought on an immediate lameness in the knee joint of that leg on which she stood. The disorder was considered as a simple sprain; and a plaster was applied round the joint. As the lameness did not diminish in the course of five or six days, I was desired to visit her.

"Upon comparing the knee[s], I could perceive no difference, except that, when the limbs were placed in a state of complete extension, the ligament of the patella of the injured joint seemed to be rather more relaxed, than in that joint which had received no injury. When I moved the affected knee by a gentle flexion and extension, my patient complained of no pain; yet she could not perfectly extend the leg in walking, nor bend it in raising the foot from the floor; but moved as if the joint had been stiff, limping very much, and walking with pain.

"I thought it probable, that the sudden exertion might in some degree have altered the situation of the crossed ligaments, or otherwise have displaced the condyles of the os femoris with respect to the semilunar cartilages, so that the condyles might meet with some resistance when the flexor or extensor muscles were put into action, and thereby the free motion of the joint might be hindered, when the incumbent weight of the body pressed the thigh bone closely against the tibia; though this derangement was not so great as to prevent the joint, when relaxed, from being moved with ease.

"To remedy this derangement, I placed my patient upon an elevated seat, which had nothing underneath it that could prevent the leg from being pushed backward towards the posterior part of the thigh. I then extended the joint by the assistance of one hand placed just above the knee, while with the other hand I grasped the leg. During the continuance of the extension I suddenly moved the leg backwards, that it might make as acute an angle with the thigh as possible. This operation I repeated once, and then desired the young lady to try how she could walk. Whatever may be thought of my theory, my practice proved successful; for she was immediately able to walk without lameness, and on the third day after this reduction she danced at a private ball without inconvenience, or receiving any injury from the exercise."

FIRST DESCRIPTION OF A MENISCAL TEAR
DR. J. REID, 1834

A man died in the Infirmary. He had not complained of his knee. He did not limp.

"The fibrous tissue connecting the outer margin of the external semilunar cartilage to the edge of the head of the tibia was torn through in its anterior half, and the semilunar cartilage was found thrown inwards and backwards. The cartilage of the anterior part of the tibia, which had been exposed to the free motion of the condyle of the femur, had become rough."

Reid reported this because the writings of Hey and A. Cooper were uncluttered by pathologic descriptions.

Thomas Porter McMurray (1888–1949)

McMurray followed Robert Jones at Liverpool, and shared his rooms at 11 Nelson Street—rooms that had been built by Hugh Owen Thomas. ("Rooms" is English for office.)

He was born in Belfast, and graduated there in 1910. He then came as a house surgeon to work for Robert Jones. Later he became lecturer in orthopaedics, and in 1938 occupied the first Chair of orthopaedics in Liverpool.

McMurray was a man who threw himself into the spirit of things, whether it was relaxing in the country, playing golf, or operating. His surgery was dexterous, assured, and very quickly carried out—a meniscus would come out in its entirety in five minutes. It was his dogmatic verbal teaching and training that are remembered, rather than his literary output, which, though important, was not extensive. He wrote a small textbook of orthopaedics in 1937, and an article on internal derangements of the knee, in which he introduced his sign of a torn meniscus. He was one of the originators of osteotomy for arthritis of the hip, an operation that bears his name.

THE DIAGNOSIS OF INTERNAL DERANGEMENTS OF THE KNEE
1928

"Lesions of the outer cartilage are, undoubtedly, much more difficult of diagnosis than those of the inner cartilage, especially in those cases in which the definite snap, so typical of these lesions, is not present, and lesions of the posterior end of the internal cartilage give a much less definite train of symptoms than those of the anterior end, and for these cases I have found an accessory method of diagnosis of the greatest help.

"In using this method the knee should be flexed completely, so that the heel rests on the buttock or as near this point as possible: the ankle is then grasped in the right hand, and the joint controlled by the left hand with the thumb and fore-finger

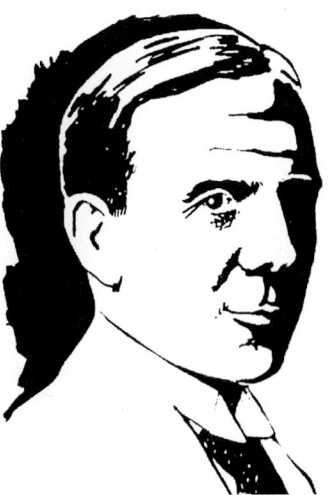

◆ Thomas Porter McMurray

firmly grasping it on either side at the level of the joint to its posterior aspect, and behind the external and internal lateral ligaments respectively. The ankle is now twisted by the right hand, so that the knee is rotated inwards and outwards to its fullest extent, and if a lesion of the external cartilage or of the posterior portion of the internal cartilage is present a definite click can be felt under the finger or thumb of the left hand. Examination of an abnormally lax knee-joint in which there is no lesion of the internal or external cartilages may give a sensation which might at first be mistaken for this click, but in such a case the click is not definite, and there is never the peculiar sliding or gliding of the femur over an apparent obstacle which is so typically present when there has been an injury to the external cartilage or posterior portion of the internal.

"As an aid in the diagnosis of doubtful knee-joint lesions this method of examination has been of the greatest help to me, because it is applicable in just those cases which are otherwise so difficult, and in which a correct diagnosis is essential. It is by this means that I have been able to diagnose correctly on many occasions an injury to the posterior end of the semilunar cartilage, which at operation on first opening of the joint appeared to be perfectly normal. This method is inapplicable to lesions of the anterior end of the internal semilunar cartilage, but this, fortunately, is of little moment, because diagnosis here is usually comparatively easy, and should give rise to little trouble if sufficient care is exercised."

Thomas Annandale (1838–1908)

Annandale was professor of surgery at Edinburgh.

AN OPERATION FOR DISPLACED SEMILUNAR CARTILAGE
THOMAS ANNANDALE, 1885

Annandale begins by saying that a peripheral detachment of the medial meniscus may heal back with rest, but if it does not and interferes with a patient's occupation or comfort, it may need

"... a new method of procedure which I successfully adopted. The excellent result obtained in this case encourages me to ex-

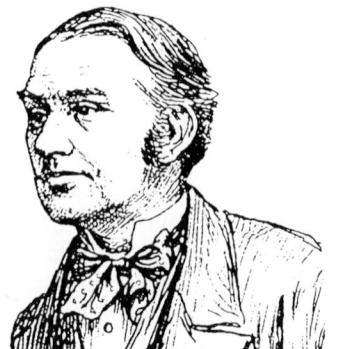

♦ Thomas Annandale

press the opinion that this, or some similar procedure, may now become an established means of treatment."

◆ CASE

"Thomas M, aged 30, miner, was sent to me on November 1st 1883. About ten months before, he was working in a kneeling position, when he felt something give way in his right knee.

"He was unable to work and had an effusion, locking, a hollow over the medial meniscus. Came to operation on 16th November 1883." [The waiting list was shorter then than it is now].

"An incision was made along the upper and inner border of the tibia, parallel with the anterior margin of the internal semilunar cartilage; and the few superficial vessels having been secured, the joint was opened. It was then seen that this semilunar cartilage was completely separated from its anterior attachments, and was displaced backwards about half an inch. The anterior edge of this cartilage was now seized by a pair of artery catch forceps, and it was drawn forwards into its natural position, and held there until three stitches of chromic catgut were passed through it and through the fascia and periosteum covering the margin of the tibia. The forceps were then withdrawn, the cartilage remaining securely stitched in position. The wound in the synovial membrane and soft textures having been closed with catgut stitches, a splint and plaster-of-Paris bandage were applied, so as to keep the joint at rest. Seven weeks after the operation, the splint and bandages were removed, and gentle movements of the joint practised.

"On January 25th, 1884, the patient was dismissed cured, the movement of the joint being good, and the limb steadily gaining strength. In April of the same year, the patient returned to show the result. He was then seen by many of our distinguished guests at the Tercentenary, who all expressed the opinion that the result was everything that could be desired. He had perfect movement in the joint, and had never had the slightest effusion or locking of the joint since he commenced to go about after the operation."

Arthroscopy

Arthroscopes are modified cystoscopes. The idea of peeking at the interior of the bladder, which originated in about 1800, could not advance until the invention of the small light bulb nearly 100 years later. Cystoscopy became an important diagnostic tool at the turn of the century. Miniaturization took another 50 years and the application of fiberoptics and video another 30 years. At first arthroscopy was used for diagnosis alone; gradually more and more complicated procedures became possible. Now there are surgeons who do nothing but arthroscopy, but they have to compete with magnetic resonance imaging in the diagnostic role.

TIMELINE OF ARTHROSCOPY

1918 In Tokyo, Kenji Takagi inspected a cadaver knee with a cystoscope and begins designing scopes. Watanabe studies with him.
1921 Eugen Bircher examined a knee with a laparoscope.
1925 Phillip H. Kreuser was the first American to use arthroscopy for diagnosis: "Semilunar cartilage disease: A plea for early recognition by means of the arthroscope."
1931 Finkelstein and Meyer did a biopsy through an arthroscope.
1931 Burman used an arthroscope in several joints while a Fellow in Germany.
1957 Masaki Watanabe's *Atlas* and model 21 arthroscope.
1962 Arthroscopic surgery begins.
1968 Robert Jackson of Toronto goes to Japan to study sarcoma and brings arthroscopy back.
1973 First instructional course is given in Philadelphia.

Eugen Bircher (1882–1956)

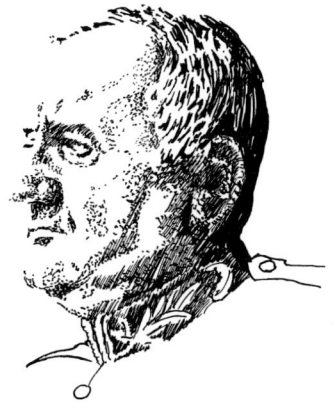

◆ Eugen Bircher

Swiss general surgeon who developed ivory intramedullary pegs for fractures and was a pioneer of arthroscopy. In 1920 he published the results of arthroscopy in cadaver knees and then in 18 patients. By 1922 he could diagnose 8 of 9 meniscus tears correctly.

"Arthroscopy is superior to all other methods of investigation and, like endoscopy of the bladder, can be used to define certain indications for surgery. It will be met with resistance but will gain in popularity and develop to the point at which it becomes indispensable."

Robert Jackson

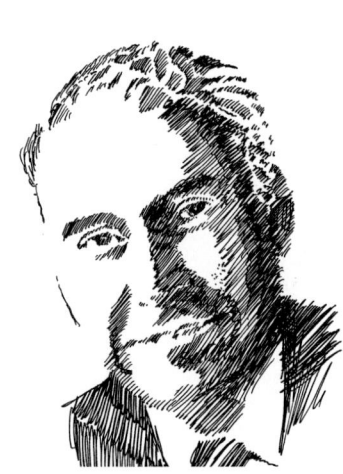

◆ Robert Jackson

Orthopaedic surgeon who practiced in Toronto. As a Fellow he spent a year in Japan in 1968, planning to study the tissue culture of bone tumors. He came back with an arthroscope and was responsible for the explosion of interest in arthroscopy in North America. He became very active in the Para-Olympics. Like many Canadian orthopaedic surgeons of his generation, he moved to the United States, where he is Chairman at Baylor College of Medicine, Houston, Texas.

ARTHROSCOPY, OR THE DIRECT VISUALIZATION OF JOINTS. AN EXPERIMENTAL CADAVER STUDY

MICHAEL S. BURMAN, 1931

"The idea first occurred to us in the latter part of the year 1929 that it might be possible to see the interior of joints directly through a proper instrument introduced into the joint. In Febru-

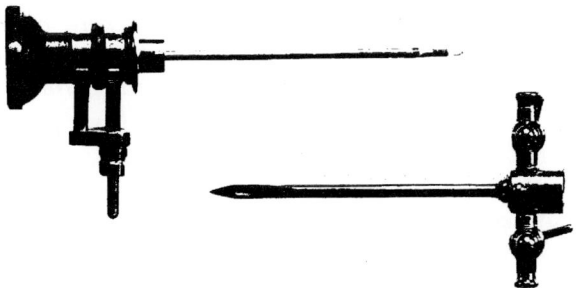

The arthroscope of Michael Burman divided into its two component parts, 1931. Why did he not pursue this idea? From Burman M: J Bone Jt Surg 1931, 13, 669, Fig. 1. Used with permission.

ary 1930, we consulted with Mr. Reinhold Wappler concerning the construction of an instrument for this purpose. An instrument was devised according to our particular requirements. At that time, Mr. Wappler told us that he had not heard of any instrument for such a purpose, nor had he ever made any similar instrument. We first began work in March 1930 in the Anatomy Laboratory of the New York University Medical School, through the kindness and interest of Dr. Harold Senior, Professor of Anatomy. Material being so limited we were asked by Dr. Senior to delay further work until autumn of the same year, at which time a greater abundance of material was sure to be available. In September 1930, however, we sailed to Europe, and it was not until February 1931 that we again resumed work in the Pathologic Institute of the Krankenhaus der Friedrichstadt-Dresden, through the great courtesy of Dr. Georg Schmorl. The following is a complete report of the work done both in New York and in Dresden. . . .

"It was not until we had completed our work that we were informed that Bircher had preceded us. Priority should be awarded to him, since his work was done in 1922. A brief survey of the highlights of his work, which was incidental to his study of meniscal injuries, is necessary. He used the Jacobaeus laparoscope in a joint filled with oxygen or nitrogen gas. On the basis of a few cadaver experiments, he believed that only the knee joint was suitable for examination. He reported twenty clinical cases which were examined through his instrument, with the findings subsequently confirmed by operation. He saw changes in the meniscus (such as hemorrhage and tears), osteochondritis of the femur, and synovial tuberculosis, etc. In a foot-note, he says that he examined fifteen other cases, in addition to the twenty described. His work does not seem to have received any support. In 1925, in a speech in Holland, Bircher again affirmed the value of this endoscopy of the knee joint, especially in the diagnosis of meniscal lesions.

"We have also received word from Dr. Leo Meyer that Dr. H. Finkelstein and he have also been working, on this same problem, during a period of time coincident, in general, with our work.

"The term 'arthroscopy' is self-evident, and everyone to whom the idea is mentioned coins the term spontaneously. It is thus natural to designate the instrument as the arthroscope."

Bircher called the process variously endoscopy of the knee joint, arthro-endoscopy, and arthroscopy.

Burman used the arthroscope for the shoulder and said this was the easiest joint. He used it also for the wrist, hip, and knee.

Kenji Takagi (1888–1963)

"Dr. Kenji Takagi, the surgeon of primacy in the development of the arthroscope, encouraged Masaki Watanabe to perfect and attract the interest of orthopaedic surgeons to arthroscopy. Takagi was Emeritus Professor at Tokyo University. Owing to lack of funds in the 1930s, it was not possible to publish color photographs of his work. The task remained for his pupil Watanabe to publish two editions of an atlas of superbly photographed arthroscopies performed in the interval between 1957 and 1969. Takagi not only designed the arthroscope but also made it available for practical use. His design included 11 types of optical tools and several designs of trochar, as well as various accessories. In 1932, Takagi succeeded in photographing on black and white film through the arthroscope operations on the inside of the knee joint, and in 1936 Takagi and associates made color photographs and motion pictures through the arthroscope. One version of the film was released with a sound track of symphony orchestra music. The instruments were on display at the International World exhibit in Paris in 1937. Takagi's arthroscope was eventually approved as a pan-endoscope for cavities other than the knee joint. In fact, Takagi employed it for myeloscopic purposes in cases of spina bifida, as well as those involving nearly every joint in the body. He continued to make improvements in the instruments until he died in 1963." Marshall R. Urist, M.D.

ARTHROSCOPE
KENJI TAKAGI, 1939

"The first application of endoscopy, cystoscopy, was introduced by Max Nitze in 1877 and in 1886. His studies stimulated further interest in the use of endoscopy for organs other than the bladder, e.g., the larynx, stomach, colon and vagina, in which the lumen consisted of soft tissue. In 1910, Thorakolaparoskop used thoracoscopy and cauterization to treat pleural adhesions (the Jacobaeus operation). But despite these advancements, the use of endoscopy to visualize the interior of joints, i.e., arthroscopy, did not develop because of the following characteristics of skeletal articular structures: (1) joints have a relatively small lumen; (2) the internal joint surfaces are complex; and (3) the internal joint surface is nonextensible. Between tightly machined surfaces a small arthroscope would be easily damaged or destroyed.

"In 1918, I first attempted to directly visualize joints in cadaver specimens using a cystoscope, but failed. In 1920, I

developed a primitive arthroscope, but the diameter was equal to that of a cystoscope, and with the external accessories attached, it was not clinically applicable. Only in one exception, an elderly woman who had tuberculous fistula arthritis of the knee, was this primitive arthroscope successfully inserted from the external orifice of the fistula. We tried to visualize the internal joint surface but fluid leakage through the fistula prevented our ballooning the lumen. Clearly, the successful use of arthroscopy required some consideration of articular structure. I therefore proposed that the arthroscope must fulfill the following requirements: (1) at 1 cm from the arthroscope, the object must be visualized as actual size; (2) the length of schadliche must be within 1 cm; and (3) the width of the distal part of the arthroscope must be as slender as possible so that the light sheath does not require suture after puncture.

"During my stay in Doutch, I tried to stimulate interest in arthroscopy, but my ideas were not well received. Thus, on return to Japan, I exclusively studied arthrography using iodine contrast medium and gas. But with arthrography, neither the pathologic changes of synovial color, changes of vascular channels, nor pathologic fine changes in the articular surface could be identified. Therefore, my attention returned to arthroscopy.

"In 1931, I designed a Charriere No. 10.5 arthroscope (3.5 mm diameter) and gained confidence in the clinical application of arthroscopy. The first results with its use were presented at the 64th Orthopaedic Meeting in Japan, June 19, 1932 (J. Jap. Orthop. Assoc. 7:241, 1932). In 1933, at the 8th meeting of the Japanese Orthopaedic Association, I reported additional results and presented a 16 mm motion picture film using arthroscopy (J. Jap. Orthop. Assoc. 7:132, 1932; Tokyo Med. J. 2824:21, 1932). I showed that the arthroscope could be applied to visualize the inside of joints destroyed by tuberculous arthritis, Charcot hip joint arthrosis, osteoarthritis, dislocation of the patella, fibrillation of knee joints, and ligamental changes. We also demonstrated that a giant cell sarcoma of the distal femur had proliferated near cruciate ligaments and invaded cartilage tissue. Whereas we could not observe the changes using only roentgenography, by means of the arthroscopy, we could easily visualize such lesions as spina bifida and osteitis fibrosa cystica. Entering from within the nasal cavity, we could observe the movement of the soft palate in exercises of pronunciation before and after a cleft palate operation. At this same meeting, Sabrolino, a member of my orthopedic department, demonstrated the arthroscopic anatomy of normal joints.

"In 1937, the focus adjustable arthroscope (No. 4) and accessories were displayed at the international exposition in Paris. Arthroscopy did not further improve until recently because at first we could not correctly interpret the arthroscopic anatomy of the joints. There were also technical problems with designing a slender light sheath. Arthroscopy was technically difficult to perform. With time, however, I have been able to overcome most of these problems."

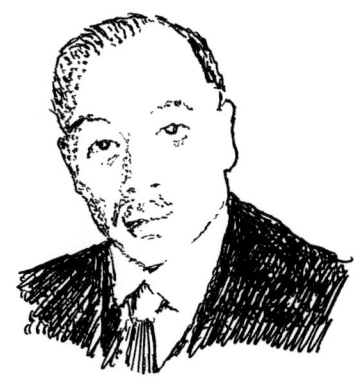

◆ **Kenji Takagi**
Professor at Tokyo University. He was disappointed by arthrography and started using a cystoscope for cadaver knees in 1918. He reported arthroscopy in 1932 and later used cine-. He also did arthroscopy of other joints and myeloscopy in spina bifida.

THE FORMATION OF ABNORMAL SYNOVIAL CYSTS IN CONNECTION WITH THE JOINTS

W. MORRANT BAKER, 1877 AND 1885

After describing cases at some length Baker writes that the following conclusions may be drawn:

"1. That abnormal synovial cysts may be formed in connection, not only with the knee, but in connection with the shoulder, the elbow, the wrist, the hip, and the ankle joints.

2. That the manner of formation of these synovial cysts probably resembles that which has been proved to occur in connection with the knee-joint, namely, that the synovial fluid on reaching a certain amount of tension by accumulation within the joint, finds its way out in the direction of least resistance, either by the channel by which some normal bursa communicates with the joint, or, in the absence of any such channel, by forming first a hernia of the synovial membrane. In both cases, should the tension continue or increase, the fluid at length escapes from the sac, and its boundaries are then formed only by the muscles and other tissues between and amongst which it accumulates.

3. That in the case of the shoulder-joint the abnormal synovial cyst may be found either in front a little below the clavicle, or in the upper arm in the region of the biceps muscle.

4. That in connection with the elbow-joint the cyst is usually placed on the inner side, a little above the internal condyle of the humerus.

5. That in the case of the wrist-joint the synovial cyst may be either in front or behind.

6. In the only case in connection with the hip of which a note has been preserved, the swelling was in the upper part of Scarpa's triangle.

7. In the one case in connection with the ankle-joint the synovial cyst was in front and to the outer side.

8. That the apparent want of direct communication between the joint and the abnormal synovial cyst is frequently deceptive, and should not lead to the inference that no such communication exists.

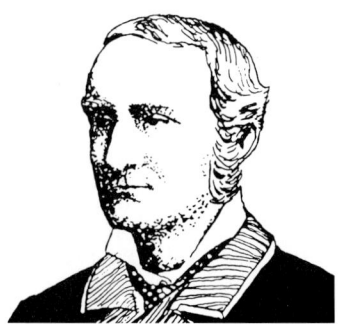

◆ William Morrant Baker

◆ William Morrant Baker (1839–1896)

Born at Andover, the son of a solicitor, William Baker, after being apprenticed to a local surgeon, studied at St. Bartholomew's Hospital, London. He was a very mature student; he passed the Fellowship at the age of 25, and married the anesthetist's sister, but he did not get on to the staff as a full surgeon until the age of 43. He passed the intervening years as casualty surgeon, assistant to out-patients, and assistant to Paget in private practice. At one time he was in charge of the skin department, and was for a long time an anatomy lecturer.

He was a general surgeon, who entered the era of antiseptic surgery without being attracted to it, and was regarded as a "good opinion" rather than a good operator. He wrote widely on general surgery and examined for several boards; rubber tracheostomy tubes were his invention, and he is immortalized by his two papers on synovial cysts.

He retired before his time on account of locomotor ataxy which led to his death.

9. That the caution given in the previous communication, not to interfere by operation with these synovial sacs without good reason, has been justified by increased experience.

"Hitherto I have not discovered any relationship between the form of osteoarthritis with which some of these synovial cysts are associated and locomotor ataxy, but I suspect that in some of them a relationship will be found to exist."

HEMOPHILIA
F. KONIG, 1892

Konig connected hemophilia and swollen joints. He wrote his article because a patient of his had died after incision of a swollen joint.

"We must differentiate between: 1. The stage of the first bleeding, the hemarthrosis of the bleeder: 2. the inflammatory stage, panarthritis of the bleeder's joint; 3. the regressive stage which causes permanent deformity of the bleeder's knee, the contracture of the joint."

ANTERIOR KNEE PAIN
- 1888 Cesar Roux of Lausanne describes an operation for recurrent dislocation of the patella.
- 1891 Osgood Schlatter's disorder is described by Paget.
- 1903 Osgood describes it.
- 1921 Christian Sinding-Larsen and Sven Johansson independently describe traction tendinitis of the lower pole of the patella.
- 1921 Fairbank—apprehension test

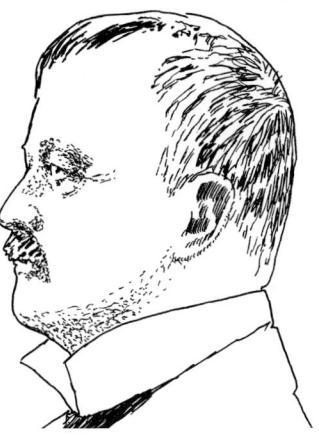

◆ Christian Sinding-Larsen

Apophysitis of the Tibial Tubercle

This seems to have been the only variety of osteochondritis that was appreciated before the era of X-ray diagnosis. In the last 30 years of the 19th century, there were half a dozen accounts of this condition, and that of Paget is included here. R. B. Osgood and Carl Schlatter (1864–1935) independently described the X-ray appearances.

Osteochondritis has been described in most epiphyses, starting with the coming of X-rays.

PERIOSTOSIS FOLLOWING STRAINS
SIR JAMES PAGET, 1891

"Much more common are the enlargements of the tubercle of the tibia which are often seen in young people much given to athletic games. They complain of aching pain at or about the part, especially during and after active exercise, and the tubercle

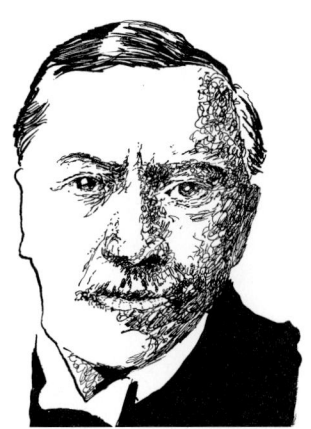

◆ Carl Schlatter

may be felt enlarged, and is often too warm. The pain often continues more or less for many months, and there may be enlargement of the bursa under the ligamentum patellae, and the tubercle may remain too prominent; but common as are these cases, especially in our public schools, I have never known grave mischief ensue in any of them, and they get well of themselves. They may represent one of the least degrees of periostosis due to strain; the increase of the prominence of the bone is only just beyond that which may be deemed the normal limit for the attachment of vigorous muscles."

Robert Osgood (1873–1956)

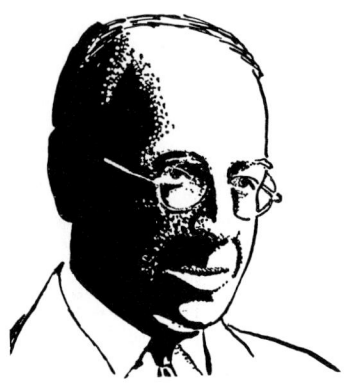

◆ Robert Osgood

Osgood had a great capacity for getting on well with people. After World War I had brought English and American orthopaedic surgeons together, he encouraged this unity and assisted Robert Jones in inaugurating the British Orthopaedic Association.

He was born in Salem, Massachusetts, and graduated from Harvard in 1899. At this time X-rays were the latest thing. As an intern at Massachusetts General Hospital, Osgood helped the hospital pharmacist run the pioneer X-ray service. The following year he became roentgenologist to the Boston Children's Hospital and wrote his first paper, on the disease which now bears his name. Fortunately his interest in radiology dwindled after this—the pharmacist subsequently developed X-ray cancers and eventually died, and Osgood himself developed many skin cancers, but several operations prevented a fatal outcome.

After this paper he went to England to study and worked with Robert Jones. He returned to Massachusetts General Hospital as an orthopaedic surgeon and studied the virology of polio, among other things. With Goldthwait and Painter he wrote an orthopaedic textbook.

He suffered at one time from a tennis elbow. It did not improve with conservative measures so he was stimulated to think about its possible cause.

Thinking it might be due to a bursa lying between the muscles and the radiohumeral joint, he went to the anatomy department where he found such a bursa in a cadaver. He had his own elbow explored under local anesthetic and a bursa was excised. He never had any trouble again.

During World War I he went to France with Harvey Cushing and later worked at headquarters in London with Robert Jones, who was directing the orthopaedic war effort.

LESIONS OF THE TIBIAL TUBERCLE OCCURRING DURING ADOLESCENCE
ROBERT B. OSGOOD, 1903

"Fractures of the tubercle of the tibia have for many years been recognized and have been considered almost as curiosities. The reported cases are nearly all those of fracture and marked separation, and are undoubtedly rare. There are, however, other

lesions representing less severe forms of injury to the tubercle. These are interesting because they have apparently been seldom recognized and because of their comparatively frequent occurrence; because of the old difficulty of diagnosis and our present simple and accurate means; and because of their relation to the development of the tubercle.

"The tubercle of the tibia develops ordinarily from the upper epiphysis of the tibia by the ossification of a tongue-like process extending downwards over the anterior surface of the diaphysis.

"To the tip of a tongue-like process of bone, or to a separate bone center, is attached the tendon of one of the most powerful muscle groups in the body. This tongue or bone center is at the age at which the lesions occur separated from the strong shaft of bone by a layer of cartilage, and the first strain of the contraction of the quadriceps transmitted by the patella tendon comes on the tibial tubercle.

"**Dissection.** In a knee the skin and subcutaneous tissues were dissected back. The dissection was then carried upwards and the quadriceps muscle isolated. Traction upon this extended the knee, and the strain appeared to be taken first by the patella tendon, almost immediately followed by a tightening of these bands of accessory tendons.

"With a chisel, the tibial tubercle was then fractured, leaving the patella tendon still attached to it.

"The conditions were now analogous to a complete fracture of the tubercle, and a detachment of the patella tendon from its point of pull.

"The knee was flexed, and barely a quarter of an inch separation of the tubercle from its original situation occurred. The tubercle was then replaced and held loosely in position. By traction on the isolated quadriceps it was found that the knee could be practically fully extended without any difficulty, and that about one fourth of an inch displacement of the tubercle occurred. The first pull was transmitted mainly to the patella tendon and tubercle, and when that had yielded barely one fourth of an inch, it was adequately taken by the lateral expansions of the tendon of the quadriceps. The dissection made evident the strength of these expansions and their ability to act as tendons of insertion with a detached patella tendon, and also the fact that the knee could readily be extended with the attachment of the patella tendon gone.

"We now come to lesions of the tubercle occurring during adolescence. These consist in a solution of continuity between the tubercle and the tibial shaft. They vary in severity from a complete avulsion of the tubercle to a slight separation of the epiphysis.

"**Separation of a fragment**. It would seem from the experimental dissections that the first pull in a violent contraction of the quadriceps extensor comes on the fibres of the patella tendon, and is then taken also by the lateral expansions of the tendon of the quadriceps. In the complete avulsions and fractures, as stated above, we must suppose these accessory tendons to be torn from their attachments together with the tubercle and the patella tendon.

> "It is possible, however, to have a partial separation of the tubercle and the interference with normal function be so slight that the condition is often unrecognized and the diagnosis made of a bursitis or a periostitis, or even a joint fringe.
>
> "**(1) Clinical Picture.** These lesions occur in boys at or shortly after the age of puberty, when the epiphyseal growth is most rapid and a layer of cartilage intervenes between the epiphysis and the tibial shaft. In eight of the ten cases collected the boys were between fourteen and fifteen years of age; one was thirteen and the other sixteen. The boys were all active, athletic and well-developed muscularly. The histories and clinical pictures are very similar. . . .
>
> "In the gymnasium, in running, in a football game, or in some athletic sport, the knee is 'strained'. This so-called strain is usually found on questioning to have been caused by the sudden violent extension of the leg; namely, by the strong contraction of the quadriceps. More rarely there is associated a fall on the flexed knee which would, of course, bring a sudden involuntary strain on the patella tendon, associated with trauma.
>
> "At the time of the injury there is felt acute pain in the knee referred to below the patella. There is often slight swelling, either general, or pretty definitely localised over the region of the tubercle. There is distinct tenderness at this point. The ability to use the leg is only slightly diminished, and the acute pain is soon replaced by a feeling of weakness on strong exertion. Sharp pain is present on violent extension or extreme flexion of the leg, and the patient usually consults the surgeon because of this pain, the annoying weakness and the continued localised swelling or tenderness.
>
> "The condition presents no complete loss of function, but a severe handicap to the active, athletic life which this class of patients wish to lead.
>
> "Ordinarily treatment directed toward lessening the pull of the patella tendon and restricting motion is adequate for the relief of the symptoms. . . .
>
> "**(4) Prognosis.** The prognosis with treatment has been uniformly good as to relief of pain and restoration of function."

Anterior Cruciate Ligament

TIMELINE OF ANTERIOR CRUCIATE LIGAMENT

- 170 Galen described the presence of the ligaments.
- 1850 Stark—rupture described—treated with a brace
- 1900 Battle: first surgical repair described
- 1903 Mayo Robertson reports an 8-year follow-up of a direct repair of both cruciates. The patient continued to work in a mine.
- 1913 Goetjes describes five patients he treated by direct repair.
- 1917 Hey Groves' first article decribes using tensor fascia lata threaded through a tunnel in the tibia to replace the anterior cruciate ligament.

1918 Alwyn Smith reviews the subject and announces the first failure with a synthetic graft.
1936 Willis Campbell describes the terrible triad and uses patellar tendon as a graft.
1950 O'Donaghue points out the frequency and importance of this injury in college athletes.
1972 Pivot shift test of Galway and MacIntosh
1976 John Lachman: test for cruciate instability

David MacIntosh

This Toronto orthopaedic surgeon was an expert on the injured knee before arthroscopy and magnetic resonance imaging. He invented the "over the top" repair and described the pivot shift test with Robert Galway, who trained with him, in 1972.

THE LATERAL PIVOT SHIFT: A SYMPTOM AND SIGN OF ANTERIOR CRUCIATE LIGAMENT INSTABILITY
H. R. GALWAY AND D. L. MACINTOSH, 1980

"The pivot shift is both a clinical phenomenon that gives rise to the complaint of giving way, and a physical sign that can be elicited upon examination of the injured knee.

"The pivot shift is characterised by anterior subluxation of the lateral tibial plateau on the femoral condyle as the knee approaches extension, and the spontaneous reduction of the subluxation during flexion.

"We would like to state unequivocally that the sine qua non of the lateral pivot shift phenomenon is a torn anterior cruciate ligament.

The Pivot Shift Test

"The leg is picked up at the ankle with one of the examiner's hands, and if the patient is holding the leg in extension, the knee is flexed by placing the heel of the other hand behind the fibula over the lateral head of the gastrocnemius. It is essential that the patient be completely relaxed. If relaxation cannot be obtained, then examination with the patient under anesthesia is justified when there is a high index of suspicion of an occult tear of the anterior cruciate ligament.

"As the knee is extended, the tibia is supported on the lateral side with a slight valgus strain applied to it. The femur falls backwards, as the knee approaches extension, and the tibial plateau subluxes forward. In fact, this subluxation can be slightly increased by subtly internally rotating the tibia, with the hand that is cradling the foot and ankle. A strong valgus force is placed on the knee by the upper hand. This impinges the subluxed tibial plateau against the lateral femoral condyle, jamming the 2 joint surfaces together, preventing easy reduction as the tibia is flexed on the femur. At approximately 30° of flexion, and occasionally

more, the displaced tibial plateau will suddenly reduce in a dramatic fashion. At this point, the patient will jump and exclaim, 'That's it!'

"The authors are able to reproduce a pivot shift test in the presence of anterior cruciate insufficiency in almost all instances. This holds true not only for the knee with chronic anterior cruciate insufficiency, but even more so for knees with acute injury. In fact, the authors now place more reliance on the pivot shift test in diagnosing acute anterior cruciate ligament injuries than they do on the drawer test and other tests of anterior cruciate laxity."

REPAIR OF THE CRUCIATE LIGAMENTS
BATTLE, 1898

"The patient, a married woman aged 50, was admitted to St Thomas's Hospital on July 23, 1898, and left on October 8 of that year. She was admitted for an injury to the right knee sustained during an attempt to enter a train in motion. . . . There was a curious appearance of the limb . . . complete rupture of the internal ligament . . . the crucial ligaments were ruptured."

[It was irreducible.]

"On August 5 a free incision was made across the front of the joint dividing the ligamentum patellae, and the interior of the joint exposed. [An anterior band was divided to allow reduction] . . . The crucial ligaments came into view: the anterior one had been torn away from its attachment to the femur, leaving sufficient ligamentous structure attached to admit of sutures being inserted; the posterior was not completely torn off. Silk sutures were passed to restore these ligaments, and afterwards the internal lateral ligaments and the ligamentum patellae were sutured also with silk.

"Recovery was for a time retarded by suppuration in the inner side of the wound, but it remained localised.

"The knee is apparently normal as regards its ligaments, can be flexed to a right angle, and the patient walks well."

RECONSTRUCTION OF THE CRUCIATE LIGAMENTS
E. W. HEY GROVES, 1920

"In all my cases the ligaments have been so destroyed, or torn out of their bony attachments, that direct suture would have been utterly impossible.

"In 1917 I first operated upon this condition, using the iliotibial band to replace the lost anterior crucial.

"*Anatomy and Physiology*

"It is especially necessary to emphasize the obliquity of both crucial ligaments in the sagittal plane, because it is this obliquity which gives them their most important function, viz., the checking of forward displacement of the tibia by the anterior, and of backward displacement by the posterior, ligament. There is no

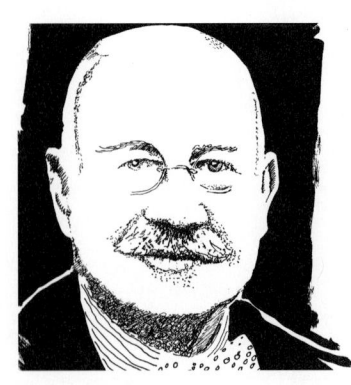

◆ Hey Groves

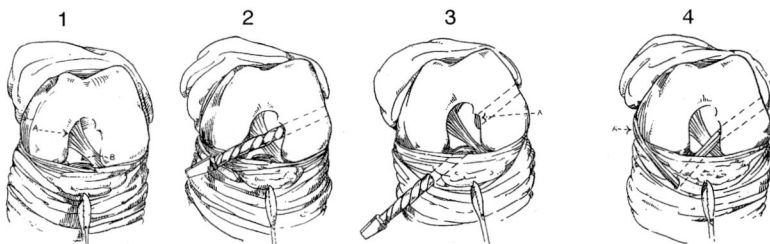

Hey Groves: Repair of the anterior cruciate ligament, 1920.

other structure in the knee-joint which serves as a check to this forward or backward displacement. The lateral ligaments have a vertical direction, and will, in the absence of the crucials, allow of the tibia being displaced forwards or backwards.

The importance of recognizing the check rein action of the crucial ligaments as being dependent upon their oblique direction, has a definite relationship to the operation proposed for their repair. Any new ligament which is used to replace them should be given this oblique direction, even in exaggerated degree....

"Symptoms of Anterior Crucial Injury

"On passive manipulation, the head of the tibia can be moved forwards on the femur. In active exercise, when the foot is put forward and the weight of the body pressed on the leg, then

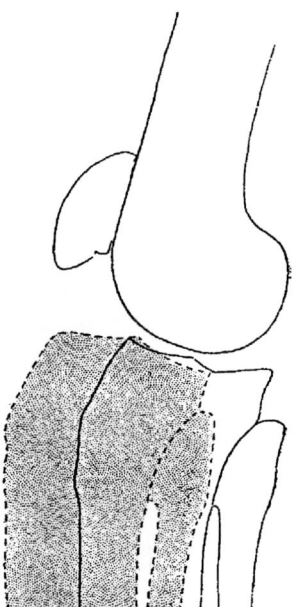

Hey Groves: Drawings constructed by the superimposition of two X-ray films, showing the extent of forward displacement of the tibia that is possible when the anterior cruciate ligament is missing, 1920.

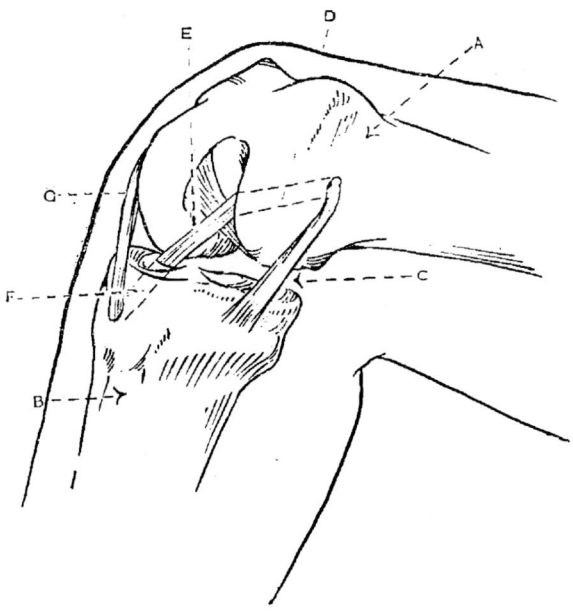

Repair of the anterior cruciate ligament.

the tibia slips forwards. Sometimes this forward slipping occurs abruptly with a jerk: often it is under the patient's control. This man could walk deliberately quite well, but if he hurried or forgot to control his knee, the subluxation would suddenly occur, giving him a sense of insecurity, or actually throwing him down.

"Symptoms of Posterior Crucial Injury

"On passive manipulation, the head of the tibia can be displaced backwards on the femur. On walking, at the end of the step when the leg is just about to be raised from the ground, the posterior displacement occurs."

[The operation was done through a large U-shaped incision. The tibial tubercle was taken off and turned up. The tensor was passed through drill holes as shown in the illustrations. After operation a cast was used for 6 weeks and then a cast brace. He could only give a few results because these were military patients.]

"Of the 14 cases operated upon, none were made worse by the operation: 4 cases showed no benefit; 4 were benefited to some degree; 4 were cured to such an extent that the men could return to active service . . . 2 were only operated on 6 months ago . . ."

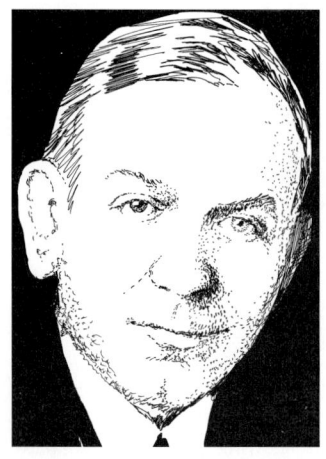

♦ Willis C. Campbell

Willis C. Campbell (1880–1941)

Campbell went to Memphis as a pediatrician/anesthetist and couldn't make a go of it, so he left and studied orthopaedics. In 1911 he founded the University Department at Memphis, Tennessee, and the Campbell Clinic, Memphis, in 1921. He was successful in many ways. In 1939 the first edition of *Operative Orthopaedics* was published, which has remained the number one reference for orthopaedic surgeons around the world.

The writing style has been one of the many reasons for its success. Operative descriptions are written in the active voice: *Begin the incision 2 inches proximal . . .* , instead of *The incision should be made . . .* or *Smith recommended that . . . .*

REPAIR OF LIGAMENTS OF THE KNEE

WILLIS C. CAMPBELL, 1936

"When there is a rupture of a ligament or undue relaxation following partial rupture, there is in most instances displacement or fracture of one of the cartilages. Impairment of the anterior crucial and mesial ligaments is associated with injuries of the internal cartilage, while impairment of the posterior crucial and lateral ligament is associated with injuries of the external semilunar cartilage."

He replaced the anterior cruciate ligament with a strip of quadriceps/patellar tendon.

Don O'Donaghue (1901–)

He was born and studied in Iowa, before moving from junior resident to chairman of the department of Orthopaedics in Oklahoma. He wrote a book on sports injuries and played a big role in making sports medicine an accepted specialty. He put an end to the practice of leaving sports injuries to the trainees for care. Lipmann Kessel was a trainee at the Royal National Orthopaedic Hospital in London when he was told that he was in charge of the Medical Services for the 1948 Olympic Games.

THE TERRIBLE TRIAD
DON O'DONAGHUE, 1950

"For many years the author has had the privilege of attending to the major injuries of a large number of athletes, not only of college, but also of high school age. None are so pleasant to treat and so eager to get back to the fray as these students. It is a problem to keep them from recovering too soon for their own good.

"Only one goal is permissible in the care of the young athlete—namely, complete recovery: for if the recovery is not complete, the patient is no longer an athlete.

"One particular injury which apparently has not received excellent, or even very good, treatment throughout the years is that injury caused primarily by abduction and external rotation of the tibia on the femur, with that unhappy triad (1) rupture of the medial collateral ligament, (2) damage to the medial meniscus, and (3) rupture of the anterior cruciate ligament."

He observed that immediate diagnosis was easier than late diagnosis and allowed repair of all structures rather than reconstruction.

"The habit of seeing Saturday's injuries on Monday is not conducive to early diagnosis and prompt definitive treatment.

"Surgery should not be reserved for those cases in which conservative treatment has failed.

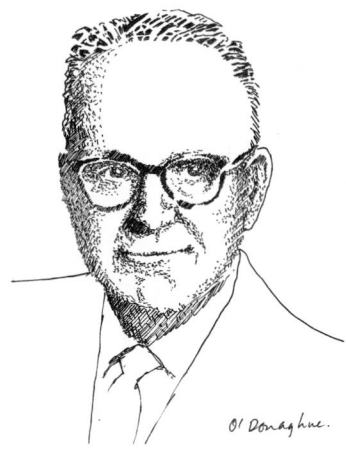

◆ Don O'Donaghue

Loose Bodies

> 1558 Paré removes a loose body from the knee of Jean Bourlier.
> 1867 Brodhust reports on 36 arthrotomies for loose bodies.
> 1888 Konig describes osteochondritis dissecans.

Deformity

> Rickets affected the majority of children until food was supplemented with vitamin D in the 1920s. Knockknee and bowleg were much commoner then than now. Furthermore, spontaneous recovery was not to be expected as it is today in children. Many children required osteotomy.
> 1853 Mayer: osteotomy for knockknee
> 1878 Macewen: in 7 years he performed 1800 osteotomies.
> 1937 Blount popularizes tibia vara.
> 1952 Langenskiold classifies tibia vara.

Walter Blount

His mother was a physician and surgeon and his father a science teacher. He studied at the University of Illinois and in Wisconsin and Europe. He wrote a travelogue in the Journal of Bone and Joint Surgery in April, 1929. He became widely known for his skills and was president of the American Academy of Orthopaedic Surgery in 1956.

He was well known for a number of important developments. In 1937 he coined the name tibia vara, which many surgeons call Blount's disease. The Milwaukee brace was devised by Dr. Blount and Dr. Albert Schmidt in 1945; it was the subject of a paper in 1958 and a book in 1973.

Blount developed hip osteotomies and wrote, *"Don't throw away the cane,"* about the mechanics of the hip. In 1949 he described epiphyseal stapling to achieve leg length equality. A big claim to fame was a book on fractures in children published in 1954. He was a charming person.

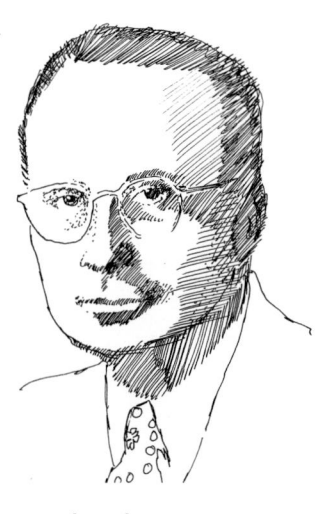

◆ Walter Blount

TIBIA VARA
W. P. BLOUNT, 1937

"1. Thirteen new cases; and fifteen from the literature illustrate the occurrence of an osteochondrosis similar to coxa plana and Madelung's deformity, but located at the medial side of the proximal tibial epiphysis.

    2. *The resulting abrupt angulation into varus with backknee and internal rotation of the leg is usually confused with rickets.*

    3. *The roentgenographic and pathological changes are like those of coxa plana and similar to those of chondrodysplasia, but quite different from those of rickets.*

    4. *The changes may appear in the first year or two of life (infantile type) as a developmental exaggeration of the normal, with sloping epiphysis and beaklike metaphysis.*

    5. *A similar deformity may occur just before puberty (adolescent type), secondary probably to local trauma or possibly to infection.*

    6. *The age at which the deformity is observed is more important than the causative factor in determining the roentgenographic appearance.*

    7. *The roentgenographic findings of the infantile type gradually change to those of the adolescent, so that the two can be distinguished later only by the history.*

    8. *Treatment should be directed toward the mechanical relief of strain until the deformity is stationary or until the epiphysis is closed.*

    9. *A simple osteotomy is desirable in the correction of marked deformity. If it is done before the amount of angulation has become stationary, some degree of recurrence may be anticipated."*

Arthritis of the Knee

> **OSTEOARTHRITIS**
>
> 1860 Verneuil begins about 100 years of largely unsuccessful interposition arthroplasty—newcomers to the field pinned their hopes on different materials.
> 1890 Themistocles Gluck: knee replacement (for infection)
> 1900 Mignon: synovectomy for posttraumatic arthritis
> 1925 Lexer achieves some impressive results with joint transplantation.
> 1932 Key invented the idea of compression arthrodesis to secure a certain fusion. Arthrodesis had been attempted since the days of White, almost a century before.
> 1941 Magnusson: debridement
> 1949 McKeever: patella prosthesis
> 1950 Majoni D'Intignano: acrylic hinge knee prosthesis
> 1953 Shiers: metal hinge prosthesis
> 1954 Moeys in Germany puts a hinge into a dog.
> 1957 Walldius hinge in acrylic, which he changed to vitallium in 1958
> 1958 Waugh realignment osteotomy. Much later Waugh wrote a wonderful biography of Charnley and a history of the British Orthopaedic Association.
> 1966 MacIntosh: tibial plateau prosthesis
> 1971 Gunston: polycentric knee replacement

Resurfacing with all kinds of materials had been used for the arthritic knee with little success. Lexer wrote a whole book in 1917 on free transplantation of joints, and he was especially proud of his knee results. Arthrodesis had been the only reliable treatment for pain—but the price was a knee that wouldn't bend. Shiers wrote from Tilbury, England, about the first hinge prosthesis for the knee. The Shiers was never satisfactory—the long stems broke, it came apart, and the load-bearing surfaces were so small that the prosthesis settled into the bone. Its faults made it the best possible start for a new generation of designs. Hemiarthroplasty was better than nothing. Charnley was too busy with the hip to think about the knee. Then Frank Gunston, a Canadian who was working with him, started to design knees and made them in his home workshop. From this beginning came a whole industry.

ARTHROPLASTY OF THE KNEE
L. G. P. SHIERS, 1954

"Indications for operation. It is merely suggested that if arthrodesis of the knee is contemplated for instability due to injury, or for pain from osteoarthritis, this method be given a trial."

He described four cases. The first formed "a solid bony coffin" around the prosthesis. The others were good at 9 years and 3 years and 3 months.

"If conclusions are to be of any value they must be definite, and one cannot draw definite conclusions from less than, say, fifty cases followed up for at least five years. However, few surgeons will ever see fifty patients requiring arthroplasty of the knee, let alone operate on them, even in five years."

References

Chapter references are located in Chapter 26.

◆ Chapter Twenty-three

The Shoulder

For years the shoulder was the forgotten joint. Ernest Codman was one of the first to start a shoulder service and devote a book to the subject. However, he confessed his interest in the shoulder only in middle age. *"I feared that if I wrote a book on this subject, my friends (competitors) would specialize me. It is far more interesting when you get up in the morning to realize that today you may remove a gall bladder, a stomach or colon, or do a circumcision in a millionaire's family, than it is to know that you will painstakingly do a fussy little shoulder operation just like the one you had done the day before, and the day before that, and the day before that."*

Famous People

Winston Churchill had a recurrent dislocation of the shoulder. The first dislocation put an end to his polo playing as a cavalry officer in Bombay. Perhaps without this he would never have entered politics.

The Birth of Wilhelm II of Germany. He was the grandson of Queen Victoria. He was found to be in a breech presentation at the last minute, and the left arm was trapped behind the head. It could not be hooked down and the head could not be delivered. The obstetrician pulled with all his strength—there was a crack. The arm came down and baby was delivered, scarcely breathing, and was resuscitated.

Only later was it realized that there was a brachial plexus palsy in addition to the fracture.

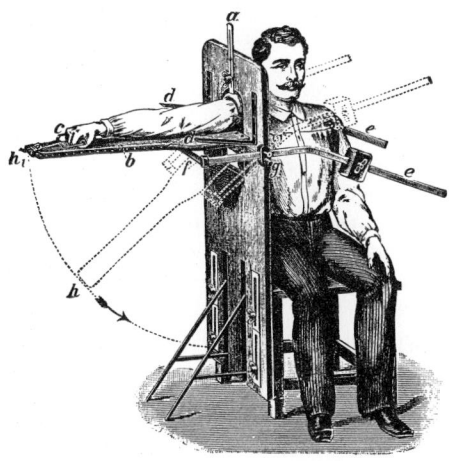

Many exercising machines were developed. This is Beely's design, in Joachimstal G (ed.). Handbuch der Orthopaedischen Chirurgie. Jena: G Fischer, 1905.

TIMELINE

Acute and Recurrent Dislocation

- 400 BC   Hippocrates: recurrent dislocation of the shoulder
- 1839   Astley Cooper describes posterior dislocation.
- 1861   Flower: bone defect in head
- 1870   Kocher reduction
- 1923   Bankart repair
- 1940   Hill-Sachs lesion
- 1948   Osmond Clarke: Putti-Platt repair

Ruptured Tendons

- 1911   Codman: rotator cuff tear
- 1931   Codman's book, *The Shoulder*

Arthroscopy

- 1972   Wiley and Older in Toronto started to use the arthroscope on cadavers and then on patients, particularly to distend the joint in frozen shoulder.
- 1978   Watanabe describes anterior and posterior portals.
- 1980   Widespread interest

Brachial Plexus Palsy

- 1768   Smellie: birth palsy
- 1872   Duchenne: brachial plexus palsy
- 1873   Erb: upper brachial palsy
- 1885   Dejerine-Klumpke: lower brachial palsy
- 1916   Sever: experimental brachial plexus palsy
- 1934   L'Episcopo transfer

High Scapula

- 1863   Eulenberg describes high scapula
- 1880–1883   Willett and Walsham described it at autopsy in an adult and later excised the omovertebral bone in a child. At the meeting it was thought that the excised bone was an analogue of a bone occurring normally in the skate. "*Mr. Willett introduced the child to the notice of the fellows. She now had little difficulty in lifting both arms straight above her head, and the left scapula was movable with tolerable freedom. Before the operation it was fixed, and the elbow could not be raised nearly as high as the shoulder.*"
- 1891   Sprengel has his name attached to high scapula.
- 1908   Putti repair
- 1957   Green repair
- 1961   Woodward repair

Replacement

- 1894   Pean shoulder replacement
- 1955   Neer prosthesis: "*The late results of 20 unimpacted fracture dislocations treated by reduction, excision of the head, or arthrodesis were found to be unsatisfactory. Replacement by a prosthesis presented a logical solution.*"
- 1973   Kessel total shoulder prosthesis

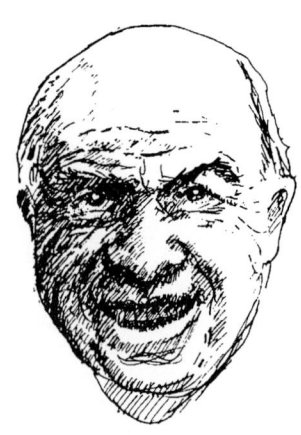

♦ Charles S. Neer, Contemporary

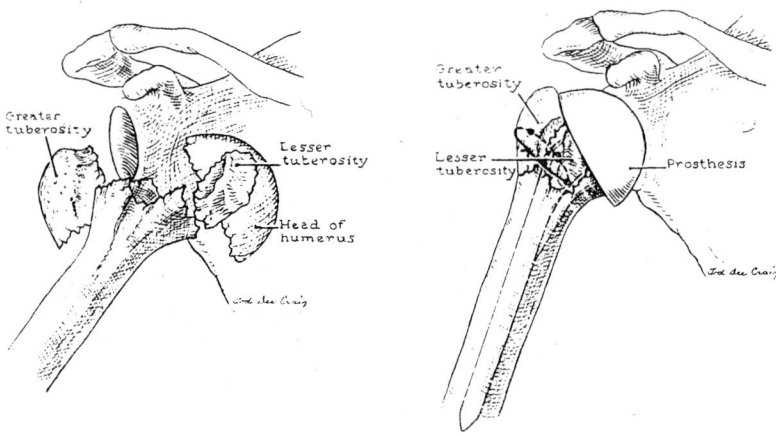

Neer's prosthesis, 1955. From Neer CS: Articular replacement for the humeral head. J Bone Jt Surg Am 1955, 37A, 217, Fig. 2A and B. Used with permission.

Original Papers

HIPPOCRATES ON RECURRENT DISLOCATION OF THE SHOULDER

"Those who are subject to frequent dislocations at the shoulder joint, are for the most part competent to effect reduction themselves; for having introduced the knuckles of the other hand into the armpit, they force the joint upwards, and bring the elbow towards the breast.

"It deserves to be known how a shoulder which is subject to frequent dislocations should be treated. For many persons, owing to this accident, have been obliged to abandon gymnastic exercises, though otherwise well qualified for therein; and from the same misfortune have become inept in warlike practices and have thus perished. And this subject deserves to be noticed because I have never known any physician treat the case properly. For many physicians have burned the shoulder subject to dislocation at the top of the shoulder, at the anterior part . . . and a little behind the top of the shoulder: these burnings, if the dislocations of the arm were upwards, or forwards, or backwards would have been properly performed; but now when the dislocation is downwards, they promote rather than prevent dislocations, for they shut out the head of the humerus from the free space above.

"The cautery should be applied thus: taking hold of the skin of the armpit, it is drawn into the line in which the head of the humerus is dislocated, and then the skin thus drawn aside is to be burnt to the opposite side. The burnings should be performed with irons. . . . When you have burnt through, it will be sufficient in most cases to make eschars only in the lower part, but if there is a considerable piece of skin between the holes, a thin spatula may be passed through the holes and the skin is let go. Then between the two eschars you should form another eschar with a slender iron, and burn through until you come in contact with the spatula.

"The following directions will enable you to determine how much skin of the armpit should be grasped—all men have glands in the armpit. The glands should not be taken hold of, nor the parts internal to the glands; for this would be attended with great danger as they are adjacent to the most important nerves. But the greater part of the substances external to the glands are to be grasped, for there is no danger from them. You should only raise the arm a little and grasp a large quantity of skin. The nerves which you ought to guard against are left within and at a distance from the operation.

"When the sores have become clean and are going on to cicatrisation, then by all means the arm is bound to the side night and day, and even when the ulcers are completely healed the arm must still be bound to the side for a long time; for thus more especially will cicatrisation take place, and the wide space into which the humerus used to escape will be contracted."

THE BANKART LESION

1923

"The head of the humerus is forced out of the joint, not by leverage, but by a direct drive from behind. In its passage forwards the head shears off the fibrous capsule of the joint from its attachment to the fibro-cartilaginous glenoid ligament. The detachment occurs over practically the whole of the anterior half of the glenoid rim. The reason why the dislocation occurs is that, whereas a rent in the fibrous capsule heals rapidly and soundly, there is no tendency whatsoever for the detached capsule to unite spontaneously with the fibrocartilage. The defect in the joint is therefore permanent, and the head of the humerus is free to move forwards over the anterior rim of the glenoid cavity on the slightest provocation."

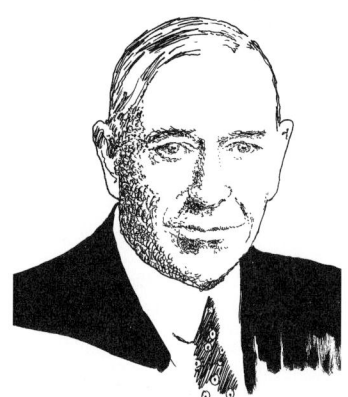

◆ **Blundell Bankart (1898–1951)**

Bankart was the first registrar at the Royal National Orthopaedic Hospital, London, England and remained there and at the Middlesex Hospital in London all his life. He believed that operating was the best part of orthopaedics. He died after operating all day, finding his car tire had a puncture, changing the tire, and driving home.

Brachial Plexus Injuries

The obstetricians are said to have been the first to observe these injuries, though I have been unable to locate Smellie's account among the hundreds of case reports that he published.

Duchenne of Boulogne introduced the subject of obstetrical palsies in 1855, and 22 years later Erb began to locate the site of the lesion by studying the pattern of paralysis. Klumpke then distinguished the different varieties of paralysis that could occur, bringing animal experiments to support her ideas of the mechanism of some of the features.

It is interesting that of the five cases Erb marshals to support his argument that brachial plexus paralyses often conform to a pattern, only one would today be called an Erb's palsy. Two of his patients appear to have had cervical spondylosis—one was a Pancoast syndrome, another is not clearly one thing or another; only his last case—included almost as an afterthought—is an Erb's palsy. It is remarkable that on the basis of these miscellaneous cases he should have accurately localized the site of a group of brachial plexus injuries, which every medical student knows as Erb's point.

I guess that Erb wrote this paper after reading the challenge that Duchenne threw out 22 years before when he described this birth injury. It explains Erb's rather obtuse title.

Duchenne described four cases of upper trunk birth palsies.

"In this kind of paralysis of the upper limb from obstetrical manipulations, the arm falls motionless along the side of the body, and is rotated inwards; the forearm remains extended, but the movements of the hand are preserved.

"I leave to others the study of the anatomical cause, and to say why in these cases the same muscles (deltoid, infraspinatus, biceps and brachialis) are always paralysed."

CONCERNING AN UNUSUAL LOCALISATION OF BRACHIAL PLEXUS PARALYSES

WILHELM ERB, 1877

"When reviewing the case histories of my material with reference to peripheral paralyses of the upper extremity there was remarkable uniformity of the muscles affected by the paralysis. The paralysis was not exclusively localised to one of the main branches of the brachial plexus but to lesser branches with the exception of the ulnar nerve. The paralyses of the various branches of the brachial plexus are sufficiently known and their effects have been sufficiently studied; however this is not true of paralyses of the individual roots which form the brachial plexus (the anterior branches of the cervical nerves).

"It would be desirable to understand the localisation and effects of the various syndromes that can occur. It must be assumed that each root is always composed of the same motor and sensory fibres; then one is in a position to determine the site of the lesion in one or other of the roots on the basis of the motor and sensory deficit."

He describes four cases to demonstrate this.

◆ CASE 1

"Konrad Sauer, 52 years old, a ropemaker. The condition had been present for 5 weeks after carrying a heavy load on his head. It began with pain and stiffness on the left side of the neck and of the left shoulder radiating down the arm to the fingers. At the same time a feeling of numbness affected the thumb and index fingers; there was such a degree of weakness of the arm that the patient could no longer lift it. On examina-

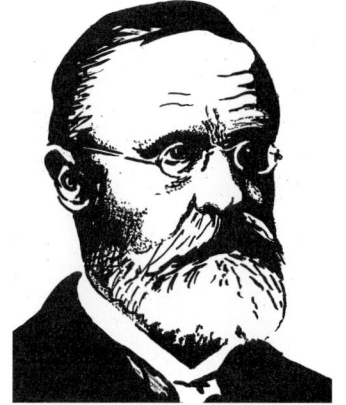

◆ Wilhelm Heinrich Erb (1840–1921)

"Erb's fame was made possible by hard work over a long period of time, with close attention to detail."

The son of a woodsman in the Black Forest, Erb studied at Heidelberg. His interest in clinical neurology developed when he worked for Friedreich. Erb was a prolific writer; on returning from his holidays, he usually produced a nice piece of work. In all he wrote 237 papers and several books, one on peripheral nerve diseases, a textbook of spinal cord disease, and another on electrotherapy. In 1880 he succeeded Friedreich at Heidelberg. He founded a journal, and was first president of the Society of German Neurologists.

Erb did much to give clinical examination of the nervous system its present form. He pointed out the significance and value of pupillary and tendon reflexes. He is remembered for his account of brachial plexus injuries.

In manner he was brusque and intense, and offended people by language unusual in academic circles; he was more respected than loved. Medical administration, education, and local politics were subsidiary interests. He died, it is said, while listening to his favorite symphony, the Beethoven Eroica.

tion there was complete paralysis of the left deltoid, biceps, brachialis, and brachioradialis. The supinator also appeared much weakened. The remaining shoulder muscles, triceps, all the forearm muscles and all the small muscles of the hand were normal.

"The sense of touch of the thumb and index finger was slightly reduced. Electrical examination revealed an incomplete reaction of degeneration. The muscles were slightly tender on palpation and atrophied during the course of the disease.

"Treatment: The patient was treated by galvanism, and was discharged cured after 7 weeks. This case was evidently a traumatic neuritis of a part of the brachial plexus."

His second case developed after a fall in which the patient's shoulder received a little of the impact. The neurologic deficit was the same as that of the first case. "Satisfactory" improvement occurred after six months.

The third case was of spontaneous onset.

The fourth case presented with the same neurologic deficit and hard supraclavicular glands. The patient died soon afterward from carcinomatosis. The fact that these four cases had a similar neurologic deficit led him to suggest that the lesion was at the same place in all.

"It is probable that the lesion in the cases mentioned was localised to the fifth or sixth cervical roots or their anterior branches or at the junction of them both."

He recalls that similar cases are found in the newborn, caused by birth injury, and were first described by Duchenne. Biceps, brachialis, deltoid, and sometimes infraspinatus muscles are paralyzed. Secondary contractures develop, giving rise to a very characteristic deformity of the arm.

"I have myself observed a case in an infant which had been delivered two months before—after a version and subsequent extraction. I found the arm rather mobile, flaccid, and lay extended by the side of the trunk, in a position of full internal rotation, the wrist and fingers were flexed and moved little. More precise observation, which is so difficult in infants, showed complete paralysis of the deltoid, biceps, brachialis, and possibly of brachio-radialis and infraspinatus. There was marked weakness of all the muscles innervated by the radial nerve. Finally there was a secondary contracture of the pectoralis major."

He thought that it was most likely that the plexus was compressed during this difficult delivery. The lesion must be high up in the neck in the region of the scalene muscles. He considered the paralysis of the infraspinatus an important clue to the localization of the lesion and one which should be carefully looked for in the future.

Klumpke's Paralysis

CONTRIBUTION TO THE STUDY OF RADICULAR PARALYSES OF THE BRACHIAL PLEXUS
1885

"The paralysis of the upper roots, generally known as Erb's palsy, is certainly the best studied and most widely recognised of all the radicular paralyses of the brachial plexus.

"At other times, however, one has to deal with a total paralysis of the upper limb in which the group of muscles affected in the Duchenne-Erb paralysis recover leaving the whole of the lower part of the arm paralysed: this is a paralysis of the lower roots of the brachial plexus.

"Then what constitutes this complete brachial plexus paralysis, which can remain the same or at a given moment can change into the upper type or become lower type? Like the upper palsy, it is produced by violent injury—a fall, after a blow on the shoulder, after a gunshot wound, or following reduction of a dislocated shoulder.

"Here the palsy affects the hand and forearm as well as the shoulder; it is flail; but while the sensory loss is slight or missing in the upper type, it is practically never absent in the combined or lower varieties. The anaesthesia is complete for the forearm and hand. In the majority of cases it extends for one or two finger-breadths above the elbow, limited there by a more or less irregular boundary. Occasionally it extends over the arm, but it is always the outer and posterior aspect up to the level of the deltoid insertion that are affected by this sensory disturbance. The skin of the inner aspect of the arm and that of the shoulder always remains unaffected, since the lesion is definitely limited to the brachial plexus. The sparing of the inner aspect of the arm is easily explained since it is innervated by the intercosto-brachial nerve and branches of the medial cutaneous nerve of the arm; the former takes its origin from perforating branches of the second and third intercostals and the latter receives anastomotic branches from the same source.

"Depending on the severity of the injury, the motor and sensory disturbances may be slight or may, on the other hand, be accompanied by the complications of serious injuries of the peripheral nerves: muscular atrophy, loss of electrical reactions, trophic changes, glossy skin, loss of sweating, cyanosis, increase or reduction of skin temperature, subcutaneous adiposity, fibrous ankylosis, etc., etc.

"There is another sign mentioned in all communications, a sign pathognomonic of lower root paralysis, a sign that is not found in complete plexus palsies which are to become the Duchenne-Erb variety: this is the oculo-pupillary phenomenon.

"This sign, which is constant in all true lower root palsies, is characterised by myosis, narrowing of the palpebral fissure, and in some cases by the eyeball retracting and becoming smaller.

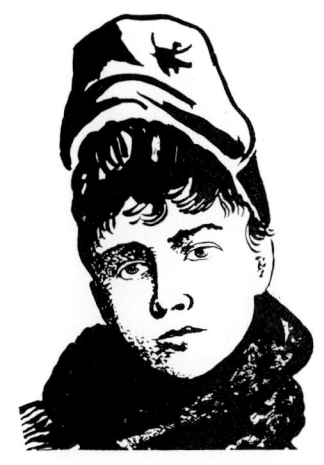

◆ **Madame Auguste Dejerine-Klumpke (1859–1927)**

Auguste Klumpke was one of the first woman doctors in Paris. While a student, she described the brachial palsy that bears her name. She must have eased the way for women who wished to follow her.

She was born in San Francisco, educated in Lausanne, and, with her sisters, arrived in Paris at the age of 18 determined to overcome the hostility that women who wished to study medicine met with at this time. Her sisters all achieved distinction; one as a musician, another as an artist, and the third as a Doctor of Science.

In her final year as a student she married Jules Dejerine, who later achieved fame as a neurologist at the Salpêtrière. Auguste helped him with his study of neuroanatomy, and when he died in 1917 founded an institute to commemorate him and allow his work to go on.

Furthermore in three cases one has noticed flattening of the cheek on the side corresponding with the paralysis."

ROTATOR CUFF TEAR
ERNEST CODMAN, 1934

"Certain conditions, symptoms and signs which indicate complete rupture of the supraspinatus tendon and which should be present within twenty-four hours after the accident:

"(1) Occupation—labor.
(2) Age—over 40.
(3) No symptoms in shoulder prior to accident.
(4) Adequate injury—usually a fall.
(5) Immediate sharp, brief pain.
(6) Severe pain on following night.
(7) Loss of power in elevation of the arm.
(8) Negative X-ray.
(9) Little, if any, restriction when stooping.
(10) Faulty scapulo-humeral rhythm.
(11) A tender point,
(12) a sulcus, and
(13) an eminence
(14) at the insertion of the supraspinatus,
(15) which cause a jog,
(16) a wince and
(17) soft crepitus as the tuberosity
(18) disappears under the acromion when the arm is elevated, and usually also, as it reappears during the descent of the arm.

"Here are eighteen conditions to be fulfilled—an especially exacting syndrome. If such a syndrome is present I do feel that not only is exploration indicated but that it should be strongly urged, for immediate suture should be a simple and successful operation. Delay means retraction of the tendon and a much more serious problem.

"I have operated on 37 cases. Two out of every three were successful in that the results enabled the patients to return to work.

"In Massachusetts the cost in compensation for this disability in an individual case is as great as from any major injury. To the man incapacitated it is a major injury. One hundred such neglected cases cost us more than the entire gross income of the average doctor during his lifetime."

References

Chapter references are located in Chapter 26.

◆
◆
◆ PART FOUR

Finale

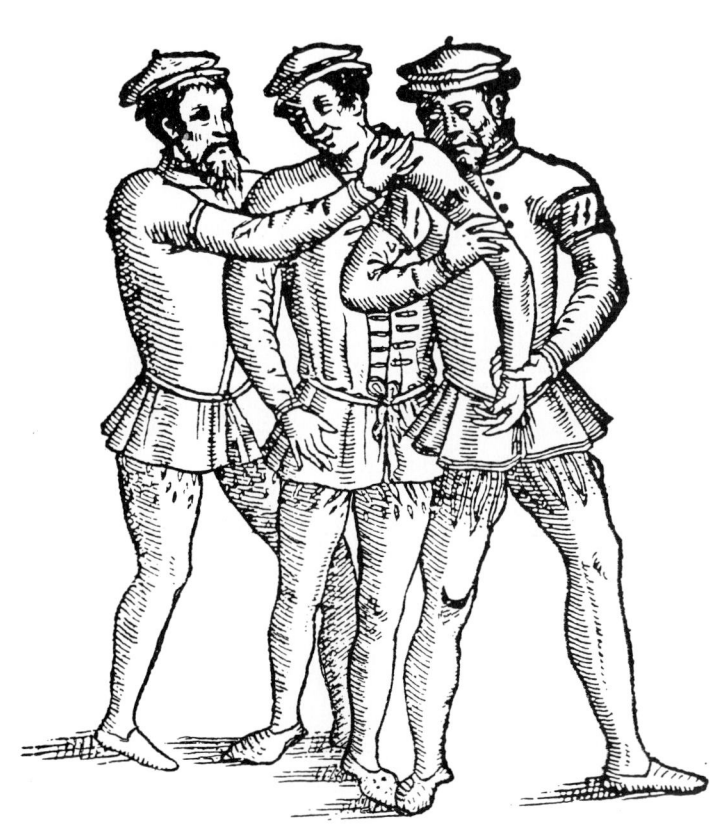

◆ Chapter Twenty-four

Hospitals and the Organization of Care

Public hospitals had better be abandoned—the frequent occurrence in them of hospital gangrene has rendered them a scourge rather than a benefit to humanity.   Poutreau, 1787

Hospitals were originally places for the poor to die. When a patient showed signs of recovery from one condition, another fatal condition took its place. If a patient was expected to recover, the first step was to leave the hospital for home and hire a doctor. People used to go to the hospital at the end of a disease—now they go at the beginning.

Some hospitals were religious institutions—perhaps because medicine was a priestly function at one time—and they aimed at providing patients with a good death, meaning that religious obligations were fulfilled.

Some hospitals were homes for the elderly.

Children's hospitals grew out of foundling hospitals—places where unwanted children were dumped. The first was Montpellier in 1181. Every city came to have a place to leave unwanted children, but these provided such bad care that most children died, creating a moral dilemma. For example, the Foundling Hospital in Dublin admitted 12,786 children during the 7-year span 1791-1797. This was about 2000 a year or about 5 a day for a small city. Of these only 135 lived—1%. An editorial of the time suggested that a banner be hung over the entrance: *Children murdered here at the public expense.*

Great Leaps Forward

The hospitals in 18th century France were terrible. They were investigated by Tenon. The revelations in his 1788 Report led the Revolutionary Government to start funding hospitals—leading to the era of the great French clinicians. Tenon called hospitals "Machines for Health."

Florence Nightingale. She was named after the Italian city of her birth. She changed hospitals forever in the English-speaking world.

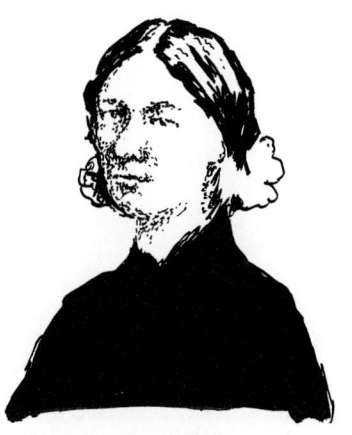

◆ Florence Nightingale

Before her, nurses had been under religious orders looking after the poor, so there was no money to put into nursing. St. Vincent de Paul and St. Louise de Marillac founded the Sisters of Charity in 1633, and this was a model for hospitals. Pastor Theodore Fliedner started a Deaconess School—the Protestant equivalent—on the Rhine, which Florence Nightingale visited. It served as her inspiration. About the same time Elizabeth Fry had created the Sisters of Charity to visit prisoners in 1848 and later changed the name to Nursing Sisters to avoid the religious connection. But to this day the head nurse in Britain is called Sister.

Florence Nightingale cleaned hospitals up. She gave the nursing staff training and status, but she was more of an administrator than a nurse. She promoted the huge ward with more than thirty beds in a single room; it was easier for a solo nurse to see what was happening everywhere, ventilation was improved, and the cost of construction was least. It is interesting that she did not believe in contagion and would have little to do with Lister. She founded her school of nursing in 1860. The original nurse's uniform was chosen by the board of directors to resemble that of a Victorian domestic servant. No wonder North American nurses threw it out.

As hospitals became larger and better organized during the hospital revolution, the number increased enormously. In the United States there were 178 in 1872, more than 4000 in 1910, and now there are 7300 in 1997.

The Origin of the Orthopaedic Hospital

We have seen that orthopaedics in its present form started with X-rays, anesthesia, and aseptic surgery a little over a hundred years ago. Before that there were gymnasium-based centers, such as Venel's in Switzerland in 1780, spa-based centers that go back to the earliest times, and bracing establishments such as the Schott brothers ran for scoliosis in the 1650s, but none of these were places for surgery. Then for the terrible 50 years between the invention of anesthesia and the invention of asepsis, a bevy of orthopaedic hospitals were founded in Europe. There was a strong spirit of entrepreneurship and breakaway to secularism.

The army hospitals and the reforms of health care were a later influence and model. The idea of huge orthopaedic hospitals in the country came about because tuberculosis of the bone and joint was common. Patients were isolated as a public health measure in a sanatorium.

The organization of a separate orthopaedic service started earlier in the United States because general surgeons were less powerful and there was a spirit of experimentation.

In the United Kingdom, Girdlestone and Jones returned from the army in 1918 and set up a military-style system for orthopaedics, using peripheral clinics, follow-up nurses, and a central unit with a nonpersonal doctor where the surgical work was done. This model focused everyone's energy and brain power and led to

In the era after World War I there were attempts to provide orthopaedic services to all. This was a successful scheme, described by Girdlestone, helped by Mrs. Hey Groves.

many advances in orthopaedics. But as orthopaedics became more complicated, this model lacked the advantages of integration and cross-fertilization from a general hospital.

Medical Insurance

In the days of Hippocrates, and through the first millennium, doctors were paid by the municipality to look after the poor. Medieval guilds provided mutual aid on payment of a subscription, and the poor were cared for by the monasteries. In Britain, Henry the Eighth abolished the monasteries, and the government later enacted the Poor Law of 1601, leading to a basic state welfare system and health service. A private system of Friendly Societies and a charity system of voluntary hospitals provided coverage for different segments of the population.

In Europe, there were many local sickness funds—families paid for stamps every week and could see the panel doctor—a forerunner of managed care.

In the United States, the first compulsory prepaid medical care program was started by the United States Congress in 1798 for merchant seamen to pay for the upkeep of hospitals. In 1847, The Massachusetts Health Insurance Company was formed, and Blue Cross had its beginnings in 1929 at Baylor.

Funding was the key to the expansion of orthopaedic services. Bismarck, Prussian Chancellor, started a welfare system for workers in 1883, and this spread through Friendly Societies to the national plans of today. Bismarck's idea was to prevent poverty due to sickness—this contrasted with the public health idea of preventing sickness due to poverty. His plan paid workers while they were sick. Since the object was to replace earnings and to produce a happier workforce, it was not available to the poor. Other countries followed: Austria in 1888, Hungary in 1891, Norway in 1909, Serbia in 1910, Britain in 1911, Russia in 1912, and later many national systems of health insurance were introduced.

In the United States, medical groups and business interests opposed these, partly because of anti-German feeling. Only when the medical costs of sickness exceeded the value of lost wages in the 1920s and 1930s did interest waken. People came to be viewed as capital—worth more well than sick or dead. Health spending made economic sense.

Funding specially allocated to orthopaedics began with military spending in World War I.

Evolution of Qualifications

There was a need for qualifications in the knowledge business that did not exist in the goods business. Buyers of a chair could see whether it was well made by looking at it, but buyers of orthopaedic information would learn too late whether it was any good. Hence orthopaedic examinations to measure knowledge. Medical education was very variable until the landmark report by

Flexner in 1910. *"For the past 25 years there has been an enormous over-production of uneducated and ill trained medical practitioners,"* he wrote. *"This has been in absolute disregard of the public welfare and without any serious thought of the interests of the public."*

Many medical schools were shut down.

LOUIS BAUER LECTURES ON ORTHOPAEDIC SURGERY
NEW YORK, 1868

"The country abounds with quacks and pretenders, who victimize and fleece the community at a fearful rate. There is no law to arrest their illegitimate invasion of the professional domain."

TIMELINE OF QUALIFICATIONS
Roman times MD and licensing of doctors
1743 Academy of Surgery in France—François La Peyronie
1745 Royal College of Surgeons, London
1934 American Boards
1990s United Kingdom Boards

Professional Organizations

The 19th century saw a rise in the status, power, and wealth of doctors. They organized and took up technology. Orthopaedics was swept up in this movement. Orthopaedic societies started, and members no longer saw themselves as general surgeons. They shared knowledge, set common goals, and generally improved the prognosis of the patient with an orthopaedic problem. When a group with a special interest gets together, the members provide the critical mass to push their subject forward.

The American Orthopaedic Association began in 1887 and is the oldest orthopaedic society in the world. It had a restricted membership because meetings were held in the home of the president. Subsequently, various traveling clubs met, with the idea of seeing famous clinics at work. In 1931, Willis Campbell thought that a group for all orthopaedic surgeons was needed. The Academy was founded in 1933 and has gone from strength to strength.

The British Orthopaedic Society was founded in 1894 and floundered 4 years later. In 1918, the British Orthopaedic Association was formed with postwar enthusiasm.

The Italian Society began in 1892, Netherlands in 1898, Germany in 1901, France in 1918, Scandinavia in 1919, Belgium in 1921, Switzerland in 1942—one of the last to break free from general surgery. This is surprising because the first orthopaedic hospital in the world was started in Switzerland.

Subspecialty societies—heralding the breakup of general orthopaedics—began with the American Society for Surgery of the

Hand in 1948, the Hip Society in 1968, and many others about this time.

Informed Consent

This is a recent idea—largely invented by lawyers as a way of getting round the difficulty of successfully prosecuting doctors for poor work.

Hippocrates wrote nothing about informed consent. In the Middle Ages a doctor's job was to give the patient hope, not to offer new causes for worry.

HENRI DE MONDEVILLE
13TH CENTURY

"Promise a cure to every patient, but tell the parents or friends if there is any danger."

JOHN WOODALL
THE SURGEON'S MATE, 1617

Advice to a surgeon preparing for an amputation.

"Let first your patient to be well informed of the imminent danger of death, prescribe him no certainty of life and let the work be done of his own free will and request and not otherwise. Let him prepare his Soul as a ready sacrifice to the Lord by earnest prayers craving mercy and help unfainedly...."

Obviously anesthesia brought about a change in ideas about consent—there must have been few patients who weren't screaming "stop" when they were having an operation without an anesthetic.

The first case in which informed consent was an issue was Slater vs. Drs. Baker and Stapleton in 1767. The doctors were expected to change the dressing on a partially healed fracture of the leg. Instead they broke it and reset it.

In 1871, Carpenter vs. Blake, there was some kind of unorthodox treatment of a dislocated elbow, and the doctor was held negligent because of lack of explanations.

AMERICAN LAW REPORTS
1932

"The general rule seems to have become well established that a surgeon must obtain consent."

FREDRICK COTTON
1933

Dr. Cotton was an early advocate of a signed written consent to operation.

"Signature of a paper stating the kind of treatment proposed, the risks involved, the necessary limitations of success, even the

chance of partial failure, seems to have no argument against it. Though rarely used it would seem as minimising the chance of honest misunderstanding."

The Good Samaritan law was introduced in the early 1960's after a woman was left unattended by several doctors on the ski slopes following an injury.

Medical Records and Outcome Studies

Records started as memory aids to guide day-to-day care and then became a way of allowing multiple people to cooperate in care. They allowed new diseases to be documented and were the basis of research. Old doctors published their case books. Records were a defense against malpractice. Only recently have standardized forms been developed to be sure that the information is complete.

Théophraste Renaudot (1584-1653) was among the first to implement this pro forma in 1642. This little booklet was designed to let the sick in the country get advice through the mail. They ticked off symptoms and marked diagrams to show where it hurt.

How is the work of a doctor or hospital measured? In the early days an occasional success was enough, and this resulted in

Summary of Eleven Cases of Secondary Excision of the Head of the Femur for Shot Injury.

[table of cases]

Condensed Summary of Two Hundred and Fifty-nine Amputations in the Leg for Disease or Miscellaneous Injuries.

[Recoveries, 1—180; Deaths, 181—258; Result undetermined, 259.]

[table of cases]

Early outcome studies. Records of the War of the Rebellion published in 1883 name the patient, name the surgeon, and describe the outcome. This would be considered unacceptable today, but what a powerful tool! The amputation specimens, surgical notes, contemporary photographs, and long-term results can be viewed at the National Museum of Medicine and Health, Washington, DC.

the testimonial approach. Then came crude mortality statistics. Pierre Louis (1787–1872) used mathematics to evaluate treatment. But this pioneer of outcome studies gave up because none of the treatments of his day were of benefit. He did show that bloodletting was harmful. As results improved, the quality of treatment was measured in the 20th century using follow-up studies that often focused on one feature, such as a radiologic angle.

Then came rating scales combining a salad of measurements. Gradually the emphasis is changing from assessment by the physician to assessment by the patient and patients comparing their quality of life with that of the general population.

Outcome studies are much in the news and were started by the eccentric Codman in about 1920. It did not endear him to his colleagues and he left the hospital.

Some of the most detailed studies are found in the history of the American Civil War. There is no attempt at confidentiality.

Ernest Amory Codman (1869–1940)

He had three professional passions in life—the shoulder, a bone sarcoma register, and the end result idea. He must have been a fascinating man. As a student on an elective in Vienna, he had been introduced to the subacromial bursa—a structure thought to have no clinical significance in Boston. He diagnosed patients with bursitis as a resident and found enough material to give a paper that attracted interest.

He graduated from Harvard in the year Roentgen discovered X-rays. He took to this and, like others, made a new discovery every week. His enthusiasm was dampened after he wrote an essay for a prize on all the new and exciting clinical uses for this technology. His essay was passed over for a boring paper on a moribund operation. His description of Codman's triangle dates from this time. Afterward he thought his rejection may have saved his life. Most X-ray pioneers died of radiation cancers.

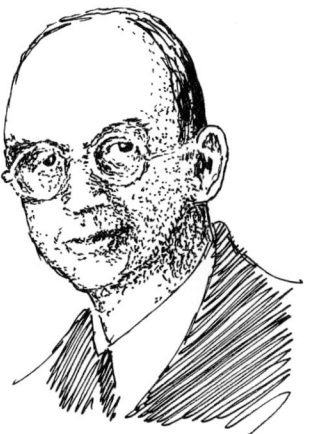

◆ Ernest Amory Codman

He became a general surgeon at Massachusetts General Hospital and took an interest in perforated duodenal ulcers but kept coming back to the shoulder. For a time he combined a clinical interest in the shoulder with the personal experience of a duodenal ulcer.

His book on the shoulder was self-published in 1934. It included operations for ruptured rotator cuff and the first description of chondroblastoma.

Another interest was the end result idea, *"which was merely the common sense notion that every hospital should follow every patient it treats, long enough to determine whether or not the treatment has been successful, and then to enquire 'if not, why not?' with a view to preventing similar failures in the future."* He started tracking his own patients in 1900 and later analyzed the results of upper abdominal operations for each surgeon at the Massachusetts General Hospital. He started his own hospital where the idea could be put to use. He gained allies when the American

College was founded and he became chair of the Hospital Standardization Committee in 1912.

Codman advocated a "Tel-U-Where System" to ensure that doctors would would know where to send patients so that they would get the best care.

Here is Codman's report of one of his campaigns for outcome studies.

"The opening gun was fired at Philadelphia on May 14, 1913. Edward Martin, by adroit advertising, gathered an enormous audience in the great ballroom of the Academy of Medicine and I spoke on "The Product of a Hospital." (Surg. Gyn. and Obst., April, 1914, pp. 491–496.) There was much that seemed very radical in this address, and the audience showed itself not only interested, but stirred. I asked and discussed such questions as these:

'For whose primary interest is it to have the hospital efficient?

'For (1) The patient who seeks relief.

(2) The public who support the hospital and in return expect [a] high standard of knowledge on the part of their own private doctor.

(3) The Hospital itself which, as an institution, has an individuality of its own.

'Who represents or acts for these interests? Strangely enough the answer is: No one; it is for the interest of no one. It is the duty of no one. For instance: For whose interest is it to investigate what is the actual result to the patient operated on? For whose interest is it to insist on the resignation of incompetent old Doctor So-and-So, who is one of the best fellows that ever lived? Who will warn the largest contributor that his agreeable classmate, Doctor So-and-So, is totally unfitted to remove his stomach? There is a difference between interest and duty. You do your duty if it is for your interest.

'Let us make attention to the medical and surgical efficiency of the hospital the duty of some one.'

"I closed the address with the following suggestions:

'That each prominent hospital in this city appoint an efficiency committee consisting of a trustee, a member of the staff, and a superintendent. That these committees inquire into the efficiency of their own Hospitals with a view to answering the questions which are sure to come from the Carnegie Foundation (which had just then agreed to help with the movement).

'That an example of this kind set by the Philadelphia Hospitals would lead to the establishment of similar committees in other cities, and eventually lead to a national organization representing the patient, the public and the individual institutions.'

"The surgeons of Pennsylvania rose to the occasion and, under the leadership of Dr. Edward Martin, set a grand example. Dr. Baldy did heroic work, and, for a time, Pennsylvania was the shining light of this new form of hospital housecleaning."

Soon afterwards Codman resigned from the Massachusetts General Hospital and ran a meeting at which he produced a huge cartoon comparing Harvard to a goose laying golden eggs for its surgeons and comparing the surgeons to an ostrich with its head in the ground as far as outcome was concerned. For a time he was in disgrace and his wife had to explain him daily to their friends. When he published his book on hospital efficiency he could not give it away.

He joined up in World War I and put his end result study to good use. He was chief surgeon with 500 beds. An orderly carried the box of cards—one card for each soldier—and he kept track of everyone. When the war was over he returned in debt to his closed hospital. "*I had patched up too many fine young men to feel much enthusiasm about keeping the aged and infirm alive, or listen with any pretense of sympathy to even the nicest lady's description of the daily behaviour of her digestion. I determined to be a money-maker until I paid off my debts, and for two years charged most of my patients three times as much as formerly.*"

He drifted into an interest in the organization of a registry of bone sarcoma because one of his best patients had a bone tumor. Codman treated about six patients in 13 years but thought bone sarcoma would be a good model for his end result idea. He charged nothing and eventually registered 1500 cases.

He believed in advertising in a curious way. If a few patients received poor treatment because their doctors did not keep track of their efficiency, the cost to the community was more than the doctors' income. He proposed that each doctor would take on a special interest and become an expert on something. He would write about it and this would advertise his skill so that wise general practitioners would know where to send their cases.

Codman had a few pithy sayings:

I am not a believer in socialism but in aristocracy.

I believe that if we worked for the general good for one day in seven, we should need no religion.

END RESULTS AND THE FOLLOW-UP IN ORTHOPAEDIC SURGERY
W. A. ROGERS, 1927

"*During the past year an End-result clinic has been held at the Massachusetts General Hospital. The plan of its organization is as follows: one Sunday morning in each month is designated as the time to report for all cases operated on during that month of the preceding years, inviting the patient to the hospital. A card is sent.*

"*The results obtained: 75% of the cases reported. Out of 532 cases operated upon, almost 400 were examined by the staff as a whole.*"

History of Statistics

The word *statistic* comes from "state." Figures were collected about trade, population, and so on, of relevance to the state.

The English Domesday Book (socioeconomic survey) started it, and by the 17th century the causes of death in towns were being recorded.

Around 1800 the word *statistics* got its contemporary meaning.

In 1788, Tenon collected statistics in Parisian hospitals. The conditions were so bad that the Revolutionary Government started to run hospitals. For example, the general mortality was 1 death in 4½ admissions at the Hôtel Dieu. There were several patients in the same bed. In 1774 this hospital received 1334 foundlings—newborns abandoned by their mothers—and 1097 were dead within a month. Only 76 were still alive 4 years later. The system that replaced this was so successful that French medicine came to lead the world.

Statistics became important for public health and were used to track down the source of cholera in Soho, London, to one particular water pump. On September 7, 1854, Dr. John Snow (a leading London anesthetist) took off the handle of the Broad Street pump and cholera left the community.

Today everyone knows that any discussion requires people to use words that have a universally accepted meaning. Diseases need classifications and definitions. This began with Linnaeus classifying plants in 1763. Just a few years later, in 1768, diseases were classified into classes and species by François Bossier de Sauvages de la Croix, and this system continued until recently.

TIMELINE

- **1662** John Gaunt: large numbers display patterns/regularities not seen in small numbers.
- **1763** Thomas Bayes' posthumous *"An essay towards solving a problem in the doctrine of chances"* becomes the basis of a Bayesian analysis—choosing management on the probability of the best outcome.
- **1785** Marquis de Condorcet: "application of mathematics to decision analysis"
- **1793** In Philadelphia, Benjamin Rush claims to cure yellow fever by bleeding and purging but does not present figures. William Cobbett, a politician, examines the mortality figures and concludes that the cure was "one of those great discoveries which have contributed to the depopulation of the earth."
- **1795** Pierre-Simon Laplace: it is possible to reason from the frequency of events to the probable cause. He invents sampling.
- *circa* **1800** Phillippe Pinel used numbers to assess treatment.
- **1801** Friedrich Gauss describes the bell-shaped normal distribution curve.
- **1809** Statistical Society of Paris founded. Others follow in the United Kingdom (1834) and United States (1839).
- **1829** Francis Bisset Hawkins' book, *Elements of Medical Statistics,* is the first book about statistics in English.

1835 Statistics about bloodletting published by Pierre Louis (1787-1872). He also correlated physical signs with pathology and founded the Society for Medical Observation.
1842 Chadwick's report on life expectancy in Britain, and in France Louis Villermé (1782-1863) used numerical methods for the mortality in different classes.
1888 Sir Francis Galton introduces the words *regression* and *correlation*.
1894 Karl Pearson introduces *standard deviation* and in 1900 the *chi squared test*.
1908 The *"Student" T test* developed by W. Gosset.
1945 Frank Wilcoxon publishes *Individual Comparisons by Ranking Methods*. Born in Ireland, he worked on insecticides in the United States.

What does Guinness have in common with an experimental farm?

William Gosset was working for the Guinness Brewery in Dublin in the early 1900s and had to investigate the effect of hops and barley from different sources on the final product. He developed a statistical test to relate the size of the sample to its reliability. Guinness had a policy of no publications for fear that it would help the competition, but allowed, for the first time, publication under a pseudonym. Gosset chose the name Student.

Sir Ronald Fisher was a mathematical genius, graduating from Cambridge in 1913. He was unfit for the war and filled a number of unsatisfying jobs until he was given a job at Rothamsted Experimental Station to study the 60-year accumulation of data on the effect of manure and weather on crop yields. From this unpromising start in farming trials, he worked out just about all that we know about the organization and analysis of clinical trials, publishing *Statistical Methods for Research Workers* in 1925 to bad reviews. He didn't stop, writing *The Design of Experiments* in 1935. He was knighted and became president of the Royal Statistical Society.

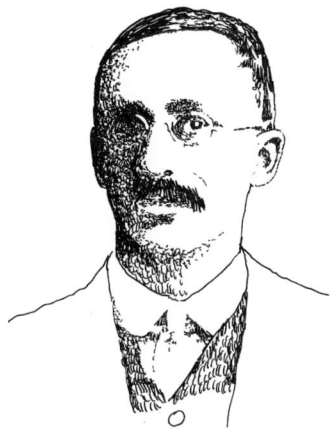

◆ William Gosset

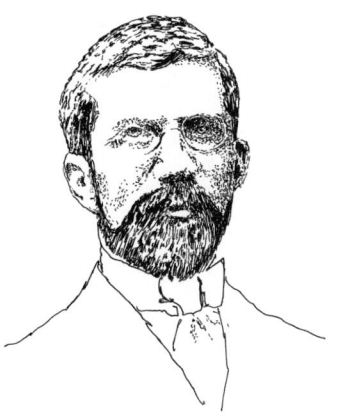

◆ Sir Ronald Aylmer Fisher

Third World

Today, only about half the population of the world benefits from all the advances in orthopaedics. The belt of poverty around the globe leaves many people without orthopaedic care. They go without housing, safety, clean water, transportation, food, and education in varying degrees as well. In some countries less than $10 a year per person is allocated to health care, compared with $1000 to $2000 in NATO countries.

Doctors went first to the Third World with explorers to treat explorers. Later they went as missionaries to trade health knowledge with the inhabitants for conversion to christianity. Many went because these were the only jobs. Later they treated the sick slaves as a way of avoiding a lost investment, making productive work possible in a bad climate and to make money for absentee landlords. This interesting evolution of motive included some scientific curiosity and desire for social justice later.

In colonial times governments provided some kind of health service and posted Europeans to the Third World. With self-government, this link was broken, and newly independent countries ran health plans with their own people and some outside help, mostly with about 1% of the per capita expenditure of the developed world. It is said that today one third of the world's population receives no health care.

In the 1950s and 1960s an orthopaedic surgeon could go to the Third World and use much the same technology as in London or Toronto. The growth of technology in the 1980s and 1990s has placed a huge gulf between the two worlds, making it difficult to wander between the two.

GROWING NUMBERS OF ORTHOPAEDIC SURGEONS (MEMBERSHIP OF THE BRITISH ORTHOPAEDIC ASSOCIATION)

Year	Members
1918	24
1923	80
1944	370
1957	698
1967	1145
1975	1060
1991	2637 (1462 associates and fellows)
1998	3289 members

Until World War I there were very few orthopaedic surgeons in Europe and America, and in the rest of the world musculoskeletal surgery was undertaken by general surgeons.

The question of orthopaedic surgeons for the developing world really came up only at the end of World War II. For the first time there were a number of orthopaedic surgeons in the developed world. The old colonial health services were giving up; new universities were starting up. Many trainees from the ex-colonies came to Europe to gain qualifications. There were a lot of challenges. Tuberculosis and leprosy had become treatable for the first time.

However, there were not a lot of orthopaedic surgeons to spare for working overseas, and there was no financial or career incentive.

In 1945, Sir Herbert Seddon suggested that the British Orthopaedic Association send staff to spend time overseas, and various schemes started—in Kano, Nigeria, in 1958, Sudan in 1962, and Burma in 1965. The Australians provided encouragement in Indonesia.

A few orthopaedic pioneers came to the fore: John Golding in Jamaica, Ron Huckstep in Uganda, Gunn in Singapore. These people achieved much more than they could have done in Britain. In

Britain the doctor treating patients had as much chance of initiating change as a fly on flypaper. The developing countries were looking for leaders, who would develop organizations and training programs.

In 1970 Ron Huckstep held a meeting at Oriel College, Oxford, which led to the formation of World Orthopaedic Concern. This started an era of volunteerism and writing grants for overseas aid money. Rotary International funded a campaign to eradicate polio by the year 2000.

In the United States, Care Medico became Orthopaedics Overseas, which has provided care to large parts of the world. Project Hope sent a ship carrying volunteer orthopaedic surgeons to ports around the world.

The emphasis was on training and start-up projects. Some of the projects have developed their own momentum, but many flounder without support.

The World Health Organization (WHO) is favoring funding of primary health care only—a return to the state of affairs many years ago.

The Trend to Day Surgery

In the past, orthopaedics was linked to long-stay care—producing huge hospital wards. The treatment of tuberculosis proceeded at glacial speed, then there was slow correction of deformities, and after operation prolonged recumbency was frequent. Often there was the feeling that this was the only way to ensure compliance with treatment. It was not uncommon for patients to marry their nurses, whom they got to know so well. How times have changed!

Yet the forces we feel today are not entirely new, as the next quotes show.

IN-PATIENT TRACTION FOR FRACTURES
JOHN DUNLOP, 1939

John Dunlop was an orthopaedic surgeon in Pasadena, California. He introduced traction in extension for children with supracondylar fractures in 1939. He believed that anatomic reduction was essential for a good result and that traction was the best way to maintain it at that time—better than sending the child home with a flexed elbow. Obviously he was contending with the same pressures as we do today because he finishes his article with these remarks:

"Do not be influenced by the parents' desire to take the child home immediately after reduction.

"Do not let the additional cost of hospitalization and frequent roentgenographic examinations influence you in your choice of method. In the end, the additional hospital expense is trivial in comparison to a deformed elbow joint for life.

"Do not be hurried in the removal of the traction in order to get the child out of hospital."

SPINA BIFIDA. ITS OPERATIVE TREATMENT AMONGST OUT-PATIENTS
J. H. NICOLL, GLASGOW, 1902

"The patient was brought to Glasgow Children's Hospital at the age of 2 months. The spina bifida appeared to be a pure meningocele.

"The tumour was excised in the outpatient clinic and the child was sent home in the care of its mother. Convalescence was uneventful. The child was nursed throughout by its mother, aided by an aunt, and instructed by the Surgical Sister, who visited the patient daily."

He concludes, *"I am conscious of a growing belief that infants of tender age operated on for these and various other surgical affections fare at least as well in the care of their mothers as in the wards of a hospital, however well conducted and efficient in the treatment of older beings."*

Prevention

The improvement of medical practice, which will become more efficacious with the progress of reason and of social order, will mean the end of infectious and hereditary diseases and illness brought on by climate, food or working conditions. Marquis of Condorcet (1743-1794)

Preventive Versus Reactive Orthopaedics

Most of us are practicing reactive orthopaedics—reacting to problems we see in the clinics. However, over the years this approach has been less successful than taking a proactive approach.

My hypothesis is that orthopaedics has been changed more by prevention strategies developed by nonorthopaedists, than by the invention of better methods of treatment by orthopaedists. Look at some examples.

Infections

Polio stimulated the fertile imagination of orthopaedists and resulted in the invention of bracing, leg lengthening, and epiphyseodesis, arthrodesis, tendon transfer.

It played a big part in establishing the specialty of orthopaedics.

All this knowledge was made redundant as far as polio was concerned, by polio vaccine. The knowledge was put to other uses.

Formerly, polio care was a large part of the work of orthopaedic surgeons. However, they did not make the crucial breakthrough.

Tuberculosis caused 25% of deaths but with pasteurization of milk, better living conditions, segregation of active cases, tracing of contacts, and most of all streptomycin, the disease has been virtually eradicated.

Osteomyelitis used to be a lifelong disease. But with improved pediatric care, septicemia is becoming infrequent. A few years ago I used to drain quite a lot of osteomyelitis abscesses and thought that early drainage was conquering the disease. I have not drained a bone abscess for a long time. It must be that children are healthier and are given antibiotics early, preventing septicemia.

Injury Prevention

Injuries used to be called "accidents," as if they were just bad luck. The change of name is a step toward understanding that they are a failure of safety behavior.

Industrial safety. Hand injuries from unguarded machines become less frequent. Safety codes are written up everywhere. Industrial insurance rates are tied to the rates of injuries in the past.

When children were pressed into factories during the Industrial Revolution, they were frequently injured until employers had to pay for the health care of children injured on the job.

Transportation injury has always been a major cause of injury—sailors drowned, horsemen were thrown, walkers were attacked. Automobiles just focused interest. Mandatory seat belts and car design have done much for safety. Speed limits reduce the severity and frequency of injury. Bike helmets reduce cycle deaths.

The rapid provision of **trauma life support** and transportation that came from the Vietnam War has been translated into paramedics, who resuscitate the injured on the spot and evacuate them quickly to reduce mortality.

There have been **lifestyle changes**—less drinking and driving—reducing road deaths.

Prevention of war. A movement to ban land mines and efforts by United Nations and organizations opposed to nuclear war have perhaps achieved more to prevent orthopaedic misery than all the orthopaedic surgeons who have ever lived. In the past, wartime deaths wiped out the pride of a generation.

Children's Diseases

Screening for developmental dysplasia of the hip and scoliosis have not succeeded in making operative treatment obsolete.

Spina bifida and cerebral palsy—these are expensive diseases for the community, and many patients never repay the costs in taxes. Prevention has had some impact.

Genetic diseases—counseling helps now, and in the future gene therapy may offer more.

Rickets used to affect up to 90% of children and is now a thing of the past due to vitamin D in milk.

The conclusion is that orthopaedic surgery owed its origins to tuberculosis, polio, osteomyelitis, rickets, malunited fractures, clubfeet, and scoliosis. Now only the last two remain in significant numbers. In the past prevention transformed orthopaedics; today joint replacement is transforming it again.

It took about 2000 years for surgeons to separate from doctors and 200 years for orthopaedic surgeons to separate orthopaedics from general surgery. It is taking 50 years for general orthopaedics to disappear into subspecialties.

Triumphalist Orthopaedics

This book, like most history books, is written in a triumphant style. Knowledge triumphs over ignorance. The good guys have one success after another. Achievements increase. Mistakes and errors are washed clean, and all is for the greater good of humanity.

But not everyone agrees. For example, the alternative medicine groups and Ivan Illich who looks at iatrogenic disease. Then there are those who say we are polluting our planet so that it will become unlivable. Often the course of orthopaedics has taken long rambles sideways before getting back on track.

But even the cynic must see that there is a lot to celebrate.

References

Chapter references are located in Chapter 26.

◆ Chapter Twenty-five

Conclusions

The great number of deformed persons of both sexes who are daily to be seen in every district of the metropolis, must surely tend to impress the public mind with the idea that distortions are incapable of being cured or prevented, or that the branch of surgery to which they belong is in a very imperfect state.   John Bishop, 1852

The Rise and Fall of Orthopaedics

Orthopaedics began as a name 250 years ago but really only became useful 100 years ago when three inventions were in place—aseptic surgery, anesthesia, and X-rays. Orthopaedics began as a subdivision of general surgery but is now bigger than general surgery. In the future, it may suffer the same fate as general surgery—fragmentation. Already in some countries residency training for children's orthopaedics is distinct from that for adult orthopaedics. Orthopaedics may disappear into subspecialties: joint replacement surgery, upper limb surgery, sports medicine, trauma care, and so on.

We may now, after 100 years, be seeing the first signs of the atrophy of general orthopaedics. Increasing control by third-party payers, domination by the medico-industrial complex, and fragmentation are changing us. It may be a good time to look back and see what has been achieved.

What Has Been the Impact of Orthopaedics on Everyday Life?

- Fewer cripples are seen in the streets here than in the Third World—partly due to living standards, social welfare, and treatment.
- Gone are the huge, long-stay orthopaedic hospitals—a change comparable to the extinction of mental hospitals. Gone are homes for crippled children.
- Many musculoskeletal diseases have almost disappeared. The major problems are no longer infection, malunited fractures, rickets, and polio. A lot of the fear of being handicapped has disappeared. Even in the 1950s, summer meant outbreaks of

polio; public swimming pools were viewed with suspicion; newspapers tracked epidemics.
- Children grow up straight; the elderly are more mobile with less arthritis.

As more and more people reach old age, the need for orthopaedic care has increased, and there are more orthopaedic surgeons than ever. Some of the emphasis has moved from tissue repair to tissue replacement. Old age talk is about golf and hip replacements instead of crutches and live-in maids.

Trauma care has gone beyond a sip of brandy and smelling salts for the injured. "Fractures," I was advised when I was starting, "are just work for surgeons who cannot build an elective practice." This is no longer the case. Fracture care has become respectable and attracts the best brains. Gone are the days when an ankle fracture made a patient unemployable for life.

What Has Been the Impact of Orthopaedic Diseases on History/Social Progress?

If orthopaedics is so important, one might expect it to have an effect beyond the individual patient. What, if any, is the group effect?

Travel and Exploration

Scurvy limited long distance travel to about three weeks—the length of time the body could store vitamin C. The vitamins made immigration and settling new lands safe.

Government

Genetic diseases affecting the musculoskeletal system had an impact on the course of history—such as

- *Russian Revolution.* The descendants of Queen Victoria in Russia carried the gene for hemophilia. One of the factors contributing to the Russian Revolution was that the Tsar was torn between looking after his hemophilic son and the Russian people. The Tsarina only made things worse because she would stop at nothing to care for her son. The ineptitude of Tsar Nicholas during the childhood of his hemophilic son led to the Russian Revolution of 1917. Perhaps without hemophilia the history of the world would have been different.

    Only recently has the question been asked: How did Victoria come to be a carrier of hemophilia, since no one in the family before Victoria had hemophilia? One possibility is that her father had a 1:50,000 random mutation. Another possibility is that she was the illegitimate daughter of a man with hemophilia. Or that some kind of baby swap took place at the time of her birth.

In the past our rulers were kings and queens; sons succeeded fathers so that genetic diseases were important. Democracy has reduced the significance of genetic disease in hereditary leaders.

- *American War of Independence.* Porphyria and George III: The gene for porphyria causes attacks of peripheral neuritis, insanity, and abdominal pain. Its presence in the British Royal Family has been tracked. Porphyria was responsible for the madness of George III, which contributed to the American War of Independence.
- *The Inquisition.* King Philip of Spain suffered from gout, and he was assured that the pain of gout was like the pains of hell promised to sinners. So when he was dealing with heretics it seemed only rational to allow them to experience the same pains as he himself had experienced.

Communism

During the Victorian era, Henry Mayhew, a journalist with the London Times interviewed London's poor and published the articles as a book, which had a huge impact. Mayhew included pictures of arthrogryposis. Karl Marx read this book, and it became a reason for trying to change the way the world worked.

Trauma and Death

Care for the injured runs contrary to the goals of war. Killing has been the military means to resolve conflict. But until about 1900, dysentery had more impact on the outcome of battles than infliction of injury because dysentery resulted from herding people together in an army. Treating the injured has been an orthopaedic obligation, but it has not swung the results of a battle. Even today orthopedic surgeons have little impact on the outcome of war.

Assassination has been used to change leadership and policy. Even here we have done little. The wounds that kill are outside our domain.

What Has Been the Impact of Social Progress on Orthopaedics?

The impact has been enormous.
Increasing general wealth has
—*made orthopaedic care accessible to many, through insurance.* All kinds of Friendly Societies have assisted in the costs of medical care for more than 100 years.

In Canada, Medicare was started in 1958 by the Premier of Saskatchewan, Tommy Douglas. When he was a poor immigrant boy, he had severe osteomyelitis of the tibia. While he was in a charity hospital awaiting amputation, a group of students from the local medical school visited him on rounds. As a result, he was taken to the teaching hospital for sequestrectomy. He healed and kept his leg. "That's the last I am having to do with charity medicine," he said, and when he became premier he was in a position to abolish charity medicine for ever; Tommy Douglas introduced universal health care.

—*provided money to do research.* One hundred years ago, research was just a hobby for the inquisitive; now it's everywhere. There were no granting agencies, as there are now.

—*increased commercialization.* For example, hip replacements and for profit hospitals. On the one hand, implants would not have attracted much development if there were no profit to be made, but on the other hand, the old simple relationship between doctor and patient has been blown apart by big business.

Now more orthopaedic surgeons are working at one time than there were in the whole of history before.

Partly this is because *everything takes longer.* In the early days, lists of twenty cases in a morning were not unusual. Osteotomies without fixation took only a few minutes. Tenotomies were quick. There were no scoliosis cases or complex ligament reconstructions. Anesthesia was basic without monitors. All the instruments were boiled up at the beginning of the day and kept sterile in one corner of the operating room, ready for use. There was no computer to occupy the circulating nurse.

There are more diseases we can treat. Backache, arthritis, and nerve compression, for example, were untreated in days gone by.

Partly there are more orthopaedic surgeons now *because we get paid.* There used to be a lot of unpaid work, or work paid in chickens—competition to get into medical school was unknown in those days. In the past, residents in training were not paid, and this limited applicants.

Orthopaedics has become more attractive. Walking around 100 beds peopled with tuberculous patients, writing up braces for impoverished children with polio, or having half the clinic space set aside to change dressings on draining sinuses would not appeal to today's generation of orthopaedic surgeons. Today there is more job satisfaction from the kind of work and the likelihood of curing patients. The intrusions of health insurers now fall on us, whereas in the past the economic controls fell on patients, keeping them from care.

Social progress has imposed **standards,** such as examinations, training requirements. In its wake come litigation and higher expectations.

What Problems Remain to Be Solved?

Uneven Distribution. There are currently about 15,000 orthopaedic surgeons in the United States and few in the Third World. The ratio of orthopaedic surgeons to patients in Equatorial

Africa is about 1 to 6 million. If this ratio were applied to the United States, there would be less than 50 orthopaedic surgeons for the whole country.

New Answers to Disease. Perhaps the biggest problem needing an answer is postmenopausal osteoporosis, the cause of so many fractures. Preventable trauma needs social answers. Spinal cord injuries must have a better answer than a wheelchair.

Bird's Eye View. We all tend to choose treatment that works for us. If the choice were dictated, there would be little progress. But it should be possible to learn more from this huge, continuing experiment. Epidemiologists have looked at regional differences and found that some operations are done more frequently in some communities than in others. Some doctors are more gung-ho than others.

What is the best treatment for a condition? Some have said that the distinguishing feature of orthopaedics is not the difficulty of making a diagnosis but the difficulty of choosing the best management. How do we do this now? How do we compare one treatment with another? New methods of care are based on studies of just a few patients. The big picture is something only occasionally studied. There is no system to enroll every patient in a study so that we learn fast. Evidence-based practice is still largely a dream. Perhaps we can learn from the business world.

Money is a value system that has been adopted by civilization to put value on diverse services and goods. We need a value system in orthopaedics to measure outcome. Is the SF 36 (a popular measure of health) the answer?

Does History Change?

When I first wrote a book about orthopaedic history 30 years ago, the topics which were important enough to discuss were different. Joint replacement results were unimpressive, and the subject was less important than arthrodesis. Arthroscopy was just a paper or two written in the twenties that led nowhere. Fracture fixation was basic. Traction was big. The whole focus has changed. History changes like everything else.

Why Study History?

It answers our curiosity about the past. It does not help make discoveries in the future or see the direction that the future will take. It does tell us that having a good idea is not enough—promotion is important. History does explain why things are as they are.

Aphorisms

Our name is really Greek for child—not Latin for foot.   Anonymous

Study principles rather than methods. A mind that grasps principles will devise its own methods. Bruce Gill, quoted by EJ Nangle: Instruments and apparatus in orthopaedic surgery. Oxford, Blackwell: 1951, p 1

All unsuccessful operations bring a certain degree of discredit on surgery. Anonymous, Med Chir Rev 1833, 18, p 237

The conditions necessary for a surgeon are four: first, he should be learned. Second, he should be expert. Third, he must be ingenious. Fourth, he should be able to adapt himself. Guy de Chauliac: Art of Surgery, Introduction. The first European book on surgery, 1363. Rightly, there is nothing here about being good with the hands.

In treating this disease, I must own myself considerably at a loss. James Latta: Practical System of Surgery, Vol 1. 1795, p 44. There are many diseases we could say the same about today, but Latta was writing about tetanus.

An operation should not only bring relief or health to the patient, but should give a glow of keen delight to the artist himself, a thrill of joy and a sense of complete satisfaction to a critical observer.

Every operation is an experiment in bacteriology. Sir Berkeley Moynihan: The ritual of a surgical operation. Br J Surg 1920-1921, 8, p 27-28

Unfortunately, to the great bulk of the people, the word orthopaedic has no conceivable meaning. Annual Report of the City Orthopaedic Hospital, London, England, 1869

I was never much attached to operative surgery, which I considered as requiring far less of intellectual accomplishments than the diagnosis of disease and treatment of it in other ways. Benjamin Brodie: Autobiography, 1865, p 89

Often it takes longer to convince the patient that he does not need a procedure than it would to post the operation and proceed with the surgery. The excuse is often given that "If I don't do it, some other surgeon will." This is the most illogical of reasons. Why should you make the other surgeon's mistakes? Harold Boyd

Do not be wedded to one method. The good surgeon, like the good golfer, has many clubs in his bag and goes to great pains to use the correct one for each shot. Harold Boyd

Adieu, Goodbye. Thank you, Dear Reader, for reaching this point.

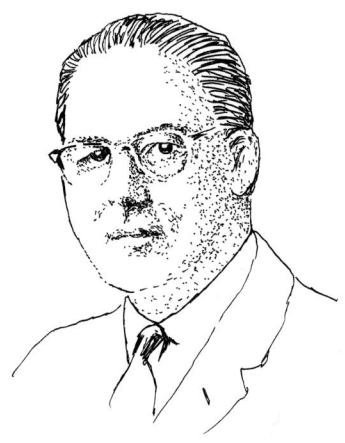

◆ **Harold Boyd (1904–1981)**

He was a master surgeon and thinker at the Campbell Clinic, Memphis, Tennessee. Of his many original papers, the one on Boyd's approach will be used the longest.

References

Chapter references are located in Chapter 26.

◆ Chapter Twenty-six

References

Finding Old References

There is no lack of history. You will find a lot of references here and in other books of orthopaedic history, such as Peltier and Le Vay. Many current articles begin with a historical review. The series "Classics" in Clinical Orthopaedics and Related Research has more than 350 classic articles, biographies, and portraits.

The *Index Medicus* began in 1879, and this is helpful, particularly for foreign language papers. The earliest purely orthopaedic list of references is by Hoffa; it is cited in the references for Chapter One. Hoffa went right back to the beginning. Blencke and then Witte brought it up to 1935. There are copies at the Wellcome Library. In 1965 the National Library of Medicine in Washington, D.C., started to publish a *Bibliography of the History of Medicine,* which has a heading for Orthopaedic Surgery and has a history of medicine database, as well as 60,000 historical images on line. A chronology of medicine can be found in F. H. Garrison's *History of Medicine,* 4th ed., Philadelphia: W. B. Saunders, 1929.

There are many libraries with large historical collections. I used those of the University of Toronto, The Academy of Medicine Collection at the Toronto Hospital, and The Royal College of Surgeons of England, as well as the Wellcome Library in London.

The references are written in this order: journal, year, volume, page. The obituaries are listed under the name of the deceased.

General Reading

A list of books about the history of orthopaedics appears in Chapter One.

Chapter One—Introduction

Sources of Quotes

Alcock T: On the disinfection of inhabited wards of hospitals, etc. London, 1827
Anonymous: Surgical use of X rays. Br J Photography Mar 20, 1896, p 180
Editorial: Fear during operations. Lancet 1836, 2, 311
Lister J: On the antiseptic principle in Surgery. Lancet 1867, 2, 353
Macfarlane RG: Russell's viper venom. Br J Haematol 1967, 13, 437
Mayer L: Orthopaedic surgery in the USA. J Bone Jt Surg Br 1950, 32B, 461 (the initial quote) (the whole issue is historically based)
Moynihan B: Br J Surg 1920, 1, 8, 27

Spencer Wells T: Some causes of excessive mortality after surgical operations. Br Med J 1864, 2, 384

References

Blencke A, Gocht H: Die orthopädische Weltliteratur 1903-1930. Stuttgart: Verlag, 1936

Chadwick Report, 1842 (life expectancy in Britain was 22 years for laborers, 30 years for tradesmen, and 43 years for the gentry)

Duraiswami PK, Tulli M: 5000 years of orthopaedics in India. Clin Orthop Rel Res 1971, 75, 269-280 (pictures of Suśruta and instruments)

Griffiths DL: Some classics of British orthopaedic literature. J Bone Jt Surg Br 1950, 32B, 676-693

Hoffa A, Blencke A: Die orthopädische Literatur. Stuttgart: Verlag, 1905

Lonsdale E: Analysis of 3000 orthopaedic cases treated. Lancet 1855, ii, 188, 218

Osmond-Clarke H: Half a century of orthopaedic progress in Great Britain. J Bone Jt Surg Br 1950, 32B, 620-675

Platt H: Orthopaedics in continental Europe. J Bone Jt Surg Br 1950, 32B, 570

Starr P: Social Transformation of American Medicine. New York: Basic Books, 1982

Webb S: The Watching of Shadows. The Origins of Radiological Tomography. Bristol: Adam Hilger, 1990 (origin of CT)

Witte E: Die orthopädische Weltliteratur 1931-1935. Stuttgart: Verlag, 1938

Chapter Two—Adult Hip

Sources of Quotes

Albee F: End result study of intracapsular non impacted fractures of the neck of the femur over the age of 60 years. J Bone Jt Surg 1930, 12, 966

Campbell WC, Orr HW, Osgood RB: Commission report of American Orthopaedic Association—End result study of intracapsular fractures of the neck of the femur. J Bone Jt Surg 1930, 12, 966

Charnley J: Arthroplasty of the hip. Lancet 1961, 1, 1129

Cooper A: Fractures and Dislocations. London: 1822, p 128

Girdlestone GR: Acute pyogenic arthritis of the hip. An operation giving free access and effective drainage. Lancet 1943, 1, 419. See also Proc R Soc Med 1945, 38, 363, a discussion of pseudarthrosis for osteoarthritis

Hey Groves EW: J Bone Jt Surg 1930, 12, 1 (on negligence)

Johansson S: On the operative treatment of medial fractures of the femoral neck. Acta Orthop Scand 1932, 3, 362

Leadbetter GW: A treatment for fracture of the neck of the femur. J Bone Jt Surg 1933, 15, 931-940

McMurray TP: Osteoarthritis of the hip. Br J Surg 1934, 22, 716

McMurray TP: Osteoarthritis of the hip. J Bone Jt Surg 1939, 21, 1-11

Moore AT, Bohlman HR: A metal hip joint. A case report. J Bone Jt Surg 1943, 25, 688

Park H, Moreau PF: Cases of the Excision of Carious Joints. Glasgow: 1806 (joint excision arthroplasty using Jeffray's chain saw to cut the bone without soft tissue damage. He also excised protruding bone in open fractures)

Pauwels F: Biomechanics of the Normal and Diseased Hip (English translation). New York: Springer-Verlag, 1976, pp 29, 271

Pean JE: Des moyens prosthetiques destines a obtentir la reparation de parties ossueses. Paris: Gaz Hôp 1894, 67, 291; On prosthetic methods intended to repair bone fragments (trans by EM Bick). Clin Orthop Rel Res 1973, 94, 4

Senn N: The treatment of fractures of the neck of the femur by immediate reduction and permanent fixation. Am Med Assoc J 1889, 13, 150-159, and Trans Am Surg Assoc 1881, 3, 1

Smith-Petersen M: Arthroplasty of the hip: a new method. J Bone Jt Surg 1939, 21, 269-288

Smith-Petersen M: Evolution of mould arthroplasty of the hip joint. J Bone Jt Surg Br 1948, 30B, 59-75

Smith-Petersen M, Cave EF, Vangorder GW: Intracapsular fractures of the neck of the femur. AMA Arch Surg 1931, 23, 715-759 (triflanged nail combined with open reduction for fractures of the neck of femur)

Thompson FR: NY Med J 1952, 52, 3011-3018 and Two and a half years' experience with a vitallium hip prosthesis. J Bone Jt Surg Am 1954, 36A, 489-500

Wescott HH: A method of internal fixation of transcervical fractures of the femur. J Bone Jt Surg 1934, 6, 372

Wiles P: The surgery of the osteoarthritic hip. Br J Surg 1958, 45, 488-497

References

Baer W: Symposium on Arthroplasty. Arthroplasty with the aid of animal membrane. Am J Orthop Surg 1918, 16, 1, 94 and 171 (reports on 100 patients using allograft interposition)

Charnley J: Anchorage of the femoral head prosthesis to the shaft of the femur. J Bone Jt Surg Br 1960, 42B, 28-30

Charnley J: Clean air. Br J Surg 1964, 51, 195

Charnley J: Acrylic Cement in Orthopaedic Surgery. Edinburgh: Livingstone, 1970

Charnley JC: Postoperative infection after total hip replacement with special reference to air contamination in the operating room. Clin Orthop Rel Res 1972, 87, 167

Charnley J: Low Friction Arthroplasty of the Hip. Theory and Practice. Berlin: Springer Verlag, 1979

Cuthbertson H: Excision of the large joints of the extremities. Philadelphia: Collins, 1876

Delbert: Bull Soc Nat Chir 1903, 24, 1172 (hip replacement)

Gluck T: Berlin, Klin Wochenschr 1890, 19, 732, and Arch Klin Chir 1891, 41, 186 and 234 (ivory replacement of upper tibia and hip). Berlin: Klin Wochenschr 1890, 27, 421 (ivory ball)

Harboush EJ: Arthroplasty of the hip based on biomechanics, photo-elasticity, fast setting acrylic cement and other considerations. Bull Hosp Jt Dis 1953, 14, 242-277

Hey Groves EW: Arthroplasty. Br J Surg 1923, 11, 234

Hey Groves EW: Some contributions to the reconstructive surgery of the hip. Br J Surg 1927, 14, 486 (replaces hip with ivory ball and stem)

Hey Groves EW: Treatment of fractured neck of femur with especial regard to results. J Bone Jt Surg 1930, 12, 1-11

Hey Groves EW: The surgical treatment of osteoarthritic hip. Br Med J 1933, 1, 3 (osteotomy to relieve pain and deformity)

Hulbert J: Biomed Mater Res 1970, 4, 433 (ceramics)

Jewett EL: One-piece angle nail for trochanteric fractures. J Bone Jt Surg 1941, 23, 803-810

Judet R, Judet J: J Chir (Paris) 1949, 65, 17-24

Judet J, Judet R, LaGrange J, Dunoyer J: Resection-reconstruction of the hip. Arthroplasty with an acrylic prosthesis. Edinburgh: Livingstone, 1954 (published in French in 1952)

Kiaer S: Experimental investigation on the tissue reactions to acrylic plastics. 5th Congress Int Chir Orthop, Stockholm, 1951. Published Brussels, 1953

Langenbeck 7th Congress Verh Dtsch Ges Chir 1878, 1, 92 (ivory pegs failed)

Malkin SAS: Femoral osteotomy in osteoarthritic hip. Br Med J 1936, 1, 304 (osteotomy to relieve pain and deformity)

Martin, King: New Orleans Med Surg J 1922, 75, 710 (see Surg Gynecol Obstet 1914, 18, 260; introduces closed fixation with nail and x-ray)

McKee GK: Artificial hip joint. J Bone Jt Surg Br 1951, 33B, 465

McKee GK: Development of total prosthetic replacement of the hip. Clin Orthop Rel Res 1970, 72, 85 (shows early prototypes)

McKee GK, Farrar JW: Replacement of arthritic hips by the McKee-Farrar prosthesis. J Bone Jt Surg Br 1966, 48B, 245

Murphy JB: Arthroplasty for ankylosed hips. Trans Am Surg Assoc 1913, 31, 67 (reprinted in Clin Orthop Rel Res 1986, 213, 4) (uses fat and fascia as an interposition for arthroplasty and goes on to use this for hip, knee, elbow, and jaw)

Ollier L: Experimental and Clinical Treatise on Regeneration of Bone (in French). Paris: Masson et Cie 1867 (studied joint repair after damage)

Pugh A: A self-adjusting nail plate for fractures about the hip joint. J Bone Jt Surg Am 1955, 37, 1085-1093 (sliding nail plate)

Senn N: Experiments on animals with hip fractures. Trans Am Surg Assoc 1883, 1, 167-170 and 333-452. Is this the longest paper ever published?

Senn N: JAMA 1889, 13, 150-159

Waugh W: John Charnley: The Man and the Hip. New York: Springer, 1990 (biography)

Whitman R: Med Rec NY 1904, 65, 441-447 (plaster is the standard)

Whitman R: J Bone Jt Surg 1925, 7, 374-391

Chapter Three—Child's Hip

Sources of Quotes

Barlow TG: Early diagnosis and treatment of congenital dislocation of the hip. J Bone Jt Surg Br 1962, 44B, 292-301

Chiari K: Medial displacement osteotomy of the pelvis. Clin Orthop Rel Res 1974, 98, 55-71

Le Damany P: La Luxation Congenitale de la Hanche. Paris: Flammarion, 1923 (trans by Dr. Andrew Howard).

Dupuytren G: Injuries and Diseases of Bone (trans by F LeGros Clark). London: New Sydenham Society, 1847, pp 174-180

Golding JSR, MacIver JE, Went LN: The bone changes in sickle cell anaemia and its genetic variants. J Bone Jt Surg Br 1959, 41B, 711

Legg AT: An obscure affection of the hip-joint. Boston Med Surg J 1910, 162, 202-204. Legg wrote several other articles: Surg Gynecol Obstet 1916, 22, 307; Am Orthop Surg 1918, 16, 448-452; the last article was in J Bone Jt Surg 1927, 9, 26-34

Muller E: (translated by EM Bick). Beitr Klin Chir 1889, 4, 137. On deflection of the femoral neck in childhood. Clin Orthop Rel Res 1966, 48, 7

Ortolani M: Paediatria 1937, 45, 129-136 and La Lussazione Congenita del'Anca (trans at Royal National Orthopaedic Hospital). Bologna: Capelli, 1937

Paré A: The Collected Works. Reprint of the 1634 English edition. New York: Milford House, 1968. Of dislocations: 16th book, p 593 (regarding slipped epiphysis)

Petit J-L: A Treatise of the Diseases of Bones (translated into English). London: 1926

Poggi A: Contribution to the radical treatment of congenital unilateral coxa-femoral dislocation (trans by J Ferrara). Bologna: 1890 and reprinted in Clin Orthop Rel Res 1974, 98, 5

Reclus Paul: Rev Med Chir 1878, p 17

Salter RB: Innominate osteotomy in the treatment of congenital dislocation and subluxation of the hip. J Bone Jt Surg Br 1961, 43B, 518

Trendelenburg F: Dtsch Med Wochenschr 1895, 21, 21-24

Verneuil A: Paralytic dislocation of the hip. 1866

Waldenström H: On necrosis of the joint cartilage by epiphyseolysis capitis femoris. Acta Chir Scand 1930, 67, 936

Watson Jones R: Spontaneous dislocation of the hip. Br J Surg 1926-1927, 14, 36

References

Adams W: Observations on the so-called congenital dislocation of the hip joint. Br Med J 1885, 2, 859

Albee F: Bone Graft Surgery. Philadelphia: WB Saunders, 1917; NY Med J 1915, 102, 433

Barlow TG: Early diagnosis and treatment of congenital dislocation of the hip. J Bone Jt Surg Br 1962, 44B, 292-301

Bouvier H: Disorders of locomotor system. 1858 Book—Leçon cliniques, Paris. Gaz Hôp 1864, 10

Brodhurst BE: St. Georges Hosp Reports 1866, 1, 217

Brown B: Boston Med Surg J 1885, 62, 541 (report on Guérin's methods) and Malgaigne commented in a report on the treatment of Jules Guérin (in French). Paris: 1848

Caillard-Biloniere AJ: Thesis. Amsterdam: 1828 (treatment of 8 year old by extension bed in a single case succeeds)

Carnochan JM: A Treatise on the Etiology, Pathology and Treatment of Congenital Dislocation of the Head of the Femur. New York: Wood, 1850

Colonna P: An arthroplastic operation for congenital dislocation of the hip. A two stage procedure. Surg Gynecol Obstet 1936, 63, 777-781

Colonna P: Arthroplasty of the hip for congenital dislocation in children. J Bone Jt Surg 1947, 29, 711 (deepened acetabulum)

Le Damany P: Life. *In* Dickson JW: Proc R Soc Med 1969, 62, 575; Z Orthop Chir 1908, 21, 129; and Rev Chir (Paris) 1910, 45, 502

Le Damany P: La Luxation Congenitale de la Hanche. Paris: 1912

Dickson FD: The shelf operation in the treatment of congenital dislocation of the hip. J Bone Jt Surg 1935, 17, 43

Dupuytren G: Mémoire sur un déplacement originel ou congénital de la tête des fémurs. Répert Gén Anat Physiol Path Clin Chir Paris 1826, 2, 82

Frejka B: Präevention der angeboren Hüftverrenkung durch Abductionspolster. Wien Med Wochenschr 1941, 91, 523-524 (pillow splint)

Ghormley RK: Use of the anterior spine and crest of the ilium in surgery of the hip joint. J Bone Jt Surg 1931, 13, 784

Gill AB: Operation for old or irreducible congenital dislocation of the hip. J Bone Jt Surg 1928, 10, 696

Gill AB: Plastic construction of an acetabulum in congenital dislocation of the hip—the shelf operation. J Bone Jt Surg 1935, 17, 48

Guérin JR: Research on congenital dislocation of the hip. Book. Paris, 1841

Hey Groves EW: Some contributions to the reconstructive surgery of the hip. Br J Surg 1927, 14, 486 (femoral shortening to assist reduction)

Hey Groves EW: The treatment of congenital dislocation of the hip-joint. *In* The Robert Jones Birthday Volume. London: Oxford University Press, 1928

Hey Groves EW: Obituary. J Bone Jt Surg 1945, 27, 340

Hilgenreiner H: Med Klin 1925, 21, 1425-1429 (line)

Hilgenreiner H: Obituary. Z Orthop Chir 1954, 84, 502

Hoffa A: Arch Klin Chir 1896, 53, 3 (open reduction)

Humbert F: reported 1835 in French: Essay and observations on the method of reduction. Bar-le-duc and Paris: 1871

Klein A, Joplin R, Reidy JA, Hanelin J: Slipped capital femoral epiphysis—Early diagnosis and treatment facilitated by "normal" roentgenogram. J Bone Jt Surg Am 1952, 34, 233-238 (Klein's line)

Koenig: Verh Dtsch Ges Chir, 20th Congress, 1891, p 75

Lorenz A: Wien Klin Wochenschr 1919, 41 (femoral osteotomy)

Lorenz A: My Life and Work. New York: Scribner's, 1936

Margary: Arch Ortop Milan 1884, 381 (deepened acetabulum)

Mustard WT: Iliopsoas transfer for weakness of the hip abductors. J Bone Jt Surg Am 1952, 34A, 647 and J Bone Jt Surg Br 1959, 41B, 289

Ortolani M: Paediatria (Naples) 1937, 45, 129

Paci A: Closed Reduction. Genoa: 1888

Palletta JB: Adversaria Chirurgica. Milan: 1783, and Exercitationes Pathologicae. Milan: 1820 (pathology in 15 day old child)

Pavlik A: Z Orthop 1958, 8, 341 (harness)

Pavlik A: Obituary. Ortop Traumatol Protezirovanie 1992, 23, 94

Pemberton PA: Pericapsular osteotomy of the ilium for the treatment of congenital subluxation and dislocation of the hip. J Bone Jt Surg Am 1965, 47A, 65-86 (pelvic osteotomy)

Perkins G: Signs by which to diagnose congenital dislocation of the hip. Lancet 1928, 1, 648

Perkins G: Obituary. J Bone Jt Surg Br 1980, 62B

Perthes G: Zbl Chir 1920, 47, 123-125

Petrie G: Obituary. J Bone Jt Surg Br 1982, 64B, 614-615

Phemister DB: Obituary. J Bone Jt Surg Am 1952, 34A, 746-747; Arch Surg 1921, 2, 221

Poggi A: Arch Ortop 1880, 7, 105 (reports open reduction and deepening of acetabulum in 12 year old girl)

Pravaz CG: Reports are presented to Academy of Science in 1838 and 1839

Pravaz CG: Bull de L'Acad 1841, 7 and book about 19 cases from Lyons, 1847

Pravaz CG: Traite theorique et pratique des luxation; 1847 commission looked at his claims

Putti V: Early treatment of congenital dislocation of the hip. J Bone Jt Surg 1929, 11, 798-809

Schanz: Münch Med Wschr 1922, 69, 930 (femoral osteotomy)

Sharrard WJW: Posterior iliopsoas transplantation in the treatment of paralytic dislocation of the hip. J Bone Jt Surg Br 1964, 46B, 426

Von Rosen S: Early diagnosis and treatment of congenital dislocation of the hip. Acta Scand Orthop 1956, 26, 136-155

Vrolik G: (1755-1859): Essai due les effets produit dans le Corps humain par la luxation congénitale et accidentelle nonréduite du fémur, Amsterdam. 1839. (Illustration of pathology of developmental dislocation of the hip)

Chapter Four—Foot

Sources of Quotes

Brown JB: Boston Med Surg J 1842, 25, 12-14 and 53

Browne D: Modern methods of treating club-foot. Br Med J 1937, 2, 570 (splints—boots and bar)

Camper P: Dissertation on the best form of shoe. London: 1781. English translation, 1861

Davies-Colley N: On contraction of the M-P joint of the great toe. Trans Clin Soc Lond 1887, 20, 165-171

Dupuytren G: Exostosis of the Ungual Phalanx; Injuries and Diseases of Bones (trans by F LeGros Clark). London: New Sydenham Society, 1847.

Flaubert G: Madame Bovary (trans by G Wall). London: Penguin Books, 1992

Harris RI, Beath T: Etiology of peroneal spastic flat foot. J Bone Jt Surg 1948, 30B, 624-634

Keller W: NY Med J 1904, 80, 741-742 and 1912, 95, 696-698

Lane A: Clin Journal Aug 7, 1895

Little WJ: Treatise on the nature of club foot. Preface. London: 1839

Morton TG: A peculiar and painful affection of the fourth MP articulation. Am J Med Sci 1876, 71, 37-45

Ryerson EW: Arthrodesing operation on the feet. J Bone Jt Surg 1923, 5, 453. Reprinted in Clin Orthop Rel Res 1977, 122, 4-9

Whitman R: Observations on 45 cases of flat foot with particular reference to etiology and treatment. Boston Med Surg J 1888, 118, 598

References

Adams W: Clubfoot, its cause, pathology and treatment. 1866 (dissects 30 clubfeet and describes talar deformity)

Brockman EP: Modern methods of treatment of clubfoot. Br Med J 1937, 2, 572-574 (describes pathology)

Browne D: The problem of Byron's lameness. Proc R Soc Med 1960, 53, 440 (describes Byron's foot based on an orthosis he wore)

Guérin J: Plaster mold. Lancet 1836, 2, 648-649

Harris RI, Beath T: John Hunter's specimen of talocalcaneal bridge. J Bone Jt Surg Br 1950, 32, 203

Kite H: The treatment of congenital clubfoot. JAMA 1932, 99, 1156 (88% treated nonoperatively)

Kite H: Principles involved in the treatment of congenital club-foot. J Bone Jt Surg 1939, 21, 595 (popularizes serial casting for clubfeet)

Lambrinudi G: New operation on dropfoot. Br J Surg 1927, 15, 193 (triple arthrodesis)

Lamy L, Weissman L: Congenital convex pes planus. J Bone Jt Surg 1939, 21, 79-91

Ogston A: A new principle of curing club-foot in severe cases in children a few years old. Br Med J 1902, 1, 1524-1526 (starts to remove ossific nucleus to avoid problem of compressing bone)

Phelps AM: Med Rec 1890, 38, 593-598 (reviews the results of 161 operations for clubfoot and illustrates a long-lever machine for forcible correction)

Ritsila VA: Talipes equinovarus and vertical talus produced experimentally in newborn rabbits. Acta Orthop Scand 1969, Suppl 121 (this article has a wealth of historic references)

Schwartz RP: Arthrodesis of subtalus and midtarsal joints of the foot. Historical review, etc. Surgery 1946, 20, 619

Sloman N: On coalitio-calcaneonavicularis. J Orthop Surg 1921, NS 3, 586

Stewart SF: Footgear: Its history, use and abuses. Clin Orthop Rel Res 1972, 88, 119-130

Tubby AH: Deformities, including diseases of the bones and joints. London: 1896 (two volumes)

Chapter Five—Hand

Sources of Quotes

Bowlby A: Injuries and Diseases of Nerves. London: Churchill, 1889, pp 127-128

Brand P: Paralytic claw hand. J Bone Jt Surg Br 1958, 40B, 618

Cline H: *In* Elliot D: The early history of contracture of the palmar fascia. J Hand Surg 1988, 13B, 246-253 and 371-378; also in Windsor J: Lancet 1834, 2, 501

Darrach W: Partial excision of the lower shaft of ulna for deformity following Colles's fracture. Ann Surg 1913, 57, 764. Reprinted in Clin Orthop Rel Res 1992, 275, 4

de Quervain F: Concerning a form of chronic teno-vaginitis (trans by D Pevsner). Korresp Bl schweiz Arz 1895, 25, 389-394

Dupuytren G: Lancet 1834, 2, 222-225

Froment J: Signe de Pouce (trans by H Rang). Presse Med 1915, 23, 409

Haighton J: An experimental inquiry concerning the reproduction of nerves. Philos Trans R Soc Lond 1795, part 1, Read 26 Feb 1795

Heberden W: Commentaries on the history and cure of diseases. London: Payne, 1802, pp 148-149

Kienbock R: Fortschr Geb Roentgenstrahlen 1910, 16, 78-103

Kienbock R: Concerning traumatic malacia of the lunate (trans by L Peltier.) Clin Orthop Rel Res 1980, 149, 4-8

Madelung O: Spontaneous anterior subluxation of the hand (trans by D Pevsner). Verh Dtsch Ges Chir 1878, 7, part 2, 259-275

Malt RA, McKahn CF: Replantation of severed arms. JAMA 1964, 189, 716 and Clin Orthop Rel Res 1978, 133, 3

Mitchell SW, Moorehouse GR, Keen WW: Gunshot wounds and other injuries of nerves. Philadelphia: Lippincott, 1864.

Omerod JA: On a peculiar numbness and paresis of the hands. St Bart's Hosp Rep 1883, 19, 17-26

Paget J: Lectures on Surgical Pathology, Vol 1. London: Longmans, 1853, p 43

Pulvertaft RG: Tendon grafts for finger flexor injuries in the fingers and thumb. J Bone Jt Surg Br 1956, 35B, 175-194

Rank BK, Wakefield AR: Surgery of the Repair as Applied to Hand Injuries, 2nd ed. Edinburgh: Livingstone, 1960

Seddon H: Surgical Disorders of the Peripheral Nerves. Edinburgh: Churchill Livingstone, 1975

Seddon H: A classification of nerve injuries. Br Med J 1942, 2, 237

Tinel J: Nerve Wounds (trans by F Rothwell). London: Balliere, 1917

References

Adamson JE, Wilson JN: The history of flexor tendon grafting. J Bone Jt Surg Am 1961, 43A, 709-716

Beck C: The Crippled Hand and Arm. Philadelphia: Lippincott, 1925

Bunnell S: Surgery of the Hand. Philadelphia: Lippincott, 1944

Carrell A: Macrotechnique for experimental replantation. Am J Med Sci 1906, 131, 297

Cooper PA: A Treatise on Dislocations. . . . London: Longman, 1822, p 524 (briefly describes contracture of palmar fascia)

Cruickshank C: Experiments on nerves. Philos Trans 1795, 85, 1777

Darrach: Ann Surg 1912, 56, 802-803 (distal radioulnar joint problems, procedure)

Duchenne G: Physiology of Motion. 1855

Elliot D: The early history of contracture of the palmar fascia (in three parts). J Hand Surg, 13B, 1988, 246-253 and 371-378

Esser: Island flaps. NY Med J 1917, 106, 264

Finochetti R: Ischemic contracture of small muscles of the hand. Boll Trabajos Soc Cir Buenos Aires 1920, 4, 31-37

Flourens MJP: Experimental Research on the Nervous System. Paris: 1824

Foerster: Münch Med Wschr 1916, 63, 283

Gelberman RH: History of microsurgery. AAOS Symposium on Microsurgery, 1977

Gratz CM: The history of tendon suture. Med J Rec 1928, 127, 156-157 and 213-215

Keith A: Menders of the Maimed. Huntington, NY: Kreiger, 1975 reprint (a wonderful chapter on nerve research)

Manske PR: Flexor tendon healing J Hand Surg 1988, 13B, 237-245 (wonderful review of old and new ideas with references)

Mason M, et al: Tendon and graft repair. Arch Surg 1932, 25, 615

Mitchell SW: Injuries of Nerves and Their Consequences. Philadelphia: 1872

Mitchell SW, Moorehouse GR, Keen WW: Gunshot Wounds and Other Injuries of Nerves. Philadelphia: Lippincott, 1864

Morrison J: Synostosis—excised the radial head. Br Med J 1892, 2, 1337

Paul of Aegina: Collected Works. London: New Sydenham Society, 1846 (ganglion)

Pfeffer GB, Gelberman RH, Boyes JH, Rydevik B: The history of carpal tunnel syndrome. J Hand Surg 1988, 13B, 28-34

Pulvertaft RG: Obituary. J Bone Jt Surg Br 1987, 69, 145

Robson M: A case of tendon grafting. Trans Clin Soc Lond 1889, 22, 289

Schulte: Trigger finger in the German Army. Boston Med Surg J 1900, 142, 226 (experiments supported division of pulley)

Seddon H: Surgical Disorders of the Peripheral Nerves. Edinburgh: Churchill Livingstone, 1975

Simmons BP, Southmayd WW, Riseborough EJ: Congenital radio-ulnar synostosis. J Hand Surg 1983, 8, 829-838 (many old references)

Stiles HJ, Forrester Brown M: Treatment of Injuries of the Peripheral Spinal Nerves. Oxford: 1922 (Maud Forrester Brown was one of the early female orthopaedic surgeons)

Waller AV: Philos Trans R Soc Lond 1850, 140, 423-429

Chapter Six—Spinal Deformity

Sources of Quotes

Adams W: Curvature of the Spine, 2nd ed. London: 1882

Anonymous: Operation for lateral curvature of the spine (myotomy). Boston Med Surg J 1841, 24, 46

Anonymous: Book review of Bauer. Boston Med Surg J 1868, 78, 139

Anonymous: Infirmary for the cure of distortions of the spine and limbs. Boston Med Surg J 1841, 24, 187-189

Anonymous: Division of muscles of the back. Boston Med Surg J 1841, 24, 273

Austin RT: Robert Chessher. First English Orthopaedist. Leicestershire County Council Libraries and Information Service, 1981

Bigg HH: Orthopaxy. London: 1865. Other books in 1880, 1882, 1905

Boni T, Ruttimann B, Dvorak J, Sandler A: Historical perspectives—Jean-Andre Venel. Spine 1994, 19, 2007-2011

Brockbank W: The crookedness clinic of Nicholas and Peter Schott Bros. J Bone Jt Surg Br 1959, 4B, 413, and Br Med J 1903, 2, 89-90

Dale PM: Medical Biographies. University of Oklahoma Press, 1952 (Catherine the Great)

Freke J: Myositis ossificans progressiva. Philos Trans 1740, 41, 369-370

Harrington PR: The treatment of scoliosis. J Bone Jt Surg Am 1962, 44, 591-610

Harrington PR: Obituary. J Bone Jt Surg Am 1981, 63, 857

Hibbs RA: A report of 59 cases of scoliosis treated by fusion operation. J Bone Jt Surg 1924, 6, 3-37

Moe J: A critical analysis of the methods of fusion for scoliosis. J Bone Jt Surg Am 1958, 40, 529

Report of Research Committee of AOA: End result study of the treatment of idiopathic scoliosis. J Bone Jt Surg 1941, 23, 963-977

Risser JC: The iliac apophysis. Clin Orthop Rel Res 1958, 11, 111

Risser JC, Fergusson AB: Scoliosis: its prognosis. J Bone Jt Surg 1936, 18, 667

Scheuermann H: Kyphosis dorsalis juvenalis (trans by Dr. Hirsch). Z Orthop Chir 1921, 51, 305-317

Schulthess W: Die Pathologie und Therapie der Ruckgratsverkrummungen. *In* Handbuch der Orthopaedischen Chirurgie (Georg Joachimstal, ed). Jena: Gustav Fischer, 1905-1907

Smith Petersen MN, Larson CB, Aufranc OL: Osteotomy of the spine. J Bone Jt Surg 1945, 27, 1-11

Stafford RA: The Stoop. The Injuries, the Diseases and Distortions of the Spine. London: Longmans, 1832

References

Brackett EH: The school in its effect upon the health of girls. Boston Med Surg J 1902, 145

Bradford EH: The seating of schoolchildren. Trans Am Orthop Assoc 1899, p 12

Cobb J: Treatment of scoliosis. Conn Med J 1943, 7, 467

Cobb J: Outline for the study of scoliosis. AAOS Instructional course. Vol 5. 1948, pp 261-275

Cobb J: Obituary. J Bone Jt Surg Am 1968, 50A, 1074

Guérin J: Gaz med Paris 1839, pp 403-404 (Guérin conflict)

Hada BE: Med Times Register 1891, 22, 423; also, Biography in Clin Orthop Rel Res 1961, 21, 32

Hibbs R: JAMA 1917, 69 (started joint excision plus cancellous graft)

Klapp B: Das Klapp'sche Kreichverfahren. Stuttgart: Georg Thieme, 1955

Lange F: Support for the spondylitic spine by means of buried steel bars, attached to the vertebrae. Am J Orthop Surg 1910, 8, 344. Also in Clin Orthop Rel Res 1986, 203, 3-6

Lovett RW: The mechanics of lateral curvature of the spine. Trans Am Orthop Assoc 1900, 13, 251 (he studied curves in a cadaver)

Malgaigne JF: J Chir (Paris) 1843, 1, 256-265 (Guérin conflict)

Paget J: Studies of old casebooks. London: Longmans, 1891, p 25

Peltier LF: Guérin versus Malgaigne: a precedent for the free criticism of scientific papers. J Orthop Res 1983, 1, 115-118

Rocyn Jones A: Biography of William Adams. J Bone Jt Surg Br 1951, 33B, 124

Sayre L: Spinal disease and spinal curvature. London: Smith Elder, 1877

Scheier H, Dvorak J, Sandler A: Historical Perspectives—Wilhelm Schulthess. Spine 1994, 19, 2239-2243

Sheldrake T: An Essay on the Various Causes and Effects of the Distorted Spine. 1773 book (he advertised as a trussmaker)

Chapter Seven—Spinal Pain

Sources of Quotes

Barr J: Lumbar disk lesions in retrospect and prospect. Clin Orthop Rel Res 1977, 129, 4

Burman M: Myeloscopy. J Bone Jt Surg 1931, 13, 695

Calvé J: A localised affection of the spine. J Bone Jt Surg 1925, 7, 41-46

Cotugno D: A treatise on the Nervous Sciatica. London: Wilkie, 1775

Dandy WE: Loose cartilage from the intervertebral disc simulating tumor of the spinal cord. Arch Surg 1929, 19, 660-672

Forst JJ: Contribution à l'ètude de la sciatique (trans by H Rang). Thèse pour la Doctorat de Médecin. Paris, No 33, 1881

Goldthwait JE: The lumbo-sacral articulation. Boston Med Surg J 1911, 164, 365-372

Middleton GS, Teacher JH: Injury to the spinal cord due to rupture of an intervertebral disc during muscular effort. N Engl J Med 1934, 211, 210-214; also Glasgow Med J 1911

Mixter WJ, Barr JS: Rupture of the IV disc with involvement of the spinal cord. N Engl J Med 1934, 211, 210

Nicholas JA, Burstein CL, Umberger CJ, Wilson PD: Management of adrenocortical insufficiency during surgery. AMA Arch Surg 1955, 71, 737–741

Neugebauer FL: A new contribution to the history and etiology of spondylolisthesis. 1882. Reprinted in London: New Sydenham Society and published in Clin Orthop Rel Res 1976, 117, 2

Putti V: Pathogenesis of sciatic pain. Lancet 1927, July 9, p 53

Smith-Petersen MN, Rogers WA: End result study of arthrodesis of the sacro-iliac joint for arthritis. J Bone Jt Surg 1926, 8, 118

Verbeist H: A radicular syndrome from developmental narrowing of the lumbar vertebral canal. J Bone Jt Surg Br 1954, 36, 230

References

Bailey P, Casamajor L: Osteoarthritis of the spine as a cause of compression of the spinal cord and the roots. J Nerv Ment Dis 1911, 38, 588–609

Bailey P, Elsberg CA: Spinal decompression. JAMA 1912, 58, 675

Brailsford JF: Br Med J 1932, 827 (relation of x-ray to pain)

Brodie B: Diseases of Joints, 5th ed. 1850, p 353

Dandy WE: Loose cartilage from intervertebral disc simulating tumor of the spinal cord. Arch Surg 1929, 19, 1660

Fagge: Trans Path Soc Lond 1877, 28, 201

Gilbert RE: The Mortal Presidency. New York: Basic Books, 1992

Jacquod S: Les Paraplegias et L'Atorie du Mouvement. Paris: Adriene Delahoye, 1864

Jenkins JA: Spondylolisthesis. Br J Surg 1936, 24, 80 (reduction of spondylolisthesis)

Kirkaldy-Willis WH, Paine KWE, Cauchoix J, McIvor G: Lumbar spinal stenosis. Clin Orthop Rel Res 1974, 99, 30

Lane A: Case of spondylisthesis associated with progressive paraplegia; Laminectomy. Lancet 1893, 1, 991 (decompresses a degenerative spondylolisthesis with relief)

Lindblom K: Diagnostic puncture of IV disks in sciatica. Acta Scand Orthop 1948, 17 suppl 4, 231

Lyons PM: A remarkable case of rapid ossification of the fibrocartilaginous tissues or pure general ankylosis. Lancet 1831, 1, 27

Parkes HL, Adson AW: Compression of the spinal cord and its roots by hypertrophic osteoarthritis. Surg Gynecol Obstet 1925, 41, 1

Peterson D, Wiese G: Chiropractic; An Illustrated History. St. Louis: Mosby, 1995

Portal A: Cours d'anatomie medicale ou elemens de l'anatomie de l'homme. Paris: Baudoin, 1803

Sachs B, Fraenckel L: Progressive ankylotic rigidity of the spine. J Nerv Ment Dis 1900, 37, 661 (early description of spinal stenosis)

Sarpyener MA: Congenital stricture. J Bone Jt Surg 1945, 27, 70

Schmorl G: Atlas of Spine in Health and Disease. 1932

Sicard, Forestier: Lipiodol myelography. Rev Neurol 1921, 37, 1264

Smith L: Enzyme dissolution of the nucleus pulposus. Nature 1963, p 198

Sumita M: Beitrage zur Lehre von de Chondrodystrophia Foetalis. Dtsch Z Chir 1910, 107, 1–110 (describes the narrow canal in achondroplasia)

Watkins MB: Postero-lateral fusion of the lumbar spine. J Bone Jt Surg Am 1953, 35A, 1014 (introduces posterolateral fusion)

Williams DH, Kenning J: Microsurgical lumbar discectomy. Preliminary report of 83 consecutive cases. Neurosurgery 1979, 4, 140

Wiltse LL, Newman PH, Macnab I: Classification of spondylolysis and spondylolisthesis. Clin Orthop Rel Res 1976, 117, 23

Chapter Eight—Cervical Spine

Sources of Quotes

Camps W: Railway Accidents. London: 1866

Collie J: Malingering and Feigned Sickness. London: Arnold, 1913

Davis AG: Injuries of the cervical spine. JAMA 1945, 127, 149

Erichsen JE: On Railway and Other Injuries of the Spine. London: Walton, 1886

Johnson JG: Compensation. New York, 1883

Klippel M, Feil A: A case of absence of cervical vertebrae. Nouv Iconogr Salpêtrière 1912, 25, 223

Klippel M, Feil A: A case of absence of cervical vertebrae with the thoracic cage rising to the base of the cranium (trans by EM Bick). Reprinted in Clin Orthop Rel Res 1975, 109, 3-8

Macnab I: AAOS Instructional Course: Acceleration injuries of the neck. J Bone Jt Surg Am 1964, 46, 1797-1799

Syme J: On compensation for Railway injuries. Lancet 1867, 1, 2-3

References

Allen CD: Neurology of cervical spondylotic myelopathy. *In* Saunders RL, Bernini PM: Cervical Spondylotic Myelopathy. Oxford: Blackwell, 1992

Brain R, Northfield D, Wilkinson M: Neurological manifestations of cervical spondylosis. Brain 1952, 75, 187-225

Gowers WR: A Manual of Diseases of the Nervous System; Diseases of the Spinal Cord and Nerves. Vol 1. Philadelphia: 1886, p 8

Jaccoud S: Étude de pathogenie et de semiotique; Les paraplegies et l'ataxie du mouvement. Paris: 1864, pp 222-223 (disc degeneration and paraplegia)

Key CA: Guys Hosp Reports 1838, 3, 17 (disc degeneration and paraplegia)

Krag MH: (A good account of C1-2 fusion technics). *In* Frymoyer JW: The Adult Spine, 2nd ed. Philadelphia: Lippincott, 1997, p 1096 on

Luschka H: Die Halbergelenke des Menschlichen Korpers. Berlin: 1858, p 144 (disc degeneration)

Lane WA: Some points in the physiology and pathology of the changes produced by pressure in the bony skeleton of the trunk and shoulder girdle. Guy's Hosp Reports 1886, 3, suppl 28, 321-434 (disc degeneration)

Leyden E: Klinik der Ruckenmarks-Krankheiten. Berlin Band 1 1874, 270-278 (disc degeneration and paraplegia)

Olliver CP: De la Moelle Epiniere et des Maladies. Paris: 1824, p 213 (disc degeneration and paraplegia)

Rokitansky C: Handbook of Pathological Anatomy. Vol 2. 1844, p 285 (disc degeneration)

Stookey B: Compression of the spinal cord due to ventral cervical chondroma. Arch Neurol Psychiatr 1928, 20, 275

Wenzel C: Uber Krankheiten am Ruckgrathe. Bamberg, 1824 (disc degeneration)

Wiltse LL: The history of spinal disorders. *In* Frymoyer JW: The Adult Spine, 2nd ed. Philadelphia: Lippincott, 1997

Chapter Nine — Infection

Sources of Quotes

Brodie BC: An account of some cases of chronic abscess of the tibia. Med-Chir Trans 1832, 17, 239

Gravenstein JS: The book shelf: Richard von Volkmann-Leander. Surg Gynecol Obstet 1962, 115, 776-778

Hippocrates: Genuine Works of Hippocrates (trans by F Adams). London: New Sydenham Society, 1849

Pott P: Remarks on that kind of palsy of the lower limbs. Chirurgical Workes of Pott. London: Wood & Innes, 1808. Also published as pamphlet in 1779

Smith T: On the acute arthritis of infants. St Bart's Hosp Reports 1874, 10, 189-204

References

Altemeier WA, Helmsworth JA: Penicillin therapy in acute osteomyelitis. Surg Gynecol Obstet 1945, 81, 138 (reports on 22 months' experience in Cincinnati in 34 patients)

Becker: Wein Med Wschr 1883, 6, 1410-1412 and Dtsch Med Wschr 1884, 10, 35 (cultures organisms from osteomyelitis)

Bonnet A: Book, Paris, 1845 (injects cadaver joints with fluid to discover what position the joint takes up and where the site of rupture lies)

Burr CW: Med News Phil 1893, 63, 539 (pathology of tuberculous cord)

Butler RW: Paraplegia in Pott's disease with especial reference to the pathology and treatment. Br J Surg 1935, 22, 738

Capener N: The evolution of lateral rachotomy. J Bone Jt Surg Br 1954, 36B, 173 (the aim of this was to decompress the cord, whereas costotransversectomy developed by Menard in 1900 and Alexander and Dott in 1946 was to drain the vertebral abscess)

Charcot J-M: Gaz Höp (Paris) 1883, 56, 483 (TB paraplegia)

Chipault A: Paris Med Moderne 1896, 11, 465 (spine fusion for TB)

Dalechamps: Chirurgie Françoise, 3rd ed. Paris: 1610 (TB paraplegia)

David JP of Paris writes description of spine tuberculosis in a book. Rouen, 1779 (see Ridlon: Boston Med Surg J 1916, 175, 3316-3338 for comment)

Eggers GWN: Hadra biography. Clin Orthop Rel Res 1961, 21, 32

Fleming A: Antiseptics and chemotherapy. Proc R Soc Med 1940, 33, 127

Gibney VP: Compression paraplegia in Pott's disease of the spine. J Nerv Ment Dis 1897, 24, 195 (pathology of TB cord)

Girdlestone GR: Tuberculosis of Bones and Joints. Oxford, 1940

Hall C: Med Phil Comment. London 1779, 6 vi 71-74 (TB paraplegia)

Hibbs RA: An operation for Pott's disease of the spine. JAMA 1912, 59, 433 (he fractured the spinous processes inferiorly to secure fusion)

Hibbs RA: Treatment of vertebral TB by fusion operation. Report of 210 cases. JAMA 1918, 71, 1372 (posterior fusion)

Hilton J: Rest and Pain. On the influence of mechanical and physiological rest in the treatment of accidents and surgical diseases. London: Bell and Daldy 1863

Hodgson AR, Stock FE: Anterior spinal fusion. A preliminary communication on the radical treatment of Pott's disease and Pott's paraplegia. Br J Surg 1956, 44, 266-275

Hodgson AR, Stock FE, Fang HSY, Ong GP: Anterior spinal fusion. The operative approach and pathological findings in 412 patients with Pott's disease of the spine. Br J Surg 1960, 48, 172

Ito H, Tsuchiya J, Asami G: A new radical operation for Pott's disease. A report of 10 cases. J Bone Jt Surg 1934, 16, 504 (starts anterior debridement and strut grafting)

Johnson RW, Hillman JW, Southwick WO: The importance of direct surgical attack upon lesions of the vertebral bodies, particularly in Pott's disease. J Bone Jt Surg Am 1953, 35, 17 (anterior surgery)

Key A: Compression arthrodesis of the knee. South Med J 1932, 25, 909

Lane A: Br Med J 1989, Oct 31 (laminectomy for TB)

Lange F: Support for the spondylitic spine by means of buried steel bars attached to the vertebrae. Am J Orthop Surg 1910, 8, 344 (uses rods to fuse spine)

Lehmann J: PAS in the treatment of tuberculosis. Lancet 1946, 251, 15 (this 1-page paper introduces PAS which revolutionized the treatment of tuberculosis—there is no connection between a paper's length and its importance)

Lexer E: Arch Klin Chir 1896, 52, 576 (experimental bone abscesses begin in metaphyses after IV injection of bacteria)

Macewen W: On surgery of the brain and spinal cord. Br Med J 1888, 2, 302 (laminectomy for TB and for posterior hemivertebra)

Menard V: Orthopédie et tuberculose chirurgicale, 1914 (Book on TB surgery)

Michaud: Paris thesis, 1871 (TB paraplegia)

Moreau PF: Observations pratiques relatives à la résection des articulations affectées de carie. Paris: Farge, 1803 (Book on joint excision)

Orr W: The treatment of osteomyelitis and other infected wounds by drainage and rest. Surg Gynecol Obstet 1927, 45, 446

Park H, Moreau PF: Cases of the Excision of Carious Joints. Glasgow: University Press, 1806 (biography of Park by Sir D'Arcy, Br J Surg 1936, 24, 205)

Rosenbach J: Dtsch Zeit Chir 1878, 10, 369-393 (experimental production of osteomyelitis)

Rosenheim S: Johns Hopkins Bull 1898, 9, 240 (pathology of TB cord)

Seddon HJ: Pott's paraplegia. Prognosis and treatment. Br J Surg 1935, 22, 769 (classification of TB paraplegia)

Senn N: Tuberculosis of the Bones and Joints. Philadelphia: F. A. Davis, 1901, p 463

Severinus: De Recondite Abscessum Natura. Naples: 1610 (TB paraplegia)

Smith N: Medical-Surgical Memoirs. Baltimore: Francis, 1831, pp 98-100 (on osteomyelitis—a good clinical description)

Sorrel E, Sorrel Dejerine C: Rev Neurol (Paris) 1923, 2, 88 and book in 1925 (classification of TB paraplegia)

Spiller WG: Johns Hopkins Hosp Bull 1898, 9, 125 (pathology of TB cord)

Starr CL: Acute haematogenous osteomyelitis. Arch Surg 1922, 4, 567 (advocates drainage of osteomyelitis)

Wilensky AO: Osteomyelitis. New York: Macmillan, 1934

Wilson JC, McKeever FM: Hematogenous acute osteomyelitis in children. J Bone Jt Surg 1936, 18, 328 (25% died with early bone surgery)

Chapter Ten—Neuromuscular Disease

Sources of Quotes

Brown C: The Story of Christie Brown. New York: Simon and Schuster Pocket Books. Reprint Ontario: Richmond Hill, 1971, pp 14-15

Duchenne G: Selections from the Clinical Works of Dr Duchenne de Boulogne (trans by GV Poore). London: New Sydenham Society, 1883

Freud S: Infantile Cerebral Palsy (trans by LA Russin). Coral Gables, Fla: University of Miami, 1968

Howell M, Ford P: The True Story of the Elephant Man. London: Allison & Busby, 1983

Little WJ: On the influence of abnormal parturition. Trans Obstet Soc London 1862, 3, 293

Mayhew H: London Labour and London Poor. 1861. Dover reprint 1968, vol 1, p 330

Monteggia GB: Istituzione chirurgiche. Milan: 1813. Translation of paragraph on p 558 in Peltier L: Orthopaedics. San Francisco: Norman Publishing, 1993

Morgagni GB: The seats and causes of diseases investigated by anatomy (trans by B Alexander). London: 1796

Smith RW: A Treatise on the Pathology, Diagnosis and Treatment of Neuroma. Dublin: Hodges, 1849

Underwood M: A Treatise on the Diseases of Children, 2nd ed. London: 1788

References

Banta JV: The orthopaedic history of spinal dysraphism—1: The early history. Dev Med Child Neurol 1996, 38, 848-854

Gowers WR: A Manual of Diseases of the Nervous System. Diseases of the Spinal Cord and Nerves. Philadelphia: 1886

Gowers W: Br Med J 1902, 2, 89

Maloney WJ: Michael Underwood: A surgeon practicing midwifery from 1764-1784. J Hist Med 1950, 5, 289-314

Miller DS, Davis EH: Shakespeare and orthopaedics. Surg Gynecol Obstet 1969, 128, 358-366

Chapter Eleven—Arthritis

Sources of Quotes

Adams R: A Treatise on Chronic Rheumatic Gout. London: Churchill, 1857

de Baillou G: New researches on articular rheumatism. 1836

Charcot JM: Lectures on diseases of the nervous system (trans by G Sigerson). London: New Sydenham Society, 1881, 2, 49-61

Marie P: Sur la spondylose rhizomelique (trans by H Rang). Rev Med 1898, 18, 285-315

Still GF: On a form of chronic joint disease in children. Med Chir Trans 1897, 80, 47-59

Strümpell A: Lehrbuch der speziellen Pathologie und Therapie der inneren Krankheiten (trans by M Rang). Leipzig: Vogel, 1884

Swanner GM: Saratoga, Queen of Spas. Utica, NY: North Country Books, 1988

Sydenham T: The Works of Sydenham (trans by RG Latham). London: New Sydenham Society, 1850

References

Adams R: A Treatise on Rheumatic Gout or Chronic Arthritis of All the Joints. London: 1857 (first to separate rheumatoid arthritis from osteoarthritis)

Applebloom T, de Boelpaepe C, Ehrich GE, Famaey JP: Rubens and the question of antiquity of rheumatoid arthritis. JAMA 1981, 245, 483

Buck G: Osteotomy for deformity due to arthritis. Med Classics 1939, 3, 800 (first clinical photograph published)

Caughey DA: The arthritis of Constantine IX. Ann Rheum Dis 1974, 33, 77-80

Christopher Columbus. . . . JAMA 1894, 27, 647

Connor B: Phil Trans 1695, 19, 21-27, published in Rheims (first account of ankylosing spondylitis)

Copeman WSC: A Short History of Gout. Berkeley: University of California Press, 1964

Copeman WSC: Historical aspects of gout. Clin Orthop Rel Res 1970, 71, 14-22

Garrod AB: Reprint from A Treatise on Gout. Clin Orthop Rel Res 1970, 71, 3-13

Ingram GIC: The history of haemophilia. J Clin Pathol 1976, 29, 469-479

Landre-Beauvais AJ: (Account of rheumatoid arthritis.) Acta Med Scand 1952, 142 (Suppl), 115

Scott JT: Historical. Copeman's Textbook of Rheumatic Disease, 6th ed. Edinburgh: Churchill-Livingstone, 1986 (lots of references)

Chapter Twelve—Tumors

Sources of Quotes

Bloodgood JC: The conservative treatment of giant-cell sarcoma. Ann Surg 1912, 56, 210-238

Boyer A: The Lectures of Boyer upon Diseases of the Bones (trans by M Farrell). Arranged into a Systematic Treatise by A. Richerand. London: 1804

Broders AC: Squamous-cell epithelioma of the lip. JAMA 1920, March 6, 656

Codman EA: The registry of cases of bone sarcoma. Surg Gynecol Obstet 1922, 34, 335-343

Codman EA: The Shoulder. Boston: 1934, p 427

Enneking WF, Spanier SS, Goodman MA: A system for surgical staging of musculoskeletal sarcoma. Clin Orthop Rel Res 1980, 153, 106-120

Ewing J: Diffuse endothelioma of bone. Proc NY Pathol Soc 1921, 21, 17

Phemister DB: Conservative surgery in the treatment of bone tumors. Surg Gynecol Obstet 1925, 40, 355-364

References

Abernethy J: Surgical Observations on Tumours. London: 1804

Berger P: Bull Soc Chir Paris 1893, 9, 656 (forequarter amputation)

Boyer A: The Lectures of Boyer upon Diseases of the Bones (trans by M Farrell). Arranged into a Systematic Treatise by A. Richerand. London: 1804

Bracegirdle B: A History of Microtechnique. Ithaca, NY, Cornell University Press, 1978

Burrows HJ: Presidential Address: Major prosthetic replacement of bone; Lessons learnt in 17 years. J Bone Jt Surg Br 1968, 50B, 225 (prosthetic replacement for tumor)

Cade S: J R Coll Surg Edin 1955, 1, 79 (radiation and amputation in survivors of osteosarcoma)

Campanacci M, Costa P: Total resection of the distal femur or proximal tibia for bone tumors. Autogenous bone grafts and arthrodesis in 24 cases. J Bone Jt Surg Br 1979, 61B, 454 (salvage surgery for malignant tumors)

Codman EA: Chapter in Keen WW: System of Surgery. 1909, 5, 1170 (Codman's triangle)

Codman EA: Bone sarcoma registry. Surg Gynecol Obstet 1922, 34, 335 and Surg Gynecol Obstet 1924, 38, 712

Codman EA: Epiphyseal chondromatous giant cell tumors of the upper end of the humerus. Surg Gynecol Obstet 1931, 52, 543-548 (chondroblastoma)

Cooper AP, Travers B: Surgical Essays. Part 1, 169. London: 1818 (classifies tumors, discusses exostoses)

Enneking WF, Shirley PD: Resection arthrodesis for malignant and potentially malignant lesions about the knee. J Bone Jt Surg Am 1977, 59, 223

Ewing J: Proc NY Pathol Soc 1921, 21, 17-24 (Ewing's tumor). Textbook of Pathology, 1919

Ferguson A: Treatment of osteogenic sarcoma. J Bone Jt Surg 1940, 22, 92 (radiation and amputation of survivors of osteosarcoma)

Girard C: Lyon Med 1894, 75, 507 (hindquarter amputation)

Gordon Taylor G: A further review of the interinnomino-abdominal operation. 11 personal cases. Br J Surg 1940, 27, 643

Gordon Taylor G, Wiles P, Patey DH, Turner-Warwick W, Monro RS: The interinnomino-abdominal operation. J Bone Jt Surg Br 1952, 34B, 14 (hindquarter amputation had a 60% mortality)

Gross S: Sarcoma of the long bones, based on a study of 165 cases. Am J Med Sci 1879, 78, 2-57, 338-377

Jaffe N: Osteogenic sarcoma. State of the art with high dose methotrexate treatment. Clin Orthop Rel Res 1976, 120, 95

Jaffe N, Frei E, Traggis D, Bishop Y: Adjuvant methotrexate and citrovorum rescue factor treatment of osteogenic sarcoma. N Engl J Med 1974, 291, 994

Kirklin BR, Moore C: Roentgenologic manifestations of giant-cell tumor. Am J Roentgenol Rad Ther 1932, 28, 145 (first paper to distinguish giant cell tumor from osteosarcoma)

Kotz R, Salzer M: Rotationplasty for childhood sarcoma of the distal part of the femur. J Bone Jt Surg Am 1982, 64A, 959

Lebert H: Book—Physiologie pathologique des recherches cliniques, experimentales, et microscopiques. Paris: J B Ballière, 1845 (used microscopy to classify tumors)

MacCarthy EF: Giant-cell tumor of bone: An historical perspective. Clin Orthop Rel Res 1980, 153, 14-25

Marcove RC, Lyden JP, Huvos AG, Bullough PB: Giant cell tumors treated by cryosurgery. J Bone Jt Surg Am 1973, 55A, 1633

McClellan G: Principles and Practice of Surgery. 1848, p 412 (forequarter amputation)

Müller starts histologic study. Book in German, 1838

Pack GT, Ariel IM: Tumours of the Somatic Soft Tissues. New York: Hoeber-Harper, 1958

Pringle JH: The interpelvic-abdominal operation. Br J Surg 1916, 4, 283 (hindquarter amputation)

Récamier JC: Research on the Treatment of Cancer by the Compression Method. Paris: Gabon, 1829 (distinguishes between primary and secondary bone tumors, coining the word metastasis)

Seddon HJ, Scales JT: A polyethylene substitute for the upper 2/3 of the shaft of the femur. Lancet 1949, 2, 795 (prosthetic replacement for cartilaginous dysplasia/tumor, which was combined with an above-knee amputation)

Salvage Surgery

Borggreve J: Femoral rotationplasty. Arch Orthop unfall Chir 1930, 28, 175-178

Clutton excises giant cell tumor of radius. Trans Clin Soc Lond 1894, 27, 86

Lexer E: Transfer of whole joints. Arch Klin Chir 1908, 86, 939 and Surg Gynecol Obstet 1925, 40, 782

Lexer E: Obituary. Plast Reconstr Surg 1962, 29, 141 and 1962, 30, 670

Linberg BE: Interscapulo-thoracic resection for malignant tumors of the shoulder joint region. J Bone Jt Surg 1928, 10, 344

Mikulicz J: Arch Klin Chir 1895, 50, 660

Moore AT, Bohlmann HR: A metal hip joint. J Bone Jt Surg 1943, 25, 688-692 (hip prosthesis for giant cell tumor)

Morris H: Editorial: Conservative surgery. Lancet 1876, 1, 440 (distal forearm resection for giant cell tumor)

Mott V: Excision of the clavicle for osteosarcoma. Am J Med Sci 1828, 3, 100 (patient died)

Sauerbruch F: Turnup plasty of distal femur. Dtsch Zeit Chir 1922, 169, 9-10
Van Nes CP: Rotationplasty for congenital defects of the femur. J Bone J Surg Br 1950, 32B, 12-16
Volkmann curettes bone tumors (Krause). Verh Dtsch Ges Chir 1889, 18, 198

Chapter Thirteen—General Bone Diseases

Sources of Quotes

Albright F, Reifenstein EC: The Parathyroid Glands and Metabolic Bone Disease. Selected Studies. Baltimore: Williams & Wilkins, 1948
Bartholomeus Anglicus, 1230: Quoted in de Mause L (ed): A History of Childhood. NJ: Aronson, 1995
Cartier J: On a strange and cruel disease. Reprinted in Major RH: Classic Descriptions of Disease, 3rd ed. Springfield, Ill: Charles C Thomas, 1948, p 587
Glisson F: De Rachitide. 1650
Glisson F, Bate G, Regemorter A: A Treatise of the Rickets (trans by P. Armin). London: Peter Cole, 1651
Jean, Sire de Joinville: *In* Major RH: Classic Descriptions of Disease, 3rd ed. Springfield, Ill: Charles C Thomas, 1948, p 586
Ollier L: Dyschondroplasia (trans by H Rang). Lyon Med 1900, 93, 23-25
Paget J: On a form of chronic inflammation of bones. Med Chir Trans 1877, 60, 37-64 and 1882, 65, 225
de Vitry J: Scurvy. *In* Major RH: Classic Descriptions of Disease, 3rd ed. Springfield, Ill: Charles C Thomas, 1948, p 585
Whistler D: The Disease of English Children. Thesis, Leyden, 1645

References

American Pediatric Society: Report on Scurvy. Boston Med Surg Soc 1898, 138, 605
Barlow T: Med Surg Trans 1883, 6, 159-219 (distinguishes between acute scurvy and acute rickets)
Barlow T: Obituary. Lancet 1945, 1, 131
Bodin W, Hershey B: The World of Midgets. London: Jarrolds, 1935
Escherich T: Compt Rendu du 12 congre Int Med 1899, 3, section 6 (in Vienna: 97% of infants aged 9-15 months have rickets)
Goldthwait JE: Boston Med Surg J 1889, 71, 336 (osteotomy)
Hess A: Rickets. Philadelphia: 1929 (75% of children in New York have rickets)
Hess A, Unger LJ: Prophylactic therapy for rickets in a negro community. JAMA 1917, 69, 1583-1586 (rickets affected 90% of children in New York; they set up rickets clinics and describe prevention with cod liver oil or by ultraviolet radiation)
Lind J: A Treatise on Scurvy. Edinburgh: Sands, Murray and Cochran, 1753
Macewen W: Osteotomy with an Inquiry into the Etiology and Pathology of Knock Knee, etc. London: 1880
McCollum EV et al: Studies on experimental rickets 21. J Biol Chem 1922, 53, 293 (vitamin D identified)
McCune: Am J Dis Child 1949, 112-113 (vitamin D-resistant rickets)
Morse JL: The frequency of rickets in Boston and vicinity. JAMA 1900, 34, 724-726 (80% of infants under 2 years have rickets in Boston)
Parsons LJ: Scurvy treated with ascorbic acid. Proc Soc Med 1933, 23, 1533 (uses ascorbic acid for scurvy with success; 350 mg was all it took in a 9 month old girl. A half-page paper that transformed the world)
Parsons LG: Biography. J Pediatr 1956, 48
Rocyn Jones A: Francis Glisson biography. J Bone Jt Surg Br 1950, 32B, 425-428
Roddis LH: James Lind, founder of nautical medicine. London: Heinemann, 1951
Szent-Gyorgi A: Biochem J 1928, 22, 1387-1409 (ascorbic acid synthesized)
Volkmann AW: Edinburgh Med Surg J 1875, 10, 740 (osteotomy)

Syndromes

Apert E: Bull Mem Soc Med Hôp Paris 1906, 23, 1310-1330
Archard EC: Bull Mem Soc Med Hôp Paris 1902, 19, 834-840

Cooperman EM: Marfan's and Sherlock Holmes. Can Med Assoc J 1975, 112, 423 (a villain appears to have this condition)
Danlos H: Bull Soc Fr Derm Syph 1908, 19, 70-72
Down JLH: Lond Hosp Reports 1866, 3, 250
Ehlers E: Derm Zschr 1901, 8, 173-175
Klippel M, Feil A: A case of absence of cervical vertebrae with the thoracic cage rising to the base of the cranium (translated by EM Bick). Reprinted in Clin Orthop 1975, 109, 3-8
Klippel M, Trenaunay P: Arch Gen Med 1900 (series 9), 3, 641-672
Larsen LJ, Schottstaedt ER, Bost FC: J Pediatr 1950, 37, 574-581
Mafucci A: Movimento Med Chir Nap 1881, 3, 399-412 and 565-575
Marfan A: Bull Mem Soc Med Hôp Paris 1896, 13, 220-226
Ollier L: Lyon Med 1900, 93, 23-25
Otto AW: A human monster with inwardly curved extremities (trans from Latin by BA Victor). Reprinted in Clin Orthop Rel Res 1985, 194, 4-5 (arthrogryposis)
Petit JL: Mem Acad R Sci Paris 1773, p 17 (absent radius)
Poland A: Guys Hosp Reports 1841, 6, 191-193
Quan L, Smith DW: The VATER association. J Pediatr 1973, 82, 104-107
Von Recklinghausen F: Reprinted in Adv Neurol 1981, 29, 259-275

Chapter Fourteen— Amputations and Prostheses

Sources of Quotes

Ellis H: Surgical Case Histories of the Past. London: RSM Press, 1994, pp 90-96 (Admiral Nelson)
Melville H: Whitejacket. 1850
Pirogoff N: Resection of bones and joints and amputations and disarticulation of joints (trans by TI Malinen). Reprinted in Clin Orthop Rel Res 1991, 266, 3
Syme J: Amputation at the Ankle. Observations in Clinical Surgery, 2nd ed. Edinburgh: 1862
Weiss M: Myoplastic amputation, immediate prosthesis, and early ambulation. Washington, National Institutes of Health, undated

References

Epstein S: Art history and the crutch. Ann Med Hist 1937, 9, 304
Girard: Cong Franc Chir 1895, 9, 823 (hindquarter amputation)
Jaboulay: Lyon Med 1894, 75, 507 (hindquarter amputation)
Pirogov N: Questions of Life: Diary of an Old Physician. Canton, Mass: Science History Publications, 1991. (very thick)
Smith N: Am Med Rev 1825, 2, 370 (through-knee amputation)
Stokes: Med Chir Trans 1870, 53, 175
Velpeau: Arch Gen Med 1830, 84, 44 (through-knee amputation)

Chapter Fifteen—Orthopaedic Treatment Methods

Sources of Quotes

Albert E: Some cases of artificially produced ankyloses in paralysed limbs (trans by D Pevsner). Wien Med Presse 1882, 23, 725
Barton JR: On the treatment of ankylosis. North Am Med Surg J 1827, 3, 279-292, 400
Barton JR: Corrective osteotomy. Am J Med Sci 1837, 21, 332-340
Esmarch JFA: On the artificial emptying of blood vessels. German clinical lectures selected by Volkmann. London: New Sydenham Society, 1876
Jones R: Arthrodesis and tendon transplantation. Br Med J 1908, 1, 728

Lexer E: Joint transplantation. Surg Gynecol Obstet 1925, 40, 783
Little WJ: A Treatise on the Nature of Club Foot. London: Longmans, 1839
Macewen W: Antiseptic osteotomy. Lancet 1878, 1, 449-450
Macewen W: Observations concerning transplantation of bone. Proc R Soc London 1881, 32, 232 and Ann Surg 1909, 1, 959
Mayer: Quoted by Bonney. Lancet 1853, 1, 557-558
Moreau PF: Tract in Library of Royal College of Surgeons, London
Park H: An Account of a New Method of Treating Diseases of Joints of the Knee and Elbow in a Letter to Mr Percivall Pott. Tract at Royal College of Surgeons, London, 1781
Park H, Moreau PF: Cases of the Excision of Carious Joints. Glasgow, 1806
Syme J: On the Diseases and Injuries in Which Excision May Be Performed. A Treatise on the Excision of Diseased Joints. Edinburgh: Black, 1831
Watson Jones R: J Chartered Soc Physiotherapy 1944, 29, 72
Watson Jones R: Fractures and Joint Injuries, 2nd ed. Edinburgh: Livingstone, 1955
White A, White C: *In* Chelius MJ: A System of Surgery (trans by JF South). Vol 2. London: Renshaw, 1847, p 979

References

Anderson M, Green WT, Messner MB: Growth and predictions of growth in the lower extremities. J Bone Jt Surg Am 1963, 45A, 1
Bankart ASB: A case of pathological dislocation of the hip—and what happened to an epiphyseal transplant. Proc R Soc Med 1944, 38, 618 (transfer of fibula to replace hip)
Bertelsen A, Capener N: Fingers, compensation and King Canute. J Bone Jt Surg Br 1960, 42B, 390-392
de Boer HH: A history of bone grafting. Clin Orthop Rel Res 1988, 226, 292-298
Bowman AK: The Life and Teaching of Sir William Macewen. London: 1942 (complete bibliography)
Boyer MI, Bray PW, Bowen CVA: Epiphyseal plate transplantation: An historical review. Br J Plast Surg 1994, 47, 563-569
Christensen NO: Growth arrest by stapling. Acta Orthop Scand 1973, Suppl 151 (a good source of references)
Great teachers of surgery in the past. Bristol: John Wright, 1969. Reprints of articles from Br J Surg (Robert Jones' operating list)
Ilizarov GA: Clinical application of the tension-stress effect for limb lengthening. Clin Orthop Rel Res 1990, 250, 8
Jozsa LG, Kannus P: Human tendons. Anatomy Physiology and Pathology. Champaign, Ill: Human Kinetics, 1997
Kenwright J, White SH: A historical review of limb lengthening and bone transport. Injury 1993, 24 Suppl 2, S2-19
Macewen W: The growth of bone. Glasgow: 1912 (thick book on many experiments)
May H: Lexer biography. Plast Reconstr Surg 1962, 29, 141-152
Nickel VL: Orthotics in America: Past, present and future. Clin Orthop Rel Res 1974, 102, 10-17
Paterson D: Leg-lengthening procedures. A historical review. Clin Orthop Rel Res Rel Res 1990, 250, 27-33
Phelps: Med Rec 1891, 39, 221
Phemister D: Surg Gynecol Obstet 1914, 19, 303
Ritt MJPF, Stuart PR, Naggar L, Beckenbaugh RD: The early history of arthroplasty of the wrist. J Hand Surg 1994, 19B, 778-782
Taylor GI: Plast Reconstr Surg 1975, 55, 533 (vascularized fibula graft)

Chapter Sixteen—Injury

Sources of Quotes

Adams F: Works of Areteus. London: 1956
Clarke WA: History of fracture treatment up to the 16th century. J Bone Jt Surg 1937, 19, 50 (Hippocrates quote)

Dupuytren G: On the formation of callus. *In* Injuries and Diseases of Bone (trans by F Le Gros Clark). London: New Sydenham Society, 1847, pp 40-44

Editorial: The dangers of the 'cycle. Lancet July 11 1896, reprinted in JAMA 1896, 27, 654

Hall M: Medical Essays. London: 1825, pp 37-40

Hall M: Researches Principally Relative to the Morbid Effects of Loss of Blood. London: Seeley & Burnside, 1830, p 108

Holland CT: A radiological note. Proc R Soc Med 1929, 22, 695-700

Jepson PN: Ischemic contracture. Ann Surg 1926, 84, 785

Lister J: On the antiseptic principle in Surgery. Lancet 1867, 2, 353

London Times for Tuesday, September 17, 1830

Macleod GHB: Notes on the Surgery of the War in the Crimea. London: 1858, p 281

Volkmann R: Ischemic muscular paralyses (trans by JD Wicht). Zentralbl Chir 1881, 8, 801-803

Wilson E: Diary. Quoted in Freedman BJ: Dr E. Wilson of the Antarctic. Proc R Soc Med 1953, 47, 7-13 (I am grateful to Dr. Scott Mubarak for finding this) and Mubarak SJ, Hargens AR: Compartment Syndromes. Philadelphia: WB Saunders, 1981

References

Aitken AP, Magill HK: Fractures involving the distal femoral epiphysis. J Bone Jt Surg Am 1952, 34A, 96 and Clin Orthop Rel Res 1965, 41, 19 (growth plate injuries: their type 1 is Salter-Harris type 2; 2 is 3, and 3 is 4)

Blount W: Notes on a visit to Orthopaedic Clinics in Europe. J Bone Jt Surg 1929

Blount W: Fractures in Children. Baltimore: Williams & Wilkins, 1955

Blount W: Tribute to a contemporary. Orthop Rev 1979, 8, 19

Diamond LK: A history of blood transfusion. *In* Wintrobe MM: Blood, Pure and Eloquent. New York: McGraw-Hill, 1980

Dupuytren G: Bull Fac Med Paris 1811, 2, 152-160 (bending fractures in children)

Foucher JTE: Annales du Congres medical de Rouen, 1863, and Cong Med de France, Paris, 1863, tom 1 pp 63-72 (growth plate injury). Reprinted in Clin Orthop Rel Res 1984, 188, 3

Hart J: Partial fracture of the long bones in children. Dublin Med Chir Rev 1832, 16, 588-590

Holland CT: Obituary. Br Med J 1941, 1, 139; Lancet 1941, 1, 165

Hutchinson J: Growth arrest. *In* Bryant T. The Practice of Surgery. London: Churchill, 1872. Growth arrest also described by Dittmayer (These de Würtzburg, 1887); Stehr (These de Tübingen, 1889)

Maisonneuve J-G: Gaz med de Paris 1853, p 592 (gas gangrene)

Marriott HL, Keswick A: Continuous drip blood. Lancet 1935, 1, 977 (the drip chamber comes in)

Ogden JA: Skeletal Injury in the Child, 2nd ed. Philadelphia: Saunders, 1990 (a prolific source of references)

Pirogoff NI: Grundzüge der allgemeinen Kriegschirurgie. Leipzig: 1864, pp 867, 1006 (gas gangrene)

Poland J: Traumatic separation of the epiphyses. London: 1898

Salmon PA: Thesis, Paris, 1845 (separating the distal humeral epiphysis)

Salter RB, Harris WR: Injuries involving the epiphyseal plate. J Bone Jt Surg Am 1963, 45, 587

Welch W: Medical Classics 1941, 5, 823-885 (gas gangrene)

Chapter Seventeen — Lower Limb Fractures

Sources of Quotes

Adams F: Works of Areteus. London: 1856

Burgess A: Little Wilson and Big God. New York: Weidenfeld and Nicolson, 1987, p 244

Freiberg AH: Infraction of the second metatarsal bone. Surg Gynecol Obstet 1914, 19, 191-193

Hodges: Voluntary dislocation of the hip. Boston Med Surg J 1865, 72, 470

Hunter J: Clift transcript. Cases in Surgery. Vol II, No 147. Works of J Hunter. London, 1737

Latta LL, Sarmiento A, Tarr RR: The rationale of functional bracing of fractures. Clin Orthop Rel Res 1980, 146, 28-36

Lincoln A, in Heath C: How Abraham Lincoln dealt with a malpractice suit. N Engl J Med 1976, 259, 735-736

Lister J: An address on the treatment of fracture of the patella. Br Med J 1883, 2, 855

Malgaigne JF: *In* Peltier L: Joseph François Malgaigne and Malgaigne's fracture. Surgery 1958, 44, 777

Paget J: Studies of Old Casebooks. London: Longmans, 1891

Paré A: Ten books of Surgery (trans by RW Linker and N Womack). Athens, GA: University of Georgia Press, 1969

Peltier L: Dupuytren fracture. Surgery 1958, 43, 868

Pilcher LS: Ann Surg 1896, 24, 79

Pott P: Remarkes on Fractures and Dislocations. Chirurgical Works of Pott. London: Wood & Innes, 1808, pp 325-329

St. Ignatius: Autobiography (trans by FJ O'Callaghan). New York: Harper Torchbooks, 1974

Waugh W: John Charnley. London: Springer-Verlag, 1990, p 19 (this reference to the climbing accident is a short episode in a great biography)

References

Dehne E: The weight bearing principle in the treatment of lower extremity fractures, 1885-1972. J Trauma 1972, 12, 539

Dehne E: Ambulatory treatment of the fractured tibia. Clin Orthop Rel Res 1974, 105, 192

Editorial: Ambulant treatment of fractures. Ann Surg 1896, 24, 69-79

Gilbert RE: The Mortal Presidency. New York: Basic Books, 1992, p 181

Lauge N: Fractures of the ankle. Analytic historic survey. Arch Surg AMA 1948, 56, 259-317

Lister J: An address on the treatment of fracture of the patella. Br Med J 1883, 2, 855

Sarmiento A, Latta LL: Closed Functional Treatment of Fractures. Berlin: Springer, 1981

Smith H: On the treatment of ununited fractures. Am J Med Sci 1885, 29, 102 (he was one of the first to use a weight-bearing brace)

Spiegel AD, Kavaler F: America's first malpractice crisis, 1835-1865. J Community Health 1997, 22, 283-308

Chapter Eighteen—Spine Fractures

Sources of Quotes

Beatty W: Authentic Narrative of the Death of Lord Nelson. London: 1807

Brodie B: On injuries of the spinal chord (sic). Med-Chir Trans 1836, p 20

Chance GQ: Note on a type of flexion fracture of the spine. Br J Radiol 1948, 21, 452

Hadra E: Wiring of the vertebrae as a means of immobilisation in fractures and Pott's disease. Med Times Register 1891, 22, 423

Jefferson G: Fracture of the atlas vertebra. Br J Surg 1920, 7, 407

References

Ashurst J: Injuries of the Spine. Philadelphia: 1867

Bohler L: The Treatment of Fractures, 5th English ed. New York: Grune, 1956, p 300

Crutchfield WG: South Surg 1933, 2, 156 (tongs for traction)

Denis F: The three column spine and its significance in the classification of acute thoraco-lumbar injuries. Spine 1983, 8, 817

Eggers GWN: Biography of Hadra. Clin Orthop Rel Res 1966, p 21

Gallie W: Skeletal traction in the treatment of fractures and dislocations of the cervical spine. Ann Surg 1937, 106, 770 (ice tongs)

Guttman L: Textbook of Sports for the Disabled. Aylesbury: HM&M Publishers, 1976

Guttman L: Spirit of Stoke Mandeville. The Story of Sir Ludwig Guttman. London: Collins, 1986

Holdsworth FW: Fractures, dislocations and fracture dislocations of the spine. J Bone Jt Surg Br 1963, 45B, 6

Lange F: Am J Orthop Surg 1910, 8, 334 (instrumentation)

Nickel VL, Perry J, Garrett A, Heppenstall M: The halo. J Bone Jt Surg Am 1968, 50A, 1400

Nuck A: Surgical Operations and Experiments. Leiden, 1696 (cervical traction)

O'Donnell R: Case of a fracture of the spine in which the operation of trephining was performed. Reprinted in Clin Orthop Rel Res 1984, 189, 3-11

Paul of Aegina: Fracture book in his Epitome. Venice: Aldine, 1528. Trans for the Sydenham Society by F Adams, 1834-1847 (laminectomy)

Perry J, Nickel V: Total cervical spine fusion for neck paralysis. J Bone Jt Surg Am 1959, 41, 37

Reyburn R: Clinical history of the case of President James A. Garfield. JAMA 1894, 22, 411 (the pathologic findings are illustrated in other papers in JAMA. He died of infection after a bullet wound to the spine and pancreas. His doctors did not gain prestige)

Watson Jones R: The treatment of fractures and fracture dislocations of the spine. J Bone Jt Surg 1934, 16, 30

Chapter Nineteen — Upper Limb Fractures

Sources of Quotes

Barton JR: Views and treatment of an important injury of the wrist. Med Examiner 1838, 1, 365

Bennett EH: Fractures of the metacarpal bones. Dublin Med Sci J 1882, 73, 72-75

Colles A: On fracture of the carpal extremity of the radius. Edinburgh Med Surg J 1814, 10, 182-186

Cooper A: A treatise on dislocations and on fractures of the joints. London: Longmans, 1822

Editorial on Peel: Lancet 1850, 2, 55

Galeazzi R: Arch Orthop Unfallchir 1934, 35, 557-562 (trans by D Pevsner)

Heister L: Fractures. 1719

Hippocrates: Reduction of a dislocated shoulder. Genuine Workes of Hippocrates (trans by F Adams). London: New Sydenham Society, 1849

Kocher T: (trans by Dr. Hirsch) Berl Klin Wochensch 1870, 7, 101-105

Lucas-Championnière JMM: Bull Acad Natl Med 1904, 75, 209 (chauffeur's fracture)

Monteggia GB: (Trans by H Rang.) Instituzione Chirurgiche. Milan: Maspero, 1814, 5, 130.

Payne R: The Rise and Fall of Stalin. New York: 1965, pp 37-38 (Stalin had a supracondylar fracture which left him with some stiffness and features of Volkmann's contracture)

Smith RW: Fracture of the lower extremity of the radius. A Treatise on Fractures in the Vicinity of Joints. Dublin: Hodges & Smith, 1847, p 162

Thomas HO: Pulled Elbow. The Principles of Treatment of Diseased Joints. London: Lewis, 1883, p 77

References

Cotton FJ: J Boston Soc Med Sci 1897-8, 72, 171 (experimental Colles fracture)

Peltier LF: Eponymic fractures. Barton's fracture. Surgery 1962, 29, 141-152

Peltier LF: Fractures of the distal radius. An historical account. Clin Orthop Rel Res 1984, 187, 18

Chapter Twenty — Fracture Treatment

Sources of Quotes

Allgower M, Spiegel PG: Internal fixation of fractures. Clin Orthop Rel Res 1979, 138, 26-29

Amesbury J: Practical Remarks on the Nature and Treatment of Fractures of the Trunk and Extremities. London: Longmans, 1831

Anderson R: An automatic method of treatment for fractures of the tibia and fibula. Surg Gynecol Obstet 1934, 58, 639–647

Bagby GW, Janes JM: The effect of compression on the rate of fracture healing using a special plate. Am J Surg 1958, 95, 761–771

Bagby GW: Compression bone plating: Historical considerations. J Bone Jt Surg Am 1977, 59A, 625–631

Ballingall G: Outline of Military Surgery, 4th ed. Edinburgh: Black, 1852

Bennett W: Lectures on the Use of Massage and Early Movements in Recent Fractures, 5th ed. London: Longmans, Green, and Co., 1910

Buck G: New treatment for fractures of the femur. NY Acad Med 1860, 1, 181–182

Charnley JC: The Closed Treatment of Common Fractures, 3rd ed. Edinburgh: Livingstone, 1970 (introduction, p 10)

Danis R: Theory and Practice of Osteosynthesis (trans by S Perren). Paris: Masson, 1949

Danis R: Obituary. Rev Chir Orthop Reparatrice Appar Mot 1962, 48, 764–765

Dowden JW: The Principle of Early Active Movement in Treating Fractures of the Upper Extremity. 1924

Eggers GWN, Schindler TO, Pomerat CM: The influence of contact compression factor on osteogenesis in surgical fractures J Bone Jt Surg Am 1949, 31A, 693

Eton W: Survey of the Turkish Empire. London: 1798, p 218

Gallie WE: The transplantation of bone. Br Med J 1931, 2, 840–844

Jones J: Plain, Concise, Practical Remarks on the Treatment of Wounds and Fractures: To Which Is Added an Appendix on Camp and Military Hospitals. New York: Holt, 1775

Jones R: Crippling due to fractures. Its prevention and remedy. Br Med J 1925, 1, 909–913

Kuntscher G: The intramedullary nailing of fractures. Clin Orthop Rel Res 1968, 60, 5

Lane WA: A method of treating simple oblique fractures. Trans Clin Soc Lond 1894, 27, 167–175

Lane WA: The Operative Treatment of Fractures. London: Medical Publishing Company, 1904

Lewis KM, Breidenbach L, Stader O: The Stader reduction splint. Ann Surg 1942, 116, 623–636

Lucas-Championnière J: Précis on the Treatment of Fractures by Massage and Movement. 1910

Lurie AS: The female bone setter of Epsom (Mrs Mapp). Surg Gynecol Obstet 1959, 108, 122

Mathysen A: Du Bandage Platre (trans by H Rang). Liege: Grandmont-Donders, 1854

Mowlem R: Cancellous chip bone grafting. Lancet 1944, 2, 746–748

Paré A: Workes (trans by T Johnstone). London: 1665, p 285

Parkhill C: A new apparatus for the fixation of bones. Trans Am Surg Assoc 1897, 15, 251. Reprinted in Clin Orthop Rel Res 1983, 180, 3

Phemister DB: Splint grafts. Surg Gynecol Obstet 1931, 52, 376–381

Pott P: Chirurgical Workes. London: Wood & Innes, 1808, p 313

Rush LV, Rush HL: Evolution of medullary fixation of fractures. Am J Surg 1949, 78, 324–333

Russell RH: Fracture of the femur. Br J Surg 1924, 11, 491–502

Thomas HO: Hip, Knee and Ankle, 2nd ed. Liverpool: Dobbs, 1876, p 98

References

Dehne E: J Trauma 1961, 1, 514–533 (promoted aggressive, early weightbearing)

Krause F: Dtsch Med Wschr 1891, 17, 457–460 (cast with little padding and a cast shoe)

Lane WA: Cardiac massage. Lancet 1902, 2, 1397

McCabe J: Tallyrand. London: Hutchinson, 1906 (Preface and p 1)

Editorials: Ann Surg 1895, 21, 187; Brooklyn Med J 1895, 9, 285; and Ann Surg 1896, 24, 69 (on ambulant treatment of lower limb fractures)

Reclus P: Bull Mem Soc Chir Paris 1897, 23, 267 (used the proximal flare to take most of the weight)

Sarmiento A: A functional below-the-knee cast for tibial fractures. J Bone Jt Surg Am 1967, 49A, 855 (patellar tendon-bearing cast)

Books on Fractures

3000 BC	Edwin Smith papyrus, Egypt
400 BC	Hippocrates, Cos, Greece
circa 800 BC	Suśruta, India
25-50 AD	Celsus, Rome
circa 200	Galen, Greece
circa 600	Paul of Aegina, Greece
circa 1000	Albucasis, Arab Spain
1275	William of Salicet, Italy
circa 1296	Lanfranc, Italy—France
1306-1316	Henri de Mondeville, Montpellier
1363	Guy de Chauliac, France
1465	Le Premier Manuscript, Persia
1497	Hieronymus Braunschweig, Strasbourg—good illustrations
1543	Vesalius, Padua
1544	Guido Guidi (Vidius), France—illustrations of the ancients
1564	Ambroise Paré, first book in French—a huge amount of new information
1676	Richard Wiseman, England
1718	Lorenz Heister, Germany
1733	William Cheselden, London—osteology
1765	Percivall Pott, London
1775	John Jones, first American fracture book
1813-1816	Giovanni Monteggia, Milan
1813	John Syng Dorsey, Philadelphia
1822	Astley Cooper, London—dissections and experiments
1823	Joseph Wattman, Austria—mechanical models to practice reduction of dislocations
1828	Adolph Leopold Richter, Prussia—atlas
1830	Samuel D. Gross, Philadelphia
1832	Dupuytren, France
1847	Robert William Smith, Dublin
1847	Joseph Francis Malgaigne, Paris—statistics
1852	Antonius Mathijsen, Holland—plaster bandages
1860	Frank Hastings Hamilton, United States
1862	Ernst Julius Gurlte, Germany
1886	Hugh Owen Thomas, Liverpool—rest: prolonged, enforced, and uninterrupted
1895	Just Lucas-Championnière, Paris—movement
1896	Theodor Kocher, Bern
1898	John Poland, London—growth plate injuries
1900	Charles L. Scudder, Boston
1905	Lewis Atterbury Stimson, New York
1905	Arbuthnot Lane, London—operative treatment
1907	Albin Lambotte, Belgium
1910	Fredric J. Cotton, USA
1915	Jean Tanton, Paris
1916	Hey Groves, Bristol
1916	Kellogg Speed, Chicago
1922	A. W. Tubby, London
1929	Lorenz Bohler, Vienna
1934	J. Albert Key, St. Louis
1940	Reginald Watson-Jones, Liverpool
1949	Danis, Belgium—compression fixation
1950	Walter Blount, Milwaukee—children's fractures
1950	John Charnley, Manchester
1963	Maurice Mueller, Switzerland—*AO Manual*

Books on Movement

Bennett WH: Lectures on the Use of Massage and Early Movement in Recent Fractures, 5th ed. London: Longmans, Green, and Co., 1910. His first paper was in the Lancet in 1898.

Dowden W: The Principle of Early Active Movement in Treating Fractures of the Upper Extremity. 1924

Lucas-Championnière J: Précis on the Treatment of Fractures by Massage and Movement. Paris: 1910. His first book was published in 1895.

Wires, Screws, and Plates

Bagby GW: J Bone Jt Surg Am 1977, 59A, 625 (compression plate)

Bérenger Féraud LJB: Immobilisation directe. Bull Acad Med Paris 1864-1865, 30, 83-87

Bérenger-Féraud LJB: Traité de L'Immobilisation Directe des Fragments Osseux dans les Fractures. Paris: Delahaye, 1870

Bircher: Arch Klin Chir 1893, 34, 410-422 (intramedullary pegs)

Charnley JC: Positive pressure in arthrodesis of the knee joint. J Bone Jt Surg Br 1948, 30B, 478-486

Cooper S: San Fran Med Press 1861, 2, 13-16

Danis R: Theory and Practice of Osteosynthesis. Paris: Masson, 1947

Eggers GWN: Internal contact splint. J Bone Jt Surg Am 1948, 30A, 40

Eggers GWN, Schindler TO, Pomerat CM: The influence of contact compression factor on osteogenesis in surgical fractures. J Bone Jt Surg Am 1949, 31A, 693

Freidenberg ZB, French G: Surg Gynecol Obstet 1952, 94, 743-748 (optimal interfragmentary pressure)

Gurlte EJ: Handbuch der Lehre von den Knochenbruchen. Berlin: 1862

Hansmann: Dtsch Ges Chir 1866, 15, 134-137

Hey Groves EW: Br Med J 1912, 2, 102-105 (intramedullary rods)

Hey Groves EW: On Modern Methods of Treating Fractures. 1916

Jacoel A: Presse Med 1901, 25 Dec, 143—staples

Key JA: South Med J 1932, 25, 909-915

Kuntscher G: The practice of intramedullary nailing. Springfield, Ill, Charles C Thomas, 1967

Kuntscher G: The intramedullary nailing of fractures. Arch Klin Surg 1935, 185, 302-319; Clin Orthop Rel Res 1968, 60, 5-12

Lambotte A: L'Intervention Opératoire dans les Fractures Récentes et Anciennes. Paris: Maloine, 1907

Lambotte: Paris Chir 1925, pp 145-148

Lambrinudi G: IM Kirschner wires in the treatment of fractures. Proc R Soc Med 1940, 33, 153-157

Lane WA: Lancet 1902, 2, 1397 (he was the first person to carry out successful cardiac massage. When he was removing an appendix, the patient's heart stopped. He massaged the heart through the diaphragm and all was well)

Lane WA: The Operative Treatment of Fractures, London: Medical Publishing Company, 1905. (article on tibia); Trans Clin Sci Lond 1894, 27, 167-175; Br Med J 1907, 1, 1037-1038; Lancet 1893, 2, 1500-1501; Clin J 1894, 5, 392-400; Surg Gynecol Obstet 1909, 8, 344-354

Lister J: An address on the treatment of fracture of the patella. Br Med J 1883, 2, 855

Maatz R: Bruns Beitr Z Klin Chir 1942, 1, 175

Matter P: History of AO and its global effect on operative fracture management. Clin Orthop Rel Res 1998, 347, 11-18 (group met with Maurice Muller, Hans Willenegger, Martin Allgower at Kantonsspital, Chur, on March 15, 1958, and held first court in 1960)

Mengaux G, Odiette D: L'Osteosynthesis au Point de Vue . . . Paris: Masson, 1936

Muller-Meernach: Zentralbl Chir 1933, 60, 1718-1723 (intramedullary nails)

Parham FW, Martin ED: Circlage band. Surg Gynecol Obstet 1916, 23, 541-544

Rush L, Rush L: Am J Surg 1937, 38, 332-333; ditto 1939, 21, 619-626; ditto 1949, 78, 324-333

Rush LV: Intramedullary fixation of the femur. Reflections on the use of the round rod after 30 years. Clin Orthop Rel Res 1968, 60, 21-27

Schone G: Munch Med Wschr 1913, 60, 2327-2328 (closed intramedullary pins)

Scudder C: Is open reduction ever justified? Boston Med Surg J 1900, 142, 289-293

Senn N: Trans Am Surg Assoc 1893, 11, 125-151 (intramedullary pegs)

Sherman WO: Surg Gynecol Obstet 1912, 14, 629-634

Townsend E, Gilfillian C: Surg Gynecol Obstet 1943, 77, 595-597 (compression plate)

Venable CS: An impacting bone plate to attain reduction. Ann Surg 1951, 133, 808 (inboard compressor on a plate)

Venable CS, Stuck: Internal Fixation of Fractures. Springfield, Ill: Charles C Thomas, 1947
Watson-Jones R, et al: Medullary nailing of fractures after 50 years with a review of difficulties and complications of the operation. J Bone Jt Surg Br 1950, 32B, 694
Zierold AA: Arch Surg 1924, 9, 365 (metal corrosion in dogs)

Traction and External Fixation

Anderson R: J Int Coll Surg 1942, 5, 458-462 and 1944, 7, 1-8
Bryant T: The Practice of Surgery. London: Churchill, 1872, p 984
Buck G: Trans NY Acad Med 1861, 2, 232-250
Codivilla A: Am J Orthop Surg 1905, 2, 352-369
Crosby: Trans Am Med Assoc 1850, 3, 382-383; NY Med J Series 2, 1851, 6, 137-138
Hey Groves EW: Br Med J 1913, 2, 1079-1080; Br J Surg 1915, 2, 429-443
Hodgen J: Am Med Times 1863, 7, 169-170
Hoffmann R: Helv Med Acta 1938, 844-880
Kirschner F: Arch Klin Chir 1927, 148, 651
Klapp R: Zentralbl Chir 1914, 41, 1209
Parkhill C: A new apparatus for the fixation of bones after resection and in fractures with a tendency to displacement. With report of cases. Trans Am Surg Assoc 1897, 15, 251-256; reprinted Clin Orthop Rel Res 1983, 180, 3
Parkhill C: Ann Surg 1898, 27, 553-570
Ransohoff J: Trans Am Surg Assoc 1912, 30, 706-715
Sisk TD: External fixation. Historic review, advantages, disadvantages, complications, and indications. Clin Orthop Rel Res 1983, 180, 15
Stader O: North Am Vet 1937, 18, 37-38 and 1939, 20, 55-59
Stader O: Ann Surg 1942, 116, 623-636
Stader O: J Bone Jt Surg 1944, 26, 471-474
Steinmann F: Zentralbl Chir 1907, 34, 938-942
Vidal J: External fixation yesterday, today and tomorrow. Clin Orthop Rel Res 1983, 180, 7

History of Plaster for Fractures

Bacon LW: On the history of the introduction of Plaster of Paris bandages as a fixation dressing. Bull Soc Med Hist 1923, 3, 122
Bremer GJ: The Plaster of Paris Bandage. Nieuwkoop, Holland: B de Graaf, 1962
Munro JK: History of Plaster of Paris in the treatment of fractures. Br J Surg 1935, 23, 257

The Treatment of Nonunion and Bone Defects

Albee FH: JAMA 1911, Aug; JAMA 1923, 81, 1429
Albee FH: Bone-graft Surgery. Philadelphia: Saunders, 1917
Amesbury J: Observations on the Nature and Treatment . . . London: Underwood, 1828, p 193 (early review)
Boyer A: Treatise on Surgical Diseases (trans by AH Stevens). New York: Swords, 1816, 2, 387
Crawford RR: A history of the treatment of non-union of fractures in the 19th century in the United States. J Bone Jt Surg Am 1973, 55A, 1685-1697 (this gives a wealth of information)
Delangenière H, Lewin P: A general method of repairing loss of bone substance and of reconstructing bones by osteoperiosteal grafts taken from the tibia. Surg Gynecol Obstet 1920, 30, 441-447 (osteoperiosteal grafts: a sliver of bone the thickness of a 10 cent piece, together with the overlying periosteum is taken and used to replace bone defects)
Gallie WE: The transplantation of bone. Br Med J 1931, 2, 840-844
Goff CW: The os purum implant. A review. J Bone Jt Surg 1944, 26, 758-767
Hey Groves EW: Methods and results of transplantation of bone. Br J Surg 1917, 5, 185
Inclan A: The use of preserved bone graft in orthopaedic surgery. J Bone Jt Surg 1942, 24, 81
Kearney Rodgers JK: A case of ununited fracture of the os brachii, successfully treated. NY Med Phys J 1827, 6, 521-523
Orell S: Surgical grafting with os purum. J Bone Jt Surg 1937, 19, 873-885

Peltier LF: A brief historical note on the use of electricity in the treatment of fractures. Clin Orthop Rel Res 1981, 161, 4-7 (beginning in 1812, success was obtained in un-united fractures)
Phemister: Splint grafts. Surg Gynecol Obstet 1931, 52, 376-381
Physick PS: Med Repository 1804, 1, 30-31 (Physick uses a nonabsorbable suture in the fracture nonunion to excite inflammation). Reprinted in J Bone Jt Surg Am 1973, 55A, 1685
Senn N: Int J Med Sci 1889, p 98
Smith HH: Am J Med Sci 1855, 29, 102-119
Taylor GI, Miller GDH, Ham FJ: The free vascularised bone graft—a clinical extension of microvascular techniques. Plast Reconstr Surg 1975, 55, 533
Taylor GI: Orthop Clin North Am 1977, 8, 425 (microvascular transfer of fibula)
Thomas HO: The Principles of the Treatment of Fractures and Dislocations. Part 6. London: Lewis, 1871, pp 40-41
White C: Cases in Surgery with Remarks. London: Johnson, 1770, Part 1, pp 79-93

Children's Fractures

Barton JR: Am Rec 1821, 4, 920
Bonnet A: Text on Diseases of Joints. Paris: 1845, vol 2, pp 178-194
Foucher: Congres med France 1867, 1, 63-72

Open Fractures

Beaumont W: Med Chir Rev London 1832, 16, 247-251
Carrel A, Dehelly G: The treatment of wounds (trans by H Childs) New York: Hoeber, 1917
Dakin HD: Br Med J 1915, 2, 318-320
Denis W: JAMA 1884, 2, 673-687
Ellis VH: Lancet 1945, 1, 524
Friedreich: Arch Klin Chir 1898, 57, 288-310
Gustilo RB, Anderson JT: Prevention of infection in the treatment of 1025 open fractures of long bones. J Bone Jt Surg Am 1976, 58, 453-458
Lister J: Lancet 1867, 1, 326, 357, 387, 507; and 1867, 2, 95
MacLeod: Notes on the Surgery of War in Crimea. London: Churchill, 1858
Ollier L: Congres Med France 1872, 11, 192-219 and 220-230
Orr W: Wounds and fractures: a guide to civil and military practice. Springfield, Ill: Charles C Thomas, 1941
Trueta J: Practice of War Surgery. St. Louis: CV Mosby, 1943
Wells TS: Br Med J 1864, 2, 384
Wiseman R: Severall Chirurgical Treatises, 1676. Reprinted and edited by J Kirkup, Bath: Kingsmead Press

Chapter Twenty-one—Sports and Medicine

Sources of Quotes

Kirby EJ: Foreign bodies in the elbow joint, "Baseball Pitchers' elbow." JAMA 1930, 95, 404-405

References

Osgood R: Radiohumeral bursitis (tennis elbow). Arch Surg 1922, 4, 420
Peltier LF: The lineage of sports medicine. Clin Orthop Rel Res 1987, 216, 4-12

Chapter Twenty-two—Knee

Sources of Quotes

Annandale T: An operation for displaced semilunar cartilage. Br Med J 1885, 1, 779; also Lancet 1879, 2, 162; reprinted in Clin Orthop Rel Res 1990, 260, 3-5

Battle WH: A case after open section of the knee joint for irreducible dislocation. Trans Clin Soc Lond 1900, 33, 232-233
Bircher E: Bruns Beitr Klin Chir 1922, 127, 329
Blount WP: Tibia vara. J Bone Jt Surg 1937, 19, 1
Burman MS: Arthroscopy. J Bone Jt Surg 1931, 13, 669 and J Bone Jt Surg 1934, 16, 225
Campbell WC: Repair of the ligaments of the knee. Report of a new operation for repair of the anterior crucial ligament. Surg Gynecol Obstet 1936, 62, 964
Galway HR, MacIntosh D: The lateral pivot shift. Clin Orthop Rel Res 1980, 147, 45-50
Hey W: Practical observations in surgery. London: Capell, 1803, chapter 8
Hey Groves EW: The crucial ligaments. Br J Surg 1920, 7, 505-515
McMurray TP: The diagnosis of internal derangement of the knee. Robert Jones Birthday Volume. London: Oxford University Press, 1928, p 305
Morrant Baker W: The formation of abnormal synovial cysts. St Bart's Hosp Rep 1877, 13, 245-261 and 1885, 21, 177-190
O'Donaghue DH: Surgical treatment of fresh injuries to the major ligaments of the knee. J Bone Jt Surg Am 1950, 32, 721
Osgood RB: Lesions of the tibial tubercle occurring during adolescence. Boston Med Surg J 1903, 148, 114-117
Paget J: Studies of Old Case Books. London: 1891, pp 6-7
Reid J: Displacement of one of the semilunar cartilages of the knee joint. Edinburgh Med Surg J 1834, 42, 377-378
Shiers LGP: Arthroplasty of the knee. J Bone Jt Surg Br 1954, 36, 553-560
Takagi K: Arthroscope. J Jap Orthop Assoc 1939, 14, 359. Translated and reprinted in Clin Orthop Rel Res 1982, 167, 6

References

Bircher E: Verh Dtsch Ges Chir 1886, 15, 130 (ivory intramedullary peg)
Bonnet A: Experimental production of tears (Traite des maladies des articulations). Vol 2. Paris: Bailliere, p 178
Brodhust: St Georges Hosp Reports 1867, 2, 141 (reports on 36 arthrotomies for loose bodies)
Bromfeild W: Chirurgical Observations and Cases. Vol 2. London: 1773 (an early account of meniscal locking)
Campbell W: Surg Gynecol Obstet 1935, 60, 214 and 1936, 62, 964 (describes the terrible triad and uses patellar tendon as a graft)
Charnley JC, Lowe HG: A study of the end-results of compression arthrodesis of the knee. J Bone Jt Surg Br 1958, 40, 633
Goetjes: Dtsch Z Chir 1913, 123, 221 (describes 5 patients he treated by direct repair of the anterior cruciate ligament)
Jackson JP: Osteotomy of osteoarthritis of the knee (abstract). J Bone Jt Surg Br 1958, 40, 826
Jackson R: Memories of the early days of arthroscopy. J Arthrop Rel Surg 1987, 3, 1-3
Key: South Med J 1932, 25, 902 (arthrodesis)
King D: The healing of semilunar cartilages. J Bone Jt Surg 1936, 18, 333-342 (peripheral experimental tears in dogs heal but not central tears)
Kreuser PH: Ill Med J 1925, 47, 290 (first American to use arthroscope for diagnosis)
Smith A: Br J Surg 1917, 2, 176 (reviews anterior cruciate ligament repairs and the first failure with a synthetic graft)
Snook GA: A short history of the anterior cruciate ligament and the treatment of tears. Clin Orthop Rel Res 1983, 172, 11-13
Watanabe M: Memories. Arthroscopy 1986, 2, 209

Chapter Twenty-three — Shoulder

Sources of Quotes

Bankart B: Br Med J 1923, 2, 1132 and Br J Surg 1938, 26, 23
Codman EA: The Shoulder. Boston: Privately published, 1931, Epilogue, pp 12 and 134

Duchenne GBA: Selection of the Clinical Works of Duchenne (trans by GV Poore). London: New Sydenham Society, 1983

Erb WH: Concerning an unusual localisation of brachial plexus paralyses (trans by Dr Hirsch). Verh naturh med Ver Heidelb NF 1877, Bd 1, 130-136

Hippocrates: Genuine Works of Hippocrates (trans by F Adams). London: New Sydenham Society, 1849

Klumpke AD: (Trans by H Rang.) Rev Med 1885, 5, 591-616, 739-790

Marx R: The birth of an Emperor. Surg Gynecol Obstet 1949, 89, 366

Prince M: The Psychology of the Kaiser. Boston: 1915

References

Cavendish ME: Congenital elevation of the scapula. J Bone Jt Surg Br 1972, 54B, 395-408

Grogan DP, Stanley AE, Bobechko WP: The congenital undescended scapula. J Bone Jt Surg Br 1983, 65B, 598-605

Manchester W: The Last Lion. Boston: Little, Brown, 1983, p 237 (Winston Churchill discussed)

Marx R: Birth of an Emperor. Surg Gynecol Obstet 1949, 89, 366-369

Osmond Clarke H: Habitual dislocation of the shoulder (the Putti-Platt operation). J Bone Jt Surg Br 1948, 30B, 19

Strafford BR, Pizzo WD: A historical review of shoulder arthroscopy. Orthop Clin North Am 1993, 24, 1-4

Waugh W: History of the British Orthopaedic Association. 1993 (biography of Blundell Bankart)

Willett, Walsham: (Description of Sprengel's deformity.) Br Med J 1883, 1, 513-514

Chapter Twenty-four — Hospitals and the Organization of Care

Sources of Quotes

Codman EA: The Shoulder. Boston: Self-published, 1934

Cotton F: N Engl J Med 1933, 208, 589

Dunlop J: Transcondylar fractures of the humerus in childhood. J Bone Jt Surg 1939, 21, 59-73

Editorial: The Foundling Hospital. Edinburgh Med Surg J 1805, 1, 319

Faden RR, Beauchamp TL: A History and Theory of Informed Consent. Oxford: Oxford University Press, 1986

Flexner A: Medical Education in the USA and Canada. New York: Carnegie Foundation, 1910, p 10

Nicholl JH: Spina bifida. Br Med J 1902, June 21, 1532-1535

Rogers WA: J Bone Jt Surg 1927, 104-107

Woodall J: The Surgeon's Mate. 1617

References

Gehan EA, Lemak NA: Statistics in Medical Research. Developments in Clinical Trials. New York: Plenum, 1994 (despite the title, this is 200 pages of the history of medical statistics, with biographies and portraits)

Chapter Twenty-five — Conclusions

Source of Quote

Bishop J: Researches into the Pathology and Treatment of Deformities in the Human Body. London: Highley, 1852

Reference

Potts DM, Potts WTW: Queen Victoria's Gene. Phoenix Mill, Stroud UK: Sutton, 1995

◆ CREDITS

The author is indebted to the following publishers and publications for permission to reproduce text and illustrations. Every effort has been made to identify material covered by copyright and I regret any oversights and offer to correct them.

The chapters in which the excerpts appear are enclosed in brackets as follows: [1].

AMA Archives of Surgery
Dandy WE: Loose cartilage from the intervertebral disk simulating tumor. AMA Arch Surg 1929, 19, 660 [7]

Nicholas JA, Burstein CL, Umberger CJ, Wilson PD: Management of adrenocortical insufficiency during surgery. 1955, 71, 737 [7]

Smith Petersen M et al: Intracapsular fractures of the neck of the femur. 1931, 23, 715 [3]

American Journal of Surgery–Cahners Publ Co
Bagby GW, Janes JM: The effect of compression on the rate of fracture healing. 1958, 95, 761 [20]

Annals of Surgery–Lippincott Williams & Wilkins
Lewis KM, Breidenbach L, Stader O: The Stader reduction splint. Ann Surg 1942, 116, 623 [20]

E Arnold Co
McMurray TP: A Practice of Orthopaedic Surgery, 3rd ed. 1949 (Figs 18, 71A&B, 72A&B) [2]

Baillière Tindall and Cox
Wood Jones F: Structure and Function as Seen in the Foot. 1944 [4]

Blackwell Scientific Publications
Nangle EJ: Instruments and Apparatus in Orthopaedic Surgery. 1951. Page 90 (Fig 79A) [2]

British Journal of Radiology
Chance GQ: Note on a type of a flexion fracture of the spine. Br J Radiol 1948, 21, 425 [18]

British Medical Journal
Browne D: Modern methods of treating club feet. 1937, 2, 570 [4]

Seddon HJ: A classification of nerve injuries. 1942, 2, 237 [5]

Gallie WE: The transplantation of bone. 1931, 2, 840 [20]

Bulletin of the Hospital for Joint Diseases
Harboush EJ: Arthroplasty of the hip based on biomechanics, photo-elasticity, fast setting acrylic cement and other considerations. Bull Hosp Joint Diseases 1953, 14, 242-277 (Figs 53 and 54) [4]

Chapman and Hall
Cholmeley JA: The History of the Royal National Orthopaedic Hospital. (Fig 3) 1985 [24]

Churchill Livingstone
Charnley JC: The Closed Treatment of Common Fractures, 3rd ed. 1970 (Text and Figs 51, 87, 104) [20]

Judet J, Judet R et al: Resection-Reconstruction of the Hip. 1954. (Text and one figure) [2]

Rank BK, Wakefield AR: Surgery of Repair as Applied to Hand Injuries, 2nd ed. 1960 [5]

Clinical Orthopaedics and Related Research–Lippincott Williams & Wilkins
Allgower M, Spiegel PG: Internal fixation of fractures. Clin Orthop 1979, 138, 26-29 [20]

Barr JS: Lumbar disc lesions in retrospect and prospect. (Address tape recorded May 1961.) Clin Orthop 1977, 129, 4-8 [7]

Chairi K: Medial displacement osteotomy of the pelvis. Clin Orthop 1974, 98, 55-71 [3]

Danis R: Theory and practice of osteosynthesis. (Translated by S Perren.) Clin Orthop 1979, 138, 25 (Original was published in Paris 1949.) Portrait [20]

Eggers G: Biography of Hadra. Clin Orthop 1966, 21, 4 [20]

Galway HR, Macintosh, D: The lateral pivot shift. Clin Orthop 1980, 147, 45 [22]

Hadra E: Wiring of the vertebrae as a means of immobilization in fracture and Pott's disease. Clin Orthop 1966, 21, 4 [19]

Keinbock: Concerning traumatic malacia of the lunate. (Translated by L Peltier—the classic.) Clin Orthop 1980, 149, 4 [5]

Kuntscher G: The intramedullary nailing of fractures. (Translated by C Andren.) Clin Orthop 1968, 60, 5 [20]

Muller: On deflection of the femoral head. (Translated by EM Bick.) Clin Orthop 1966, 48, 7 [3]

Pean JE: On prosthetic methods intended to repair bone fragments. (Translated by EM Bick.) Clin Orthop 1973, 94, 4 [2]

Pirogoff N: Resection of bones and joints. (Translated by TI Malinen.) Clin Orthop 1991, 266, 3 [14]

   Poggi A: Contribution to the radical treatment of congenital unilateral coxo-femoral dislocation. (Translated by J Ferrara.) Clin Orthop 1974, 98, 5 [3]

Risser JC: The iliac apophysis. Clin Orthop 1958, 11, 111 [6]

Rush LV, Rush HL: Evolution of medullary fixation of fractures by the longitudinal pin. Clin Orthop 1986, 212, 4-9 [20]

Takagi K: Arthroscope. (The classic.) Clin Orthop 1982, 167, 6 and Tagaki, Life by MR Urist—same reference [22]

Journal of the American Medical Association
Malt RA, McKahn CF: Replantation of severed arms. JAMA 1964, 189, 716 [5]

Kirby EJ: Foreign bodies in the elbow joint. JAMA 1930, 95, 404 [21]

Journal of Bone and Joint Surgery (American)
Bagby GW: Compression bone plating: historical considerations. J Bone Jt Surg 1977, 59A, 625-631 [20]

Blount WP: Tibia vara. J Bone Jt Surg 1937, 19, 1 [22]

Burman MS: Arthroscopy. J Bone Jt Surg 1931, 13, 669 and J Bone Jt Surg 1934, 16, 225 [22]

Burman M: Myeloscopy. J Bone Jt Surg 1931, 13, 695 [7]

Calvé J: A localised affection of the spine. J Bone Jt Surg 1925, 7, 41-46 [7]

Calvé J, Galland M, de Cagny R.: Pathogenesis of limp due to coxalgia. J Bone Jt Surg 1939, 21: 12-25 [3]

Dunlop J: Transcondylar fractures of the humerus in childhood. J Bone Jt Surg 1939, 21, 59-73 [24]

Eggers GWN, Schindler TO, Pomerat CM: The influence of the contact compression factor on osteogenesis in surgical fractures. J Bone Jt Surg 1949, 31A, 693 [20]

Hey Groves EW: Treatment of fractured neck of femur. J Bone Jt Surg 1930, 12, 1 [2]

Hibbs RA: A report of 59 cases of scoliosis treated by fusion operation. J Bone Jt Surg 1924, 6, 3-37 [6]

Ito H, Tschiya J, Asami G: A new radical operation for Pott's disease. J Bone Jt Surg 1933, 499-515 [9]

Leadbetter GW: A treatment for fracture of the neck of femur. J Bone Jt Surg 1933, 15, 931-940 [2]

Legg AT: An obscure affection of the hip-joint. J Bone Jt Surg. 1927, 9, 26-34 [3]

Moe J: A critical analysis of the methods of fusion for scoliosis. J Bone Jt Surg 1958, 40A, 529 [6]

Moore AT, Bohlman HR: A metal hip joint. A case report. J Bone Jt Surg 1943, 25, 688 [2]

Mustard W: Iliopsoas transfer for weakness of the hip abductors. J Bone Jt Surg 1952, 34A, 647 [3]

Neer CS: Articular replacement for the humeral head. J Bone Jt Surg 1955, 37A, 217 [23]

O'Donoghue DH: Surgical treatment of fresh injuries to major ligaments of the knee. J Bone Jt Surg 1950, 32A, 721 [22]

Risser JC, Fergusson AB: Scoliosis: its prognosis. J Bone Jt Surg 1936, 18, 667 [6]

Rogers WA: End results and follow-up in orthopaedic surgery. J Bone Jt Surg 1928, 10, 104 [24]

Ryerson EW: Arthrodesing operation on the feet. J Bone Jt Surg 1923, 5, 453 [4]

Smith-Petersen M: Arthroplasty of the hip: a new method. J Bone Jt Surg 1939, 21, 269-288 [2]

Smith-Petersen M: Evolution of mould arthroplasty of the hip joint. J Bone Jt Surg 1948, 30A, 59-75 [2]

Smith-Petersen MN, Rogers WA: End result study of arthrodesis of the sacro-iliac joint for arthritis. J Bone Jt Surg 1926, 8, 118 [7]

Thompson FR: Two and a half years' experience with a vitallium hip prosthesis. J Bone Jt Surg 1954, 36A, 489-500 [2]

Westcott HH: A method of internal fixation of transcervical fractures of the femur. J Bone Jt Surg 1934, 6, 372 [2]

Journal of Bone and Joint Surgery (British)

Barlow TG: Early diagnosis and treatment of CDH. J Bone Jt Surg 1962, 44B, 292-301 [3]

Brand P: Paralytic claw hand. J Bone Jt Surg 1958, 40B, 618 [5]

Golding JSR, MacIver JE, Went LN: The bone changes in sickle cell anaemia and its genetic variants. J Bone Jt Surg 1959, 41B, 711 [3]

Harris RI, Beath T: Etiology of peroneal spastic flat foot. J Bone Jt Surg 1948, 30B, 624-634 [4]

Pulvertaft RG: Tendon grafts for finger flexor injuries in the fingers and thumb. J Bone Jt Surg 1956, 35B, 175-194 [5]

Shiers LGP: Arthroplasty of the knee. J Bone Jt Surg 1954, 36B, 553-560 [22]

Verbeist H: A radicular syndrome from developmental narrowing of the lumbar vertebral canal. J Bone Jt Surg 1954, 36B, 230 [7]

Lancet
Charnley J: Arthroplasty of the hip. Lancet 1961, 1, 1129 [2]

Girdlestone GR: Acute pyogenic arthritis of the hip. Lancet 1943, 1, 41 [2]

Mowlem R: Cancellous chip bone grafting. 1944, 2, 746 [20]

CV Mosby
Eftkekhar NS: Total Hip Arthroplasty. 1963. Page 3 (Fig 1) [2]

New England Journal of Medicine
Mixter WJ, Barr JS: Injury to the spinal cord. N Engl J Med 1934, 211, 210 [7]

Jaffe N, Frei E, Traggis D, Bishop Y: Adjuvant methotrexate and citrovorum-factor treatment of osteogenic sarcoma. N Engl J Med 1974, 291, 994-997 (Fig 3) [12]

Penguin Books Ltd
Flaubert G: Madame Bovary. (Translated by G Wall.) 1992. Pages 141-142, and 151 [4]

Plastic and Reconstructive Surgery
Taylor GI, Miller GDH, Ham FJ: The free vascularized bone graft. Plastic Reconstruct Surg 1975, 55, 533-544 (Fig 6) [20]

Proceedings of the Royal Society of Medicine, London
Holland CT: A radiological note. Proc RSM 1929, 22, 695 [16]

Freedman BJ: Dr. E. Wilson of the Antarctic. Proc RSM 1953, 47, 7 [16]

Royal Society of Medicine, London
Ellis H: Surgical Case Histories of the Past. 1994. Nelson 96 [18]

Raven Press
Rang M, Wenger D: The Art and Science of Children's Orthopaedics [various]

Scandinavian University Press–Acta Orthopaedica Scandinavica
Johansson S: On the operative treatment of medial fractures of the femoral neck. Acta Orthop Scand 1932, 3, 362 [2]

Scandinavian University Press–Acta Chirurgica Scandinavica
Waldenstrom H: On necrosis of the joint cartilage. 1930, 67, 936 [3]

Simon and Schuster–Pocket Books
Brown C: The Story of Christie Brown. 1971. Pages 14 and 15 [10]

Springer-Verlag
Pauwels F: Biomechanics of the Normal and Diseased Hip. 1976. Pages 29 and 271 [2]

Surgery Gynecology and Obstetrics–American College of Surgeons
Albee FH and Kuscher: The Albee spine fusion operation in the treatment of scoliosis. SGO April 1938 (Figure) [6]

Anderson R: An automatic method of treatment for fractures of the tibia and fibula. SGO 1934, 58, 639 [20]

Lurie AS: The female bone setter of Epsom. SGO 1959, 108, 122 [20]

Phemister DB: Conservative surgery in the treatment of bone tumors. SGO 1925, 40, 355 [12]

Phemister DB: Splint grafts. SGO 1931, 52, 376 [20]

Charles C Thomas
Major RH: Classic Descriptions of Disease, 3rd ed. 1948. Pages 585, 586, 587 [13] Descriptions of vitamin C deficiency by Vitry, Joinville, and Cartier

University of Miami, Coral Gables
Freud S: Infantile Cerebral Palsy. (Translated by LA Russin.) 1968 [10]

University of Oklahoma Press
Dale PM: Medical Biographies. (On Catherine the Great) 1952 [6]

◆ INDEX

Note: Page numbers in *italics* refer to illustrations.

Abbott, E.G., 161
Acetabulum, false, Lorenz dissection of, *74*
　fracture of, 376-378
Adams, Robert, on rheumatoid arthritis, 251
Adams, William, 99, 128, 153
Adams forward bend test, 153
Adrenocortical insufficiency, management of, during surgery, 174-175
Albee, Fred, 318-319
　on carpentered cortical grafts for un-united fractures, 456
Albert, Eduard, 332
　on arthrodesis, 332-333
Allbright, Fuller, 286
　on osteoporosis, 286
Allgower, Martin, on internal fixation of fractures, 452
America, orthopaedics in, 29-30
　at end of 19th century, 8
Amesbury, Joseph, 459
　on feelings of patients with un-united fractures, 459
Amesbury's splint, *379*
Amputation, 293-305
　for tumor, 274
　timeline of, 294-300
Amputees, famous, 293-294
Anderson, Roger, on external fixation of fractures, 455
Anderson's external fixator, *455*
Andry, Nicholas, 8
Andry's tree, *13*
Anesthesia, invention of, 16-17
　timeline of, 17
Ankle, Syme's amputation at, 303-304
Ankle fractures, 384-385
　closed, early treatment of, 27
Ankylosing spondylitis, 247-251
Annandale, Thomas, on operation for displaced semilunar cartilage, 492-493
Anterior cruciate ligament, 502-507
　timeline of, 502-503
Antibiotics, 22
Arendt's automatic tissue processor, *264*
Aretus, on tetanus, 370
Arthritis, 241-259
　acute, in infants, 217-219
　famous people with, 242
　hemophilic, 255-256
　of hip, 36-38
　of knee, 510-511
　　timeline of, 510
　rheumatoid, 251-252
　　osteotomy of spine in, 250-251
　timeline for, 242-244
Arthrodesis, 330-333
　of hip, 38-39
　of sacroiliac joint, 179
　triple, for paralytic foot, 113-114
Arthrogryposis, 239-240, 290
Arthroplasty, 322-330
　excision, 324-325
　　of hip, 53-54
　joint transplantation and, 333-334
　of hip, 39-55

Arthroplasty *(Continued)*
　timeline of, 40-41
　of knee, 510
Arthroscopy, 493-499
　timeline of, 494
Aseptic surgery, 18-20
Aufranc, Otto E., on osteotomy of spine in rheumatoid arthritis, 250-251

Back pain. See also *Sciatica; Spinal pain.*
　discogenic, 177-179
　　timeline of, 178-179
　famous people with, 174
　timeline of investigations on, 175
　treatment of, timeline for, 190-191
Baer, William Stevenson, 41
Baillou, Guillaume de, 251
Baker, William Morrant, 498
　on abnormal synovial cysts, 498-499
Bandages, plaster of Paris, 430-435
Bankart, Blundell, 514
　on Bankart lesion, 514
Bankart lesion, 514
Barlow, Thomas, 70, 279
Barlow's test, 70
Barr, Joe, on diagnosing a disc, 187-190
Barton, John Rhea, 311
　on Barton's fracture, 406
　on corrective osteotomy, 311-315
　on treatment of ankylosis by arthroplasty, 325-330
Barton's fracture, 406
Baseball injury, 480-481
Battle, W.H., on repair of cruciate ligaments, 504
Bauer, Louis, 29, 149
　method of recording scoliosis, *155*
　on qualifications for orthopaedic surgery, 524
Beale, Lionel J., 144
Beath, Thomas, on etiology of peroneal spastic flat foot, 106-107
Beck, Carl, 423
Belchier, John, 355
Bell, Charles, 127
Bennett, Edward Hallaran, 406
Bennett's fracture, 406-407
Bérenger-Féraud, Laurent Jean Baptiste, 446, 462
Bethune, Norman, 203, 204
Biceps, rupture of long head of, *481*
Bicycle accidents, 348
Bigelow, Henry Jacob, 17
Bigg, Heather, on spinal braces, 163
Biomechanics, 481-482
Bircher, Eugene, 494
　on arthroscopy, 494
Blood transfusion, dog-to-human, *354*
Bloodgood, Joseph, 271
　on giant cell tumor, 271-272
Blount, Walter, 372, 508
　on tibia vara, 508-509
Bohler, Lorenz, 472
Bohlman, H.R., on metal hip joint, 41-42
Boillaud, Jean-Baptiste, 251

Bone, operations on, 311-318
Bone grafting, 318-321
　for un-united fractures, 456-458
　power tools for, 321-322
　timeline of, 467-468
Bone healing, compression and, 451-452
Bone scans, 25-26
Bonesetters, 427-428
Bonnet, Amédée, 218, 334
Bonnet, Grand Appareil of, 55
Borelli, Giovanni, 481
　studies of body as machine by, 482-485
Bouvier, Sauveur-Henri Victor, 147
　illustrations of scoliosis by, 148
Bowlby, A., on primary nerve suture, 122-123
Boyer, Alexis, 266
　on osteosarcoma, 266
Brace(s). See also Orthotics; Splint(s).
　for clubfoot, 101
　for polio, 224
　for torticollis, 199
　Jorg's, 199
　Scarpa's, 98
　scoliosis, 161-164
　　iron cross, 146
Brachial plexus injuries, 514-518
Brain, W.R., on neurologic manifestations of cervical spondylosis, 198
Brand, Paul, 128
British Orthopaedic Association, membership of, 532
Brockman, Ernest Phillimore, 99
Broders' classification, 265
Brodhurst, Bernard Edward, 79
Brodie, Benjamin, 216
　on Brodie's abscess, 215-217
　on treatment of spinal cord injury, 416-417
Brodie's abscess, 215-217
Bromfeild, William, 488
Brown, Buckminster, 307
Brown, Christie, on cerebral palsy, 232-233
Brown, John Ball, 30
Browne, Denis, 100
Bryant, Thomas, 436
Bryant's traction, 436
Buck, Gordon, 29, 437-438
Buck's extension, 438-440
Bunions, Keller's operation for, 110-111
Bunnell, Sterling, 115-116
　on atraumatic technique in hand surgery, 116
Burman, Michael, on arthroscopy, 494-496
　on myeloscopy, 190

Calvé, Jacques, 85
　on vertebra plana, 191-193
Campbell, Willis C., 506
　on repair of ligaments of knee, 506
Camper, Pieter, 113
　on best form of shoe, 112-113
Cancellous bone grafting, for un-united fractures, 457
Cannulated nail, for hip fracture, 63
Capital femoral epiphysis, slip of, 87-89
　chondrolysis for, 89
Carnochan, John Murray, 29, 78
Carpal tunnel syndrome, 117-119
　early treatment of, 27
　timeline of, 117
Cartier, Jacques, on scurvy, 282
Cartilage tear, types of, 487
Cast(s), for clubfoot, 101
　for scoliosis, 161-164

Cast(s) (Continued)
　for tuberculous spine, 207
　walking, for fracture of tibia, timeline of, 391
Casting materials, timeline of, 459-460
Causalgia, 124
Celsus, 468
Cement, for hip arthroplasty, 42-43
Cerebral palsy, 229-233
Cervical myelopathy, 197-199
Cervical spine, surgery for, timeline of, 198-199
　tuberculosis of, 199
Cervical spondylosis, 197-199
　neurologic manifestations of, 198-199
Chance, G.Q., on Chance fracture, 413
Chance fracture, 413
Charcot, Jean-Martin, 256
　on neuropathic joints, 256-258
Charnley, John, 47
　on hip arthroplasty, 46-52
Charnley's closed reduction of fractures, 428-429
Chauliac, Guy de, 469-470
Chemotherapy, tumor survival with and without, 273
Cheselden, William, 98, 430
Chessher, Robert, 10, 146
Chiari, Karl, on osteotomy for congenital hip dislocation, 83-84
Children's diseases, trends in treatment of, 535-536
Children's fractures, 358-360
Chlorurets, 18
Chondroblastoma, 273
Circlage, 447
Circular saw, 322
Clubfoot, 91, 92-104
　books on, 100
　famous patients with, 94-97
　timeline for, 97-100
　treatment of, 101-104
　　by tenotomy, 335-336
Cobb, John, 155
Codman, Ernest Amory, 267-268
　on outcome studies, 527-529
　on rotator cuff tear, 518
Codman's register, 267-268
Codman's triangle, 266
Colles, Abraham, 402
　on Colles' fracture, 401-404
Colles' fracture, 401-404
　closed, early treatment of, 26
　shortening of ulna after, 141
Collie, J., on malingering and feigned sickness, 197
Colonna, Paul, 80
Communism, orthopaedic diseases and development of, 541
Compartment syndrome, 366-369
　timeline of, 366
Compensation, 196, 197, 344
Compression, in bone healing, 451-452
Computed tomography, 24-25
Congenital malformations, 291
Cooper, Astley, 57, 371, 470
　on hip fracture, 57
　on reduction of dislocated shoulder, 399
Cortical grafts, carpentered, for un-united fractures, 456-457
Corticoperiosteal grafts, for un-united fractures, 457
Cotton, F., 471
　on informed consent, 525-526
Cotugno (Cotunnius), Domenico, 181
　on nervous sciatica, 181-183
Creativity, history and, 6-7
Cross, Sam W., 263

Crutches, 305

Damadian, Raymond, 25
Dandy, Walter C., 175
Danis, Robert, on osteosynthesis, 449-450
Darrach, William, on shortening of ulna after Colles' fracture, 141
David, Jean-Pierre, 205
Davies-Colley, John Neville, 110
  on hallux flexus, 109-110
Davis, A.G., on injuries of cervical spine, 196-197
Davis, Henry Gassett, 29-30
De Bastiani, G., 343
De Quervain, Fritz, 129-130
  on chronic tenovaginitis, 129-130
Death, impact of orthopaedics on, 541
Delpech, Jacques-Mathieu, 102, 145
  plaster cast recording of scoliosis by, 154
Dessault, Pierre-Joseph, 365, 470
Detmold, William Ludwig, 29
Dieffenbach, Johann Friedrich, 98
Dislocations, 366
Duchenne, Guillaume Benjamin Armand, 127, 237
  on muscular dystrophy, 237
Dunlop, John, on in-patient traction for fractures, 533-534
Dupuytren, Guillaume, 73, 112, 133
  on congenital dislocation of hip, 73-75
  on Dupuytren's contracture, 134-138
  on Dupuytren's fracture, 386-387
  on fracture healing, 356-358
  on subungual exostosis, 112
Dupuytren's contracture, 133-138
Dupuytren's fracture, 386-387
Dwyer, Alan, 168
Dyschondroplasia, 287-288

Ehlers-Danlos syndrome, 291
Elbow, baseball pitcher's, 480-481
  pulled, 400
Enneking, William, 267
  on musculoskeletal sarcoma staging, 266-267
Enneking staging, 266-267
Erb, Wilhelm, 515
  on brachial plexus paralysis, 515-516
Erichsen, John, on railway spine, 195
Esmarch, Johann Friedrich August von, 308
  on artificial emptying of blood vessels in operations, 308-310
Esmarch's tourniquet, 308-310
Ewing, James, 268
Ewing's sarcoma, 268-271
Exercises, for treatment of scoliosis, 158-159
External fixators, 452-456
  timeline of, 467

Fairbank, Thomas, 287
Feil, André, 201
  on Klippel-Feil syndrome, 200-201
Femoral head, infarction of, in Perthes disease, 84. See also *Perthes' disease.*
Femoral neck, fracture of, treatment of, 58-63
Femur, fracture of, 378-379
  traction for, 440-441
Fibula, fracture of, open reduction of, 444-449
Finger(s). See also *Hand.*
  trigger, 130
Fisher, Ronald, 531
Flat foot, 105

Flat foot (Continued)
  peroneal spastic, etiology of, 106-107
Fleming, Alexander, 22
Foot, 93-114
  biomechanics of, 113-114
  Chinese binding of, 94
  flat. See *Flat foot.*
  fractures of, 387-390
  paralytic, 113-114
Forst, J.J., on sciatic stretch test, 184-185
Fracture(s), books on, 371-372
  children's, 358-360
  first aid for, 424
  lower limb, 373-393
    ambulatory treatment of, 390-391
    famous patients with, 373-376
    timeline of, 375-376
  open, 361-366
    and gunshot wounds, 362
    timeline of, 361-362
  special kinds of, 358-360
  stress, timeline of, 360
  treatment of, 423-472
    by closed reduction, 428-443
    by open reduction and internal fixation, 443-452
    compression for, 451-452
      timeline of, 465
    external fixators for, 452-456
      timeline of, 467
    intramedullary fixation for, 450-451
    open versus closed reduction in, 427-429
    philosophy of, 425-430
    rest versus motion in, 426-427
    timeline of wires, screws, and plates for, 461-464
  un-united, treatment of, 456-459
    timeline of, 468-469
  upper limb, 395-410
    famous patients with, 395-397
    timeline of, 397
Fracture beds, 379
Fracture healing, 354-358
  compression and, 451-452
  timeline of, 355-356
Freiberg, Albert H., 387-388
Freiberg's infraction, 388-390
Frejka, Bedrich, 76
Freke, John, 172
  on myositis ossificans progressiva, 172
Freud, Sigmund, on cerebral palsy, 232
Friedrich, Paul Leopold, 361
Froment, Jules, 124-125
Froment's sign, 124-125
Fusion, spinal, for scoliosis, 164-167

Galeazzi, Riccardo, 408
  on Galeazzi fracture dislocation, 408-410
Galeazzi fracture dislocation, 408-410
Galen, 363, 469, 477
  on spinal cord injury, 414
Galen's glossocomium, 436
Gallie, W.E., 418
  on carpentered cortical grafts for un-united fractures, 457
Galway, H.R., on lateral pivot shift, 503-504
Garré, Carl, 213
Garrod, Alfred Baring, 243
Garrod, Archibald E., 243
Gas gangrene, timeline of, 370
Giant cell tumor, 271-272
Gibney, Virgil, 150

Gibson, 471
Girdlestone, Gathorne Robert, 53
　on excision arthroplasty of hip, 53-54
Glisson, Francis, 280
　on rickets, 280
Glisson's splint, *317*
Gluck, Themistocles, 44, 323, 462
Godlee, Rickmann, on Galeazzi fracture dislocation, 410
Golding, John, 90
　on bone changes in sickle cell disease, 90
Goldthwait, Joel, 186
　on the lumbosacral articulation, 186-187
Gosset, William, 531
Gout, 244-247
　famous patients with, 244
　timeline for, 242-243
Gowers, William, 237
Great toe, disorders of, 109-111
Green, William T., 342
Gross, Samuel D., 471
Guérin, Jules, *160, 334*
Guidi, Guido, 470
Gunshot wounds, open fractures and, 362
Gurlt, Ernst Julius, 461
Guttmann, Ludwig, 422

Hadra, Berthold, 168, 417
　on wiring of vertebra in spine fracture, 417-421
Haighton, John, 122
　on nerve repair, 122
Hall, Marshall, 351-353
　on effects of loss of blood, 353-354
Hallux flexus, 109-110
Ham, F.J., on free vascularized bone graft, 458
Hamilton, Frank Hastings, 471
Hamilton Russell, Robert, 440
　on fracture of femur, 440-441
Hamilton Russell traction, *441*
Hand, 115-117
　infection of, 131
Hangman's fracture, *413*
Hansmann's plates, 20, *186, 453*
Harrington, Paul, on instrumentation for scoliosis, 168-169, *169*
Harris, Robert, 107, 360
　on etiology of peroneal spastic flat foot, 106-107
Harrison, Edward, 148
Heberden, William, 138
Heberden's nodes, 138
Heine, Jacob, 223
Heine, Johann Georg, 11
Heine's osteotome, *321*
Heister, Lorenz, 470
Hemophilia, 499
Hemophilic arthritis, 255-256
Henry, Arnold K., 310
Hey, William, 488-489
　on internal derangement of knee, 489-490
Hey Groves, E.W., on reconstruction of cruciate ligaments, 504-506
Hey Groves' hip arthroplasty, *39*
Hey Groves' osteotomy, 81
Hibbs, Russell A., 164
　on spinal fusion for scoliosis, 165-167
Hilgenreiner, Heinrich, 67
Hilton, John, 207, 471
Hip, adult, 35-63
　arthrodesis of, 38-39
　arthroplasty of, 39-55
　　timeline of, 40-41

Hip *(Continued)*
　　total, *41*
　capsular arthroplasty of, *80*
　child's, 65-91
　fracture of, 55-63
　　experimental, 57-58
　　timeline of, 56-57
　hemiarthroplasty of, 41-42
　metal, 41-42
　osteoarthritis of, 36-38
　osteotomy of, 54-55
　range of movement of, *35*
　snapping, 91
Hip dislocation, developmental, 65-84
　diagnosis of, history of, 67
　screening for, 66-75
　timeline for, *66*
　treatment of, 75-84
　　results of, 82
　　timing of, 80-81
　paralytic, 90-91
　reduction of, *376, 377*
Hippocrates, 209
　on gout, 245
　on open fractures of femur and humerus, 362-363
　on recurrent dislocation of shoulder, 513-514
　on reduction of dislocated shoulder, 397-398
　on spinal tuberculosis, 209
Hippocrates' scamnum, *436*
History, change in, 543
　reasons for studying, 2-9, 543
Hoffa, Albert, 3, 79
Hoke, Michael, 114
Hospitals, 521-522
　orthopaedic, early, 30
　origin of, 10-11, 522-523
Hounsfield, Godfrey, 24-25
Humbert, François, 75, 76, 77
Hunter, John, 392, 470
　on rupture of tendo Achillis, 392-393

Ilizarov, Gavriil, 343
Immunization, 22
Inclan, Alberto, 472
Infection, 203-220
　after injury, 369-370
　control of, 18-22
　nontuberculous granulomatous, 212-220
　pyogenic, 213-214
　　timeline of, 213
　trends in treatment of, 534-535
Informed consent, 525-526
Injury, 347-372
　causes of, 347-351
　prevention of, 348, 535
Inman, Verne, 113
Instrumentation, for scoliosis, 167-169
　timeline for, 168
Internal fixation, 443-452
　for femoral neck fracture, 58-61
Intramedullary fixation, 450-451
Intramedullary nails, timeline of, 466
Intramedullary pegs, 450
Iron cross scoliosis brace, *146*

Jackson, Robert, 494
Jaffe, Henry J., 263
Jalade-Laford, Guillaume, 76
Jean, Sire de Joinville, on scurvy, 281

Jefferson fracture, *413*
Jepson, P.N., 369
Jepson's fasciotomy, 369
Johansson, Sven, on cannulated nail for hip fracture, 63
Johnson, J.G., on compensation for railway injuries, 197
Joint(s). See also named joint, e.g., *Hip.*
　operations on, 322–334
　swollen, hemophilia and, 499
Joint replacement. See also *Arthroplasty.*
　history of, 27
Joint transplantation, 333–334
Jones, John, 423
Jones, Reginald Watson, 465
　on paralytic hip dislocation, 90–91
Jones, Robert, 336–338
　on Thomas splints, 434
Jones' pseudoarthrosis of hip, *40*
Jorg, Johann Christian, 28, 199
Jorg's brace, *199*
Joseph-François, 376–377
Judet, Robert, 48
Judet prosthesis, *39*

Kanavel, A.B., 131
Keen, W.W., on gunshot wounds and other nerve injuries, 124
Keller, William, on operation for bunions, 110–111
Kenny, Sister, 226
Kienbock, Robert, 138
　on traumatic malacia of lunate, 138–140
Kirby, F.J., on baseball pitcher's elbow, 480–481
Kirschner, Martin, 437
Kite, Hiram, 99
Klapp, Rudolf, 151
Klippel, Maurice, 201
　on Klippel-Feil syndrome, 200–201
Klippel-Feil syndrome, 200–201
Klumpke, Auguste, 517
Klumpke's paralysis, 517–518
Knee, 487–510
　arthritis of, 510–511
　　timeline of, 510
　arthroplasty of, 510
　deformity of, 508
　loose bodies in, 508
Knee pain, anterior, timeline of, 499
Kneeling prostheses, *293*
Knight, James, 29, 148
Knock-knees, operation for, 316–317
Kocher, Theodor, 398
　on reduction of dislocated shoulder, 399
König, Franz, 81
　on hemophilia and swollen joints, 499
Kuntscher, Gerhard, 451
　on Kunstscher nailing, 451
Kuntscher nailing, 451, 466
Kyphosis, 170–172
　senile, 180

Lambotte, Albin, 463
Lambotte's external fixator, *454*
Lambret's extension apparatus, *455*
Lambrinudi, Constantine, 113
Laminectomy, 416
Lane, William Arbuthnot, 443–444
　on treatment of fractures of tibia and fibula, 444–449
Lane's plates, *445*
Lange, Fritz, on instrumentation for tuberculous spinal deformity, 167–168

Larrey, Dominique, 365
Larson, Carroll B., on osteotomy of spine in rheumatoid arthritis, 250–251
Lasègue, Ernest Charles, 183
Lasègue sign, 183–184
Lateral pivot shift, 503–504
Le Damany, Pierre, on screening for hip dislocation, 68–69
Le Damany's splints, *69*
Le Vacher, François-Guillaume, 199
Le Vacher, Thomas, 199
Leadbetter, Guy Whitman, 62
Leadbetter maneuver, 62
Lebert, Herman, 262
Legg, Arthur T., 85
　on Perthes disease, 85–86
Lexer, Erich, 274, 333
　on joint transplantation and arthroplasty, 333–334
Lichtenstein, Louis, 263
Limb length equalization, 340–343
　timeline for, 342–343
Lind, James, 281
Ling, Pehr Henrik, 150
Lisfranc, Jacques, 302
Lister, Joseph, 18
　on antiseptic surgery, 18–19
　on treatment of fractured patella, 380–381
　on treatment of open fractures, 365
Lister's spray, *19*
Little, William John, 102, 229
　on Little's disease, 230–232
　on tenotomy for treatment of clubfoot, 335–336
　on treatment of clubfoot, 101–104
London, Victorian, orthopaedics in, 7–8
Lorenz, Adolph, 79
Lovett, Robert, 152
Lower limb fractures, 373–393
　ambulatory treatment of, 390–391
　famous patients with, 373–376
　timeline of, 375–376
Lucas-Championnière, Just, 426
Ludloff, K., 80
Lunate, avascular necrosis of, 138–140

Macewen, William, 318
　on antiseptic osteotomy, 317–318
　on bone grafting, 319–321
Madelung, Otto, 140
Madelung's deformity, 140–141
Mafucci, Angelo, 290
Magnetic resonance imaging, 25
Malgaigne, Joseph-François, 376–377, 471
　on vertical shear fracture, 377–378
Malgaigne's claw, *437*
Malgaigne's vertical shear fracture, 377–378
Malkin, Sydney Alan Stormer, 56
Mallet, Jean-Louis, 317
Malt, R.A., on replantation, 131–133
Marey, Étienne-Jules, 233
Marfan, Bernard, 290
Marfan's syndrome, 290
Marie, Pierre, 248
　on ankylosing spondylitis, 248–250
Mathijsen, Antonius, 432
　on plaster bandages, 432–434
Mayer, L., on operation for knock-knees, 316–317
McIntosh, David, 503
　on lateral pivot shift, 503–504
McMurray, Thomas Porter, 55, 491
　on internal derangement of knee, 491–492
　on osteotomy of hip, 54–55

McMurray osteotomy, 54-55
Medical insurance, 523
Medical records, 526-529
Meniscal tears, 487-493
Menisci, timeline of, 488
Mercuriale, Geronimo, 477
Metatarsalgia, Morton's, 107-109
Microsurgery, timeline of, 131
Middleton, George Stevenson, 185
  on intervertebral disc rupture, 185-186
Miller, G.D.H., on free vascularized bone graft, 458
Mitchell, Silas Weir, 124
  on gunshot wounds and other nerve injuries, 124
Moe, John, 167
Moller, Julius, 281
Mollet's saw, *321*
Mondeville, Henri de, on informed consent, 525
Monteggia, Giovanni Battista, 407
  on Monteggia fracture, 407-408
  on polio, 227
Moore, Austin T., 42
  on metal hip joint, 41-42
Moorehouse, G.R., on gunshot wounds and other nerve injuries, 124
Moreau, P.F., 38
  on arthrodesis, 331-332
Morgagni, G.B., on myelomeningocele, 236-237
Morton, Thomas G., 107
Morton's metatarsalgia, 107-109
Motion analysis, 233
Motor vehicle accidents, 348-351
Mott, Valentine, 29
Mowlem, Rainsford, on cancellous bone grafting for ununited fractures, 457
Muller, Ernst, on slip of capital femoral epiphysis, 87-89
Müller, Maurice, 465
Murphy, John B., 40
Muscular dystrophy, 237-239
Mustard, William, 90
Mustard's psoas transfer, *91*
Muybridge, Eadweard, 233
Myeloscopy, 190
Myositis ossificans progressiva, 172
Myotomy, for scoliosis, 163-164

Natural history, history and, 6
Neer, Charles S., 512
Neer's prosthesis, *513*
Nélaton, August, 214
Nerve injuries, 119-127
  classification of, 123
  timeline of, 120-121
Nerve repair, 122-127
Neurofibromatosis, 234-235, 290-291
Neuromuscular disease, 221-240
  famous patients with, 221-222
  timeline of, 223
Neuropathic joints, 256-258
Nicholadoni, Carl, 340
Nicoll, J.H., on outpatient treatment for spina bifida, 534
Nightingale, Florence, 522-523
Northfield, D., on neurologic manifestations of cervical spondylosis, 198

O'Donaghue, Don, 507
  on knee injuries, 507
Ollier, Louis, 287
Ollier's disease, 287-288
Open fractures, 361-366

Open fractures *(Continued)*
  and gunshot wounds, 362
  timeline of, 361-362
Open wounds, treatment of, 363-366
Ormerod, Joseph Arderne, 118
  on carpal tunnel syndrome, 118-119
Orr, H. Winnett, 472
Orthopaedic diseases, impact of, on history/social progress, 540-541
Orthopaedic hospitals, origin of, 10-11, 522-523
Orthopaedics, 307-344
  beginnings of, 8-16
  early books on, 28
  eras of, 27-28
  growth of knowledge in, 13-15
  historical references in, 30-31
  history of, 1-16
  impact of, on everyday life, 539-540
    on trauma and death, 541
  impact of social progress on, 541-542
  operating room methods in, 308-318
  predecessors of, 11
  remaining problems in, 542-543
  rise and fall of, 539
  scientization of, 15-16
  specialization and, 12-13
  success of, 28-30
  surgical exposures in, 310
Orthotics, 227-228. See also *Brace(s); Splint(s).*
  timeline for, 228
Ortolani, Marino, 70
Ortolani's sign, 70
Osgood, Robert, 500
  on apophysitis of tibial tubercle, 500-502
Osteoarthritis, 258-259
  of hip, 36-38
    clinical features of, 38
    treatment of, 38
  of knee, 510-511
    timeline of, 510
  timeline of, 36
Osteoclasis, closed, 315
Osteomyelitis, 215, 535
Osteoporosis, 286
  spinal, 180
Osteosarcoma, 266-268. See also *Tumors.*
  salvage surgery for, 274-275
Osteosynthesis, 449-450
Osteotome, Heine's, *321*
Osteotomy, corrective, 311-315
  for knock-knees, 316-317
  of hip, 54-55
  of spine, in rheumatoid arthritis, 250-251
  supracondylar, 317-318
Outcome studies, 526-529
Outpatient care, trend to, 533-534

Paci, Agostino, 79
Paget, James, 283
  on apophysitis of tibial tubercle, 499-500
  on carpal tunnel syndrome, 118
  on Paget's disease of bone, 282-286
Paget's disease of bone, 282-286
Paletta, Giovanni, 66
Palmer, Daniel, 191
Paralytic foot, 113-114
Paraplegia, from tuberculous spine, 210-212
  traumatic, 411-422
Paré, Ambroise, 381
  on fracture of tibia, 381-382

Paré *(Continued)*
　　on positions for splinting limbs, 430
　　on rupture of tendo Achillis, 392
　　on slip of capital femoral epiphysis, 87
Paré's splint, *97*
Park, Henry, 38-39, 331
　　on arthrodesis, 330-331
Parkhill, Clayton, 453
　　on external fixation of fractures, 453-454
Parkhill's external fixator, *454*
Pasteur, Louis, 21
Patella, fracture of, 380-381
Pathology, history of, 264-265
Pauwels, Friedrich, 36
　　on biomechanics of hip, 36
Pauwels' principles, 36-38
Pauwels' tension band principle, *465*
Pavlik, Arnold, 76
Pean, Jules Emile, 43
　　on prosthetic repair of bone fragments, 43-46
Pean's prosthesis, *43*
Pelvis, fracture of, 376-378
Perkins, George, 67
Perthes, Georg Clemens, 86
Perthes' disease, 84-86
Petit, Jean-Louis, 207, 461
　　on slip of capital femoral epiphysis, 87
Petrie, James Gordon, 86
Phemister, Dallas, 86
　　on salvage surgery from osteosarcoma, 274-275
　　on splint grafts for un-united fractures, 457
Physick, Philip Syng, 470
Pirogoff, Nikolai, 302
Plaster, timeline of, 459-460
Plaster of Paris bandages, 430-435
Plates, for fracture fixation. See also *Fracture(s), treatment of.*
　　timeline of, 461-464
Podiatry, history of, 93-94
Poggi, Alfonso, on open reduction of congenital hip dislocation, 82-83
Poland, John, 359
Poliomyelitis, 223-227, 534-535
　　timeline of, 225-226
Portal, Antoine, 176
Posture, scoliosis and, 160-161
Pott, Percivall, 210, 382-383
　　on function of splints, 430
　　on paraplegia, 210-212
　　on Pott's fracture, 385-386
Pott's fracture, 385-386
Poutreau, Claude, 404
Pravaz, Charles Gabriel, 77, 78, 143
Pravaz Chariot, *78*
Pravaz traction, *157*
Preventive orthopaedics, 534
Professional organizations, 524-525
Prolapsed disc, early treatment of, 27
Prostheses, 293-305
　　kneeling, *293*
　　timeline of, 301-303
Pulvertaft, Guy, 128
Putti, Vittorio, 176
　　on pathogenesis of sciatic pain, 176-177
Pyogenic infection, 213-214
　　timeline of, 213

Qualifications, evolution of, 523-524
　　timeline of, 524

Railway injuries, 350-351
　　compensation for, 196, 197
Railway spine, 195-196
Rank, B.K., on hand surgery, 116-117
Reclus, Paul, on paralytic hip dislocation, 90
Rehabilitation, 343-344
Reid, J., on meniscal tear, 491
Replantation, 131-133
Rheumatoid arthritis, 251-252
　　osteotomy of spine in, 250-251
Richter, Adolph Leopold, 471
Rickets, 278-280
　　surgical treatment of, 280
　　timeline of, 279
Ridlon, John, 150
Risser sign, 156
Rizzoli, Francesco, 315
Rizzoli's osteoclast, *315*
Roentgen, Konrad, 23
Rogers, William, on arthrodesis of sacroiliac joint for arthritis, 179
　　on outcome studies, 529
Rotator cuff tears, 518
Rush, Lowry, on Rush rods, 450-451
Rush rods, 450-451
Ryerson, Edwin, 114
　　on triple arthrodesis for paralytic foot, 113-114

Sabin, Albert, 226
Sacroiliac joint, arthrodesis of, for arthritis, end-result study of, 179
Saint-Hilaire, Geoffroy, 290
Salk, Jonas, 226
Salter, Robert B., 84
　　on innominate osteotomy for congenital hip dislocation, 84
Saw(s), circular, *322*
　　Mollet's, *321*
Sayre, Lewis Albert, 149
Scarpa, Antonio, 98
Scarpa's brace, *98*
Scheuermann, Holger Werfel, 171
　　on kyphosis, 171-172
Schlatter, Carl, 499
Schmorl, Christian George, 178
Schone, Georg, 466
Schulthess, Wilhelm, 154
　　machine for recording scoliosis used by, *155*
Sciatic stretch test, 184-185
Sciatica, 177-179
　　original papers on, 181-193
　　pathogenesis of, 176-177
Scoliosis, 143-170
　　famous people with, 144-145
　　measurement of, 154-156
　　pathology of, 152-153
　　rocker exerciser for, 144
　　timeline of, 146-151
　　treatment of, 156-170
　　　　methods of, 157-169
　　　　reason for, 156-157
　　　　results of, 169-170
Scoliosis brace(s), 161-164
　　iron cross, *146*
Screws, for fracture fixation. See also *Fracture(s), treatment of.*
　　timeline of, 461-464
Scudder, Charles Locke, 463
Scurvy, 281-282
　　in new world, 281-282
　　timeline of, 281
Seddon, Herbert, 123

Seddon *(Continued)*
 on classification of nerve injuries, 123
Semmelweis, Ignaz, 20
Senile kyphosis, 180
Senn, Nicholas, 57, 463, 466
 on experimental hip fractures, 57-58
Séquard, Charles-Édouard, 414
Seutin, Louis Jean, 431
Shaffer, Newton Melman, 149
Shanz, Alfred, 81
Sharrard, 91
Shenton, Edward Warren Hine, 67
Sherman, William O'Neill, 464
Sherman's plate and self-tapping screw, 464
Shiers, L.G.P., on arthroplasty of knee, 510
Shock, 351-354
Shoes, 112-113
Short stature, 288-289
 famous people with, 288-289
Shoulder, 511-518
 famous people with problems of, 511
 original papers on, 513-514
 recurrent dislocation of, 513-514
 timeline for, 512
Shoulder dislocation, 397-400
 posterior, 399-400
Sickle cell disease, bone changes in, 89-90
Simpson, Lewis Atterbury, 471
Sinding-Larsen, Christian, 499
Skeletal dysplasias, 287-288
Skull traction, 416
Smith, Nathan, 215
 on osteomyelitis, 215
Smith, Robert William, 234
 on neuroma, 234-235
 on Smith's fracture, 405-406
Smith, Tom, 217
 on acute arthritis of infants, 217-219
Smith-Petersen, Marius, 48
 on arthrodesis of sacroiliac joint for arthritis, 179
 on osteotomy of spine in rheumatoid arthritis, 250-251
 on treatment of femoral neck fractures by internal fixation, 58-61
Smith's fracture, 405-406
Spas, 258-259
Spiegel, Phillip, on internal fixation of fractures, 452
Spina bifida, 236
 outpatient treatment for, 534
Spinal cord injury, 414-421
 experimental studies on, 414
 in modern era, 421-422
 natural history of, 415
 stabilization of spine after, 417-421
 treatment of, 415-416
Spinal fusion, for scoliosis, 164-167
 for tuberculous spine, 208
Spinal osteoporosis, 180
Spinal pain, 173-193. See also *Back pain; Sciatica.*
Spinal stenosis, 175-177
 timeline of, 176
Spine, deformity of, 143-172
 fracture of, 411-422
  famous patients with, 411-412
  in modern era, 421-422
 tuberculosis of, jury mast for, *195*
  treatment of, 207-208
Splint(s). See also *Brace(s); Orthotics.*
 Amesbury's, *379*
 for hip dislocation, *76*
 for tuberculous spine, 207, 208
 function of, 430

Splint(s) *(Continued)*
 Glisson's, *317*
 le Damany's, *69*
 Paré's, *97*
 Stader reduction, 455-456
 Thomas, *378,* 434
Splinting, positions for, 430
Spondylolisthesis, 180
 timeline of, 180
Sports, styles of, 475-476
Sports medicine, 475-485
 timeline of, 477-478
Stader, O., on Stader reduction splint, 455-456
Stader reduction splint, 455-456
Stafford, R.A., on kyphosis, 170-171
Starr, Clarence, 214
Statistics, history of, 529-531
 timeline of, 530-531
Steindler, Arthur, 106
Steinmann, Fritz, on traction for fractures, 442-443
Steinmann traction, *442*
Still, Andrew Taylor, 190
Still, George F., 253
Still's disease, 253-255
Stress fractures, timeline of, 360
Stromeyer, Georg, 103
Strümpell, Adolf, 180, 247
 on ankylosing spondylitis, 247-248
Subungual exostosis, 112
Supracondylar osteotomy, 317-318
Surgery, aseptic, 18-20
 safe, timeline of, 20-21
Surgical exposures, 310
Susruta, 460
Susruta's forceps, 11
Swaddling, *277*
Swan, Joseph, 120
Sydenham, Thomas, 247
 on gout, 245-247
Syme, James, 330
 on amputation at the ankle, 303-304
 on compensation for railway injuries, 196
 on excision arthroplasty, 330
Syndromes, 289-291
 timeline of, 290
Synovial cysts, 498-499

Takagi, Kenji, 497
 on arthroscopy, 496-497
Tarsal coalition, 105-106
Taylor, Charles Fayette, 149
Taylor, G.I., on free vascularized bone graft, 458
Teacher, John Hammond, 185
 on intervertebral disc rupture, 185-186
Team games, history of, 479-480
Tendo Achillis, rupture of, 392-393
Tendon transfer, 336-340
 Robert Jones' rules for, 339
 timeline of, 339-340
Tendons, of hand, surgery on, 127-130
 operations on, 334-340
 timeline of, 127-128
Tenotomy, 335-336
Tetanus, 369-370
Thalidomide, 303
Third world, orthopaedics in, 8, 531-533
Thomas, Hugh Owen, 400
 on pulled elbow, 400
 on Thomas splint, 435
Thomas splint, *378,* 434-435

Thompson, Frederick R., 42
Thompson prosthesis, 42
Thurstan Holland, Charles, 360
　on Thurstand Holland sign, 360
Thurstan Holland sign, 360
Tibia, fracture of, 381-382
　　early treatment of, 26
　　open reduction of, 444-449
　　walking cast for, timeline of, 391
　pseudarthrosis of, 384
　sequestrectomy of, 213
Tibia vara, 508-509
Tibial tubercle, apophysitis of, 499-502
Tinel, Jules, 125
Tinel's sign, 126-127
Tissue processor, arendt's automatic, *264*
Toe, great, disorders of, 109-111
Tonnis, Dietrich, 81
Torticollis, 199
Traction, for dislocated shoulder, *398*
　for forearm fracture, *409*
　for fracture of femur, *441*
　for fractures, 435-443
　　in-patient, 533-534
　　timeline of, 460-461
　for spinal cord injury, 415-416
　for treatment of scoliosis, 157-158
　reduction of hip dislocation by, 76-79
　skull, 416
Trauma, impact of orthopaedics on, 541
Trendelenburg, Friedrich, 71
Trendelenburg's test, 71-73
Trigger finger, 130
Trueta, Joseph, 472
Tuberculosis, 204-212, 535
　bone and joint, surgical aspects of, timeline of, 206-207
　of cervical spine, 199
　of spine, jury mast for, *195*
　　treatment of, 207-208
　social aspects of, 209
　timeline of, 205-206
Tulp, Nicolaas, 236
Tumors, 261-275. See also *Osteosarcoma*.
　Broders' classification of, 265
　famous people with, 262
　timeline of, 262-263
　treatment of, 273-275
Turco, Vincent, 100
Turner, Robert, 11

Ulna, shortening of, after Colles' fracture, 141
Ultrasound, diagnostic, for congenital dislocation of hip, 66-67
Underwood, Michael, 225
　on polio, 226-227
Upper limb fractures, 395-410
　famous patients with, 395-397
Upper limb injuries, timeline of, 397

Velpeau, Alfred, 409
Venel, Jean Andre, 147

Verbeist, Henk, on spinal stenosis, 177
Verneuil, A., on paralytic hip dislocation, 90
Vertebra plana, 191-193
Vertical talus, 104
Vitamin C deficiency, 281-282. See also *Scurvy*.
Vitry, Jacques de, on scurvy, 281
Volkmann, Richard von, 366
　on compartment syndrome, 367-368
　on hunchback, 209
Von Rosen, Sophus, 76

Wagner, Heinz, 342
Wakefield, A.R., on hand surgery, 116-117
Waldenström, Henning, 89
　on chondrolysis for slipped capital femoral epiphysis, 89
Walking casts, for fracture of tibia, timeline of, 391
Waller, Augustus Volney, 121
Walsham's elastic support, *105*
Wattmann, Joseph, 471
Weiss, Marian, 303
　on prostheses, 304-305
Westcott, H. Heywood, on internal fixation of transcervical fractures of femur, 62-63
Whiplash, 195-197
　contemporary, 196-197
Whistler, Daniel, 280
　on rickets, 280
White, Anthony, on excision arthroplasty, 324-325
White, Charles, 322
Whitman, Royal, 63
Whitman plate, *105*
Wild, John J., 67
Wiles, Philip, 38
Wilkinson, M., on neurologic manifestations of cervical spondylosis, 198
Willard, De Forest, 151
Willard's wheeled crutch, *228*
Wilson, Edward, on exertional compartment syndrome, 368-369
Wires, for fracture fixation. See also *Fracture(s), treatment of*.
　timeline of, 461-464
Wiseman, Richard, 206, 470
Wolff, Julius, 36, 95
Woodall, John, on informed consent, 525
Wood-Jones, F., 100
Wound irrigation, *364*
Wrist fractures, 401-410

X-rays, 22-26

Zander, Jonas, 150, 478
Zander's velocipede, *479*

ISBN 0-7216-7141-1